The Control of Tumour Growth and its Biological Bases

DEVELOPMENTS IN ONCOLOGY

F. J. Cleton and J. W. I. M. Simons, eds., Genetic Origins of Tumor Cells
ISBN 90-247-2272-1
J. Aisner and P. Chang, eds., Cancer Treatment Research
ISBN 90-247-2358-2
B. W. Ongerboer de Visser, D. A. Bosch and W. M. H. van Woerkom-Eykenboom, eds., Neuro-oncology: Clinical and Experimental Aspects
ISBN 90-247-2421-X
K. Hellmann, P. Hilgard and S. Eccles, eds., Metastasis: Clinical and Experimental Aspects
ISBN 90-247-2424-4
H. F. Seigler, ed., Clinical Management of Melanoma
ISBN 90-247-2584-4
P. Correa and W. Haenszel, eds., Epidemiology of Cancer of the Digestive Tract
ISBN 90-247-2601-8
L. A. Liotta and I. R. Hart, eds., Tumour Invasion and Metastasis
ISBN 90-247-2611-5
J. Bánóczy, ed., Oral Leukoplakia
ISBN 90-247-2655-7
C. Tijssen, M. Halprin and L. Endtz, eds., Familial Brain Tumours
ISBN 90-247-2691-3
F. M. Muggia, C. W. Young and S. K. Carter, eds., Anthracycline Antibiotics in Cancer
ISBN 90-247-2711-1
B. W. Hancock, ed., Assessment of Tumor Response
ISBN 90-247-2712-X
D. E. Peterson, ed., Oral Complications of Cancer Chemotherapy
ISBN 90-247-2786-3
R. Mastrangelo, D. G. Poplack and R. Ricardi, eds.,
Central Nervous System Leukemia: Prevention and Treatment.
ISBN 0-89838-570-9
A. Polliack, ed.: Human Leukemias. Cytochemical and Ultrastructural Techniques in Diagnosis and Research.
ISBN 0-89838-585-7

The Control of Tumour Growth and its Biological Bases

edited by

W. DAVIS
International Agency for Research on Cancer
Lyon, France

C. MALTONI
Institute of Oncology 'Felice Addarii'
Bologna, Italy

S. TANNEBERGER
Central Institute of Cancer Research
Academy of Sciences
Berlin, DDR

1983 **MARTINUS NIJHOFF PUBLISHERS**
a member of the KLUWER ACADEMIC PUBLISHERS GROUP
BOSTON / THE HAGUE / DORDRECHT / LANCASTER

Distributors

for the United States and Canada: Kluwer Boston, Inc., 190 Old Derby Street, Hingham, MA 02043, USA

for Hungary, Albania, Bulgaria, China, Cuba, Czechoslovakia, German Democratic Republic, Democratic People's Republic of Korea, Mongolia, Poland, Rumania, Soviet Union, Democratic Republic of Vietnam and Yugoslavia: Akademie-Verlag, Leipziger Strasse 3—4, 1086 Berlin, DDR

for all other countries: Kluwer Academic Publishers Group, Distribution Center, P. O. Box 322, 3300 AH Dordrecht, The Netherlands

Library of Congress Cataloging in Publication Data
Main entry under title:

The Control of tumour growth and its biological bases.

   (Developments in oncology; v. 15)
   Papers delivered at the Ninth International Symposium on the Biological Characterization of Human Tumours, held in Bologna, Sept. 1981.
   1. Tumors—Treatment—Congresses. 2. Tumors—Chemotherapy—Congresses. 3. Antineoplastic agents—Testing—Congresses. 4. Cancer cells—Growth—Regulation—Congresses. I. Davis, Walter, Ph. D. II. Maltoni, Cesare. III. Tanneberger, S. (Stephan) IV. International Symposium on the Biological Characterization of Human Tumours (9th: 1981: Bologna, Italy) V. Series.
[DNLM: 1. Neoplasma invasiveness—Congresses. 2. Neoplasm metastasis—Congresses. 3. Neoplasms—Drug therapy—Congresses. 4. Receptors, Endogenous substances—Congresses. 5. Antineoplastic agents—Congresses. 6. Drug screening—Methods—Congresses. W1 DE998N v. 15 / QZ 267C764 1981]
RC270.8.C64   1983   616.99′406   83-17473
ISBN 0-89 838-603-9

Book information

Joint edition published by: Martinus Nijhoff Publishers, Boston, USA and Akademie-Verlag Berlin, DDR

PRINTED IN GDR

Introduction

During the last decades there have been enormous efforts to improve the survival of cancer patients through the use of improved cancer surgery, new approaches to radiotherapy and, particularly, by application of the very rapid developments in cancer chemotherapy. Nevertheless, only a disappointing 30% of patients developing a new cancer will survive longer than 5 years. In the case of lung or stomach cancer less than 10% of the patients will be cured. Therapeutic approaches which fundamentally change the treatment situation in cancer can be developed only by understanding the biological bases of tumour growth regulation. Treatment modalities must be adapted to the specific characteristics and the metabolic profile of target tumour cells.

Precisely this was the philosophy of the Ninth International Symposium on the Biological Characterization of Human Tumours held in Bologna, September 1981. Treatment approaches have been discussed in relation to biological cell targets taking tinto consideration such important fields of tumour cell biology as invasion, metastasis and cell surface. Cancer chemotherapy especially has been in need of more scientific background for drug development and less empiric approaches. The symposium was a very important and realistic step forwards to more scientific cancer chemotherapy research. Leading cancer research workers from both the laboratory and clinic attended the Bologna Symposium. Subsequentely these researchers from North America and Europe were invited to contribute to the present book. It is meant as a collective effort to understand growth mechanisms in neoplastic tissues, and it will, hopefully, contribute to the development of more scientific cancer therapy approaches. A number of individuals supported the editors in preparing this book. With many thanks we would like to mention Dr. PROJAN (Berlin), Mrs. GRUNOW (Berlin), Mrs. DALLÜGE (Berlin) and Mrs. DECHAUX (Lyon).

W. DAVIS
St. TANNEBERGER

Contents

Invasion and Metastasis as Targets for Tumour Therapy

K. E. Kuettner and B. U. Pauli: Primary Invasion: Natural Inhibitors 15

G. Atassi, P. Dumont and M. Vandendris: Effect of Deacetyl Vinblastine Amide Sulphate or Vindesine (VDS) against the In-Vivo Invasion and Formation of Tumour Metastasis 23

P. Hilgard and K. Hellmann: Invasion and Metastases as Targets for Tumour Therapy. An Overview 33

L. de Ridder, O. D. Laerum and S. Mörk: Invasiveness of Brain Tumour Cells in Vivo and In Vitro 42

M. Mareel, G. Storme, G. De Bruyne, R. van Cauwenberge and C. Dragonetti: Anti-invasiveness of Microtubule Inhibitors is due to Interference with the Cytoplasmic Microtubule Complex 47

T. Giraldi, G. Sava, R. Cherubino, L. Lassiani, G. Bottiroli and G. Mazzini: Metastasis: Mitostatic Drugs 55

L. R. Zacharski: Anticoagulant Treatment of Cancer 63

M. Nuti, Y. A. Teramoto, R. Marani-Constantini, P. Horan Hand, D. Colcher and J. Schlom: Reactivity of a Monoclonal Antibody (B72.3) with Fixed Sections of Human Mammary Carcinomas 66

W. A. Boggust and S. O'Connell: Polyamine Oxidation in Relation to Tumour Growth and Metastasis 71

K. Elgjo, G. Isaksson-Forsén, K. Reichelt and O. P. F. Clausen: Partial Purification of an Epidermal Growth Inhibitor (Chalone) 83

Hormone Receptors

E. Heise and M. Görlich: Estradiol Receptors in Human Breast Cancers and Prognosis . . . 87

A. Piffanelli, S. Fumero, D. Pelizzola, G. Giovannini and L. Ricci: External Quality Assessment Scheme of Estradiol Receptors Assay: An Italian Survey 93

I. Számel, B. Vincze, E. Svastits, J. Tóth, S. Kerpel-Fronius and S. Eckhardt: Methodological and Clinical Studies of the Steroid Receptor Assay in Primary Breast Cancer . . 99

Z. Pazko, H. Padzik, F. Pieńkowska, S. Chrapusta, B. Wasowska and E. Kwiatkowska: The Value of Hormone Receptor Assays for Prediction of the Effectiveness of Endocrine Therapy in Breast Cancer 104

The Cancer Cell Surface as a Target for Tumour Therapy

B. F. Deys: Normal and Pathological Cell Communication 113
H. Grunicke, H. Putzer, F. Scheidl and E. Wolff-Schreiner: The Cell Surface as a Target for Alkylating Agents 119
D. A. L. Davies: The Synergistic Effect of Drugs and Antibodies 127
A. Pihl and Ø. Fodstad: Cancerostatic Lectins 134
F. Stirpe and L. Barbieri: Ribosome-Inactivating Proteins as Possible Chemotherapeutic Agents 142
K. A. Krolick, W. Uhr and E. S. Vitetta: Selective Targeting of Ricin A Chain to a B Cell Tumour by Anti-Immunoglobin Antibodies 147

Development of New Drugs

C. Auclair, B. Meunier and C. Paoletti: The Generation of Reactive Molecular Species during the Oxidation of 9-Hydroxyellipticine Derivates. Interest of Prooxidant Compounds in the Design of Anticancer Drugs. 159
P. Workman: Development of Nitroimidazoles 166
M. Micksche, M. Colot, A. Fritsch, E. M. Kokoschka, R. Kolb, R. Lenzhofer, Th. Luger, K. Moser, H. Rainer, P. Sagaster and A. Uchida: Development of New Drugs — Immunomodulating Agents 173
C. J. Rutty, D. R. Newell, J. R. F. Muindi and K. R. Harrap: Development of Potential Clinical Alternatives to Hexamethylmelamine 180
J. Ban, E. Olah and G. Weber: Synergistic Interaction of an Alkylating Agent (Lycurim) and an Antimetabolite (Pyrazofurin) on Heptoma 3924 A Cells in Culture 189
F. Boccardo, R. Rosso, A. Barbieri, L. Canobbio, D. Guarneri and M. Merlano: Phase II Evaluation of 4-Thiazolidine-Carboxylic Acid (Thioproline) in Advanced Epidermoid Head and Neck Tumours 194
E. Csányi, Z. Hargittay, E. Király, T. Horváth, L. Bogdány and K. Tory: The Effect of a Bifunctional N-Notrosoureido Derivative (Gyki-13324) on Experimental Metastasis Models 198
M. Habs and D. Schmähl: Long-term Toxic and Carcinogenic Effects of Cytostatic Drugs 201
E. S. Newlands: VP 16-213 (Etoposide; NSC-141540; Vepesid): A Review 210
M. J. Cleare, P. C. Hydes and C. F. T. Barnard: New Platinum Anti-Cancer Drugs . . . 214
O. Wildermuth: The Status of Proteolytic Enzymes in Oncology 225
L. Lenaz, R. Canetta and P. Hilgard: Marcellomycin: A New Class II Anthracycline . . 231

Biological Response Modifiers

K. Sikora: Interferon 239
D. A. Stringfellow and G. L. Neil: Comparative Interferon-Inducing and Antitumour Activity of Substituted Pyrimidinones 245

J. Krušić, Ž. Maričić, V. Chylak, B. Rode, D. Jušić and E. Šooš: Influence of Human Leucocyte Interferon on Squamous-Cell Carcinoma of Uterine Cervix: Clinical, Histological and Histochemical Observations 253

I. Padovan, E. Šooš and I. Brodarec: Effect of Interferon on Malignant Head and Neck Tumours 256

P. K. Bondy and Z. Nakos Canellakis: Polyamines and Neoplasia: A Review of Present Knowledge of their Function and Therapeutic Potential 258

H. Wrba and A. G. Rieger: Retinoid 269

K. Takeda, J. Minowada and A. Bloch: The Role of Drug-Induced Differentiation in the Control of Tumour Growth 275

S. D. Vesselinovitch and N. Mihailovich: Modifying Effect of the Sex Hormonal Environment on the Growth of Basophilic Foci and Hepatocellular Carcinoma 282

K. Kolarić, A. Roth, I. Jelicić and A. Matković: Phase II Clinical Trial of cis-Dichlorodiamine Platinum (cis-DDP) in Metastatic Brain Tumours — A Preliminary Report . . 287

P. Chieco and C. Maltoni: Adriamycin: Experimental Evidence of Carcinogenicity . . . 292

G. Aicardi, G. Cantell Forti, M. C. Guerra, A. M. Barbaro and G. L. Biagi: Electroreduction, Mutagenicity and Antimicrobial Activity of 5-Nitroimidazole Derivates . . . 300

G. Sava, T. Giraldi, L. Lassiani and C. Nisi: Mechanism of the Antileukemic Action of DTIC and its Benzenoid Analog DM-COOK in Mice 309

Laboratory Assessment of Therapeutic Activity

St. Tanneberger and E. Nissen: The Role of In Vitro Techniques in Assessing Antineoplastic Therapeutic Activities 315

K. Lapis and L. Kopper: In Vivo Tests — Xenografts 327

C. Maltoni, G. Cotti, L. Valgimigli and A. Madrioli: Suitable Models for Long-Term Bioassays on the Therapeutic and Toxic Effects of Antiblastic Drugs: Liver Angiosarcomas Produced in Sprague-Dawley Rats by Vinyl Chloride 339

J. Sugár, O. Csuka, I. Pályi and E. Oláh: Role of some Biological Parameters in Drug Sensitivity and Resistance of Tumour Cells 342

R. I. Freshney, F. Celik and D. Morgan: Analysis of Cytotoxic and Cytostatic Effects . 349

A. H. Calvert and K. R. Harrap: An Appraisal of Current In Vivo and In Vitro Screening Methods 359

W. Krafft, D. Brückmann, J. Brückmann, H. Behling, W. Preibsch and J. Kademann: Clinical Relevance of some Useful Methodes for In Vitro Testing of Cytostatic Sensitivity in Cases of Ovarian Cancers 366

G. P. Stathopoulos, Ch. Pathouli, A. Manouras, A. Delladetsika, K. Pratsika-Uguroglou and M. Phillipakis: Immunoglobulin Producing Cell Infiltration in Colorectal Cancer Tissues Correlated with Patients Survival 369

G. Cotti, L. Valgimigli, A. Mandrioli and C. Maltoni: Suitable Models for Long-Term Bioassays of Therapeutic and Toxic Effects of Antiblastic Drugs: Brain Tumours of Neuronal Cells and Primitive Bipotential Precursors produced in Sprague-Dawley Rats by Vinyl Chloride 376

C. Maltoni: Laboratory Assessment of Therapeutic Activity (With Particular Regard to Chemotherapy): Relevant Animal Models 379

S. Perez-Cuadrado, M. C. Moreno-Koch and A. Uson-Calvo: Biological Significance and Dose-Dependent Effect of 'Resistocell' on Peripheral Blood Leucocytes In Vitro 393

9

H. G. Schleich, W. Wiest and R. Pohl: Human Serum Ribonuclease Activity as a Marker for Therapeutic Success in Ovarian Carcinoma 401

A. L. Jackman, A. H. Calvert, G. A. Taylor and K. R. Harrap: Biological Properties of the New Quinazoline Inhibitor of Thymidylate Synthetase CB 3717 404

Miscellaneous

B. Brdar and J. Sorić: Reactivation of Alkylation-Damaged Adenovirus 3 by Cell Cultures Derived from Human Tumours 413

L. Cacciari, E. Beltrandi, M. A. Bucci, R. Parente, F. Spagnolli and F. Servadei: Effects of Surgical and Radio-Chemotherapeutic Treatment on the Immunological Pattern in Malignant Glioma Patients 418

B. M. Bombik, S. Serke and H. Gerhartz: Control of Megacaryocyte Differentiation in Healthy and Leukemic Patients 423

G. Hagner, M. Bombik, W. D. Voigt and H. Gerhartz: Cytotoxic T Lymphocytes: Various Effects on Human Myeloma Cells 426

G. Cantelli Forti, G. Aicardi, N. M. Trieff, E. Speroni, T. Rossi and G. L. Biagi: Analysis of AHH Inducibility Ratios and Distribution in Human Lymphocytes by TLC-Radioisotopic Assay 431

M. Habs, H. Habs, G. Eisenbrand and D. Schmähl: Antitumour Activity of New Nitrosoureas on Yoshida Sarcoma Ascites Cells In Vitro 438

H. J. Hohorst, L. Bielicki and G. Voelcker: The Mode of Action of Cyclophosphamide 445

Index 457

Appendix 465

The Co-ordinating Committee for Human Tumour Investigations

Austria	Professor Dr. H. Wrba	Vienna
Belgium	Professor H. J. Tagnon	Brussels
Bulgaria	Dr. Maria Boeva	Sofia
Czechoslovakia	Dr. V. Ujhazy	Bratislava
Denmark	Dr. J. Clemmesen	Copenhagen
Eire	Dr. W. Boggust	Dublin
Federal Republic of Germany	Professor C. G. Schmidt	Essen
Finland	to be elected	
France	Dr. P. Malaise	
German Democratic Republic	Professor Dr. St. Tanneberger	Berlin
Greece	Dr. G. Stathopoulos	Athens
Hungary	Professor J. Sugár	Budapest
Italy	Professor C. Maltoni	Bologna
Netherlands	Dr. B. F. Deys	Amsterdam
Norway	Professor O. H. Iversen	Oslo
Poland	Dr. Olga Mioduszewska	Warsaw
Portugal	Professor A. S. Tavares	Oporto
Romania	Professor E. Craciun	Bucharest
Spain	Professor A. Llombart-Bosch	Valencia
Sweden	Dr. B. Nordenskjöld	Linköping
United Kingdom	Dr. K. Harrap	London
USSR	Dr. D. G. Zaridze	Moscow
Yugoslavia	Professor Z. Maričič	Zagreb
Secretary:	Dr. Walter Davis International Agency for Research on Cancer 150 cours Albert Thomas 69372 Lyon Cedex 2 France	

Invasion and Metastases as Targets for Tumour Therapy

Departments of Biochemistry, Orthopedic Surgery and Pathology
Rush Medical College, Chicago, Illinois 60612, USA

Primary Invasion: Natural Inhibitors

K. E. Kuettner and B. U. Pauli

The ability to invade normal host tissues and to metastasize to distant sites are the distinguishing features of malignant tumours (1). In order to invade and metastasize, tumour cells must overcome several structural barriers presented by host tissues. These barriers consist of meshworks of extracellular structural macromolecular complexes, such as collagen, proteoglycan, glycoproteins, and elastin. Since the normal packing of these macromolecules leaves little or no space for the free movement of tumour cells, cleavage by proteinases may provide a mechanism by which tumour cells invade (2). If this concept of proteinase involvement in tumour invasion is correct, proteinase inhibitors derived from host tissues may well locally impede the invasion of malignant tumour cells. Such proteinase inhibitors may partly be responsible for the classic observation that connective tissues are unequally susceptible to invasive processes even though these tissues are composed of similar structural macromolecules, and as such, are cleaved by identical proteinases (3, 4).

We have provided evidence that hyaline cartilage, a tissue highly resistant to invasive processes (Fig. 1), contains extractable, low molecular weight inhibitors directed against a spectrum of matrix-degrading enzymes, including enzymes postulated to be involved in the breakdown of the various types of collagen and proteoglycans (5—7). Hyaline cartilage, when depleted of these proteinase inhibitors by salt extraction, loses its natural resistance to invasion by malignant tumour cells in vitro (Fig. 2). Tumour cells superficially penetrate and degrade the proteinase inhibitor-depleted cartilaginous matrix (7). However, invasion of malignant tumour cells into such extracted cartilage was abolished when low concentrations of the extractant, containing the proteinase inhibitors, were added to the culture medium (4, 7) (Fig. 3). These morphological data provide strong evidence that the non-permissiveness of cartilage to tumour invasion, is caused primarily by substances directed against the invasive apparatus of tumour cells. An anti-invasion factor (AIF), can be extracted from fresh hyaline cartilage of bovine nasal septum by salt solutions, such as 1 M guanidine hydrochloride or 1 M sodium chloride, and enriched by ultrafiltration as previously described by our laboratory (6, 8, 9). AIF expresses inhibitory activity against a variety of proteinases. Kuettner et al, (5, 6) have shown that AIF contains a cationic protein fraction which possesses inhibitory activity directed against both trypsin, and mammalian collagenases. These latter enzymes have been derived from human skin, human mammary carcinoma cells, or conditioned media of TE-85 human osteosarcoma cells. Originally, it was suggested that the inhibitory activities against both trypsin and collagenase were due to a single protein eluted from an insoluble trypsoin affinity column that had a molecular weight of approximately 11,000 daltons (5, 6). However, Roughley et al, (10) have shown that the inhibition of trypsin and mammalian collagenases resides in distinct molecules, and that bovine nasal cartilage also contains a third inhibitor, directed against thiol proteinases, such as cathepsin B and papain. By gel chromatography, the inhibitors of collagenases, thiol proteinases, and trypsin are eluted with apparent molecular weights of approximately 22,000, 13,000 and 7,000 daltons, respectively. The trypsin inhibitor appears approximately at the same elution volume as the commercially available

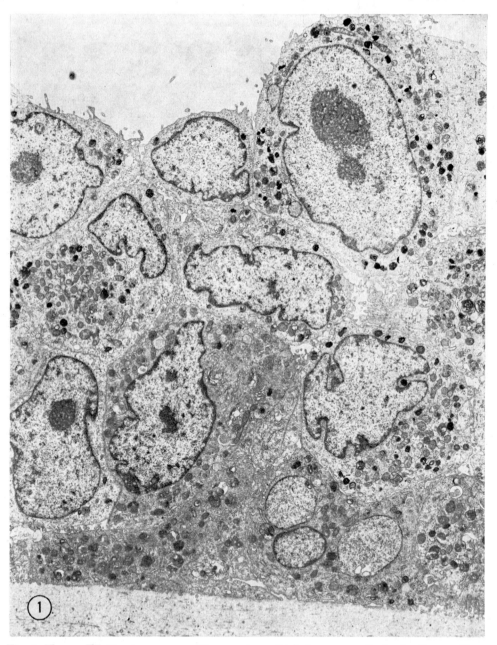

Fig. 1. Human TE-85 osteosarcoma cells grow in multiple layer on articular hyaline cartilage. Tumour cells are unable to penetrate the viable cartilagenous matrix. $\times$ 5,100

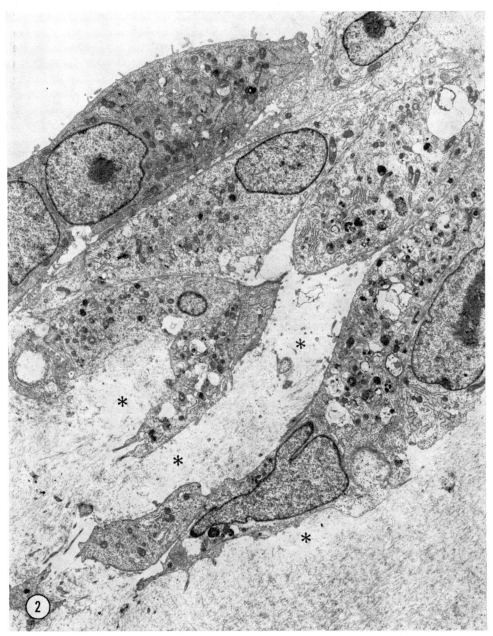

Fig. 2. Human TE-85 osteosarcoma cells penetrate the surface portion of 3M GuHCl extracted articular cartilage. Tumour invasion is associated with rarefaction (asterisk) of matrix components. × 3,700

basic pancreatic trypsin inhibitor (Trasylol[R]). It resembles Trasylol with respect to molecular weight, antigenicity, and range of susceptible proteinases, but shows slight variation in amino acid composition as reported by RIFKIN and CROWE (11). Susceptible proteinases are trypsin, chymotrypsin, plasmin, proteoglycan-degrading enzymes derived from human leukocyte extract, and tumour cell surface-associated neutral proteinases (for review see ref. 4). The similarity between the cartilage-derived trypsin inhibitor and Trasylol has motivated investigators to postulate that Trasylol and the cartilage-derived trypsin inhibitor are identical, at least in the bovine species. The presence of Trasylol in bovine cartilage could be due to synthesis by chondrocytes, or to uptake from blood plasma. The latter hypothesis seems especially intriguing, given the fact that highly anionic molecules of the cartilage matrix (the glycosamino-glycan-containing proteoglycans), may act as a sponge for low molecular weight, highly cationic molecules. By this mechanism, Trasylol could be continuously removed from the blood plasma and accumulated as this tissue ages. However, recent data obtained

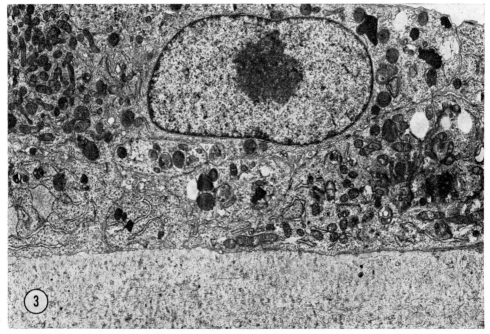

Fig. 3. Human TE-85 osteosarcoma cells are grown on 3M GuHCl-extracted articular cartilage in AIF-containing medium. There is no morphologic evidence of tumour invasion. × 7,500

in our laboratory indicate that Trasylol is synthesized by bovine articular chondrocytes in culture, and may well express a function in normal cartilage metabolism.

The cartilage-derived thiol-proteinase inhibitor described by ROUGHLY et al, (10) corresponds to the thiol-proteinase inhibitors isolated from chick egg-white, rabbit skin and rat skin. These inhibitors are rported to have similar thermal stabilities and molecular weights, and thus, may be identical. Inhibitory activity is detected against both cathepsin B and papain in a dose-dependent manner.

The collagenase inhibitory activity can be obtained as a single chromatographic fraction with an apparent molecular weight of about 22,000 daltons (10). Its electrophoretic mobility and molecular weight appear different from those of the collagenase inhibitors in serum and polymorphonuclear leukocytes, and from those of collagenase inhibitors synthesized in cultures by various explants of animal tissues. In contrast to these collagenase inhibitors, the cartilage-derived collagenase inhibitory activity resists thiol-binding reagents, and inhibits leukocyte-derived collagenases.

Recently, YASUI et al, (12) isolated and purified two collagenase inhibitors from the media of cultured metaphyseal region of embryonic chick limbs (growth cartilage)

18

by anion- and cation-exchange chromatography followed by gel filtration. The inhibitors are cationic proteins, that have molecular weights of approximately 25,000 daltons, but exhibit slight differences in molecular size. They inhibit collagenases from tadpole skin, chick bone and skin, and human granulocytes as well as gelatinases from human granulocytes and chick skin. It is noteworthy that these inhibitors also show activity against trypsin, but not bacterial collagenase.

In collaboration with Dr. LIOTTA, we have recently shown that the cartilage-derived anti-invasion factor also expresses inhibitory activities against the neutral metalloproteinases which cleave basement membrane collagens of Types IV and V (4). In a pilot experiment, using AIF at a concentration of 4 µg/ml, Type IV collagenolytic activity derived from metastatic murine PMT sarcomas was inhibited by approximately 80%. A similar degree of inhibition was observed for Type V collagenolytic activity derived from metastatic murine M-5076 reticulum cell sarcoma.

The spectrum of proteinase inhibitors, which is present in extracts of bovine hyaline cartilage, may play a significant role in the regulation of tumour invasiveness. The inhibition of major classes of matrix-degrading enzymes may prevent destruction and penetration of host connective tissue barriers by malignant tumour cells, i. e., epithelial or endothelial cell derived basement membranes. On the basis of their small molecular size, cartilage-derived proteinase inhibitors may have relatively free access to host tissue sites from which the potent, serum-derived proteinase inhibitor of $\alpha 2$-macroglobulin is excluded because of its large molecular size.

In addition to proteinase inhibitors, the anti-invasion factor (AIF) isolated from hyaline cartilage contains other small-molecular-weight cationic proteins, which may exert activity against growth and spreading of malignant tumours. One fraction of AIF possesses an anti-proliferative activity, which is directed against vascular endothelial cells in culture (8). This antiproliferative activity inhibits the proliferation of endothelial cells in a dose-dependent manner, as evidenced by both cell counts and ^{3}H-thymidine incorporation (4). SORGENTE and DOREY (13), have recently isolated and partially purified the endothelial cell growth inhibitor from an extract derived from bovine scapular cartilage by ion exchange chromatography. They observed two peaks of endothelial cell growth inhibitory activity. Each was eluted in a position distinct from the trypsin inhibitory activity. The first peak which was reported to contain about 90% of the total inhibitory activity, appeared immediately before the trypsin inhibitor, while the second peak appeared after the trypsin inhibitor. The endothelial cell growth inhibitor is non-toxic. It increases the doubling time of endothelial cells from 24 hours to 40 hours. The findings of these investigators suggest that the antiproliferative activity arrests endothelial cells in the G_1 phase.

The anti-invasion factor, derived from hyaline cartilage seems to be identical to the anti-angiogenic factor described by FOLKMAN and associates (14, 15). Using the rabbit cornea as an assay system, these investigators showed that neovascularization of tumours could be inhibited when a small piece of viable hyaline cartilage was positioned between the tumour implant and the corneoscleral junction (14). The capillary cells, which normally grew rapidly towards the corneal tumour implant, proliferated at extremely slow rates. At the end of the second week, they had only reached half of the distance which they had reached during the first week in the control experiment. A diffusable factor, isolated from a 1 M guanidinium hydrochloride-extract of bovine scapular cartilage, was recognized as being responsible for the inhibition of tumour induced vascular proliferation (15). The anti-angiogenic activity, which is probably identical to the endothelial cell growth inhibitor, may thus have significant effect on the growth of tumours by inhibiting neovascularization.

Similar low-molecular weight factors have since been prepared from extracts of other bradytrophic tissues, i.e., bovine aorta, bovine heart valve, and bovine urinary bladder mucosa. Aortic factor has been characterized by EISENSTEIN et al (16). These investigators reported that the aortic factor inhibited (a) the growth of bovine aortic endothelial cells and embryonic fibroblasts in vitro, (b) tryptic and chymotryptic activities, as demonstrated in a fibrin agar diffusion assay, (c) collagenases prepared from tadpole or human skin and (d) tumour growth in culture, and in animal hosts after systemic injection.

A low-molecular weight factor with similar biological activity has recently been isolated from extracts of bovine urinary bladder mucosa and submucosa. This factor expresses strong proteinase inhibitory activity against trypsin, and to a lesser extent, against chymotrypsin, as well as an anti-proliferative activity against endothelial cells in culture.

In summary, experimental evidence has been provided that the resistance of cartilage to tumour invasion may be due to an extractable, low-molecular weight factor, functionally defined as anti-invasion factor (9). This factor contains the following anti-invasive activities: (1) proteinase (collagenase) inhibitory activity (5, 6); (2) anti-proliferative activity directed against endothelial cells in vitro (anti-angiogenic activity) (4); and (3) tumour growth inhibitory activity (16). These activities occur in the low-molecular weight protein fractions (1,000—50,000 daltons) of a 1 M NaCl extract of hyaline cartilage, or as shown only recently, in chondrocyte cultures established from bovine articular cartilage. They may well act as local regulators for some of the major mechanistic pathways by which tumour cells are thought to invade host tissues, and metastasize to distant sites, namely by matrix-degrading enzymes as well as increased locomotion and proliferation (4). In addition, they may inhibit tumour neovascularization and control local tumour growth. On the basis of their small molecular weight, they are thought to have relatively free access to tissue sites, thus increasing their efficacy. The various protein fractions found in cartilage-derived AIF are currently being purified and biochemically characterized in our laboratories

Acknowledgements

Appreciation is expressed to the research assistants who are presently involved with the study of cartilage-derived anti-invasion factor: Mr. S. ANDERSON, Ms. J. CHARNESKY, Ms. S.-Y. CHI, Mr. R. CROXEN, Mr. G. GALL, Mr. L. MADSEN, Ms. C. SANES-MILLER, and Ms. N. WROBEL. The authors wish to thank Drs. D. SCHWARTZ, E. J.-M. THONAR, and J. C. DANIEL for helpful discussions and advice during the investigations, and Ms. P. BRIDGES and V. HEARON for preparing the manuscript.

This work was supported by NIH grants CA-21566 and CA-25034, and in part by NIH grant AM-09132, and grant numbers 1394 and 1206A from the Council for Tobacco Research-USA, Inc.

References

1. FIDLER, I. J., GERSTEN, D. M. and HART, I. R.: The biology of cancer invasion and metastasis. Adv. Canc. Res. 28 (1978), 149—250
2. STRAULI, P., BARRETT, A. J. and BAICI, A., (eds.): Proteinases and tumor invasion, Monograph Series EORTC, Vol. 6, Raven Press, New York, 1980

3. KUETTNER, K. E. and PAULI, B. U.: Resistance of cartilage to normal and neoplastic invasion. In: Proceedings, mechanisms of localized bone loss. HORTON, J. E., TARPLEY, T. M., DAVIS, W. F. (eds), Special Supplement to Calcified Tissue Abstracts, 1978, p. 251—278

4. PAULI, B. U. and KUETTNER, K. E.: The regulation of invasion by a cartilage-derived anti-invasion factor. In: Cancer invasion and metastasis, LIOTTA, L. A., HART, I. R., eds., Martinus Nijhoff Publishers, Hingham (in press)

5. KUETTNER, K. E., HITI, J., EISENSTEIN, R. and HARPER, E.: Collagenase inhibition by cationic proteins derived from cartilage and aorta. Biochem. Biophys. Res. Commun. 72 (1976), 40—46

6. KUETTNER, K. E., SOBLE, L., CROXEN, R. L., MARCZYNSKA, B., HITI, J. and HARPER, E.: Tumour cell collagenase and its inhibition by cartilage-derived protease inhibitors. Science 196 (1977), 653—654

7. PAULI, B. U., MEMOLI, V. A. and KUETTNER, K. E.: Regulation of tumor invasion by cartilage-derived anti-invasion factor in vitro. J. Natl. Cancer Inst. 67 (1981), 65—73

8. EISENSTEIN, R., KUETTNER, K. E., NEAPOLITAN, C., SOBLE, L. W. and SORGENTE, N.: The resistance of certain tissues to invasion. III. Cartilage extracts inhibit the growth of fibroblasts and endothelial cells in culture. Am. J. Pathol. 81 (1975), 337—348

9. HORTON, J. E., WEZEMAN, F. N. and KUETTNER, K. E.: Inhibition of bone resorption in vitro by a cartilage-derived anti-collagenase factor. Science 199 (1978), 1342—1345

10. ROUGHLEY, P. J., MURPHY, G. and BARRETT, A. J.: Proteinase inhibitors of bovine nasal cartilage. Biochem. J. 169 (1978), 721—724

11. RIFKIN, D. R. and CROWE, R. M.: Isolation of a proteinase inhibitor from tissues resistant to tumor invasion. Hoppe-Seyler's Z. Physiol. Chem. 358 (1977), 1525—1531

12. YASUI, Y., HISAE, H. and NAGAI, Y.: Production of collagenase inhibitor by the growth cartilage of embryonic chick bone: Isolation and partial characterization. Coll. Res. 1 (1981), 59—72

13. SORGENTE, N. and DOREY, C. K.: Inhibition of endothelial cell growth by factor isolated from cartilage. Exp. Cell. Res. 128 (1980), 63—71

14. BREM, H. and FOLKMAN, J.: Inhibition of tumor angiogenesis mediated by cartilage. J. Exp. Med. 141 (1975), 427—439

15. BREM, H., ARENSMAN, R. and FOLKMAN, J.: Inhibition of tumor angiogenesis by a diffusable factor from cartilage. In: Extracellular matrix influences on gene expression, SLAVKIN, H. C., GREULICH, R. C. (eds.), New York, Academic Press, 1975, p. 767—772

16. EISENSTEIN, R., SCHUMACHER, B., MEINECKE, C., MATIJEVITCH, B. and KUETTNER, K. E.: Growth regulators in connective tissue. Systematic administration of an aortic extract inhibits tumor growth in mice. Am. J. Pathol. 91 (1978), 1—10

Laboratoire de Chimiothérapie expérimentale et Screening,
Institut Jules Bordet, Bruxelles, Belgium

Effect of Desacetyl Vinblastine Amide Sulphate or Vindesine (VDS) against the In Vivo Invasion and Formation of Tumour Metastasis[1]

G. Atassi, P. Dumont and M. Vandendris

Abstract

Mareel and coworkers have thrown some light on the mechanisms of invasion and that of anti-invasive drugs. We assumed that it would be highly profitable to attempts to apply their findings to the prevention of invasion and metastasis in vivo. For this purpose, we used VDS, a microtubule inhibitor with anti-invasive properties in vitro. Our results show that 0.2 mg/kg of VDS administered intraperitoneally (i.p.) to mice bearing an intramuscularly implanted Lewis lung carcinoma (LLC) during 8 consecutive days did not affect the growth of the primary tumour but significantly reduced the number of metastases in the treated group (1.2 ± 0.5) as compared to that in the control group (15.37 ± 2.5 per mouse). Surgical amputation of the tumoured limb + treatment with VDS resulted not only in a significant reduction of the number of metastases but also only 2 mice out of 8 had lung metastases. This inhibitory effect on metastasis was also observed when VDS was given as a prophylactic treatment to surgery on day 9 post implant on an advanced LLC tumour. A 0.2 mg/kg dose administered i.p. during 11 days against subcutaneously (s.c.) implanted B 16 melanoma reduced the number of mice with metastases by 50 % and the number of metastases per mouse by 70 %. The same dose given from day $2-15$ after intramuscular implantation of the Madison 109 lung carcinoma reduced the number of metastases to 10 ± 5 vs. 119.2 ± 18.5 in the control group. The 2.5 mg/kg dose of VDS given intravenously on days 2, 9, 16, and 23 post implant totally inhibited the appearance of metastases. On the contrary, we did not observe any effect against lymph node metastases in the s.c. P388 model when VDS was injected i.p. to mice. The discrepancy between the latter model and the three earlier described may be due to the different local systemic mechanisms favouring or opposing the phenomena of invasion, dissemination, and the establishment of secondary malignancies and or to the difference in drug distribution. However, although our data did not permit us to conclude that VDS has a specific anti-invasive property in vivo, its inhibitory effect against secondary tumour growth is in accordance with the assumption that invasion is the first step in the establishment of metastasis and makes it worth using anti-invasive drugs for the prevention of metastasis.

Introduction

One of the most restrictive factors in the development of therapeutic agents against the establishment of metastasis is the general ignorance of many basic events and mechanisms of neoplastic invasion and spreading. The results so far obtained in the attempts to control cancer cell invasion and dissemination are either contradictory to or dependent on the experimental methods used.

Recently, invasion of malignant cells into normal cells was clearly demonstrated (1) and it was shown that invasion of malignant cells in vivo is important for the take

[1] This work was supported by Contract No. N01-CM-53850 of the NCI Liaison Office in Brussels

of a tumour transplant (2, 3). This finding supports the assumption that local invasion from a primary tumour is the first step in the formation of metastasis and makes it necessary to consider invasion as well as proliferation as a target of chemotherapy. We believed it worth investigating the antimetastatic potential of drugs with anti-invasive properties. It was reported a few years ago that microtubule inhibitors have not only an antimitotic activity but also an anti-invasive capacity in vitro (4) and in vivo (3). It was also shown that vindesine (VDS) like the other vinca alkaloids vinblastine and vincristine stops the invasion of mouse fibrosarcoma cells in vitro by interfering with the cytoplasmic microtubule complex (5—7).

To find out whether there was any correlation between the anti-invasive and anti-metastatic properties of one drug, we investigated the effect of VDS on the growth of murine primary tumour and spontaneous lung metastasis formation.

Materials and methods

Four different tumour models were used in this study:

a) the Lewis lung carcinoma (LLC) intramuscularly (i.m.) implanted in C57B1/6 or BDF$_1$ mice. In this case, pulmonary metastasization was assessed as described in (8);

b) the subcutaneously (s.c.) transplanted B16 melanoma: a tumour homogenate was prepared using 1 g of tumour and 1 ml of Hanks' balanced salt solution and 0.05 ml from this homogenate ($\pm 10^7$ tumour cells) was inoculated s.c. on day 0 in the left hind footpad of C57B1/6 mice. Lung metastases were macroscopically examined (day 18), measured as for LLC and counted;

c) the Madison 109 lung carcinoma (9) or MLC: 5×10^5 tumour cells in 0.1 ml of Hanks' balanced salt solution were inoculated i.m. (day 0) into the right hind leg of CDF$_1$ mice. The animals were sacrificed on day 28 post implant. The tumour was excised and weighed and lung metastases were counted under a stereoscopic microscope. With an other group, the antimetastatic and antitumour activity of the drug was expressed by the percent increase in lifespan (I.L.S. %) calculated from the median survival time (M.S.T.) of treated and control animals (M.S.T. of treated mice divided by that of untreated control mice, subtracting 1 and multiplying by 100).

d) the s.c. transplanted P388 leukemia: it was reported (10) that this model regularly produces lymph node metastases. One million P388 cells were inoculated into the right fore footpad of CDF$_1$ mice. VDS or 5-Fluorouracil (5-FU) was administered i.p. from day 1 to 8 post implant. One untreated group served as control. On day 8, mice were separated into two equal groups: one group was killed and their axillary lymph nodes were transferred i.p. to intact mice for evaluation of the tumour burden in the lymph nodes. The right forelimb of the mice in the other group was amputated. The median survival time of the two groups was recorded to determine the antitumour and antimetastatic activity of the drug by calculating the I.L.S. %. Fluorouracil, a well-known cytostatic agent with no anti-invasive property, was used with a view to compare its antimetastatic activity to that of VDS.

Results

A. Lewis lung carcinoma

The comparative effects of one daily i.p. injection during 9 days of 0.2 mg/kg of VDS and of 20 mg/kg of 5-FU are shown in Table 1. These doses are considered to be optimal following this schedule of treatment. Only 5-FU was able to reduce tumour weight by 36.5% in comparison with the control. VDS had no effect under the same conditions against the primary tumour while it was more effective than 5-FU in reducing the

Table 1.
Inhibitory effect of VDS or 5-FU on the growth of Lewis lung carcinoma and the formation of lung metastases

Doses mg/kg	Average tumour weight (g)	No. of mice with tumour / No. of mice in the group	No. of mice with metastases / No. of mice with tumour	Average no. of metastases per mouse	Average weight of metastases (mg)
0	10.66 ± 2	8/8	8/8	15.37 ± 2.5	48.25 ± 7.5
VDS 0.2 mg/kg	10.9 ± 1.80	7/7	6/7	1.2 ± 0.5	1.82 ± 0.2
5-FU 20 mg/kg	6.77 ± 1.2*	6/6	6/6	5.83	4.26 ± 0.52

10^6 tumour cells were inoculated i.m. on day 0. in C57B1/6 mice
VDS or 5-FU were administered i.p. from day 0 to 8.
Mice were sacrificed on day 22.
* corresponds to a 36.5% inhibition of tumour growth in comparison with the controls

Table 2.
Effect of VDS or VDS + surgery against metastases in C57B1/6 mice bearing i.m. Lewis lung carcinoma

Treatment	Average tumour weight (g)	No. of mice with metastases / No. of mice with tumour	No. of metastases per mouse	Average weight of metastases per mouse (mg)
0	8.5 ± 0.6	19/19	6.2 ± 2.5	21.5 ± 11.6
VDS 0.2 mg/kg	8.2 ± 1.2	13/13	2.7 ± 1.0	5.7 ± 1.5
surgery	–	9/9	8.1 ± 1.2	136.2 ± 30
surgery + VDS 0.2 mg/kg	–	2/8	0.13	0.25

$2 \cdot 10^5$ tumour cells were inoculated i.m. on day 0.
VDS was administered i.p. once daily from day 0 to 15.
Surgical amputation of the tumoured limb was performed on day 12.

number and weight of metastases. It was also observed that 1 mouse out of 7 in the group treated with VDS had no metastases at all.

In a second experiment with LLC, treatment with 0.2 mg/kg of VDS administered i.p. and daily from day 0 to 15 was compared to surgery where the tumour was removed under anaesthesia on day 12 and to the combination of surgery plus the above-mentioned daily administration of VDS. Again, VDS alone produced no effect against the primary tumour but significantly reduced the number and weight of metastases as compared to the controls (Table 2). Surgery alone on day 12 slightly increased the number of metastases and considerably the weight of metastases. Surgery on day 12 + 0.2 mg/kg of VDS given i.p. from day 0 to 15 strongly inhibited the appearance of lung metastases since only 2 mice out of 8 had metastases and the average number and weight of metastases were less than 1 and 1 mg respectively as compared to 8.1 metastases and 136.2 mg in the surgery group.

When VDS was administered i.v. on days 1, 5 and 9 after tumour inoculation, the 2.5 mg/kg dose was able to reduce very slightly the tumour weight and very significantly the number and weight of metastases. It should, however, be pointed out that the latter dose was toxic, 4 mice out of 9 dying before the day of evaluation. The 1.5 mg/kg dose produced no effect against the primary tumour and significantly reduced the number and weight of lung metastases.

Surgical excision of the primary tumour on day 9 induced a high increase in the number of metastases and a considerable one in the weight of metastases. Surgery on day 9 plus administration of 1.5 mg/kg of VDS on days 1, 5, and 9 were more active than VDS alone in reducing the number and weight of lung metastases (Table 3).

It seemed of interest to us to check whether a prophylactic treatment with VDS was able to prevent the increase in lung metastases after surgical treatment of advanced LLC. For this purpose, in one group of mice, the primary tumour was removed by surgical amputation of the tumoured limb 9 days after tumour transplantation. A second group received i.v. 1.25 mg/kg of VDS 1 hour before and 18 hours after surgery. A third group was treated only by VDS on day 9 and the last untreated group served as control. Table 4 shows that surgical excision of the primary tumour resulted in increasing not only the weight of metastases but also their number as compared to the untreated control mice and to the mice receiving VDS only. However, surgical removal of the primary tumour + treatment with VDS induced a reduction of the number (7.1 vs. 13 in the control group) and of the weight (26 mg vs. 38.9) of metastases, i. e. a 45.4% reduction of the number of metastases and a 33.2% reduction of their weight.

B. B16 melanoma

This tumour seemed to be much more sensitive to VDS than the Lewis lung carcinoma. Table 5 illustrates the effectiveness of VDS against B 16 melanoma. One daily i.p. administration of 0.1 mg/kg of VDS from day 1 to 11 post implant did not affect the growth of the primary tumour. When 0.2 mg/kg of VDS was administered following the same schedule, the tumour weight was reduced by 37% in comparison with untreated animals (the average tumour weight of treated mice is 0.72 ± 0.27 g vs. 1.14 ± 0.45 g for the controls). The decrease in the number and weight of metastases was also dose-dependent: 0.2 mg/kg was far more effective in inhibiting metastases formation (0.9 metastases per treated mouse instead of 3 per control mouse and 0.48 mg instead of 3.65).

Table 3.
Effect of an i.v. treatment with VDS + surgery on the growth of Lewis lung carcinoma and the formation of lung metastases

Treatment	Tumour weight (g)	Early death before day 22	No. of mice with metastases / No. of mice in the group	Average no. of metastases per mouse	Average weight of metastases per mouse (mg)
0	8.82	0	7/7	19.6	106
surgery		0	7/7	28.5	315.7
VDS 2.5 mg/kg	7.47	4/9	5/5	8	13.3
VDS 1.25 mg/kg	8.1	0	9/9	12.6	46.6
surgery + VDS 1.25 mg/kg	—	0	10/10	5.8	21.77
surgery + VDS 2.5 mg/kg	—	9/9			

$2 \cdot 10^5$ tumour cells were inoculated i.m. on day 0 in C57B1/6 mice.
VDS was administered on days 1, 5, and 9.
Surgical amputation of the tumoured limb was performed on day 9.
Metastases were counted and weighed on day 22.

Table 4.
Effect of surgery plus a prophylactic treatment with VDS on advanced Lewis lung carcinoma and lung metastases

Treatment	Average tumour weight (g)	No. of mice with metastases / No. of mice in the group	Average no. of metastases per mouse	Average weight of metastases per mouse (mg)
0	12.26 ± 0.29	14/14	13 ± 2.5	38.9 ± 6
VDS 2.5 mg/kg	11.64 ± 0.6	9/9	7 ± 0.6	21.1 ± 9
surgery	—	15/15	17.6 ± 3.8	135.66 ± 16
surgery + VS 2.5 mg/kg	—	9/9	7.1 ± 2	26.0 ± 2

$2 \cdot 10^5$ tumour cells were inoculated in BDF$_1$ mice on day 0.
Surgical amputation of the tumoured limb was performed on day 9.
A 1.25 mg/kg dose of VDS was administered twice i.v.: 1 hour before and 18 hours after surgery.

Table 5.
Effect of VDS against B16 melanoma and lung metastases

Doses mg/kg	Average tumour weight (g)	No. of mice with tumour / No. of mice in the group	No. of mice with metastases / No. of mice in the group	Average no. of metastases per mouse	Average weight of metastases per mouse (mg)
0	1.14 ± 0.45	10/10	10/10	3 ± 2	3.65 ± 1.5
0.1	1.2 ± 0.25	9/9	9/9	2.4 ± 1	1.98 ± 0.5
0.2	0.72 ± 0.27	10/10	5/10	0.9 ± 0.4	0.48 ± 0.06

0.05 ml of tumour homogenate (1 + 1) was inoculated s.c. on day 0 in the hind footpad of C57B1/6 mice.
VDS was administered daily from day 1 to day 11 post implant.
Evaluation of the number of weight of metastases on day 18.

Table 6.
Inhibitory effect of VDS on the primary tumour growth and lung metastasis formation of Madison 109 lung carcinoma

Doses mg/kg	Average tumour weight	No. of mice with tumour / No. of mice in the group	No. of mice with metastases / No. of mice with tumour	Average no. of metastases per mouse
0	7.65 ± 0.71	10/10	10/10	119.2 ± 18.5
0.1	4.8 ± 1.5	8/8	8/8	45.2 ± 13
0.2	3.46 ± 0.32	8/8	8/8	10 ± 5

$5 \cdot 10^5$ tumour cells were inoculated i.m. in CDF₁ mice on day 0.
VDS was given i.p. from day 2 to 15 post implant.
Evaluation of the inhibitory effect was performed on day 28.

C. Madison 109 lung carcinoma

Table 6 illustrates the inhibitory effect of VDS on the growth of the primary MLC and the high reduction of the number of metastases. The number of metastases per untreated animal was 119.2 ± 18.5 while 0.1 mg/kg of VDS given i.p. from day 2 to 15 post implant reduced the number of metastases to 45.2 ± 13 and 0.2 mg/kg of VDS also given during 14 days reduced it to 10 ± 5. The growth of the primary tumour (3.46 g) was reduced by 55% in comparison with the control mice (7.65 g) by the administration of 0.2 mg/kg of VDS X 14. A higher activity was observed when 1.25 and 2.5 mg/kg of VDS were given i.v. on days 2, 9, 16, and 23 post implant (Table 7). Following the latter schedule and route of treatment, 1.25 mg/kg reduced the primary tumour to 1.5 ± 0.54 g (i.e. a $80.4\pm$ reduction) as compared to $7.65 \pm \pm 0.71$ in the control group and only 1 mouse out of 10 had metastases. After the administration of the 2.5 mg/kg dose, following the same schedule and route, there was no measurable tumour at all on day 28 which is the day of evaluation and no metastases at all in this treated group. On day 33 which was the median survival time of the untreated control mice, only 2 mice out of 10 had a measurable tumour. All control mice died on day 35 and only 4 treated (2.5 mg/kg) mice had a palpable

Table 7.
Inhibitory effect of iv administration of VDS on the primary tumour and lung metastases of Madison 109 lung carcinoma

Doses mg/kg	Average tumour weight (g)	No. of mice with tumour	No. of mice with metastases	Average no. of metastases per mouse
		No. of mice in the group	No. of mice with tumour	
0	7.65 ± 0.71	10/10	10/10	119.2 ± 18.5
1.25	1.5 ± 0.54	10/10	1/10	0.20
2.5	0	0/10	0/0	0

$5 \cdot 10^5$ tumour cells were inoculated i.m. in CDF_1 mice on day 0.
I.v. treatment was administered on days 2, 9, 16 and 23 after tumour inoculation.
The evaluation was performed on day 28.

Table 8.
Effect of VDS administered i.v. on the survival of Madison lung carcinoma bearing mice

Doses	Med. S.T.	I.L.S.	Survival of tumour bearing mice
mg/kg	(days)	(%)	on day 60
0	33		0
1.25	51	54.5	1/10
2.5	> 60	81.8	6/10

$5 \cdot 10^5$ tumour cells were inoculated i.m. on day 0.
VDS was administered on days 2, 9, 16 and 23 post implant.
Med. S.T. = median survival time of 10 treated mice and 10 controls
I.L.S. = increase in lifespan: $\left(\dfrac{\text{Med. S.T. of treated mice}}{\text{Med. S.T. of control mice}} - 1 \right) \times 100$

tumour. With the increase in lifespan being used as a parameter to evaluate the effectiveness of VDS against the M109 tumour, the response was clearly dose-dependent (Table 8): 2.5 mg/kg was much more effective than 1.25 with a respectively corresponding I.L.S. of 81.8 and 54.5. Only mice dead before day 60 were used to make this evaluation.

D. P388 leukemia

Table 9 shows the effect of VDS or 5-FU against lymph node metastases of P388 transplanted s.c. Neither VDS nor 5-FU produced an antimetastatic activity under the conditions of our experiment.

Table 9.
Inhibition of lymph node metastases

Drug	Doses mg/kg	Amputation Group I.L.S. %	Lymph node recipients I.L.S. %
VDS	0.3	9	8
5-FU	10	0	0

Discussion

We have been pleasantly surprised at the clear effectiveness of VDS in preventing spontaneous lung metastases in three different models out of the four used in this study. However, our data do not permit us to conclude that VDS has a specific anti-invasive or anti-disseminative property in vivo. Indeed, there is no evidence as to whether VDS produces, like the other phase-specific anticancer drugs, an in-vivo effect which is more specific against cell population undergoing active cell replication (which is the case of metastatic cells) than against the larger cell population of the primary tumour from which the metastatic cells were derived (11−13) and to whether it prevents invasion (6). Probably, there is no clear-cut distinction between the two mechanisms and the antimetastatic effect of VDS may be due to both the anti-proliferative and anti-invasive properties of this agent. The latter assumption is supported to a certain extent by our data.

Obviously, when the tumour is rather resistant to treatment with VDS (like the Lewis lung carcinoma), VDS is not effective in inhibiting the growth of the primary tumour while it significantly inhibits the growth of lung metastases while 5-FU, a phase-specific agent with no anti-invasive property, was able to slightly reduce the primary tumour growth but was unable to reduce the number of metastases to the same extent as VDS.

An early treatment with VDS starting immediately after tumour transplantation of $2 \cdot 10^5$ tumour cells (Table 1) which reduces the number of lung metastases should induce some inhibition of the primary tumour since the tumour burden is relatively low at the beginning of the treatment. Considering that the number of metastases reflect the anti-invasive effect and their weight the proliferation, it is not unreasonable to think that VDS acts through both mechanisms.

Treatment with 5-FU was able to reduce by 36.5% the growth of the primary tumour.

It significantly inhibited the number of metastases but not so much as VDS. One may, therefore, assume that treatment with VDS interferes with the invasion of tumour cells from the site of implantation and reduces the number of metastases. Other arguments are not to be excluded.

The encouraging data obtained when VDS was used as an adjuvant to surgery (Tables 2 and 3) and when an i.v. prophylactic treatment on day 9 only was combined to surgery (Table 4) demonstrate that this microtubule inhibitor is also effective against an advanced Lewis lung carcinoma.

It is worthy of note that surgery alone increased the number of metastases — which may reflect a possible increase in the number of tumour cells invading the surrounding tissue and then disseminating to the lung where they metastasize — and the weight of metastases which reflects an increase in the proliferative rate of the metastatic cells (11). On the contrary, the use of VDS with surgery reduced the number and weight of metastases.

The effect of a treatment with VDS against B16 melanoma and Madison lung carcinoma shows that the inhibition of metastasis formation and even tumour growth is not confined to one experimental model.

With the sc P388 model, we did not observe any effect against lymph node metastases. The discrepancy between the latter model and the three earlier described may be due to the local and systemic mechanisms which may favour or oppose the phenomena of invasion, dissemination, and growth of metastases. Drug distribution may also be responsible for the absence of antimetastatic effect.

Although we may not objectively assert that VDS has an anti-invasive property, we may report the effectiveness of VDS in inhibiting tumour growth and metastasis formation does not contradict the assumption that invasion of malignant cells into normal cells is the first step to metastasis. This makes it worth using drugs showing anti-invasive activity in the treatment and prevention of metastasis.

Acknowledgements

The authors wish to thank Dr. H. DUBRUYNE for this generous supply of vindesine

References

1. MAREEL, M., KINT, J. and MEYVISCH, C: Methods of study of the invasion of malignant C$_3$H-mouse fibroblasts into embryonic chick heart in vitro. Virchows Arch. B. Cell path. 30 (1979), 95—111

2 MEYVISCH, C. and MAREEL, M.: Invasion of malignant C$_3$H-mouse fibroblasts from aggregates. transplanted into the auricles of syngeneic mice. Virchows Arch. B. cell path. 30 (1979), 113—122

3. MEYVISCH, C. and VAN CAUWENBERG, R.: Invasiveness of malignant mouse fibroblasts in vivo in: M. De Brabander (ed), Cell Locomotion and Neoplasia, Pergamon Press, Oxford, 1980, 179—185

4. MAREEL, M. and DE BRABANDER, M.: Effect of microtubule inhibitors on malignant invasion in vitro. J. Natl. Cancer Inst. 61 (1978), 787—792

5. STORM, G. and MAREEL, M.: Effect of anticancer agents on directional migration of malignant C$_3$H mouse fibroblastic cells in vitro. Cancer Res. 40 (1980), 943—948

6. STORM, G., MAREEL, M., DE BRUYNE, G., VAN CAUWENBERG, R.: Antiinvasive effect on vinca alkaloids in vitro: ultrastructural aspects and reversibility in: Brad, Bad Homburg, NAGEL and SEEBER (eds), Proceedings of the international vinca alkaloid symposium — vindesine, 1980, 7—15

7. MAREEL, M., STORM, G., DEBRUYNE, G. and VAN CAUWENBERG, R.: Anti-invasive effect of microtubule inhibitors in vitro in DE BRABANDER and DE MEY (eds), Microtubules and Microtubule Inhibitors, Elsevier, North-Holland Biomedica Press 1980, 535—544

8. ATASSI, G., DUMONT, P. and HARTEEL, J. C. E.: Potentiation of antitumor activity of 2-formyl pyridine thiosemicarbazone by metal chelation. Europ. J. Cancer 15 (1979), 451

9. MARKS, T. A., WOODMAN, R. J., GERAN, R. I., BILLUPS, L. H. and MADISON, R. M.: Characterization and responsiveness of the Madison 109 lung carcinoma to various antitumor agents. Cancer Rep. 61 (1977), 1459—1470

10. TSURNO, T., NAGANUMA, K., LIDA, H. and TSUKAGOSHI, S.: Lymph node metastasis and effects of 1 -D-arabinofurano-sylcytosine I-fluorouracil and their lipophilic derivatives in an experimental model system using P388 leukemia. Cancer Res. 40 (1980), 4758—4763

11. SIMPSON-HERREN, L., SANFORD, A. H. and HOLMQUIST, J. P.: Cell population kinetics of transplanted and metastatic Lewis lung carcinoma. Cell Tissue Kinet. 7 (1974), 349—361

12. SIMPSON-HERREN, L., SPRINGER, T. A., SANFORD, A. H., and HOLMQUIST, J. P.: Kinetics of metastases in experimental tumors in cancer invasion and metastasis: biologic mechanisms and therapy, DAY, S. B. et al. (eds) 1977, 177—133.

13. SCHABEL, F. M.: Concepts for treatment of micrometastases developped in murine systems. The American Journal of Roentgenology, Radium therapy and Nuclear Medicine 126 (1976), 500—511

Bristol Myers International Corporation, Brussels
and Department of Chemotherapy, Imperial Cancer
Research Fund, London

Invasion and Metastases as Targets for Tumour Therapy. An Overview

P. HILGARD and K. HELLMANN

Introduction

A cursory look at recent cancer statistics will immediately uncover the scale of the problem with which we are dealing in this chapter. The five-year survival rates and the disease stage at the time of diagnosis of the four leading cancers in humans are given in Table 1 (1). The failure of the currently available treatment to cure patients from their malignant disease correlates closely with the extent of tumour spread at diagnosis. Early dissemination to distant sites determines the poor prognosis of lung and stomach cancer whereas colo-rectal and breast cancer appear to metastasize comparatively late.

Table 1.
Five-year survival rates and disease stage at time of diagnosis. From (1)

	5-year survival rates (All stages)	% of cases by stage at diagnosis		
		Local	Regional	Distant
Breast cancer	65%	48%	41%	9%
Colorectal	46%	44	26%	25
Lung	13%	17	22%	48
Stomach	14%	18	28%	46

From: Cancer Statistics 1980
        American Cancer Society

Despite spectacular recent progress in the treatment of some malignant tumours by the combination of available treatment modalities, statistics give a disappointing picture of the development of the five-year survival rate for the major solid tumours listed in Table 1; no significant breakthrough in the overall survival of these malignancies has occurred since the 1940's. The results of our current approaches to cancer treatment make it clear that metastatic disease constitutes a major obstacle. As long as a malignant tumour remains localized, control and cure is possible. If, however, invasion beyond restricted local limits or distant spread occurs, the prognosis becomes considerably worse.

Chemotherapy/Immunotherapy

The realisation that a large proportion of patients with apparently localized malignant tumours present with clinically undetectable disseminated disease at the time of diagnosis, constituted the rationale for systemic treatment as an adjuvant to local therapy. Today chemotherapy and immunotherapy are the only therapeutic approaches which have experienced sufficient clinical evaluation to allow for their critical appraisal. Under experimental conditions both chemo- and immunotherapy were found to be highly effective against residual metastatic diseases and their introduction into the clinic was accompanied by great expectations. Although initial clinical data seemed to correlate well with the laboratory findings, further analysis of these studies, with longer follow-up periods, have gradually diminished the original enthusiasm (2). Both chemotherapy and immunotherapy are non-specific with regard to their target and the clinical situations in which their benefit exceeds their disadvantages have remained limited. Whilst cell proliferation — the target of chemotherapy — is a characteristic of all living cells, invasiveness and the potential to disseminate to distant sites is a more specific feature of malignant cells. Therefore a logical alternative approach to the control of cancer would be the attempt to interfere more specifically with the pathobiology of invasion and metastases formation. Despite the fact that the overall pathogenic mechanisms behind invasion and tumour dissemination are not yet fully understood, considerable knowledge has accumulated in recent years and genuine possibilities for new therapeutic measures have emerged. Since it will be impossible within the framework of this "overview" to give a comprehensive survey of all present research activities, a few examples of selective inhibition of invasion and metastases formation will be given.

Invasion and tumour vascularization

For the sake of clarity we do not want to enter into the semantics regarding the definition of the nature of invasion and metastases but rather adopt a highly simplified model which allows for the characterization of each individual step in the process of tumour dissemination (Fig. 1). Local invasion takes place at the tumour-host

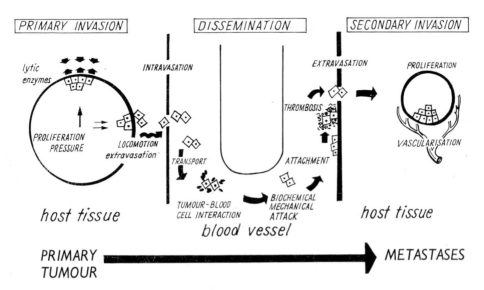

Fig. 1. Diagrammatic presentation of some pathogenic events during invasion and metastases formation from blood-borne cancer cells.

interzone and is, to a great extent, due to mechanical pressure as a consequence of uncontrolled cell proliferation.

There is, however, substantial experimental evidence that active processes such as cell motility and lytic effects derived from the cancer or induced by it in the host tissue, are important contributory factors to primary tumour invasion (3). Cancer cell locomotion has been unequivocally demonstrated in vitro as well as in vivo and its characterization has led to the discovery of pharmacological inhibitors, some of which are presented in the subsequent papers. Other properties intrinsic to the cancer cell such as decreased mutual adhesiveness and reduced contact inhibition may facilitate the initial step of the metastatic process which is the detachment of a single cell or clusters of cells from the primary tumour. The entry of the malignant cell into the vascular system may occur in the ill-defined vascular sinusoids within the primary tumour itself. Alternatively, the tumour can grow into the blood vessel and detachment may occur within the blood stream. Since detached cancer cells are capable of active locomotion, they can also migrate through interstitial spaces and gain access to the lymphatic system. The importance of the tumour blood vessels for the dissemination of cancer cells to distant sites is exemplified by the effects of drug ICRF 159 on spontaneous pulmonary metastases in the Lewis Lung Carcinoma (4). Normalisation of tumour blood vessels by long term administration of the drug inhibits the formation of lung metastases most likely by preventing the release of tumour cells into the circulation. Further experiments with ICRF 159 have indicated that the functional state of the tumour vessel might be of great importance for the antimetastatic effects. Trapping of injected carbon particles between the basement membrane and the endothelium in tumour vessels is abolished following ICRF 159 treatment. Clinical trials specifically designed to evaluate the antimetastatic effects of this compound have not yet been initiated; but in a recently terminated, randomized study ICRF 159 was administered as a cytostatic agent in an adjuvant setting in operable colorectal cancer of Dukes' stage B & C. In comparison to the untreated control group a significant recurrence advantage was found for the treatment group. Further analysis of the data with respect to recurrence site showed a striking difference between the treated and the control group in the localization of distant disease. Although the intent of this study was not primarily specific antimetastatic treatment, its results indicate that the animal data have a clinical correlate, which could be therapeutically exploited (5).

Circulating cancer cells

Having gained access to the blood or lymph stream the tumour cell or the tumour cell embolus is exposed to numerous mechanical and biochemical attacks. Experimental and clinical observation unequivocally indicate that the vast majority of circulating cancer cells fail to establish metastases and die off in the circulation. The fact that malignant cells cannot survive in the blood stream for a longer period of time has triggered experimental studies in which a prolongation of the transit time was brought about by various pharmacological manipulations. Clinical studies have shown a negative correlation between the number of circulating cancer cells found during surgical resection of the primary tumour and the frequency of subsequent tumour relapses at distant sites (6). These findings suggest that the circulating cancer cell might be an adequate target for therapeutic approaches.

In the circulation tumour cells will interact with other blood cells and considerable interest has recently focused on the interaction between the blood platelets and circulating cancer cells (7). If suspensions of viable tumour cells were injected intravenously into animals, a significant and almost immediate decrease of the peripheral

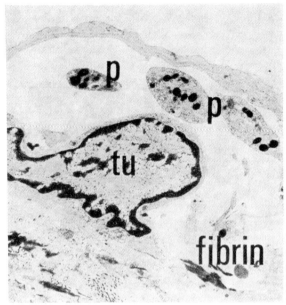

Fig. 2. EM of a Walker 256 tumour cell (tu) in a pulmonary capillary 15 min. after i. v. injection (p = platelets). From: P. HILGARD, Cancer Campaign 4 (1980), 107 (Courtesy of G. Fischer Verlag).

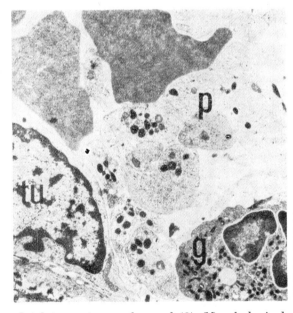

Fig. 3. EM of a Walker 256 tumour cell (tu) in a lung capillary 15 min. after i. v. injection (p = platelets, g = granulocyte). From: P. HILGARD, Cancer Campaign 4 (1980), 107 (Courtesy of G. Fischer Verlag).

platelet count was observed (8). Morphological studies revealed that these tumour cells were surrounded by clusters of platelets at the site of their primary arrest in the lung (Fig. 2 and Fig. 3). Furthermore, several experimental tumour cell lines are capable of aggregating blood platelets in vitro. GASIC's et al studies on metastases formation in thrombocytopenic animals indicated that the platelet-tumour cell interaction indeed facilitates the establishment of tumour metastases (9). It is not surprising that experiments to alter metastases formation by interference with platelet function have produced conflicting results: the mechanism by which tumour cells aggregate platelets in vitro appears to be different from other known mechanisms of platelet aggregation (10). In the light of our present knowledge concerning the possible significance of prostaglandins for tumour growth and the evolution of metastases the pharmacology of antiplatelet drugs as antimetastatic agents has to be carefully considered. The delicate balance of diametrically opposing activities of the transient metabolites of arachidonic acid, many of which are also biosynthesized by tumour cells, asks for extremely selective experimental approaches.

Tumour cell arrest, thrombosis and extravasation

The platelet-tumour cell interaction in the circulation could play an important role in the attachment of the tumour cell embolus to the vascular endothelium. The platelet-tumour cell complex is likely to have surface properties different from the original tumour cell and this could facilitate adhesion, particularly to traumatized endothelial sites. Substantial evidence however, indicates that tumour cell adhesion to the vascular endothelium occurs also in the absence of platelets and other mechanisms for this crucial step of metastases formation have to be anticipated. Electrostatic phenomena do not satisfactorily explain the interaction between the tumour cell and endothelial cell surface and more complex physico-chemical events are likely to occur. The arrest of circulating cancer cells and their escape into the interstitial space has been thoroughly studied in vivo by time-lapse cinematography in the rabbit ear chamber (11). WOOD's data have been reviewed and summarized schematically by FISHER and FISHER and are shown in Figure 4 (12). Tumour cells injected into neighbouring small arteries moved rapidly to the capillaries where they adhered to an unpredictable endothelial site in a post capillary venule (a). Within minutes, they were surrounded by a thrombus composed of fibrin and blood platelets (b). After the arrival of polymorphonuclear leucocytes and their migration through the vessel wall (c) the cancer cells penetrated the endothelial lining by diapedesis through the same opening (d). In the perivascular connective tissue the tumour cells proliferated (e) and, within 24 hours capillary buds arising from pre-existing vessels, reached the tumour. The original thrombus was frequently observed to fragment and to move down the capillary. WOOD concluded from these experiments that the failure

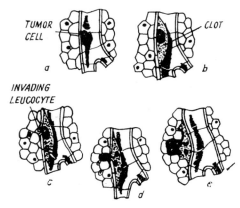

Fig. 4. Diagrammatic summary showing the conversion of tumour cell emboli to a metastatic nodule. Explanation see text (From (12). Courtesy of W. B. Saunders Comp.).

of embolic cancer cells to establish metastases may be related to their inability to attach themselves securely to the endothelium and to evoke the formation of a surrounding thrombus.

This challenging hypothesis has been tested in numerous experimental studies in which the kinetics of thrombus formation around adherent tumour cell emboli were altered by means of drugs interfering with haemostasis. The results are summarized in Figure 5. In general, deceleration of the host's coagulation mechanism by anticoagulant or fibrinolytic agents resulted in an inhibition of metastases, whereas the generation of a hypercoagulable state usually had the opposite effect. Although the experimental data have not always been as unequivocal as suggested by the graph, anticoagulants have emerged as potential antimetastatic agents into a few clinical trials. Due to design and statistical inadequacies the results of these trials however only vaguely suggest a possible benefit of this approach (13, 14). Advances in our knowledge about the coagulation mechanism and its numerous interactions with other biological systems have rendered the interpretation of experimental data increasingly difficult. The activation of the coagulation system involves numerous other biological systems which are of considerable importance in the micro-environment of tumour cell emboli. In addition, the pharmacology of anticoagulants is too complex to allow for definite conclusions concerning the role of thrombosis in metastases formation. This is exemplified by the effects of coumarin anticoagulants on the course of tumour spread. Through their action on cell locomotion and cell replication they might be considered anti-invasive drugs (15). On the other hand, coumarins are effective antimetastatic agents and indirect evidence suggests that their mode of action is partly independent from their influence on the coagulation system (16).

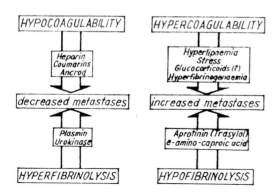

Fig. 5. Diagrammatic summary of experimental results obtained with anticoagulants in studies of metastases (From (15). Courtesy of Pergamon Press).

One of the most intriguing steps in the pathogenic sequence of extravasation of tumour cells is their interaction with the basement membrane. Collagen of type IV represents the main constituent of basement membranes and high amounts of a specific enzyme for this substrate were identified in many malignant cells. LIOTTA and co-workers found a positive correlation between the intracellular levels of type IV collagenolytic activity and the frequency with which the tumours metastasize (17). In addition, metastatic cells appear to preferentially adhere to type IV collagen. Clearly, more extensive data are needed before the tumour cell-basement membrane interaction can become a target for therapeutic approaches; the possible specificity of this phenomenon however, has opened an exciting new area for selective inhibition of invasion and metastases.

Metastasis localization and tumour cell heterogeneity

WALTHER's concept of haemodynamic factors being of primary importance for the localization of metastases is probably still valid (18). It is however well documented that the routes of dissemination of some tumours deviate from the classical ways of spreading; this has elicited speculations that "soil factors" favour the localisation of a metastatic tumour. Little is presently known about the specific interactions between the "seed" — the tumour cell — and the "soil". The relative importance of the "seed" in the localisation of metastases is supported by several experimental studies in which it was shown that the distribution of metastases forming from blood-borne malignant cells is non-random and unique to the type of tumour cell used in the experiments. NICHOLSON et al, succeeded by sequential in vivo selection to obtain B16 melanoma lines wich subsequently colonised specific organs after their trans-plantation into animals (19).

As indicated earlier, the chance of a circulating cancer cell to establish a secondary tumour is minimal. This raises the question whether or not survival of cancer cells is random and dependent on their fortuitous escape from the hostile environment of the circulation. Alternatively, the successful tumour cell can be a representative of a pre-existing subpopulation within the primary tumour which has a selective advantage for metastases. Numerous experimental and clinical reports have drawn attention to the enormous differences between primary tumours and their metastases with respect to ultrastructural, cytogenic, growth kinetic, biochemical and drug sensitivity features. It is beyond the scope of this paper to discuss the question whether the apparent differences between the primary tumour and its metastases are causatively related to dissemination or are rather a consequence of metastatic growth in a new and different environment. Heterogeneity in the metastatic potential of different cell clones within a given primary tumour was suggested by several experimentalists who succeeded in selecting cell lines with "high" and "low" metastatic efficacy from the same primary tumour (20). The general validity of these findings however, remains to be established.

Of greater immediate clinical relevance could be the recent discovery of the conformity and regularity with which haematogenous metastases formation occurs in humans. BROSS and his co-workers demonstrated by statistical analysis of metastatic sites in an autopsy survey that metastases formation involves a multistep process (21). As shown in Figure 6, generalization seldom originates from the primary tumour but rather from a few key generalizing sites which are specific for a given primary. Although there are occasional exceptions to this metastatic cascade, this concept must have substantial therapeutic implications: the generalizing sites may in many instances be considered "localized tumour" and still represent an early stage of the cascade process. The recognition of this possibility should have consequences on the management of disseminated disease by the oncologist. A more differentiated view on the kinetics of tumour dissemination will ultimately provide the rationale for new therapeutic strategies which will include specific anti-invasive and antimetastatic drugs in order to interrupt the cascade process.

The final step in the successful establishment of a metastatic tumour deposit is its connection to the vascular system of the host. Malignant tumours appear to have the property of inducing new capillaries and in the absence of this angiogenesis they remain static or will eventually die. An inhibitor of tumour angiogenesis was recently characterized and partially purified and preliminary experimental data suggest that control of tumour growth might be possible by parenteral administration of this substance (22).

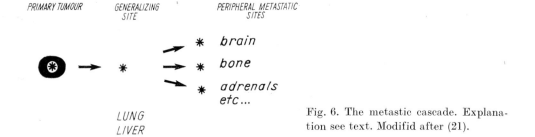

PRIMARY TUMOUR   GENERALIZING   PERIPHERAL METASTATIC
                      SITE   SITES

Fig. 6. The metastic cascade. Explanation see text. Modifid after (21).

Conclusions

Although many important areas of our present knowledge have not been covered in this survey it is hoped that it has indicated that invasion and metastases are two feature of malignant disease which are worth-while to explore from a therapeutic point of view. The frequent criticism that experimental models may not adequately reflect the clinical situation is not unique to the area of tumour invasion and tumour metastases but it is built into medical research in general. Despite "irrelevant" experimental models clinical research has progressed steadily, often to the benefit of the patient. As pointed out by HEWITT, more discouraging than the lack of appropriate experimental tools is the relative lack of interest of experimental oncologists in the mechanism and control of invasion and metastases (23). It is hoped that this conference and its proceedings will stimulate further creative thinking which hopefully results in new approaches to the management of malignant disease.

References

1. GARFINKEL, L., POINDEXTER, C. E. and SILVERBERG, E.: Cancer Statistics 1980. CA-A Cancer J. *30* (1980), 23
2. ROSSI, A., VALAGUSSA, P. and BONADONNA, G.: Combined modality management of operable breast cancer. In: Adjuvant therapies and markers of post-surgical minimal residual disease II (Ed. by G. BONADONNA, G. MATHE and S. E. SALMON). Springer, Berlin 1979 pp. 80
3. STRÄULI, P., BARRETT, A. J. and BAICI, A. (Eds.): Proteinases and tumour invasion. EORTC Monograph Series 6, Raven Press, New York, 1980
4. LE SERVE, A. W. and HELLMANN, K.: Metastases and the normalization of tumour blood vessels by ICRF 159: A new type of drug action. Brit. Med. J. *1* (1972) 597—601
5. GILBERT, J. M., HELLMANN, K., EVANS, M., CASSELL, T. G., ELLIS, H., WASTELL, C. and STOODLEY, B.: A controlled prospective randomized trial of adjuvant oral Razoxane (ICRF 159) in resectable colo-rectal cancer. In: Adj. Therapies of Can. Vol 3 (Ed. by S. E. SALMON and S. E. JONES). Grune & Stratton, New York, 1981, pp. 519—526
6. WHITE, H., GRIFFITHS, J. D. and SALSBURY, A. J.: Circulating malignant cells and fibrinolysis during resection of colorectal cancer. Proc. Roy. Soc. Med. *69* (1976) 467
7. HILGARD, P.: Platelets and experimental metastases. In: Platelets: A multidisciplinary approach (ed. by G. de GAETANO and S. GARATTINI) pp 457. Raven Press, New York, 1978
8. HILGARD, P.: The role of blood platelets in experimental metastases. Brit. J. Cancer *28* (1973), 429

9. GASIC, G., GASIC, T., GALANTI, N., JOHNSON, T. and MURPHY, S.: Platelet-tumour-cell inter-actions in mice. The role of platelets in the spread of malignant disease. Int. J. Cancer *11* (1973), 704

10. KARPATKIN, S. and PEARLSTEIN, E.: The in vitro activity of platelet aggregating material from SV-40 transformed mouse 3T3 fibroblasts. In: Malignancy and the Hemostatic System (ed. by M. B. DONATI, J. F. DAVIDSON and S. GARATTINI). Raven Press, New York, 1981, pp. 37

11. WOOD, Jr., S.: Pathogenesis of metastasis formation observed in vivo in the rabbit ear chamber. Arch. Path (Chicago) *66* (1958), 550

12 FISHER, B. and FISHER, E. R.: Host factors influencing the development of metastases. Surg. Clin. N. Amer. *42* (1962), 335

13. THORNES, R. D.: Adjuvant therapy of cancer via the cellular immune mechanism or fibrin by induced fibrinolysis and oral anticoagulants. Cancer *35* (1975), 91

14. HOOVER, Jr., H. C., KETCHAM, A. S., MILLAR, R. C. and GRALNICK, H. R.: Osteosarcoma. Improved survival with anticoagulation and amputation. Cancer *41* (1978) 2475

15. HILGARD, P. and THORNES, R. D.: Anticoagulants in the treatment of cancer. Europ. J. Cancer *12* (1976), 755

16. HILGARD, P.: Experimental vitamin K deficiency and spontaneous metastases. Brit. J. Cancer *35* (1977), 891

17. LIOTTA, L. A., TRYGGVASON, K., GARBISA, S., GEHRON, ROBEY, P. and MURRAY, J. C.: Inter-action of metastatic tumour cells with basement membrane collagen. In: Metastatic tumour growth (ed. by E. GRUNDMANN) Gustav Fischer Verlag, Stuttgart, 1980 pp. 21

18. WALTHER, H. E.: Krebsmetastasen. Schwabe Verlag, Basel, 1948

19. NICOLSON, G. L., BRUNSON, K. W. and FIDLER, I. J.: Specificity of arrest, survival and growth of selected metastatic variant cell lines. Cancer Res. *38* (1978), 4105

20. FIDLER, I. J. and KRIPKE, M. L.: Metastasis results from pre-existing variant cells within a malignant tumour. Science *197* (1977), 893

21. BROSS, I. D. Z. and BLUMENSON, L. E.: Metastatic sites that produce generalized cancer: identification and kinetics of generalizing sites. In: Fundamental aspects of metastasis (ed. by L. WEISS). North-Holland Publishing Co., Amsterdam, 1976

22. LANGER, R. and FOLKMAN, J.: Angiogenesis inhibitors. In: Molecular actions and targets for cancer chemotherapeutic agents (ed. by A. C. SARTORELLI, J. S. LAZO and J. R. BERTINO). Academic Press, New York, 1981 pp. 511

23. HEWITT, H. B.: Animal tumour models: the intrusion of artefacts. In: Metastasis, clinical and experimental aspects (ed. by K. HELLMANN, P. HILGARD and S. ECCLES). Martinus Nijhoff, The Hague, 1980 pp. 18

* Laboratory of Experimental Cancerology, Department of Radiotherapy and Nuclear Medicine, University Hospital, De Pintelaan 135, B-9000 Ghent, Belgium,

and

+ The Gade Institute, Department of Pathology, University of Bergen, N-5016 Haukeland Hospital, Norway

Invasiveness of Brain Tumour Cells In Vivo and In Vitro

L. de RIDDER*, O. D. LAERUM+ and S. MÖRK

The malignant character of a brain tumour is expressed by its invasiveness, that is, its capacity to replace progressively the surrounding normal tissue. The invasion of tumour cells into the surrounding central nervous tissue is the main cause of death of the brain cancer patient. On the other hand, metastasis of a brain tumour is an exception. To analyse these characteristics of brain tumours, we employed an in vitro technique by which the invasion and the pattern of invasion of a tumour can be correlated with its situation in vivo.

We used cells of a number of chemically-induced glial rat tumours and studied: 1. The correlation of invasiveness of cells in vitro and their ability to form tumours in syngeneic hosts in vivo; 2. the comparison of the histologic pattern of invasive brain cells in vivo and in vitro. The results indicated that this in vitro model allows the expression in a constant way of the morphological characteristics of the different brain tumour cells. This means that the model may be useful in evaluating the effects of drugs and other therapies on brain tumour cells.

Material and methods

Malignant cells

Twelve neurogenic cell lines were examined in vivo and in vitro.

1. Three of them were derived from brain tumours of the offspring of pregnant BD IX rats. These brain tumours were induced transplacentally by a single i. v. injection of ethylnitrosourea (EtNU) on the 18th day of gestation of the rats (1).
   Cell lines were started in vitro from explanted tumour fragments.
2. The other 9 cell lines (BT lines) originated from foetal rat brain cells transferred to a monolayer culture after exposure to EtNU in vivo. Normal cells, untreated foetal brain cells, cultured in monolayer for a short period, served as controls (1).

Tumorigenicity in vivo

10^6 cells were injected subcutaneously into 5- to 10-days-old syngeneic rats. The cells were suspended in phosphate buffered saline and 0.1 ml was injected per animal. The latency period for tumour formation varied between 32 and 100 days (2).

All tumours were examined microscopically on 7 μm thick HE stained sections after fixation in Zenker solution.

Invasiveness in vitro

The invasiveness of the neurogenic cell lines in vitro was evaluated by the method of MAREEL et al (3).

This multiple step method may be summarized as follows:

1. Aggregates of all the neurogenic cell lines are prepared by incubating a suspension of 10^6 neurogenic cells in 50 ml Erlenmeyer flasks on a gyratory shaker at 70 rpm. Aggregates are formed gradually and after 24 h, they reached their final diameter between 0.1—0.45 mm. The cells forming the aggregates were taken from the same culture passage as those which were tested for tumourigenicity.

2. At the same time freshly-cut heart fragments from 9-day-old embryonic chicks were incubated on a gyratory shaker for 3 days to obtain precultured heart fragments. Their mean diameter was 0.4 mm. The core of heart muscle cells was surrounded by a few layers of fibroblastoid cells.

3. The next step consisted of the confrontation of precultured heart fragments with the aggregates of neurogenic cells. They attached firmly to each other after 2 h of contact on a semi-solid medium. Then they were transferred to 10 ml Erlenmeyer flasks filled with 2 ml Eagle-Dulbecco's medium supplemented with 10% inactivated newborn calf serum. The confrontations were incubated at 120 rpm for 1, 4, 6 and 7 days on the gyratory shaker. Fixation in Zenker and embedding in paraffin to be sectioned in 7 μm sections, followed.

   All sections were stained with haematoxylin and eosin. In all experiments heart fragments alone were used as controls. The cell lines were coded and invasiveness was scored on serial sections.

Results

Tumourigenicity in vivo

All cell lines injected subcutaneously with exception of the normal brain cells, gave rise to progressively growing tumours (Fig. 1). Histological analysis showed invasion of the individual cells into the surrounding connective, fatty and muscle tissue. The

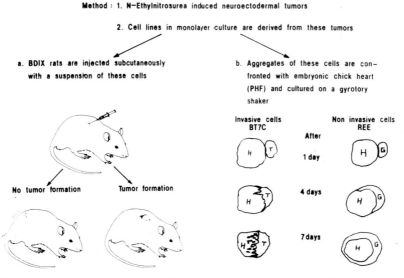

Fig. 1. Schematic representation of method and results in vivo and in vitro.

borderline between surrounding tissue and the formed tumour was unsharp. Variable amount of necrotic material was seen in the border zone. The pattern of invasion, i.e. the manner in which a group of tumour cells became progressively distributed in the host tissue, was rather stable for the individual cell lines. Two main pattern were seen:

1. The predominantly neurinoma—like pattern, characterized by bundles of parallelly—oriented cells.
2. The anaplastic or glioma—like, pattern, characterized by a mixture of polygonal and some spindle—shaped cells.

Invasiveness in vitro

All cell lines, forming a tumour in vivo, showed invasion into the heart tissue in vitro (4). After seven days, invasive cells occupied the heart muscle and were seen as single cells or strands of cells (fig. 1). The invasion was progressive and, in some cultures, complete replacement of the heart fragment by the invasive cells was found. The borderline between the two components was never well-delineated.

The untreated foetal brain cells were non-invasive in vitro and non-tumourigenic in vivo. The invasion in vitro of the aggregates from the neuroectodermal tumours occurred by similar cellular phenotypes as in the tumour transplants in vivo. The 10 cell lines originating from the foetal brain cells exposed to EtNU, showed similar histological types of the individual cells in vitro as in the subcutaneous transplants in vivo. Three main patterns were seen:

a. solitary distribution of invading cells
b. piling up in layers around the heart fragment
c. wedge shaped distribution of the invading cells (Fig. 2).

Solitary invading cells showed polymorphism (Fig. 2), filiform cells were dominant in a wedge-shaped tumour mass. All cell lines showed replacement of the heart cell during incubation.

The aggregates of foetal brain cells were only seen at the periphery of the fragment. In most confrontations, the normal foetal brain cells were no longer visible after 6 or 7 days of incubation.

Discussion

Although not a necessary property for tumour formation, invasiveness is a prerequisite for malignant growth in the body. This is even the case in malignant conditions of the nervous system where the growth is illdefined and does not lead to formation of a localized tumour, i.e. gliomatosis cerebri (5).

In the present investigation there was a good correlation between the malignant growth of neurogenic tumour lines in vivo and invasiveness in confronting cultures with chick heart fragments on gyratory shaker. In this organ culture, even the histological and cytological characteristics of the neurogenic rat cells observed in vivo were partly retained (6). Hence, this model makes it possible to correlate the in vitro properties of the cells with their malignant behaviour in vivo, enabling direct studies on the complex interaction between invasive cells and host tissues (for review, see 7). The advantage is that admixture of other cell types seen in vivo (e.g. inflammatory cells, fibroblasts, and also endothelial cells forming capillaries), does not complicate the picture. However, since immunological mechanisms may be responsible for tissue resistance against early invading cells (8), the interpretation of such data should not be based on in vitro studies alone.

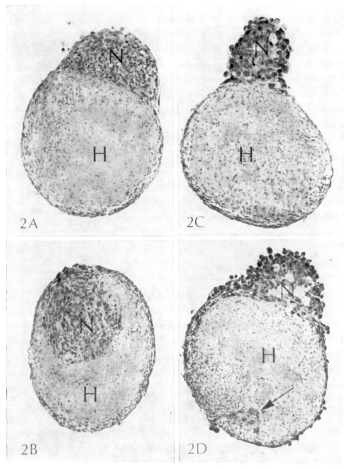

Fig. 2. Light micrographs of 7 μm thick sections of confronting cultures of precultured heart fragments (H) with invasive rat brain cells (N) in vitro.

A. Confrontation after 2 h contact on semisolid medium. BT1 cells.

B. After 4 days in culture, invading BT1 cells show wedge shaped distribution

C. Confrontation after 2 h contact on semisolid medium. BT3 cells.

D. After 4 days in culture, BT3 cells express a pattern of solitary invasion (arrow) and a piling up in layers of the bulk.

References

1. LAERUM, O. D. and RAJEWSKY, M. F.: Neoplastic transformation of fetal rat brain cells in culture after exposure to ethylnitrosourea in vivo. J. Natl. Cancer Inst. 55 (1975), 1177—1187
2. LAERUM, O. D., RAJEWSKY, M. F., SCHACHNER, M., STAVROU, D., HAGLID, K. G. and HAUGEN, A.: Phenotypic properties of neoplastic cell lines developed from fetal rat cells in culture after exposure to ethylnitrosourea in vivo. Z. Krebsforsch. 89 (1977), 273—295

3. MAREEL, M., KINT, J. and MEYVISCH, C.: Methods of study of the invasion of malignant C3H-mouse fibroblasts into embryonic chick heart in vitro. Virchows Arch. B Cell Pathol. *30* (1979), 95—111

4. DE RIDDER, L. and LAERUM, O. D.: Invasion of rat neurogenic cell lines into embryonic chick heart fragments. J. Natl. Cancer Inst. *66* (1981), 723—728

5. RUSSELL, D. S. and RUBINSTEIN, L. J.: Pathology of Tumours of the Nervous System. Fourth ed., E. Arnold Ltd, London, 1977

6. DE RIDDER, L., MÖRK, S. J. and LAERUM, O. D.: Invasive pattern and phenotypic properties of malignant neurogenic rat cells in vivo and in vitro. Anticancer Res. (Submitted).

7. MAREEL, M. M.: Recent aspects of tumour invasiveness. Int. Rev. Exp. Pathol. *22* (1980), 65—129

8. TERZAGHI, M., NETTESHEIM, P. and WILLIAMS, M. L.: Repopulation of denuded tracheal grafts with normal, preneoplastic and neoplastic epithelial cell populations. Cancer Res. *38* (1978), 4546—4553

Laboratory of Experimental Cancerology, Department of
Radiotherapy and Nuclear Medicine, Academic Hospital,
De Pintelaan 135, B-9000 Gent, Belgium

Anti-invasiveness of Microtubule Inhibitors is due to Interference with the Cytoplasmic Microtubule Complex[1]

M. Mareel, G. Storme[2], G. De Bruyne, R. Van Cauwenberge and C. Dragonetti

Abstract

We review here previous data and present new experiments about the antiinvasive effect of microtubule inhibitors on MO_4 mouse fibrosarcoma cells in vitro. Our findings support the opinion that
the antiinvasiveness of microtubule inhibitors is due to their effect on the cytoplasmic microtubule complex. A functional cytoplasmic microtubule complex is necessary for directional migration, presumed to be a vital activity of invading cells. Other chemotherapeutic drugs or ionizing
irradiation, which leave the microtubules unaltered, permit invasion at doses that inhibit growth.

Invasion determines malignancy in most solid tumours (for review see Mareel, 1980).
Inhibition of invasion may, therefore, contribute to the antitumoural activity of some
drugs. Invasion is attractive as a target of therapy in tumours that proliferate slowly
and that are not expected to respond to antiproliferative agents.

Invasion in organ culture

The effect of drugs on the invasiveness of malignant cells is difficult to assess in vivo.
In vitro models, that are relevant to at least some aspects of invasion, have been
used by various authors (for review see Mareel, 1979). They consisted of the confrontation of a fragment of normal tissue with malignant cells in organ culture. Invasion
was inferred from the histology of the confronting pairs, fixed after various periods
of incubation. Unfortunately, methods for quantitative evaluation of invasion are
not available.

We have developed an in vitro assay of invasion, that proved to be useful for the screen-
ning of potential antiinvasive agents. Precultured fragments of 9-day-old embryonic
cardiac muscle were confronted with spheroidal aggregates of malignant cells, and
individual confronting pairs were incubated in fluid medium on a gyratory shaker at
120 rpm (Mareel et al, 1979). The following observations indicated that invasion in
this assay was relevant to invasion in vivo: 1) The same criteria applied to both invasion in vivo and in vitro: Invading cells occupied neighbouring tissues; invasion was
accompanied by degeneration of the invaded tissues; both occupation and degeneration were progressive in time. 2) For a number of cell lines, the histopathology of the
confronting pairs in the in vitro assay for invasion resembled that of the tumours
obtained by implantation of the cells in appropriate animals in vivo (Mareel et al,

[1] Supported by the Kankerfonds van de Algemene Spaar- en Lijfrentekas, and by a Grant (3.009.80)
from the N.F.W.O., Brussels, Belgium.

[2] On leave from the Oncologic Center-Radiotherapy, Free University Brussels, Belgium.

in press). 3) With families of animal cell lines that were examined before and after malignant alteration, a correlation was found between invasiveness in organ culture and the capacity to form invasive tumours in syngeneic animals (MAREEL et al, 1975; KIELER et al, 1979; DE RIDDER and LAERUM, 1981).

Inhibition of invasion by microtubule inhibitors

For the study of the effect of anticancer agents on invasion in organ culture, MO_4 cells were used. MO_4 cells are virally-transformed C3H mouse fibroblastic cells (BIL-LIAU et al, 1973). Aggregates of MO_4 cells (diameter = 0.2 mm) where malignant by all standards, since they produced invasive and metastasizing tumours after subcutaneous implantation into syngeneic mice (MEYVISCH and MAREEL, 1979; MEYVISCH et al, 1980). When an aggregate of MO_4 cells was confronted with a fragment of chick cardiac muscle (diameter = 0.4 mm), the MO_4 cells progressively occupied the cardiac muscle and completely replaced it within 4 to 5 days (Fig. 1). Addition of microtubule inhibitors, at appropriate concentrations to the culture medium, prevented invasion of the MO_4 cells into the chick cardiac muscle. Confronting pairs fixed after 4 days showed a cap of MO_4 cells at the pole of attachment and no MO_4 cells were found inside

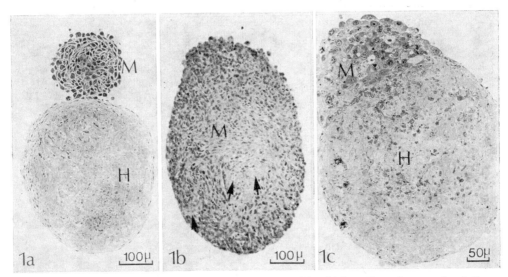

Fig. 1. Light micrographs of 2 µm (1a and 1c) and 8 µm (1b) thick sections from confrontations of an MO_4 cell aggregate (M) with a fragment of chick cardiac muscle (H). Fixed after 1 h (1a), and 4 days (1b and 1c). 1c: in presence of 0.3 µg/ml podophyllotoxin. Staining with haematoxylin and eosin. Arrows indicate remnants of cardiac muscle.

the cardiac muscle (Fig. 1c). Inhibition of invasion was demonstrated using the following microtubule inhibitors: colchicine, demecolcine, Nocodazole, vinblastine and vincristine (MAREEL and DE BRABANDER, 1978); vindesine (MAREEL et al, 1980); methyl [5-(2-(4-fluorophenyl)-1,3-dioxolan-2-yl)1H-benzimidazole-2-yl] carbamate (STORME and MAREEL, 1981); taxol (kindly provided by the Drug Synthesis & Chemistry Branch, Division of Cancer Treatment, National Cancer Institute, U.S.A.); podophyllotoxin (Aldrich Europe Division, Beerse, Belgium). It was unlikely that the anti-invasive effect of these drugs could be ascribed to non-specific cytotoxicity, since

MO$_4$ cells survived after mitotic arrest (De BRABANDER et al, 1976). Furthermore, at least for Nocodazole, vinblastine, vincristine and vindesine the antiinvasive effect was shown to be reversible. Differences of antiinvasive concentrations between various cell lines indicated that lack of invasion was due to the effect of the drugs on the MO$_4$ cells and not to alterations of the cardiac muscle.

In most experiments the microtubule inhibitors were added to the medium at the onset of the culture. Strictly, these experiments demonstrated that the drugs prevented invasion. Addition of vindesine to confronting pairs after 2 days, strongly suggested that microtubule inhibitors not only prevented invasion but also arrested invasion during its course.

It is obvious that in the organ culture assay, attachment of the MO$_4$ cell aggregate to the fragment of cardiac muscle is necessary to demonstrate invasion. Using a quantitative method, we have shown that microtubule inhibitors had no effect on attachment (MAREEL et al, 1980).

SCHALLIER and STORME (unpublished) have recently examined the effect of Nocodazole and of vincristine on the invasiveness of K12 rat adenocarcinoma cells in organ culture. Their results indicated that the antiinvasive effect of microtubule inhibitors was not limited to MO$_4$ mouse fibrosarcoma cells.

Antiinvasiveness and disturbance of the microtubule complex

The aforementioned antiinvasive drugs were known to affect microtubules. However, the possibility was not excluded that they acted on other structures also. The following arguments made it unlikely that the antiinvasiveness of the so-called microtubule inhibitors could be ascribed to an effect other than the disturbance of the microtubule complex:

1) Disturbance of microtubules was a common denominator of all the aforementioned antiinvasive drugs regardless of their mechanism of action (Fig. 2). Nocodazole and

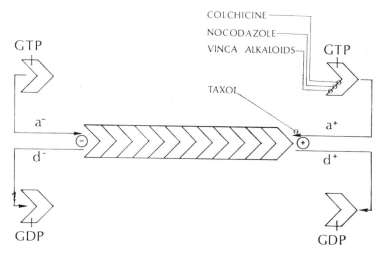

Fig. 2. Schematic representation of microtubule assembly-disassembly. GTP = guanidine triphosphate; GDP = guanidine diphosphate; a = assembly, d = disassembly; + = plus end of microtubule; − = minus end of microtubule. Modified from COTE et al, 1980.

its derivatives, colchicine, podophyllotoxin, and the vinca alkaloids inhibited the assembly of microtubules through binding to tubulin dimers. Taxol stimulated the assembly of microtubules by lowering the concentration of tubulin, that was critical for assembly.

2) Congeners of microtubule inhibitors that had lost their effect on microtubules were not antiinvasive. For example, the podophyllotoxin congeners, VP-16-213 and VM-26 (kindly provided by Laboratories Bristol Benelux, N.V., Brussels, Belgium) no longer inhibited the assembly of microtubules (LOIKE et al, 1978). VP-16-213 and VM-26 did not inhibit the invasion of MO_4 cells into the cardiac muscle in organ culture, unlike podophyllotoxin.

3) When MO_4 cells were cultured on glass in presence of antiinvasive doses of microtubule inhibitors, disturbance of the microtubule complex could be demonstrated by immunocytochemical staining with antiserum against tubulin (kindly provided by M. DE BRABANDER & J. DE MEY, Janssen Pharmaceutica, Beerse, Belgium) (Fig. 3).

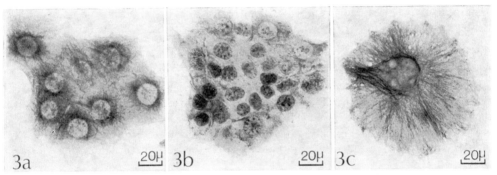

Fig. 3. Light micrographs of MO_4 cells cultured on glass and fixed in situ. 3a: control; 3b: treated with 10 µg/ml Nocodazole during 4 h; 3c: treated with 6 µg/ml taxol during 5 days. Immunocytochemical staining with an antiserum against tubulin.

4) Ultrastructural examination of confrontations between MO_4 cell aggregates and fragments of cardiac muscle in organ culture showed that inhibition of invasion was accompanied by alterations relevant to disturbance of the microtubule complex. For inhibitors of microtubule assembly these alterations are: absence or scarceness of microtubules; accumulation of 10 nm thick filaments; dislocation of the Golgi complex from its perinuclear site with hypertrophy of the smooth endoplasmic reticulum; appearance of annulate lamellae (GEORGE et al, 1965; DE BRABANDER and BORGERS, 1975). When taxol was used at antiinvasive concentrations, the cells were filled with microtubules (Fig. 4).

These observations strongly suggested that a normal assembly-disassembly of microtubules was vital for invading cells. This did not imply that an intact microtubule complex was sufficient for ivasion. We have recently obtained inhibition of invasion by dihydrocytochalasin, a substance that presumably interfered with actin filaments.

Antiinvasiveness and inhibition of growth

In interphase cells assembly of tubulin forms the cytoplasmic microtubule complex (BRINKLEY et al, 1975). At mitosis the cytoplasmic microtubule complex disappears

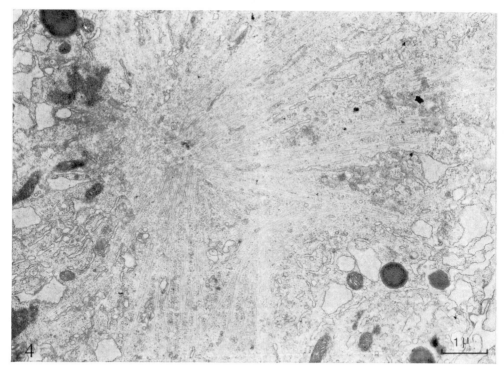

Fig. 4. Transmission electron micrograph of a MO₄ cell confronting a fragment of cardiac muscle in presence of an antiinvasive concentration (6 µg/ml) of taxol. Fixation after 4 days. Microtubules are sectioned longitudinally and transversally.

and tubulin dimers assemble into the mitotic spindle (DE BRABANDER et al, 1979). Microtubule inhibitors affected both microtubule complexes; they interefered with cell proliferation because they disturbed the formation of the mitotic spindle. This implied that, at antiinvasive doses, microtubule inhibitors arrested the growth of MO₄ cells. The following observations however, indicated that inhibition of growth was not responsible for antiinvasiveness:

1) A number of growth inhibitors that left microtubules unaltered, permitted invasion. These include cytosine arabinoside, bleomycin, 5-fluorouracil (MAREEL and DE BRABANDER, 1978); ionizing radiation (STORME and MAREEL, 1980); mitomycin-C, VM-26, VP16-213, and cisplatinum.

2) In order to exlude the possibility that lowering the number of MO₄ cells by inhibition of proliferation and by cell loss contributed to inhibition of invasion, we have confronted fragments of cardiac muscle and MO₄ cell aggregates with a diameter of 0.4 mm containing approximately the same number of cells as control aggregates after 4 days (end of the assay). Microtubule inhibitors completely inhibited invasion of MO₄ cells from such larger aggregates, as in the experiments using aggregates with a diameter of 0.2 mm.

3) Treatment with 5-fluorouracil produced a non-proliferating population of MO₄ cells, that were able to invade into the cardiac muscle in organ culture. 5-fluorouracil affected cells in S-phase and cells did not reach the phase where spindle microtubules were formed. Addition of microtubule inhibitors arrested invasion in these cultures. Clearly, in this situation, antiinvasiveness was due to disturbance of the cytoplasmic

4*

microtubule complex. Although these data strongly suggested that disturbance of the cytoplasmic microtubule complex and not growth arrest was responsible for inhibition of invasion, they did not rule out that both phenomena were involved.

Anti-invasiveness and loss of directional migration

Treatment of MO$_4$ cells or other tissue-cultured cells with microtubule inhibitors altered their migration (DE BRABANDER et al, 1977). In control cultures cells were polarized and ruffling membrane activity was largely confined to the leading edge. After treatment, ruffling membrane activity occurred all over the cell periphery, resulting in random migration of the cells. There is evidence that directional migration — i.e. migration in a direction defined by a factor outside the migrating cell — is an important activity of invading cells (for review see MAREEL, 1980). We have, therefore, examined whether the antiinvasiveness of microtubule inhibitors was due

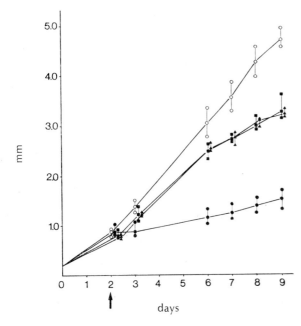

Fig. 5. Directional migration of MO$_4$ cells from aggregates explanted on glass in presence of 0.3 µg/ml podophyllotoxin (●), 10 µg/ml VP-16-213 (■) and 1 µg/ml VM-26 (▲); 0 = controls. Ordinate: mean diameter of circular area covered by MO$_4$ cells; median and extreme values from 5 cultures. Abscissa: time of culture. Arrow indicates addition of drugs.

to their effect on directional migration. Explantation of an MO$_4$ cell aggregate, and measurement of the circular area covered by cells that had migrated from the aggregate, provided us with a quantitative estimation of directional migration (STORME and MAREEL, 1980; MAREEL et al, 1981). In this assay the radial direction of migration was defined by collision with other cells resulting in inhibition of ruffling activity and migration in the opposite direction. Comparison between anti-invasive drugs and permissive drugs at concentrations that completely inhibited growth, showed striking differences in their capacity to perform directional migration (Fig. 5). With antiinvasive drugs, the inhibitory effect became visible within 24 h. With drugs that permitted invasion, a much slighter effect became obvious after 4 days. The latter was not due to the effect of the drug on directional migration per se, but could be ascribed to a decrease in the number of cells. Further, for the vinca alkaloids the dose-responsiveness was the same for both inhibition of invasion and inhibition of directional migration (MAREEL et al, 1980). These data showed that inhibition of invasion by microtubule inhibitors could be explained by their effect on directional migration. How far other cellular activities, depending on an intact cytoplasmic microtubule complex, participate at invasion remains to be elucidated.

Clinical relevance

Caution is needed in extrapolating our in vitro results with animal cell lines to the clinic.

Nevertheless, the following points might be of interest in establishing new therapeutic rationales: 1) The antiinvasive concentrations of the microtubule inhibitors in vitro might well be within achievable plasma concentrations in vivo. 2) It is conceivable that chemotherapeutic agents effectively control growth whilst a number of cells continue to invade. After a period of dormancy these cells might give rise to recurrent growth at more or less distant sites. 3) The most simple way to investigate the antiinvasiveness of microtubule inhibitors in vivo might be an examination of their effect on the number of metastases. It should, however, be accepted that inhibition of metastasis could be due to effects other than anti-invasiveness. 4) Disturbance of the cytoplasmic microtubule complex is, in many types of cells, an easily reversible phenomenon.

References

1. BILLIAU, A., SOBIS, H., EYSSEN, H. and VAN DEN BERGHE, H.: Non-Infectious Intracisternal A-Type Particles in a Sarcoma-Positive, Leukemia-Negative Mouse Cell Line Transformed by Murine Sarcoma Virus (MSV). Arch. Gesamte Virusforsch. *43* (1973), 345—351
2. BRINKLEY, B. R., FULLER, G. M. and HIGHFIELD, D. P.: Studies of microtubules in dividing and nondividing mammalian cells using antibody to 6-S bovine brain tubulin. In: Microtubules and Microtubule Inhibitors (Eds. M. BORGERS and M. DE BRABANDER), North-Holland Publ. Company-Amsterdam, 1975, pp. 297—312
3. COTE, R. H., BERGEN, L. G. and BORISY, G. G.: Head-to-tail polymerization of microtubules in vitro: a review. In: Microtubules and Microtubule Inhibitors 1980 (Eds. M. DE BRABANDER and D. DE MEY), Elsevier/North-Holland Biomedical Press-Amsterdam, 1980, pp. 325—338
4. DE BRABANDER, M. and BORGERS, M.: The formation of annulated lamellae induced by the disintegration of microtubules. J. Cell Sci. *19* (1975b), 331—340
5. DE BRABANDER, M., DE MEY, VAN DE VEIRE, R., AERTS, F. and GEUENS, G.: Microtubules in mammalian cell shape and surface modulation: an alternative hypothesis. Cell Biol. Int. Rep. *1* (1977), 453—461
6. DE BRABANDER, M., GEUENS, G., DE MEY, J. and JONIAU, M.: Light microscopic and ultrastructural distribution of immunoreactive tubulin in mitotic mammalian cells. Biologie Cellulaire *34* (1979), 213—226
7. DE BRABANDER, M. J., VAN DE VEIRE, R. M. L., AERTS, F. E. M., BORGERS, M. and JANSSEN, P. A. J.: The effect of methyl [5-(2-Thienylcarbonyl)-1H-benzimidazol-2-yl]carbamate, (R 17934; NSC 238159), a new synthetic antitumoral drug interfering with microtubules, on mammalian cells cultured in vitro. Cancer Res. *36* (1976a), 905—916
8. DE RIDDER, L. I. and LAERUM, O. D.: Invasion of rat neurogenic cell lines in embryonic chick heart fragments in vitro. J. Natl. Cancer Inst. *66* (1981), 723—728
9. GEORGE, P., JOURNEY, L. J. and GOLDSTEIN, M. N.: Effect of Vincristine on the fine structure of HeLa cells during Mitosis. J. Natl. Cancer Inst. *35* (1965), 355—375
10. KIELER, J. BRIAND, P., VAN PETEGHEM, M. C. and MAREEL, M.: Comparative studies of two types of "spontaneous" malignant alteration of ST/a mouse lung fibroblasts propagated in vitro. In Vitro *15* (1979), 758—771

11. LOIKE, J. D., BREWER, C. F., STERNLICHT, H., GENSLER, W. J. and HORWITZ, S. B.: Structure-activity study of the inhibition of microtubule assembly in vitro by podophyllotoxin and its congeners. Cancer Res. *38* (1978), 2688—2693

12. MAREEL, M. M.: Is invasiveness in vitro characteristic of malignant cells? Cell Biol. Int. Rep. *3* (1979), 627—640

13. MAREEL, M. M.: Recent aspects of tumor invasiveness. Int. Rev. Exp. Pathol. *22* (1980) 65—129

14. MAREEL, M. M., BRUYNEEL, E. and STORME, G.: Attachment of mouse fibrosarcoma cells to precultured fragments of embryonic chick heart. An early step to invasion in vitro. Virchows Arch. B (Cell Pathol.) *34* (1980), 85—97

15. MAREEL, M. M. K. and DE BRABANDER, M. J.: Effect of microtubule inhibitors on malilnant invasion in vitro. J. Natl. Cancer Inst. *61* (1978), 787—792

16. MAREEL, M., DE RIDDER, L., DE BRABANDER, M. and VAKAET, L.: Characterization of spontagous, chemical, and viral transformants of a C3H/3T3-type mouse cell line by transplantation into young chick blastoderms. J. Natl. Cancer Inst. *54* (1975), 923—929

17. MAREEL, M. M., KIELER, J. V. F., BRUYNEEL, E., VAN CAUWENBERGE, R. and DRAGONETTI, C.: Invasiveness of malignant ST/A mouse lung cells in vitro. Virchows Arch. B (Cell Pathol.), 1981 (In Press)

18. MAREEL, M., KIELER, J. and VAN CAUWENBERGE, R.: Loss of directional migration after round-cell transformation of malignant ST/A mouse lung cells. Cell Biol. Int. Rep. *5* (1981), 921—928

19. MAREEL, M., KINT, J. and MEYVISCH, C.: Methods of study of the invasion of malignant C3H-mouse fibroblasts into embryonic chick heart in vitro. Virchows Arch. B (Cell Pathol.) *30* (1979), 95—111

20. MAREEL, M., STORME, G., DE BRUYNE, G. and VAN CAUWENBERGE, R.: Antiinvasive effect of microtubule inhibitors in vivo. In: Microtubules and Microtubule Inhibitors 1980 (Eds. M. DE BRABANDER and J. DE MEY), Elsevier/North-Holland Biomedical Press-Amsterdam, 1980, pp. 535—544

21. MEYVISCH, C. and MAREEL, M.: Invasion of malignant C3H mouse fibroblasts from aggregates transplanted into the auricles of syngenic mice. Virchows Arch. B (Cell Pathol.) *30* (1979), 113—122

22. MEYVISCH, V., VAN HOORDE, P. and MAREEL, M.: Invasiveness and the metastatic potential of tumour cells. In: Metastasis, Clinical and Experimental Aspects (Eds. K. HELLMAN, P. HILGARD and S. ECCLES). Martinus Nijhoff, Den Haag, 1980, pp. 33—37

23. STORME, G. and MAREEL, M. M.: Effect of anticancer agents on directional migration of malignant C3H mouse fibroblastic cells in vitro. Cancer Res. *40* (1980), 943—948

24. STORME, G. and MAREEL, M. M.: Effect of anticancer agents on invasion of mouse fibrosarcoma cells in vitro. Oncology *38* (1981), 182—186

[1] Istituto di Farmacologia, Università degli Studi di Trieste
and
[2] Istituto di Chimica Farmaceutica, Università degli Studi di Trieste
and
[3] Centro di Studi per l'Istochimica del CNR, Università di Pavia, Italy

Metastasis: Mitostatic Drugs

T. Giraldi, G. Sava, R. Cherubino[1], L. Lassiani[2], G. Bottiroli and G. Mazzini

Introduction

The treatment of systemic metastatic diseases has recently attracted increasing attention from clinicians and from researchers working with laboratory animals. Indeed, patients with solid malignant tumours die almost invariably because of the appearance of metastases, despite successful eradication of the primary neoplastic lesion. Treatment of metastases has included alterations of the properties of the host (e.g., by anticoagulants (1) or immunostimulants (2, 3)) or use of drugs that act directly on tumour cells. Cytotoxic antitumour drugs, although found useful in several instances in laboratory animals (4—6) and in man (7), do not appear to be a general solution to the problem of treatment of metastases, and the most common human malignant neoplasms respond poorly, or have natural or acquired resistance, to such drugs (8, 9). Moreover, there appears to be no significantly exploitable difference in sensitivity to cytotoxic agents between primary and secondary tumours (10).

Recently, certain agents have been identified that capable of selectively inhibiting metastasis formation, by a mechanism different from a cytotoxic action on tumour cells. The most active compounds in this group appear to be ($\pm$) 1,2-di(3,5-dioxo-piperazin-1-yl)propane (ICRF 159) (Razoxane) (11), dimethyltriazenes such as p-(3,3-dimethyl-1-triazeno)benzoic acid potassium salt (DM-COOK) (12—14) and N-diazo-acetylglycinamide (DGA) (15—17).

This paper is a report af results recently obtained in our laboratory on the effects of the selective antimetastatic agents DM-COOK and DGA in mice bearing the spontaneously metastasizing tumour, 3 LL. The results are discussed together with those obtained using the cytotoxic antitumour agent, cycophosphamide (CP).

Experimental

Tumour implantation, surgical excision and evaluation

The 3LL tumour was maintained in C57BL/6 mice by implanting 10^6 viable tumour cells subcutaneously into the axillary region. Single-cell suspensions were prepared by mechanical dissociation of the tumour tissue, as already described (18). To study the formation of spontaneous metastases, 10^6 single viable tumour cells were transplanted subcutaneously into the axillary region of BDF1 mice. Primary tumour growth and lung metastasis formation were measured on day 15 and at sacrifice on day 21, as already reported (18). Artificial metastases were obtained by intravenous injection of 3×10^5 tumour cells; the formation of lung nodules was measured at sacrifice on day 15. For surgical studies, 5×10^5 tumour cells were implanted intramuscularly into the left hindleg; anaesthesia and amputation were performed as described previously (19).

Drug treatment

DM-COOK and DGA were synthesized by reported procedures (20, 21). The animals received 0.1 ml/10 g of body weight of freshly prepared drug solution intraperitoneally in 0.1 N NaHCO$_3$; the control groups received only the solvent.

Measurement of the number of circulating tumour cells

This determination was peformed by flow cytofluorimetric measurement of peripheral blood, following a modification of the method published by KRISHAN (22). Portions of 0.2—0.5 ml of whole blood, obtained by intracardiac puncture of the right ventricle in open-chested mice ana-esthesized with ethyl urethane (1.5 g/kg), were mixed with 5 ml sodium citrate solution in H$_2$O, 0.1% W/V, containing 250 µg propidium iodide (Cal Biochem, USA). After 10 min, the stained samples were measured by means of Cytofluorograph 4800 A (Bio-Physics System Inc., USA). A 488-nm argon-ion laser line at 10 mW was used for excitation, and the fluorescence emission above 610 nm was measured. A multichannel pulse height analyzer (Laben Spectroscope Modular 8000, Italy) was used to produce and store the DNA histogram distributions. The number of tumour cells is expressed as the population of tetraploid cells found in 10^7 nucleated cells present in the blood samples.

Results and discussion

When the effects of a purely cytotoxic antineoplastic agent, CP, and those of two selective antimetastatic agents, ICRF 159 and DM-COOK, were examined in mice bear-ing 3 LL (18), it was found that CP causes a strictly related and pronounced inhibition of the weight of the subcutaneous tumour and of spontaneous and artificial meta-stases; this behaviour is consistent with a purely cytotoxic mechanism. ICRF 159 also markedly reduces the formation of spontaneous metastases; and a dose-dependent reduction in the weight of artifical metastases was also observed: at the highest dose tolerated, artifical metastasis weight was reduced to about 5%, and subcutaneous tumour mass was significantly lowered to 40%. These effects are consistent with a combined cytotoxic and selective antimetastatic action, although the latter appears to prevail. DM-COOK, in a wide range of doses, markedly depressed the weight and number of spontaneous metastases, but had no effect on the formation of artificial metastases or primary tumour growth. The effects of these agents on the fractional incorporation of ^{3}H-thymidine into tumour cells further indicate that only DM-COOK is devoid of cytotoxic effects for pulmonary and subcutaneous tumours. In hosts pretreated with DM-COOK, no reduction in the formation of either spontaneous or artifical metastases was observed, indicating that DM-COOK acts directly on tumour cells and suggesting that it inhibits their release from the primary tumour into the blood-stream.

This suggestion was investigated by determining the influence of treatment with DM-COOK on the number of circulating tumour cells in the blood of mice bearing subcutaneous 3 LL. This research was carried out using the cytofluorimetric technique described in the experimental section, a seemingly original technique, since a search of the literature showed that research on metastasizing tumour cells is usually performed by direct morphological observation of nucleated blood cell concentrates (23—28). A cytofluorimetric technique, involving fluorescent staining of the cell membrane has been used (29), but is was employed to detect the presence of meta-stases of B 16 melanoma established in the lungs of the hosts. Our procedure allows us to measure the number of tumour cells present in samples of whole unprocessed blood, with only the addition of citrate as anticoagulant and the fluorescent stain. 3LL cells can be distinguished from other nucleated blood cells after nuclear staining because they are aneuploid (largely tetraploid); they were thus counted and expressed as the number per 10^5 diploid blood cells, since the number of leucocytes is unaffected by treatment with DM-COOK. A representative result, obtained in preliminary experiments (Table 1) shows that treatment with DM-COOK markedly reduces the number of circulating metastasizing tumour cells, in proportion to the reduction of established lung metastases formation (13, 14).

Table 1.
Effects of DM-COOK on the number of circulating tumour cells in BDF1 mice bearing 3LL[a]

Sample	Treatment schedule (days after implantation)	Tumour cells	
		Total number at peak	% control
Controls[b]	—	97	100
DM-COOK[b]	1—7	9	9.3
Controls	—	260	100
DM-COOK	1—13	7	2.7

[a] Mice were implanted intramuscularly with 3LL on day 0 and treated daily as indicated; blood collection and cell counts were performed 24 h after the last drug adminstration.
[b] The staining solution also contained 0.1% Triton X-100 V/V

In animals treated with DM-COOK, no increase in survival time is observed, since the absence of effect on the primary tumour leads to death of the treated animals at about the same time as untreated controls, in spite of the prevention of lung metastasis formation by the drug. Pre- and intraoperative treatment with DM-COOK combined with surgical removal of the primary tumour produced a large proportion of cures in mice bearing intramuscular 3LL (19, 30) and B16 melanoma (31), under conditions in which surgery alone was ineffective. In order better to examine the mechanism of action of DM-COOK under these conditions, its effects have been compared with those of similar (32) antimetastatic agent, DGA. DM-COOK and DGA reduce the formation of spontaneous lung metastases in mice bearing subcutaneous 3LL to a similar extent (13—17). In surgical experiments involving preoperative treatment of mice bearing intramuscular 3LL, DM-COOK produced about 50% of cures and a significant increase in the life span of the uncured animals, whereas DGA was completely ineffective (Fig. 1 and Table 2). A further re-implantation of the tumour into animals cured by DM-COOK and surgery produced a significantly reduced formation of spontaneous and artificial metastases (Table 3). Since a number of micrometastases persist after antimetastatic chemotherapy and surgery, it can be assumed that only with DM-COOK can the host defenses eradicate them. Indeed, 3LL is weakly immunogenic in syngeneic hosts, and treatment with the mutagenic agent N-methyl-N'-nitro-N-nitrosoguanidine increases host responses against the tumour (33). DM COOK might act as a mutagen, since mutagenic properties have been reported for a large series of structurally related 1-aryl-3,3-dimethyltriazenes (34).

These data indicate that DM-COOK is highly active, when used in combination with surgery, in reducing pre- and intraoperative haematogenous dissemination of murine

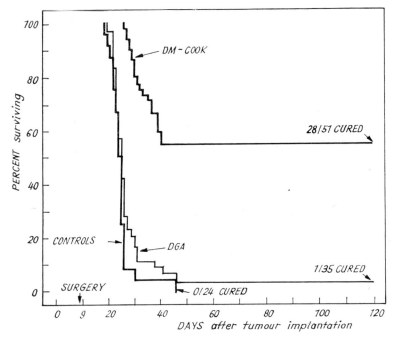

Fig. 1. Effects of treatment with 50 mg/kg DM-COOK or 300 mg/kg DGA on days 1 to 8 after surgical removal of the primary tumour in mice bearing intramuscular 3LL.

Table 2.
Mean weight of primary tumour and the mean survival time of uncured mice treated with 50 mg je kg DM-COOK or 300 mg/kg DGA on days 1 to 8 after surgical removal of the primary tumour in mice bearing intramuscular 3LL

Treatment	Primary tumour weight (g ± SE)	Mean survival time of uncured mice[a] (days ± SE)
None	1.57 ± 0.36	25.9 ± 1.0
DGA	1.51 ± 0.11	27.5 ± 0.8
DM-COOK	1.43 ± 0.05	32.9 ± 1.1*

[a] Mice surviving more than 4 months were considered to be cured
* Mean significantly different from that of controls (by Student-Newman-Keuls test (53), $p < 0.05$)

metastasizing tumours. Although CP is highly active against 3LL, it should be noted that this sensitivity is unique (35), since it is poorly or not responsive to many other clinically effective antineoplastic agents (36, 37); the situation is similar for the most common solid tumours in man (8, 9). Consequently, it appears that prophylactic antimetastatic treatment might be of great significance, particularly in the case of surgical treatment of metastasizing tumour for which no highly effective antineoplastic drugs are available. It is possible that antimetastatic agents may act on a broad spectrum of tumours, independent of the type of metastasizing tumour involved, since

58

Table 3.
Development of 3LL metastases in mice cured by preoperative chemotherapy with DM-COOK and surgery

Treatment with DM-COOK	Spontaneous metastases		Artificial metastases	
	Total $\pm$ SE	Weight (mg) $\pm$ SE	Total $\pm$ SE	Weight (mg) $\pm$ SE
—	26.0 ± 3.6	41.8 ± 8.7	20.2 ± 2.5	157 ± 20.6
+	$12.2 \pm 1.4^*$	$10.2 \pm 7.2^*$	$13.1 \pm 2.2^*$	$91.9 \pm 14.3^*$

[a] The tumour was re-implanted 4 months after amputation, and the development of metastases was measured as indicated in the experimental section. Two groups of 14 mice cured after the first tumour implantation, and two groups of 14 controls were used. Control animals without tumours underwent amputation and were implanted with the tumour after 4 months.
* Mean significantly different from that of controls, by one-way analysis of variance (52), p < 0.05.

the mechanism of metastasis formation seems to be unique for solid malignant tumours (38). The best known selective antimetastatic agent, ICRF 159, has antimetastatic effects in several animal systems (11, 39), and aryldimethyltriazenes act on all metastasizing tumours tested so far, i.e. 3LL (12—14), B16 melanoma (39) and M5 ovary carcinoma (M. D'INCALCI, personal communication).

With regard to the relevance of selective antimetastatic treatments to the clinical problems of solid tumour therapy, selective antimetastatic agents, as defined above, can be effective only in preventing metastasis formation. On the one hand, their use might thus appear of limited interest since between tumour diagnosis and treatment, a certain number of (micro) metastases are presumably already formed. On the other hand, several diagnostic and therapeutic procedures might increase metastasis formation. In experimental systems, mechanical manipulation of tumours, such as massage and biopsy, causes increased shedding of tumour cells into the blood stream (40—42). Curative local irradiation of primary tumours accelerates metastasis formation (41). The trauma of surgery as well as anaesthesia, and the use of glucose in intra- and postsurgical resuscitation decrease host resistance and augment the formation of systemic metastases (43—47). Treatment with cytotoxic agents may also increase metastasis formation, as observed with CP in animal systems (48). Although lesser of practical importance, the possibility exists that metastases can originate from tumour metastatic foci (49—50), and that this process might be the target of antimetastatic treatment (51). These data and considerations indicate that treatment with selective antimetastatic agents is therapeutically useful when combined with surgical treatment of metastasizing tumours in mice. Proposed clinical trials appear to be justified and will possibly indicate whether the integration of antimetastatic treatment(s) into combined modalities of cancer management would be useful in man.

Summary

In mice bearing 3LL, the cytotoxic antitumour drug CP causes a strictly related, pronounced inhibition of primary tumours and of spontaneous and artificial metastases. The selective antimetastatic agent, DM-COOK, markedly inhibitis the formation of spontaneous metastases, but has no effects on primary tumours or artificial metastases; ICRF 159 appears to act by a combination of cytotoxic and selective antimetastatic properties. DM-COOK markedly reduces the number of circulating tumour cells in the blood of mice bearing intramuscular 3LL. Preoperative treatment with DM-COOK of mice bearing intramuscular 3LL, followed by surgical excision of the primary tumour, causes about 50% of cures and a significant increase in the life-span of uncured mice. DM-COOK appears to increase the host's resistance to micrometastases occurring after surgery, since metastasis formation produced by further implantation of 3LL in mice cured by DM-COOK and surgery is reduced. The possibility of integrating treatment with selective antimetastatic agents into combined modalities of treatment of solid metastasizing tumours is discussed and compared with the use of cytotoxic antineoplastic drugs.

Acknowledgement

This work was supported by the Italian National Research Council, Special Project 'Control of Neoplastic Growth', contract n° 80.01562.96, and contract n° 204121/96/93251. The authors wish to acknowledge stimulating discussions over several years with Dr. C. NISI on selective treatment of metastases.

References

1. HILGARD, P. and THORNES, R. D.: Anticoagulants in the treatment of cancer. Europ. J. Cancer *12* (1976), 755—762
2. MILAS, L. and SCOTT, M. T.: Antitumor activity of *Corynebacterium parvum*. In: 'Advances in Cancer Research' Vol. 26, 257—306, Editors: KLEIN G. and WEINHOUSE, S., Academic Press, New York, 1978
3. BALDWIN, M. T. and PIMM, M. V.: BCG in tumor immunotherapy. In: 'Advances in Cancer Research' Vol. 28, 91—147. Editors: KLEIN G. and WEINHOUSE S., Academic Press, New York 1978
4. SHABEL, F. M. Jr.: Concepts for systemic treatment of micrometastases. Cancer *35* (1975), 15—24
5. SKIPPER, H. E.: Adjuvant chemotherapy. Cancer *41* (1978), 936—940
6. SHABEL, F. M. Jr.: Surgical adjuvant chemotherapy of metastatic murine tumor. Cancer *40* (1977), 558—568
7. ROSSI, A. and BONADONNA, G.: Current impact of adjuvant chemotherapy in resectable cancer. Cancer Chemother. Pharmacol. *3* (1979), 7—16
8. CARTER, S. K. and SOPER, W. T.: Integration of chemotherapy into combined modality treatment of solid tumors. I. The overall strategy. Cancer Treat. Rev. *1* (1974), 1—14
9. CARTER, S. K.: Cancer treatment today and its impact on drug development, with special emphasis on the phase II clinical trials. J. Natl. Cancer Inst. *57* (1976), 235—244
10. DONELLI, M. G., COLOMBO, T., DAGNINO, G., MADONNA, M. and GARATTINI, S.: Is better drug availability in secondary neoplasm responsible for better response to chemotherapy ? Europ. J. Cancer *17* (1981), 201—209
11. BAKOWSKI, M. T.: (±) 1,2-di(3,5-dioxopiperazin-1-yl)propane NSC-129,943; Razoxane. Cancer Treat. Rev. *3* (1976), 95—107
12. GIRALDI, T., HOUGHON, P. J., TAYLOR, D. M. and NISI, C.: Antimetastatic action of some triazene derivatives against Lewis lung carcinoma in mice. Cancer Treat. Rep. *62* (1978), 721—725
13. SAVA, G., GIRALDI, T., LASSIANI, L. and NISI, C.: Mechanism of the antimetastatic action of dimethyltriazenes. Cancer Treat. Rep. *63* (1979), 93—98
14. GIRALDI, T., GUARINO, A. M., NISI, C. and SAVA, G.: Antitumor and antimetastatic effects of benzenoid triazenes in mice bearing Lewis lung carcinoma. Pharmacol. Res. Commun. *12* (1980), 1—11

15. GIRALDI, T., NISI, C. and SAVA, G.: Antimetastatic effects of N-diazoacetyl glycine derivatives in C57BL mice. J. Natl. Cancer Inst., *58* (1977), 1129—1130

16. GIRALDI, T., SAVA, G. and NISI, C.: Mechanism of the antimetastatic action of N-diazoacetylglycinamide in mice bearing Lewis lung carcinoma. Europ. J. Cancer *16* (1980), 87—92

17. GIRALDI, T., GUARINO, A. M., NISI, C. and BALDINI, L.: Selective antimetastatic effects of N-diazoacetylglycine derivatives in mice. Europ. J. Cancer *15* (1979), 603—607

18. GIRALDI, T., SAVA, G., CUMAN, R., NISI, C. and LASSIANI, L.: Selectivity of the antimetastatic and cytotoxic effects of p-(3,3-dimethyl-1-triazeno)benzoic acid potassium salt, ($\pm$)-1,2-di(3,5-dioxopiperazin-1-yl)propane, and cyclophosphamide in mice bearing Lewis lung carcinoma. Cancer Res. *41* (1981), 2524—2528

19. SAVA, G., GIRALDI, T., NISI, C. and BERTOLI, G.: Prophylactic antimetastatic treatment with aryldimethyltriazenes as adjuvant surgical tumor removal in mice bearing Lewis lung carcinoma. Cancer Treat Rep. *66* (1982), 115—120

20. KOLAR, G. F.: Synthesis of biologically active triazenes from isolable diazonium salts. Z. Naturforsch. (B) *27* (1972), 1183—1185

21. CURTIS, T. and THOMPSON, J.: Einwirkung von salpetriger Säure auf Polyglycinester. III. Abhandlung. Einwirkung von Ammoniak auf Diazoacetylglycinester und Diazoacetyl-glycyl-glycinester. Chem. Ber. *39* (1906), 1383—1388

22. KRISHAN, A.: Rapid flow cytofluorimetric analysis of mammalian cell cycle by propidium iodide staining. J. Cell Biol. *66* (1975), 188—192

23. BUTLER, T. P. and GULLINO, P. M.: Quantitation of cell shedding into efferent blood of mammary adenocarcinoma. Cancer Res. *35* (1975), 512—516

24. SALISBURY, A. J.: The significance of the circulating cancer cell. Cancer Treat. Rev. *2* (1975), 55—72

25. LIOTTA, L. A., KLEINERMAN, J. and SAIDEL, G. M.: The significance of hematogenous tumor cell clumps in the metastatic process. Cancer. Res. *36* (1976), 889—894

26. SALISBURY, A. J., BURRAGE, K. and HELLMANN, K.: Histological analysis of the antimetastatic effect of (y)-1,2-bis(3,5-dioxopiperazin-1-yl)-propane. Cancer Res. *34* (1974), 843—849

27. LIOTTA, L. A., KLEINERMAN, J. and SAIDEL, G. M.: Quantitative relationships of intravascular tumor cells, tumor vessels, and pulmonary metastases following tumor implantation. Cancer Res. *34* (1974), 997—1004

28. MALGREN, R. A.: Studies of circulating cancer cells in cancer patients. In: "Mechanism of invasion in cancer", 108—117. Editor: DENOIX P., Springer-Verlag, Berlin, 1967

29. GRATTAROLA, M., ZIETZ, S., LESSIN, S., DESAIVE, C. and NICOLINI, C.: Early detections of micrometastases via flow microfluorimetry. Cancer Biochem. Biophys. *4* (1979), 13—18

30. GIRALDI, T., SAVA, G., CUMAN, R., NISI, C. and LASSIANI, L.: Prophylactic antimetastatic agents dimethyltriazenes, N-diazoacetylglycine derivatives and other neutral proteinase inhibitors. In: "Metastasis, Clinical and Experimental aspects", 436—440. Editors: HELLMANN, K., HILGARD P. and ECCLES S., Martinus Nijhoff Publishers, The Hague., 1980

31. GIRALDI, T. and SAVA, G.: Malignancy and tumor proteinases: effects of proteinase inhibitors. In: "Proteinases and their Inhibitors. Structure, Function and Applied Aspects", 45—56. Editors: TURK V. and VITALE Lj., Pergamon Press, Oxford 1981

32. GIRALDI, T. and SAVA, G.: Selective antimetastatic drugs (review). Anticancer Res. *1* (1981), 163—174.

33. VAN PEL, A., GEORLETTE, M. and BOON, T.: Tumor cell variants obtained by mutagenesis of a Lewis lung carcinoma cell line: immune rejection by syngeneic mice. Pro. Natl. Acad. Sci. *76* (1979), 5282—5285

34. MALAVEILLE, C., KOLAR, G. F. and BARTSCH, H.: Rats and mouse tissue-mediated mutagenicity in Salmonella typhimurium. Mutat. Res., *36* (1976), 1—10

35. DE WYS, W. D.: A quantitative model for the study of the growth and treatment of a tumor and its metastases with correlation between proliferative state and sensitivity of cyclophosphamide. Cancer Res. *32* (1972), 367—373

36. CARTER, S. K., SCHABEL, F. M., BRODER, L. E. and JOHNSTON, T. P.: 1,3-Bis(2-chloroethyl)-1-nitrosourea (BCNU) and other nitrosoureas in cancer treatment: a review. In: "Advances in Cancer Research", 16, 273—332. Editors: KLEIN, G. and WEINHOUSE S., Academic Press, New York 1972

37. OVEIERA, A. A., JOHNSON, R. K. and GOLDIN, A.: Growth characteristics and chemotherapeutic response of intravenously implanted Lewis lung carcinoma. Cancer Chemother. Rep. Part. 2 , 5 (1975), 111—125

38. ROSS, E., and DINGEMANS, K. G.: Mechanism of metastasis. Biochim. Biophys. Acta *560* (1979), 135—166

39. PIMM, M. V. and BALDWIN, R. W.: Influence of ICRF 159 and Triton WR 1339 on metastases of rat epithelioma. Br. J. Cancer *31* (1975) 62—67

40. KARLSSON, I. and PETERSON, H. I.: Preoperative intravascular tumor cell shedding. Z. Krebsforsch. *90* (1977), 115—118

41. PETERS, Lj.: A study of the influence of various diagnostic and therapeutic procedures applied to a murine squamous carcinoma on its metastatic behaviour. Br. J. Cancer *32* (1975), 355 bis 365

42. PETERSON, H. I. and RISBERG, B.: Experimental studies on the effect of induced antifibrinolysis on preoperative tumor cell shedding. Z. Krebsforsch. *86* (1976), 121—125

43. SABA, T. M. and ANTIKATZIDES, T. G.: Decreased resistance to intravenous tumor cell challenge during reticuloendothelial depression following surgery. Br. J. Cancer *34* (1976), 381—389

44. LUNDY, J., LOVETT, E. J., HAMILTON, S. and CONRAN, P.: Halothane, surgery, immunodepression and artifical pulmonary metastases. Cancer, *41* (1978), 827—830

45. LUNDY, J., LOVETT, E. J. and CONRAN, P.: Pulmonary metastases, a potential biologic consequence of anaesthetic-induced immunosuppression by thiopental. Surgery *82* (1977), 254—256

46. AGOSTINO, D. and AGOSTINO, N.: Role of operative trauma: explosive metastases of similar size following amputation of the primary leg tumor. Tumori *65* (1979), 527—538

47. RISCA, R. and TODORUTIU, C.: Influence of glucose on the development of experimental metastases. Br. J. Cancer *30* (1974), 241—245

48. DE RUITER, J., CRAMER, S. J., SMINK, T. and VAN PUTTEN, L. M.: The facilitation of tumor growth in the lung by cyclophosphamide in artificial and spontaneous metastases models. Europ. J. Cancer *15* (1979), 1139—1149.

49. KETCHAM, A. S., WEXLER, H. and CHRETIEN, P. B.: The metastatic potential of experimental pulmonary metastases. J. Surgical Res. *15* (1973), 45—52

50. SUGARBAKER, E. V. and KETCHAM, A. S.: Mechanism and prevention of cancer dissemination: an overview. Semin. Oncol. *4* (1977), 19—32

51. KETCHAM, A. S. and SUGARBAKER, E. V.: The relation of surgery to the metastatic potential of neoplastic disease. In: "Cancer Metastasis" 173—180. Editors: STANSLY, P. G. and SATO, H., University Park Press, Baltimore, 1977

52. SOKAL, R. R. and ROHLF, F. J.: Single classification analysis of variance. In: "Biometry", 204—252. Editor: FREEMAN, W. H., San Francisco. 1969

53. SNEDECOR, G. W. and COCHRAN, W. G.: In: "Statistical Methods", chap. 10, p. 258, 1967

Department of Medicine, Dartmouth Medical School and the Veterans Administration Hospital, White River Junction, VT 05001, USA

Anticoagulant Treatment of Cancer

L. R. Zacharski

The intriguing concept that blood coagulation reactions contribute to the metastatic potential of neoplastic cells has developed subsequent to observations made more than a century ago by the Viennese surgeon, Theodor Billroth. In his voluminous treatise on surgical pathology, Billroth (1878) described the occurrence of clots in association with microscopic intravascular tumour deposits.

Although this morphologic association has been confirmed on innumerable occasions in the intervening years, its significance was not considered for almost three quarters of a century. Then, in 1952, Terranova and Chiossone postulated that thrombus formation about circulating tumour cells might contribute to their lodgment within the microvasculature thus allowing them to „take root" to form metastatic foci. These authors referred to observations by DeGaetani of microthrombus formation about tumour cells lodged within the pulmonary vasculature following their intravenous injection into experimental animals. This finding was like that of human tumours as described by Billroth. These workers tested their hypothesis by infusing heparin into rats that subsequently received an intravenous inoculation of tumour cells. They found that heparin reduced the number of animals that died of malignancy and prolonged survival in tumour-retaining animals.

The ability of antithrombotic (anticoagulant and antiplatelet) agents to favorably modify the course of experimental neoplasia has been abundantly confirmed in numerous subsequent studies (Zacharski et al, 1979). It is evident that such drugs are not invariably effective in the many experimental tumour types that have been investigated, and that certain tumour types may respond to one form of antithrombotic therapy but not to another. However, overall, these studies have permitted formulation of a general hypothesis that applies to at least certain experimental tumours. According to this hypothesis, the ability of neoplastic cells to initiate coagulation reactions (for example, fibrin formation or platelet aggregation), constitutes a mechanism by which they modify their local environment in a manner that favours their perpetuation through metastatic dissemination. It is this dissemination that is the primary target of antithrombotic drugs. In a sense, the host-tumour relationship may be envisioned as a competition for survival that takes place over a period of time between the tumour cell and the host from which it has arisen and which provides the very mechanism (the coagulation mechanism) necessary for the "success" of the tumour.

The coagulation hypothesis of neoplastic spread has gained support from studies in which many different malignant cells have been demonstrated to possess clot-inducing or platelet-aggregating properties (Semeraro and Donati, 1981; Karpatkin et al, 1981). Furthermore, the occurrence of elements of clots about tumours is not restricted to the intravascular compartment. Thus, fibrin has been demonstrated by electron microscopic and immunofluorescent techniques about extravascular tumour deposits in a variety of human and experimental malignancies (DVORAK et al, 1981).

The extent to which induction of coagulation is related to the metastatic spread of human malignancy is uncertain. Although a number of attempts have been made to influence the course of human malignancy by means of anticoagulant administration, interpretation of the results has not always been easy and questions remain (ZACHARS-KI, 1981). For this reason a VA Cooperative Study Group was formed to systemati-cally evaluate anticoagulant and antiplatelet drugs by means of controlled, rando-mized clinical trials in defined tumour types. The first clinical trial undertaken by this group (VA Cooperative Study 75) began in April of 1976 and ended in May of 1981. In this study, 430 patients with malignancies of the lung, large bowel, head and neck, and prostate were entered into nine different tumour strata. All patients re-ceived conventional therapy considered to be appropriate for their tumour type and extent of disease, and were randomized to receive warfarin or no anticoagulant the-rapy.

The final results of this study are currently being formulated. However, the results obtained in patients with small cell carcinoma of the lung (SCCL) were sufficiently promising to warrant publication prior to the termination of the study (ZACHARSKI et al, 1981). Fifty patients admitted to this study who had SCCL were randomized to either warfarin-treated (25 patients) or control (25 patients) groups. Survival for warfarin-treated patients was just about double that of control patients (50 versus 24 weeks, p $= 0.026$). The survival advantage afforded by warfarin could not be attributed to difference between treatment groups in age, sex, performance status or extent of disease at randomization. Likewise, no difference between groups was noted for the amount of conventional chemotherapy given; the kinds of chemothera-peutic agents used after patients were taken off study; the average number of phy-sicians visits per month; or the mean values for leukocytes, platelets or hemoglo-bin. The survival advantage afforded by warfarin was observed in patients who had extensive disease at the time of randomization and in patients who failed to achieve a complete or partial remission from the chemotherapy and radiation therapy regi-men used. (Survival for control patients was approximately that expected on the basis of studies by others for the standard therapy used.) Although the incidence of remissions was not increased in the warfarin-treated group, the median duration of remission and the median time to first evidence of the disease progression beyond that present at the time of randomization were increased in these patients.

The results obtained so far in the VA Cooperative Study 75 do not detract from, and in fact support, the contention that the coagulation hypothesis for neoplastic spread may indeed apply to human as well as experimental tumours. Therefore, the anticoagulant approach to the clinical management of cancer would seem to merit further consideration. Since antithrombotic drugs represent a new addition to the armamentarium of the cancer therapist, it is relevant to consider certain character-istics of the anticoagulant approach to tumour management that set it apart from traditional approaches.

As currently conceived, the anticoagulant approach to the containment of malig-nancy is neither a means of enhancing host defenses that are assumed to have failed, as in immunotherapy, nor a direct toxic attack on this tumour, as in chemotherapy. Rather, anticoagulant therapy is a way of blocking specific reactions of the host that appear to be required for expression of the metastatic potential of tumour cells.

One might predict, on the basis of results in experimental tumours, that different human tumours might respond to one form of antithrombotic therapy but not to another. However, there is, at present, no way of knowing the extent to which results in experimental tumour systems can be translated to the human setting or of predicting which, if any, human tumour types will respond to which, if any, form of antithrombotic therapy. However, a variety of relatively well understood drugs having different mechanisms of action are currently available for testing. Thus, it is the well designed and carefully executed clinical trial that will provide not only an answer to the question of efficacy but also an opportunity to further define the mechanisms involved.

References

BILLROTH, T.: Lectures on Surgical Pathology and Therapeutics, translated from the 8th ed., New Sydenham Society, London, 1978

DVORAK, H. F., ORENSTEIN, N. S. and DVORAK, A. M.: Tumour-secreted mediators and the tumour microenvironment: relationship to immunologic surveillance. Lymphokines 2 (1981), 203

KARPATKIN, S., PEARLSTEIN, E., SALK, P. L. and YOGEESWARAN, G.: Role of platelets in tumour cell metastasis. Ann. N.Y. Acad. Sci. 370 (1981), 101

SEMERARO, N. and DONATI, M. D.: Pathways of blood clotting initiation by cancer cells. In: Malignancy and the Hemostatic System, pp. 65—81. Eds.: M. B. DONATI, J. F. DAVIDSON, and S. GARATTINE. Raven Press, New York, 1981

TERRANOVA, T. and CHIOSSONE, F.: Il fattore coagulazione nell' attecchimento delle cellule neoplastiche immesse in circulo. Boll. Soc. Ital. Biol. Sper. 28 (1952), 1224

ZACHARSKI, L. R., HENDERSON, W. G., RICKLES, F. R., FORMAN, W. B., CORNELL, C. J. Jr., FORCIER, R. J., HARROWER, H. W. and JONHSON, R. O.: Rationale and experimental design for the VA Cooperative Study of anticoagulation (warfarin) in the treatment of cancer. Cancer 44 (1979), 732

ZACHARSKI, L. R.: Anticoagulation in the treatment of cancer in man. In: Malignancy and the Hemostatic System, pp. 113—127. Eds.: M. B. DONATI, J. F. DAVIDSON, and S. GARATTINI. Raven Press, New York, 1981

ZACHARSKI, L. R., HENDERSON, W. G., RICKLES, F. R., FORMAN, W. B., CORNELL, C. J., Jr., FORCIER, R. J. HEADLEY, E., KIM, S.-H., O'DONNELL, J. F., O'DELL, R., TORNYOS, K. and KWAAN, H.: Effect of sodium warfarin on survival in small cell carcinoma of the lung: VA Cooperative Study 75. J. Am. Med. Assoc. 245 (1981), 831

Laboratory of Cellular and Molecular Biology
National Cancer Institute, National Institutes of Health
Bethesda, Maryland, USA

Reactivity of a Monoclonal Antibody (B72.3)
with Fixed Sections of Human Mammary Carcinomas

M. Nuti, Y. A. Teramoto, R. Mariani-Costantini, P. Horan Hand, D. Colcher and J. Schlom

Previous studies, using polyclonal sera (1—5), have described the presence of mammary tumour associated antigens. We have recently reported (6) the production of eleven monoclonal antibodies prepared against human metastatic mammary tumour cells. These antibodies have been shown to react with several human breast tumour cell lines and not with normal human cell lines. In this report we will describe in detail the reactivity of one of these monoclonals, B72.3, which displayed the most restricted range of reactivity for tumour versus normal cells. Monoclonal B72.3, of IgG_1 isotype, was shown (6) to react in solid phase radioimmunoassay with extracts of one of two breast tumour metastases to the liver and scored negative with extracts of normal liver and other tissues. In preliminary immunoperoxidase studies, B72.3 scored positive with two of four mammary tumours and one of four metastatic lesions. The antigen immunoprecipitated from mammary carcinoma cells by monoclonal B72.3 appears to be a 220K—400K glycoprotein complex (Teramoto et al, manuscript in preparation). We present here a more extensive study of both the range and the patterns of reactivities of monoclonal antibody B72.3. The materials and methods used in this report are as previously published (6). Unless otherwise specified, fixed tissue sections were used for immunoperoxidase studies.

Results

Monoclonal antibody B72.3 was used at various inputs in immunoperoxidase assays of tissue sections to determine the effect of antibody dose on the staining intensity and the percent of tumour cells stained; a range of antibody concentrations, varying from 0.02 μg to 10 μg of purified immunoglobulin per tissue section, were used. As shown in Table 1, where four representative tumours are listed, the antibody dose employed can sometimes determine if a given tumour scores positive or negative. Tumours 1 and 2 were positive only at higher concentrations of B72.3, whereas Tumour 4 was negative even at the highest antibody concentration tested. Tumour 3 remained positive even at the lowest concentration of immunoglobulin used. These results demonstrate that (a) different mammary tumours may vary in their concentration of the antigen detected by B72.3, (b) that a given mammary tumour may contain tumour cell popopulations which vary in antigen concentration (Table 1, Tumour 1), and (c) a given mammary tumour may score positive or negative depending on the dose of antibody employed (Table 1, Tumours 1 and 2).

To further characterize the range of reactivity of B72.3 the immunoperoxidase technique was used to test a variety of malignant, benign and normal human mammary

Table 1.

Dose of monoclonal antibody B72.3 vs. reactivity of human mammary carcinoma cells
Tumour staining intensity (% reactive tumour cells)

μg B72.3	Tumour 1	Tumour 2	Tumour 3	Tumour 4
10	1 + (90)	3 + (100)	3 + (80)	NEG
	2 + (10)			
4	1 + (5)	2 + (100)	3 + (80)	NEG
2	NEG	1 + (80)	3 + (70)	NEG
1	NEG	NEG	3 + (70)	NEG
0.2	NEG	NEG	2 + (50)	NEG
0.02	NEG	NEG	2 + (30)	NEG

Staining intensity: 1+ weak, 2+ moderate, 3+ strong. 0.02 μg of B72.3 is equivalent to a 1:100,000 dilution of mouse ascites fluid. Immunoglobulin in 200 μl was used per slide. Phosphate buffered saline, containing no B72.3, was used in all experiments as a control.

tissues. Two different doses (0.2 μg and 4 μg) of antibody were used for these experiments. Twelve of 51, or 23 percent, of primary mammary carcinomas and two of three of metastatic lesions of breast carcinomas were positive using 0.2 μg of antibody per tissue section. Increasing the amount of antibody to four μg per slide, however, increased the percent of positive primary breast tumours to 44 percent (17/39); 64 percent of the metastatic lesions also were positive using this antibody dose. These results are consistent with the data in Table 1 in that there is variability in terms of B72.3 reactive-antigen concentration among human breast carcinomas. Two primary mammary tumours that scored positive in fixed section were also positive in frozen section. Some other mammary tumours were negative both in fixed and frozen sections. Several histologic types of primary mammary tumours were included in those that were scored positive; these include infiltrating duct, infiltrating lobular and comedo carcinoma. Many of the in-situ elements present in the above lesions also stained. None of six medullary carcinomas scored positive. Metastatic breast carcinoma cells were also positive in axillary lymph nodes and at distal sites such as skin, liver, lung, pleura and mesentery.
Monoclonal B72.3 was also tested against normal breast tissue and normal lactating breast from non-cancer patients and showed no reactivity. This was closely surveyed in six breast tumours that contained normal ducts adjacent to tumour cells in the same section. In one case, a few cells from apparently normal ducts immediately adjacent to the tumour showed some faint staining. No staining was observed in normal mammary epithelium of 26 patients whose mammary carcinoma cells did not stain. Occasionally, the histiocytes or the polymorphonuclear leukocytes present in the stroma surrounding breast tumour cells showed positive cytoplasmic staining; this may be due to the reaction of B72.3 with antigen shed by tumour cells and phagocytized by the reactive cells. Fifteen benign breast lesions were also tested with the immunoperoxidase technique using monoclonal B72.3; these included fibrocystic disease, fibroadenomas and sclerosing adenosis. Two specimens showed positive staining: one case of fibrocystic disease where just a few cells in some ducts were faintly positive, and a case of intraductal papillomatosis and sclerosing adenosis with the majority of cells staining strongly. To define the range of reactivity of monoclonal B72.3 a variety of non-breast cells and tissues were tested. These experiments where

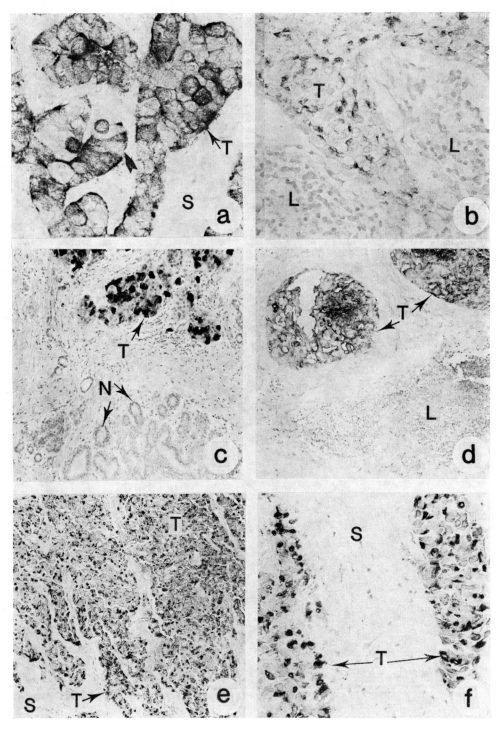

see page 69 below

carried out using both a live cell radioimmunoassay (6) and the immunoperoxidase technique. Monoclonal B72.3 was negative for binding to the surface of a number of human cell lines including uterus, breast, and fetal lung, skin, testis, kidney, thymus, bone marrow, and spleen. A variety of sarcoma and melanoma cell lines were also negative. Experiments using the immunoperoxidase technique were performed using B72.3 at concentration of 4 µg per slide against a variety of apparently normal tissues from non-cancer patients. These included two livers, two spleens, three lungs, two bone marrows, five colons, one stomach, one salivary gland, five lymph nodes and one kidney. All cell types in the above tissues scored negative. Other primary tumours were also tested for reactivity with B62.3 in immunoperoxidase. These included four colon carcinomas, two benign colon tumours, four lung carcinomas, two kidney carcinomas, one prostata carcinoma, one bladder carcinoma, one melanoma, two lymphomas and two sarcomas. Of the above, four colon carcinomas and two of four lung carcinomas were positive at four µg per slide. The reactivity to selected non-breast carcinomas raised the possibility of B62.3 being an anti-CEA antibody. We have previously shown (6), however, that monoclonal B62.3 does not react with purified CEA.

The differential distribution of the antigen recognized by monoclonal B72.3 among different mammary carcinomas was manifested by the various patterns of reactivity observed using the immunoperoxidase technique. The majority of breast carcinomas showed the reddish-brown diaminobenzidine precipitate intensely localized in the membrane, with a lesser degree of staining of the cytoplasm of tumour cells (Figure 1a). Some mammary tumours, on the other hand, showed a "focal" staining pattern (Figure 1b and 1f) with intensely concentrated areas of stain in the cytoplasm of the tumour cells. A third pattern of reactivity was also observed in some mammary tumours in which staining was localized on the luminal edge of carcinoma cells. All of the above three patterns of staining were also observed in metastatic mammary tumour cell populations (Figure 1e, and 1f). An example of the differential staining between normal ducts and malignant cells in a given section is shown in Figure 1c, where intense stain is localized in the tumour cells and not in adjacent normal mammary epithelium. As mentioned above, both infiltrating (Figure 1a—c) and in-situ (Figure 1d) breast tumour lesions stained positively with monoclonal B72.3; note that both stroma and lymphocytes surrounding tumour cells do not stain. Two kinds of heterogeneity were observed in most of the breast tumours tested. The first kind is a "patchwork" effect seen within a given mass, i.e., stained tumour cells that possess the antigen are immediately adjacent to negative tumour cells (see Figure 1a, broad arrow, and 1f). The second kind of heterogeneity was observed between different areas of the same tumour, i.e., in one area of a given tumour virtually all tumour cells stained, while in another area of the same tumour mass, most tumour cells scored

Fig. 1. Immunoperoxidase staining of fixed tissue sections of primary and metastatic mammary carcinomas with monoclonal antibody B72.3. (a) Infiltrating duct carcincma; note the intense membrane staining and faint cytoplasmic staining of tumour cells (T) and the negative stroma (S). The broad arrow indicates a negative tumour cell flanked by positive tumour cells. 540×. (b) Infiltrating duct carcinoma. Note negative lymphocytes (L) surrounding tumour cells. 330×. (c) Infiltrating duct carcinoma. Note the intense staining of tumour cells and adjacent normal mammary ducts (N) scoring negative. 130×. (d) In situ element (T) of an infiltrating duct carcinoma. 130×. (e) Breast tumour metastasis in the pleura. 130×. (f) Higher magnification of "e". Note focal staining of tumour cells. 330×.

69

negative. Heterogeneity was also observed with mammary tumour cell lines in culture. Tumours obtained from the MCF-7 cell line transplanted into nude mice also displayed this phenomenon, i. e., clusters of cells stained intensely while others scored negative.

Discussion

The reason or reasons for the antigenic heterogeneity observed in mammary carcinoma cell populations are uncertain at this time. At least three explanations merit consideration: (a) the antigens detected by B72.3 are differentially expressed in different phases of the cell cycle, (b) there are differences in cell surface receptors for growth factors or hormones in different cell populations which are manifested in differential antigen expression, or (c) there are inherent genotypic or phenotypic variations among tumour cell populations.

It is important to point out that not all mammary carcinomas react with antibody B72.3. Indeed, the percent of positive tumours changed from 23 percent to 44 percent when the amount of purified B72.3 immunoglobulin used was varied from 0.2 to 4 µg per slide. These results and those of Table 1 (Tumours 1 and 2) indicate that in many mammary tumours the antigen reactive with monoclonal B72.3 may be present in low amounts. Whereas none of the apparently normal human tissues or cell lines (from adult and fetal tissues) tested scored positive using high doses of B72.3, it would be naive to state that this or any other monoclonal antibody is "specific" for tumour cells. To make such claims, one would have to test every known cell type of numerous adults and fetuses. Even then, one could not be sure that the antigen sought is not below the limits of detection of the assay or assays used. It is thus sufficient to say at this point that monoclonal B72.3 appears to have a restricted range of reactivity for normal tissues. Studies are now underway to determine if the detection of, or intensity of, the antigen reactive with monoclonal B72.3 in various benign breast diseases and carcinomas is of prognostic value. The fact that the reactive antigen is not destroyed by fixation makes these studies feasible since sections of primary tumours of patients known to have remained disease free, versus those in remission, can now be compared for reactivities with monoclonal antibody B72.3.

References

1. MESA-TEJADA, R., KEYDAR, I., RAMANARAYANAN, M., OHNO, T., FEOGLIO, C. and SPIEGEL-MAN, S.: Proc. Natl. Sci. Acad. USA 75 (1978), 1529—1533
2. LEUNG, J. P., BORDIN, G. M., NAKAMURA, R. M., DEHEER, D. H. and EDGINGTON, T. S.: Cancer Res 39 (1979), 2057—2061
3. HOWARD, D. R. and TAYLOR, C. R.: Cancer 43 (1979), 2279—2287
4. YU, G. S. M., KADISH, A. S., JOHNSON, A. B. and MARCUS, D. M.: Am. J. Clin. Pathol. 74 (1980), 453—457
5. SCHLOM, J., WUNDERLICH, D. and TERAMOTO, Y. A.: Proc. Natl. Acad. Sci. USA 77 (1980), 6841—6845
6. COLCHER, D., HORAN HAND, P., NUTI, M., and SCHLOM, J.: Proc. Natl. Acad. Sci. USA 78 (1981), 3199—3203

Acknowledgements

We wish to thank R. FITZGERALD, J. CROWLEY, D. POOLE, L. OTSBY, and C. CHRZAN for excellent assistance. This work was supported, in part, by a contract from the National Cancer Institute.

Cancer Research Unit, Department of Experimental Medicine, Trinity College and Saint Luke's Hospital, Dublin, Ireland

Polyamine Oxidation in Relation to Tumour Growth and Metastasis*

W. A. Boggust and S. O'Connell

Introduction

I.C.R.F.-159 (Razoxane), 5-fluorouracil and other drugs are reported (9, 16, 17, 20, 28) to inhibit secondary tumour formation in mice carrying the Lewis 3 LL carcinoma which normally metastasises fatally to the lungs. No mechanism for the protective action of these drugs has so far been accepted. I.C.R.F.-159 also has an antimetastatic affect in WHT/Ht mice (24) carrying the 'G' carcinoma which likewise produces multiple secondary nodules in the lungs.

We here extend earlier findings (3, 5, 11, 23, 31, 33) that I.C.R.F.-159, 5-FU and compounds including anti-depressants and amine oxidase inhibitors increase polyamine levels by blockade of enzyme which would otherwise degrade them in mammalian sera, HeLa cells and tissues including tumours.

We have confirmed the protective action of I.C.R.F.-159 in WHT/Ht mice inoculated with tumour (7) and now show that intraperitoneal injections of the polyamine growth regulators putrescine, spermidine and spermine have a pronounced antimetastatic effect in this system and also control the rate of primary tumour growth. We further show that the oxidation product obtained from putrescine with diamine oxidase is more effective when injected than unreacted putrescine and that changes in the numbers of tumour macrophages, a source of polyamine oxidase, in the tumour inoculum, affect the growth of tumours in mice receiving polyamines.

The proliferation of He-La cells was accelerated or retarded according to circumstances by changes in polyamine levels induced by direct addition of putrescine and spermidine, of amine oxidase or amine oxidase inhibitor (4). Growth is now shown to be increased at specific concentrations of putrescine oxidation product added to the cultures and also by critical numbers of mouse peritoneal macrophages.

Accordingly we propose a mechanism for the antimetastatic effect of I.C.R.F.-159 related to the role of polyamines as substrates for the amine oxidase activity of macrophages in a para-immunological response to tumour.

Experimental

Methods. The inbred albino WHT/Ht mice and the spontaneous syngeneic squamous 'G' carcinoma were supplied by Dr. H. Hewitt, King's College Hospital Medical School, London. This tumour metastasises consistently and fatally to the lungs and mediastinum. The procedures and

* Supported by The Medical Research Council of Ireland, Saint Luke's Cancer Research Fund and The Irish Tobacco Manufacturers' Advisory Committee.

tumour characteristics have been described (24). The tumour was maintained by subcutaneous passage at 14 day intervals and by storage at −75 °C. For use, intradermal inoculations of 1.5 × 10^5 viable cells in 0.02 ml of 0.25% carboxy-methyl cellulose in sterile saline, located in the right flank of 3 month female mice, gave rise to discoid tumours which were excised on the 12th day when 5 × 5 mm in diameter. Correct placing of the tumour inoculum was confirmed by histological examination of tumour section.

Test substances as sterile solutions or suspensions in CMC-saline or CMC-saline only as controls were injected intraperitoneally into mice each day from 4 hours before inoculation until excision of the tumours. The characteristics of primary tumour growth and mouse survival after tumour excision of untreated control tumour inoculated mice are presented in Table 1. The effects on primary tumour growth and survival of putrescine. 2 HCl, spermidine · 3 HCl, spermine · 4 HCl and ±1,2 bis (3:5 dioxopiperazin-1-yl) propane (I.C.R.F.-159; Razoxane, I.C.I.) supplied by Dr A. Creighton, Imperial Cancer Research Fund Laboratories, London (7) are shown in Figures 1, 2, 3 and 4.

Table 1.
Characteristics of 12-day primary intradermal tumour of tumour-inoculated WHT/Ht mice receiving daily i. p. injections of C.M.C.-saline

Number of mice	45
Number of viable tumour cells inoculated	150,00
Survival (days)	39.5 ± 4.0 (S.D.)
Weight of tumour (mg)	176.5 ± 49

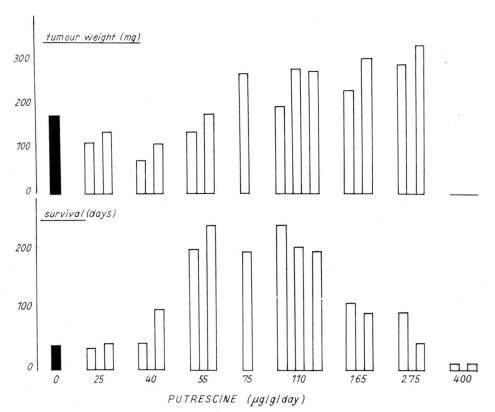

Fig.1. Survival and tumour weights of mice receiving putrescine.

72

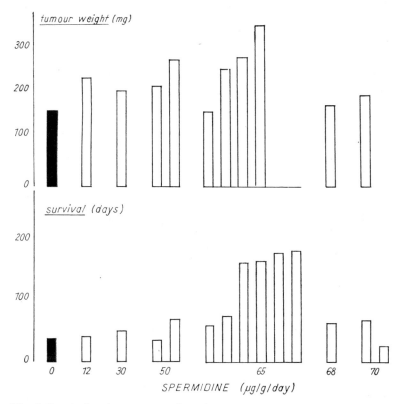

Fig. 2. Survival and tumour weights of mice receiving spermidine.

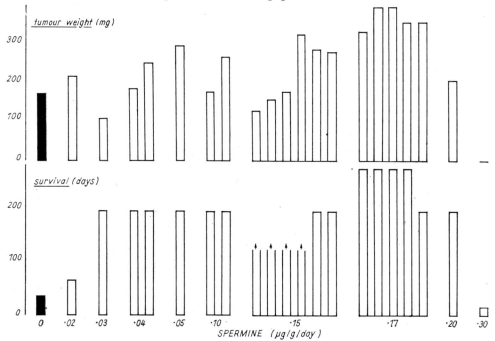

Fig. 3. Survival and tumour weights of mice receiving spermine.

Putrescine oxidation product for injection was prepared by incubating put · 2 HCl (33 mg) with hog kidney diamine oxidase (360 mg) in 3.6 ml Ringer's solution for 20 hours at 37 °C; the mixture was heated for 2 mins. at 100 °C to coagulate enzyme protein. The supernatant was sterilised by Millipore filtration and diluted in CMC-saline before injection to produce the concentrations stated. Mouse survival and primary tumour growth after inoculation with standard preparations of 150,000 viable tumour cells are shown in Figure 5.

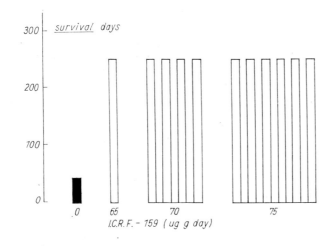

Fig. 4. Survival after tumour excision of mice receiving. I.C.R.F.—159.

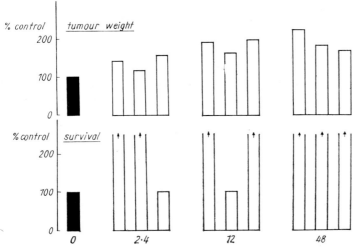

Fig. 5. Survival and tumour weights of mice receiving putrescine oxidation product.

Macrophage-depleted tumour cell suspensions were obtained by incubating standard preparations in glass bottles at 37 °C. After allowing 30 mins. for macrophage attachment, the tumour cells and remaining macrophages in the supernatant were again counted. Peritoneal macrophages obtained from tumour-bearing WHT/Ht mice by lavage with 5 ml portions of growth medium (34) containing 1% inactivated calf serum were counted and recombined in the numbers stated with macrophage-depleted suspensions containing 150,000 viable tumour cells for inoculation into mice. The effects on growth of primary tumours are shown in Figure 6.

For inhibition of amine oxidase activity by drugs, 20 µg portions of putrescine spermidine and spermine (as HCl salts) were incubated in Ringer's solution to make total volumes of 3 ml with human serum (1.5, 0.25 and 0.1 ml), with calf serum (1.0, 0.25 and 0.1 ml) and with hog kidney diamine oxidase (50, 100 and 140 µg) respectively. Test substances in Ringer's solution were added at the

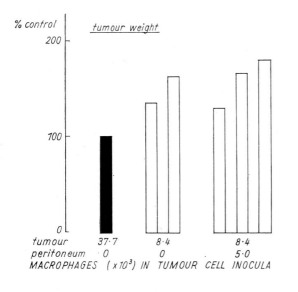

Fig. 6. Tumour weights of mice receiving spermine with standard and macrophage-depleted inoculations and with peritoneal macrophages.

Table 2.

Degradation of polyamines by human serum at 37 °C showing inhibition by drugs

Putrescine (μg) recovered after 20 hours

pargyline (μg/ml)	0	100	200
(n = 4)	8.7 ± 0.5 SD.	15.1 ± 0.4	19.1 ± 0.5
iproniazid (μg/ml)		100	200
(n = 4)		15.1 ± 0.5	17.9 ± 0.5
control, put. recovered at 0 hours.	20.2 ± 0.6	(n = 4)	

Spermidine (μg) recovered after 20 hours

paragyline (μg/ml)	0	30	100
(n = 4)	8.0 ± 0.5	16.0 ± 0.5	20.4 ± 0.4
iproniazid (μg/ml)		30	100
(n = 4)		13.1 ± 0.3	16.9 ± 0.4
control, spd. recovered at 0 hours.	20.1 ± 1.0	(n = 4)	

Spermine (μg) recovered after 20 hours

pargyline (μg/ml)	0	30	100
(n = 4)	5.7 ± 0.6	10.6 ± 0.8	16.6 ± 0.7
iproniazid (μg/ml)		30	100
(n = 4)		9.2 ± 0.9 (n = 3)	14.4 ± 0.4
control, spn. recovered at 0 hours.	19.2 ± 0.6	(n = 3)	

put., putrescine; spd., spermidine; spn., spermine; S.D., standard deviation

Table 3.
Degradation of polyamines by calf serum at 37 °C showing inhibition by drugs

Putrescine (µg) recovered after 20 hours

pargyline (µg/ml)	*0	30	100
(n = 5)	3.5 ± 0.3 SD.	6.7 ± 0.5	10.0 ± 0.5
iproniazid (µg/ml)	0	30	100
(n = 4)	7.7 ± 0.6	17.5 ± 0.5	20.6 ± 0.5
isoniazid (µg/ml)		30	100
(n = 4)		16.4 ± 0.7	20.1 ± 0.4
sodium azide (µg/ml)		50	150
(n = 4)		17.6 ± 0.6	19.5 ± 0.5
control, put. recovered at 0 hours.	19.7 ± 0.6	(n = 4)	

* Different specimen of serum assayed.

Spermidine (µg) recovered after 20 hours

pargyline (µg/ml)	0	20	50
(n = 4)	7.6 ± 0.7	11.4 ± 0.6	16.1 ± 0.8
iproniazid (µg/ml)		10	30
(n = 4)		9.6 ± 0.9	12.3 ± 0.4
isoniazid (µg/ml)		10	30
(n '4)		10.3 ± 0.3	12.7 ± 0.4
sodium azide (µg/ml)		50	150
(n = 4)		12.5 ± 0.3	14.1 ± 0.3
control, spd. recovered at 0 hours	20.7 ± 1.0	(n = 4)	

Spermine (µg) recovered after 20 hours

pargyline (µg/ml)	0	10	30
(n = 4)	2.1 ± 0.8	10.4 ± 0.6	18.6 ± 0.6
iproniazid (µg/ml)		10	30
(n = 3)		9.6 ± 0.8	19.9 ± 0.5
isoniazid (µg/ml)		10	30
(n = 4)		6.3 ± 0.9	12.4 ± 0.5 (n = 3)
sodium azide (µg/ml)		10	100
(n = 3)		5.5 ± 0.1	9.5 ± 0.9
control, spn. recovered at 0 hours.	22.0 ± 1.8	(n = 4)	

concentrations stated. After incubation for 20 hours at 37 °C, unreacted polyamine was assayed by ion-exchange and high voltage elektrophoresis (3). The results are shown in Tables 2, 3 and 4. HeLa cells were layer cultured as described (4) with a seeding rate of 10^4 cells per ml. Sterile solutions of test substances in Ringer's solution were added after seeding at the concentrations stated.

Table 4.

Degradation of polyamines by hog kidney diamine oxidase at 37 °C showing inhibiticn by drugs

Putrescine (µg) recovered after 20 hours

	0	50	100	200
I.C.R.F.-159 (µg/ml)	0	50	100	200
(n = 4)	9.2 ± 0.2 SD.	12.5 ± 0.8	15.8 ± 0.4	20.7 ± 0.3
5-FU (µg/ml)		50	100	200
(n = 5)		13.6 ± 0.6	16.4 ± 0.1	20.5 ± 0.6
doxorubicin (µg/ml)		0.5	2.0	5.0
(n = 4)		13.5 ± 0.7	16.4 ± 0.5	20.4 ± 0.4
pargyline (µg/ml)		50	—	200
(n = 4)		14.3 ± 0.9	—	20.0 ± 0.1
iproniazid (µg/ml)		50	—	200
(n = 4)		14.1 ± 0.2	—	20.1 ± 0.3
isoniazid (µg/ml)		50	100	200
(n = 4)		14.4 ± 0.6	16.2 ± 0.6	20.5 ± 0.9
control, put. recovered at 0 hours.		20.9 ± 0.5	(n = 5)	

Spermidine (µg) recovered after 20 hours

	0	50	200
pargyline (µg/ml)	0	50	200
(n = 4)	9.9 ± 0.3	13.7 ± 0.3	19.7 ± 0.1
iproniazid (µg/ml)		50	200
(n = 4)		13.4 ± 0.8	19.1 ± 0.5
control, spd. recovered at 0 hours	19.8 ± 0.4	(n = 4)	

Spermine (µg) recovered after 20 hours

	0	50	200
pargyline (µg/ml)	0	50	200
(n = 4)	8.1 ± 0.6	14.0 ± 0.4	18.8 ± 0.5
iproniazid (µg/ml)		50	200
(n = 4)		13.1 ± 1.0	17.7 ± 0.7
control, spn. recovered at 0 hours.	19.5 ± 0.8	(n = 4)	

Proliferation rates, defined as the factors by which cell counts increased during a 4-day period at 37 °C, are shown as mean values with standard deviations. The effects of polyamine, hog kidney diamine oxidase and iproniazid (4) are shown in Tables 5, 6 and 7.

Putrescine oxidation product for addition to HeLa cultures was prepared by incubating put · 2 HCl (183 µg) with hog kidney diamine oxidase (1.0 mg) in 2 ml Ringer's solution for 20 hours at 37 °C followed by coagulation at 100 °C, centrifugation and addition to cultures (table 8). Complete oxidation of putrescine to products was demonstrated by dansylation and TLC assay by the method of Seiler (30). Enzyme controls without putrescine had no effect on cultures.

Suspensions of peritoneal macrophages from normal WHT/Ht mice, prepared as above, were added to HeLa cultures in the presence of putrescine (0.05 µg/ml), together with the cell-free Millipore filtrate as controls. A typical result is shown in table 9.

Results

Untreated control mice with standard inoculations of 150,000 tumour cells produced primary tumours weighing 176.5 ± 49 mg when excised after 12 days' growth. Mice receiving solvent only survived for 39.5 ± 4 days after inoculation and on autopsy showed multiple metastatic nodules in the lungs. With putrescine injections over the range 40—275 µg/g/day, survival was increased, being indefinitely extended over 200 days in the optimum range between 55 and 110 µg/g/day so that experiments were terminated by decision. Primary tumour weights increased with dosage of putrescine and reached almost 200% of control value at the highest levels tolerated. With spermidine, survival was more critically related to concentration, being extended to 186 days at 65 µg/g/day. Tumour weights increased irregularly with rising spermidine levels to over 200% of control value at 65 µg/g/day. With spermine, the effective concentration range was from 0.02 to 0.2 µg/g/day. Primary tumour weights increased with increasing dosage of spermine to over 200% of control value at the highest levels tolerated. In the range 0.03 to 0.2 µg/g/day survival was recorded for 200 days or longer before experiments were terminated by decision.

Table 5.
Proliferation rate of HeLa cultures as % of control showing acceleratory and inhibitory effect of polyamines (putrescine 9 + spermidine 1) ($\pm$ S.D., n = 4, 6)

µg/ml medium

0	0.01	0.03	0.04	0.05	0.06	0.10	0.20
100	80 ± 3.3	99 ± 9.3	109 ± 3.2	122 ± 10.6	108 ± 4.6	87 ± 6.1	77 ± 2.8

Table 6.
Proliferation rate of HeLa cultures as % of control showing increase in cell counts induced by hog kidney diamine oxidase ($\pm$ S.D., n = 6)

µg/ml medium

0	2	5	10
100 ± 8.1	117 ± 20	128 ± 8.1	145 ± 7.1

Table 7.
Proliferation rate of HeLa cultures as % of control showing decrease in cell counts induced by iproniazid ($\pm$ S.D., n = 5)

µg/ml medium

0	0.2	0.8	2.0
100 ± 13.7	93 ± 14.7	88 ± 11.7	67 ± 14.7

At lower dosages of P.A., survival approximated to that of untreated control mice, while at higher levels, death from toxicity intervened. The maximum daily dose tolerated over a 12-day period (7) was highest with putrescine, intermediate with spermidine and lowest and most critical with spermine which is nephrotoxic (27). The most rapidly proliferating tumours were more haemorrhagic around the periphery than control tumours, especially with putrescine. With I.C.R.F.-159 (7), haemorrhage was absent and survival at $65-75$ µg/g/day was limited only by termination of the experiments.

Putrescine oxidation product was active at much lower concentrations than unchanged putrescine. Mice continued to be alive and well 100 days after tumour inoculation at levels of product corresponding to 2.4, 12 and 48 µg/g/day of original putrescine. Tumour weights exceeded 200% of control value at the highest levels administered.

Reduction of tumour macrophage numbers per 150×10^3 tumour cells inoculated from 37.7×10^3 to 8.4×10^3 increased tumour proliferation by over 50% relative to normal controls. Addition to inocula of 5×10^3 and 100×10^3 peritoneal macrophages from tumour-bearing WHT/Ht mice induced little further in increase tumour growth rate.

The results of drug inhibition of mammalian amine oxidase extend previous findings (3, 5, 23). Degradation of putrescine, spermidine and spermine by human serum was inhibited by pargyline and iproniazid and in calf serum by pargyline, iproniazid, isoniazid and sodium azide. Hog kidney diamine oxidase with putrescine substrate was inhibited by I.C.R.F.-159, 5-fluorouracil, doxorubicin, pargyline, iproniazid and isoniazid, and with spermidine and spermine substrates by pargyline and irponiazid.

Table 8.
Proliferation rate of HeLa cultures as % of control showing acceleratory effect of putrescine — hog kidney diamine oxidase product ($\pm$ S.D., n = 5)

µg/ml medium

0	0.001	0.002	0.003	0.004	0.005	0.010	0.030
100	105 ± 6.9	111 ± 7.0	134 ± 10.9	123 ± 17.7	100 ± 7.4	94 ± 32	102 ± 10.8

Table 9.
Proliferation rate of HeLa cultures as % of control showing increased cell counts with and without putrescine in presence of added normal mouse peritoneal macrophages and macrophage-free lavage fluid.

macrophages per ml medium ($\times 10^3$)

	0	1.2	2.4	3.6	6.0	12.0
with putrescine	100	155	217	214	80	53
without put.	100	104	157	161	73	37
equivalent lavage fluid with putrescine	100	68	75	135	87	64

He-La proliferation was progressively inhibited by increasing levels of polyamines except over a critical range about 0.05 µg/ml when growth was increased up to 134% of control value. With hog kidney diamine oxidase, proliferation increased to over 150% of control at 10 µg/ml. With the amine oxidase inhibitor iproniazid, proliferation was reduced to approximately 50% of control at 2.0 µg/ml. Putrescine oxidation product was more active than unchanged putrescine and enhanced proliferation at concentrations from 0 to 0.03 µg/ml. Marked acceleration of growth was repeatedly demonstrated at 0.03 µg/ml of unchanged putrescine.

Normal mouse peritoneal macrophages increased HeLa cell proliferation markedly in the presence of added putrescine. Maximum increase was always at about 3.0×10^3 macrophages per ml medium above which higher concentrations reduced proliferation. Washed macrophages produced a lesser increase whereas equivalent amounts of Millipore-filtered macrophages produced a lesser increase whereas equivalent amounts of Millipore-filtered macrophage-free fluid, though positive, were much less active. This suggested that macrophages were a source of diffusible polyamine oxidase activity responsible for the release of products from putrescine or other polyamines which regulate proliferation.

Discussion

As I.C.R.F.-159, 5-FU and other drugs increase polyamine concentrations relative to normal by blockade of amine oxidase activity in serum and tissues including tumours (3, 5, 11, 23, 31), the antimetastatic effects of I.C.R.F.-159 and 5-FU in 3LL and WHT/Ht tumour-bearing mice may be attributable to this rise in polyamine levels. This interpretation is supported by the demonstration of increased mouse survival in the presence of injected putrescine, spermidine and spermine.

Similarly, just as critical levels of these drugs increased HeLa cell proliferation (6) the relationship between increased primary tumour growth and reduced metastasis in tumour-inoculated mice injected with polyamines and increased proliferation of HeLa cultures with added polyamines correspond to and confirm the growth-promoting and growth-retarding properties of polyamines in vivo and in vitro (8, 13, 15, 21) which also are related to polyamine concentration and cell numbers (25). The existence of limiting concentrations above which polyamines do not promote increased cell proliferation but demonstrate chalone-like cytostatic or cytotoxic properties in the presence of serum amine oxidase is in agreement with several findings (1, 2, 10, 18, 19, 32) and also with reports (14, 29) that in some cases, anticipated cytotoxicity, lymphocyte transformation or inhibition of cell proliferation by polyamines was not observed.

Although the growth-inhibitory properties of polyamines are generally attributed to the release by amine oxidase of compounds which are toxic above certain concentration levels, the evidence that polyamines increase proliferation in mouse tumours and in fibroblasts and HeLa cells below critical concentrations and our finding that the product of oxidative deamination is more active both in vivo and in vitro than the precursor polyamine, support the view that an unidentified polyamine metabolite enhances cell proliferation at very low concentrations. Possibly growth acceleration and inhibition shown by polyamines form opposing phases of a homeostatic control system.

The enhancement of proliferation in HeLa cultures by mouse peritoneal macrophages resembles the effects of amine oxidase from kidney and serum described above. As we have confirmed the presence of a diffusible amine oxidase in peritoneal macrophages from normal and tumour-bearing WHT/Ht mice corresponding to the activity previously reported (22), we propose that oxidation products released from intrinsic and added polyamine are responsible for the effects observed in cultures.

As polyamine oxidase activity has not been found in serum of WHT/Ht mice, the tumour growth-promoting effects of injected polyamines are attributed to the release of oxidation products by the amino oxidase of macrophages which form a significant proportion of total tumour cells. The observation that a reduction in the number of macrophages in the tumour cell inoculum induces increased tumour proliferation with injected spermine confirms the existence of a macrophage-polyamine interaction. Conventionally, this change in growth equilibrium may be due to a reduction in the level of cytotoxic polyamine products in the tumour cell environment, or alternatively, to a change in the metabolic activity of the cell inoculum arising from pre-treatment before injection. The inefficacy of peritoneal macrophages added to the inoculum, but not to HeLa cultures, may be similarly interpreted.

Promotion of primary tumour growth in mice by polyamines and suppression of metastasis resemble the effects of mild immunological stimulation (26) whereby small numbers of immunologically active cells accelerated growth but larger numbers were inhibitory. The killing of tumour cells by macrophages has been shown (12) to involve independent stages of immunologically specific tumour recognition and associated but non-specific lethal action. It is now proposed that the character of the second para-immunological phase may be dependent on the concentration and identity of polyamine metabolites released by macrophage amine oxidase activity.

Depending on macrophage location, a concentration gradient around the tumour periphery could be low inside and favourable to cell proliferation but high outside and toxic to metastasising cells about to leave the tumour. Alternatively a high level of macrophage amine oxidase activity might be toxic for all tumour cells.

Summary

1. In WHT/Ht mice inoculated syngeneic primary tumour growth is increased and metastatic secondary tumour formation decreased by intraperitoneal injections of putrescine, spermidine and spermine.
2. The growth of He-La cells is regulated by changes in polyamine levels induced by
    a) direct addition of P.A. which inhibit growth except at low concentrations which increase proliferation.
    b) amine oxidase in serum and tissues which enhance proliferation.
    c) inhibitors of amine oxidase which inhibit proliferation.
3. The inhibition of metastasis by I.C.R.F.-159 and 5-FU is attributed to increased P.A. levels following inhibition of amine oxidases in serum and tissues including tumours.
4. Various drugs used in clinical practice which inhibiti amine oxidase may indirectly affect the growth and metastasis of tumours.
5. Increased He-La growth with diamine oxidase may be due either to removal of inhibitory P.A. or release of an acceleratory product. Increased proliferation was obtained by addition of preformed putrescine oxidation product at low concentrations.
6. In mice primary tumours were increased and metastatic secondaries were inhibited by injection of preformed putrescine oxidation product.
7. Macrophages release amine oxidase activity capable of reacting with P.A.
8. Macrophages added to He-La cultures containing P.A. increase and decrease cell proliferation according to their numbers.
9. Inoculated primary tumour growth rate and metastasis are regulated by changes in the macrophage content of the tumour cell inoculum.
10. Para-immunological events concerning promotion and retardation of tumour growth and metastasis may be interpreted in terms of macrophage numbers and P.A. concentration.

Acknowledgement

We thank Professor M. O'HALLORAN, Medical Director, Saint Luke's Hospital, Dublin and Mr. P. WILSON, Manager, Wellcome Research Animal Laboratories, Trinity College, Dublin, for facilities.

References

1. ALARCON, R.: Arch. Biochem. Biophys. *137* (1970), 365—372
2. ALLEN, J. C., SMITH, C. J. and CUNY, M. C.: Nature *267* (1977), 623—625
3. BOGGUST, W. A.: In: Characterisation and Treatment of Human tumours, pp. 106—112. Editors: Davis and Harrap, Excerpta Medica, Amsterdam, 1978
4. BOGGUST, W. A.: I.R.C.S. Med. Sci. *8* (1980), 600—601
5. BOGGUST, W. A., MORIARTY, M. and O'CONNELL, S.: Irish J. Med. Sci *148* (1979), 210—222
6. BOGGUST, W. A. and O'CONNELL, S.: In: Human Cancer, its Characterisation and Treatment, pp. 374—386. Editors: Davis, Harrap and Stathopoulos, Excerpta Medica, Amsterdam, 1980
7. BOGGUST, W. A., O'CONNELL, S., CARROLL, R. and WILSON, P.: I.R.S.C. Med. Sci. *8* (1980), 597—598
8. BOYLAND, E.: Biochem. J. *35* (1941), 1283—1288
8. BURRAGE, K., HELLMANN, K. and SALSBURY, A. J.: Brit. J. Pharmacol. *39* (1970), 205—206
10. BYRD, W. J., JACOBS, D. M. and AMOSS, M. S.: Nature *267* (1977) 621—623
11. CALDARA, C. M., BARBIROLI, B. and MORUZZI, G.: Biochem. J. *97* (1965), 84
12. EVANS, E. and ALEXANDER, P.: Nature *236* (1972), 168—170
13. FLEMING, D. E. and FOSHAY, L.: Bacteriol. Proc. (Soc. Am. Bacteriol) Abstr. M141 *106* (1957)
14. GAUGAS, J. M.: In: Polyamines in Biomedical Research, pp. 343—362. Editor: GAUGAS, John Wiley & Sons, New York, 1980
15. HAM, R. G.: Biochem. Biophys. Res. Commun. *14* (1964), 35—38
16. HELLMANN, K. and BURRAGE, K.: Nature *224* (1969), 273—275
17. HELLMANN, K. et al.: In: Chemotherapy of Cancer Dissemination and Metastasis, pp. 355—359 Editors: GARATTINI and FRANCHI, Raven Press, New York, 1973
18. HIRSCH, J. C.: J. Exp. Med. *97* (1953), 323—325; 327—344
19. HIRSCH, J. C. and DUBOS, R. J.: J. Exp. Med. *95* (1952), 191—208
20. LE SERVE, A. W. and HELLMANN, K.: Brit. Med. J. *1* (1972), 597—601
21. MIYAKI, K. et al: Chem. Pharm. Bull. *8* (1960), 933
22. MORGAN, D. M. L., FERULGA, J. and ALLISON, A. C.: In: Polyamines in Biomedical Research, pp. 303—308. Editor: GAUGAS, Wiley & Sons, New York, 1980
23. O'CONNELL, S.: Changes in polyamine levels and their relevance to tumours. M. Sc. Thesis, University of Dublin, 1980
24. PETERS, L. J.: Brit. J. Cancer *32* (1975), 355—365
25. POHJANPELTO, P. and RAINA, A.: Nature New Biology *235* (1972), 247—249
26. PREHN, R. T.: Science *176* (1972), 170—171
27. ROSENTHAL, S. M., FISHER, E. R. and STOHLMAN, E. F.: Proc. Soc. Exp. Biol. N.Y. *80* (1952), 432—434
28. SALSBURY, A. J., BURRAGE, K. and HELLMANN, K.: Brit. Med. J. *4* (1970), 344—346
29. SCHAUENSTEIN, E., ESTERBAUER, H. and ZOLLNER, H.: Aldehydes in Biological Systems. Pion, London, 1977
30. SEILER, N.: Methods in Biochemical Analysis *18* (1970), 259—337
31. SEILER, N. and RICHENTOPF, B.: Biochem. J. *152* (1975), 201—210
32. TABOR, C. W., TABOR, H. and BACHRACH, U.: J. biol. Chem. *239* (1964), 2194—2203
33. TAYLOR, J. D., WYKES, A. A., GLADISH, Y. C. and MARTIN, W. B.: Nature *187* (1960), 941 — 942
34. TOLNAI, S.: Tissue Culture Association Manual *1* (1975), 17—19

Institute of Pathology, University of Oslo, Rikshospitalet, Oslo 1, Norway

Partial Purification of an Epidermal Growth Inhibitor (Chalone)

K. Elgjo, G. Isaksson-Forsén, K. Reichelt and O. P. F. Clausen

A large number of factors can influence the rate of cell proliferation in different cell populations. The majority of such factors has, however, been tested only in vitro, and we know little or nothing about their physiological role in an organism. Most of the factors that have been studied have a stimulating effect on cell proliferation in vitro. In vivo, the situation seems to be the opposite. The data we have indicate that cell populations, or organs, that are integrated in a living organism regulate their rate of cell renewal according to a negative feedback principle. Thus, the communication between maturing cell and the proliferating cells in a tissue seems to be mediated by certain endogeneous substances that act as inhibitors of cell division. Such endogeneous, tissue-specific inhibitors have been named chalones.

It has been difficult to purify and characterize biochemically such endogenous inhibitors and thus prove their existence. The first part of this lecture reports some limited success we have had in purifying one such inhibitor. The second part presents some findings that demonstrate why it is so difficult to purify and test such substances.

Previous work has shown that there are at least two different growth regulators in normal epidermis (Elgjo 1973, Natl. Inst. Monogr. *38*, 71—76). They have different biochemical properties and act at different phases of the cell cycle. One of them was first shown to act on epidermal cells in the G2 phase and is called the epidermal G2 inhibitor, or G2 chalone. The other was first shown to act on cell in the late part of the G1 phase and is called the epidermal G1 inhibitor, or G1 chalone. We have concentrated our work on the epidermal G2 inhibitor.

In our purification experiments we have tested the various batches for G2 inhibitory activity in vivo, using hairless mouse epidermis as the assay organ. We stick to a rigid test system for reasons that will become clear shortly. We have used water extracts of hairless mouse epidermis or cod fish epidermis as starting material. First, we used ordinary Sephadex chromatography and ultrafiltration and found that the epidermal G2 inhibitor seemed to be a peptide with a molecular weight of less than 10,000 Daltons. Extracts from other organs and tissues were used as controls (Isaksson-Forsén et al, 1981, Cell Biol. Intern. Rep. *5*, 195—199). We then modified the purification procedures and used reverse phase high pressure liquid chromatography. This technique has given us a very high degreee of purification so that a dose of only several nanograms will inhibit significantly the mitotic rate in hairless mouse epidermis. The active substance is, however, still not completely pure. It is a small peptide but we don't know the exact molecular weight. It is a difficult stuff to work with because it sticks to the surface of the glass or plastic vials when in solution.

For some years we thought that the G2 inhibitor acted only or mainly on epidermal G2 cells, and the G1 inhibitor only or mainly on epidermal G1 cells. Quite recently the situation has become much more complex. We have been able to show that crude epidermis extracts act on cells in several phases of the cell cycle. Furthermore, the effect of an extract depends strongly on the time of the day when it is given (ELGJO et al 1981, Cell Tissue Kinet. *4*, 21—29). These experiments were made by combining several cell kinetics methods, like pulse label autoradiography, double labelling autoradiography, the Colcemid technique, and flow cytometry combined with cell sorting.

Hairless mouse epidermis has a pronounced circadian rhythm (CLAUSEN et al 1979, Cell Tissue Kinet. *12*, 319—337). The influx to the S phase shows only minor variations over a 24-hour period, but the efflux from S, the mitotic rate, and the phase durations exhibit wide circadian variations. This circadian pattern determines the effect of a single injection of skin extract. In accordance with the almost constant influx to S, the effect of a single injection of extract is about the same whatever time is chosen for injection. After a period of inhibition there is an overshoot at 8—11 hr after the treatment. The situation is different for the other parameters. Thus, the mitotic rate is only moderately inhibited when the extract is given in the morning when the mitotic rate is high, whereas the inhibition is much stronger in the evening when the rate is slow — when the brake already is on, so to speak. The same applies to the efflux from S. When the extract is given at a time of the day when the efflux is decreasing and low, the inhibition is very pronounced but is followed by an overshoot. If the extract is given when the efflux is increasing, the inhibition is less pronounced the first 7 hr, but it lasts several hours longer.

These results have demonstrated a couple of points. First, a single injection of skin extract inhibits epidermal cells at several phase transitions. We do not know if this is accomplished by the two known inhibitors or if there are more than two. Second, the results of a single injection of extract depend critically on the time of the day when it is administered, due to the circadian rhythm that is present in most organs. Third, purification and testing of endogenous inhibitors are complicate not only because of their biochemistry but because of the difficulties in testing them. Lastly, the fact that the effect of the inhibitors is dependent on the circadian rhythm strongly indicates that several factors act together to achieve the final results, which is a balanced rate of cell renewal.

84

Hormonal Receptors

Central Institute for Cancer Research,
Academy of Sciences of German Democratic Republic, Berlin

Estradiol Receptor in Human Breast Cancers and Prognosis

E. Heise and M. Görlich

There is no doubt that the determination of the estradiol receptor (ER) activity in the cytoplasm of human breast cancers can be used successfully to predict the hormone responsiveness of these cancers (1). This clinical experience has led a number of investigators to look for further correlations between ER activity in breast cancers and other clinical or paraclinical parameters of the patient, or the tumour which are known to characterize the course of the disease. Studies by Heuson (2), Elston (3), Cooke (4) and others all showed that there was a better prognosis for ER-positive cancers compared with those that were ER-negative. This paper deals with investigations of correlations between the ER status of the breast cancer in pre- and postmenopausal patients and some clinical parameters which are known to define the prognosis of the disease.

Materials and methods

ER determinations were performed in breast cancers and metastatic axillary lymph nodes of more than 350 pre- and postmenopausal patients, who were operated at the Robert-Rössle-Institute in Berlin-Buch during the last 5 years. In a few cases, ER determinations were also performed in distant metastases and recurrent tumours. The ER determination in the tumour specimen was done following the recommendations of the E.O.R.T.C. Breast Cancer Group (5) using dextran-coated charcoal for separating free and proteinbound hormone. In summary: tissue to be investigated was either worked up immediately or stored in frozen condition at $-70\ °C$ for not longer than 2 weeks. The homogenization was performed using 0.01 M TRIS-buffer, pH 7.4 in a porcelain mortar, cooled with liquid nitrogen. After thawing, the homogenate was centrifuged at 20000 g for 1 hr. Thereafter, the cytosol obtained was incubated with ^{3}H-labelled estradiol to give a final concentration of 10^{-9} molar, at $0\ °C$ for 18 hrs, in the presence or absence of cold estradiol or nafoxidin in 1000-fold excess, to compete for ER-binding sites and, therefore, to differentiate between specific and unspecific binding. For separation of free and protein-bound hormone, a suspension of dextran-coated charcoal (0.5% Norit A, 0.05% dextran T and 0.1% gelatine in homogenization buffer) was added to the cytosol in a ratio 1:1. The mixture was allowed to stand for 30 min interrupted by two 15 sec intervals of shaking and thereafter centrifuged for 15 min. The bound radioactivity was measured by liquid scintillation counting. The receptor activity was expressed as femtomoles estradiol bound per mg cytosol protein after subtraction of the unspecific binding. Estradiol binding higher than 10 femtomoles was classified as ER-positive and binding less than 3 femtomoles as ER-negative. Binding activities between 3 and 10 femtomoles were classified as ER-positive if there was also a significant inhibition of the estradiol uptake by nafoxidin. The significance was calculated according to the Student's t-test. Protein was determined by the method of Lowry (6).

Results and Discussion

Fig. 1 shows the ER status of breast cancers related to the menopausal status of the patients. The patients were grouped into three categories: 1. premenopausal patients, 2. patients within 5 years of the last menstruation, 3. patients with more than 5 years after the last menstruation. This classification seems to be important, because the success of a hormone therapy generally, and the kind of hormone therapy which should be used in the special case, depend largely on the menopausal status of the patient being treated. Clinical experience has shown that patients within 5 years of menopause respond very poorly to hormone-therapy and therefore it seemed to be

Fig. 1.

Patients investigated: 379

Menopausal status	Patients	ER+	%	ER−	%
premenopausal	164	59	36.0	105	64.0
postmenopausal within 5 years	47	25	53.0	22	46.8
postmenopausal more than 5 years	168	80	47.6	88	53.4

ER status and menopausal status of the patients

justified to separate this group of patients from the two others. The results obtained show a lower percentage of ER-positive cancers among premenopausal patients than among postmenopausal patients, which is in agreement with the findings of other authors (7, 8). On the other hand, the percentage of ER-positive breast cancers in patients within 5 years of last menstruation was unexpectedly high despite the already-mentioned clinical experience of the relatively low hormone sensitivity of breast cancers in these patients. Moreover the average ER concentration was found to be significantly higher in postmenopausal than in premenopausal patients (data not shown). It is well known that the course of the disease is decisively defined by the stage of the disease at the time of clinical detection. Therefore it seemed useful to look at the ER status in breast cancers in relation to the stage of the disease. The results obtained are shown in Fig. 2. The stage classification followed the recommendations of UICC (9). It can be seen that there is a gradual decrease of the percentage of ER-positive cancers from stage II to IV and a corresponding increase of the percentage of ER-negative cancers. Whereas the distribution of ER-positive and ER-negative cancers is nearly

Fig. 2.

Patients investigated: 347

Clinical stage	Patients	ER+	%	ER−	%
I	23	9	39.1	14	60.9
II	95	52	54.7	43	45.3
III	192	77	40.1	115	59.9
IV	35	8	22.9	27	77.1

ER status and clinical stage of the disease

equal in stage II, the probability of finding a ER-negative cancer in stage IV is more than three times that of finding a ER-positive cancer. The ER status of stage I patients, however, differs remarkably from this generalization. Despite the well-known favourable prognosis of these patients, their ER status resembled that of stage III patients, who from clinical experience have a worse prognosis. Because the distribution of pre- and postmenopausal patients in stage I did not differ from that found in the other stage groups, the reason for this unexpected behaviour cannot be explained by an altered menopausal status in the stage I group. Neither did the mean age of the stage I patients differ significantly from that found in the other groups.

Besides the clinical stage of the disease, nodal involvement is also known to be an important parameter in defining the prognosis of breast cancers. If there is a correlation between ER status and prognosis, one would expect a lower incidence of ER-positive primary tumours with metastatic axillary lymph nodes than in cancers without nodal involvement. By clinical experience, a nodal involvement of more than 7 metastatic lymph nodes has an especially unfavourable prognosis, whereas breast cancers with no metastatic lymph nodes or with an involvement of less than 7 positive lymph nodes are known to have a relatively good prognosis.

The results found from comparing ER status and nodal involvement are shown in Fig. 3. The patients were grouped into three categories according to the nodal involvement and the ER status of the primary tumours registered. It can be seen that the percentage of ER-negative tumours is higher in the group of patients with the highest nodal involvement although no difference of ER status could be detected in the other two groups.

Fig. 3.
Patients investigated: 346

Nodal involvement	Patients	ER+	%	ER−	%
No nodal involvement	82	40	48.8	42	51.2
Less than 7 metastatic lymph nodes	146	74	50.7	72	49.2
More than 7 metastatic lymph nodes	118	41	34.7	77	65.3

ER status and nodal involvement

Prognosis is generally characterized by the duration of the period (free interval) between the removal of the primary tumour and the metastatic axillary lymph nodes and the appearance of recurrences, and also detection of the cancer and death of the patient, independently of the kind of therapy used. If ER status is a suitable marker for evaluating prognosis, one would expect a close correlation between these parameters and ER status. From Fig. 4, it can be seen that the average free interval for patients with ER-positive breast cancers is significantly longer than that for patients with ER-negative primary tumours. Because a few patients received adjuvant chemo- and/or hormone-therapy after removal of the primary tumour the influence of this therapy on the free intervall in relation to the ER status was also investigated. Adjuvant therapy unexpectedly and dramatically decreased the free interval for patients with ER-positive primary tumours, but it was not changed for patients with ER-negative cancers, which eliminated any significant difference between ER-positive and ER-negative cancers for the whole group. On the other hand there was a statis-

Fig. 4.

Patients investigated: 93

ER status	Patients	Free interval (months) $M \pm S_D$	Significance
ER+	35	23.2 ± 12.2	$P < 0.05$
ER−	58	17.2 ± 14.7	
With adjuvant therapy			
ER+	7	13.1 ± 5.4	NS
ER−	17	18.9 ± 19.4	
Without adjuvant therapy			
ER+	28	25.7 ± 12.2	$P < 0.01$
ER−	41	16.5 ± 12.2	

ER status and free interval

Fig. 5.

Patients investigated: 93

ER status	Patients	Survival time (months) $M \pm S_D$	Significance
ER+	28	40.1 ± 25.3	$P < 0.001$
ER−	65	22.2 ± 13.8	
With adjuvant therapy			
ER+	9	36.3 ± 36.5	NS
ER−	20	18.9 ± 12.3	
Without adjuvant therapy			
ER+	19	41.9 ± 18.9	$P < 0.001$
ER−	45	23.7 ± 14.3	

ER status and survival time

Fig. 6.

Patients investigated: 195 = 100%

ER status Primary tumour	ER status Lymph node	Patients	%
+	+	90	46.2
−	−	67	34.4
+	−	14	7.2
−	+	24	12.3

ER status in primary tumours and
metastatic lymph nodes

tically significant difference between the free interval for patients with ER-positive and ER-negative cancers, who did not receive any adjuvant therapy. Although these results might be of great interest in evaluating the role of adjuvant therapy for patients with ER-positive breast cancers, it is too early to draw any conclusion, because of the small number of patients investigated.

Similar results were obtained from comparing survival time and ER status (Fig. 5). The survival time of patients with ER-positive cancers was significantly longer than that of patients with ER-negative cancers, but here again, survival was reduced for patients with ER-positive breast cancers who received adjuvant chemo- and/or hormone-therapy; in the group of patients with ER-negative cancers, a slight decrease of the survival time was also observed. However, the difference of the survival time between the two groups was not significant. Among patients, who did not receive adjuvant therapy, those with ER-positive cancers showed a significantly longer survival time than those with ER-negative cancers.

Of great interest for therapy planning, is the comparability of the ER status of the primary tumour with the ER status in metastatic lymph nodes or in distant metastases and recurrent tumour which appeared months or years later. Generally, the ER status of primary tumours and of metastatic lymph nodes determined at the same time have been found to be comparable by several authors (10). The results abtained in the present study (Fig. 6) confirmed this. More important, however, seems to be a comparison of ER status of the primary tumour with that of distant metastases and recurrent tumours which appeared later. Because it is rather difficult to obtain sufficient biological material from distant metastases or recurrent tumours, the number of cases

Fig. 7

Patient	ER status Primary tumour	ER status Metastasis	Time interval (months)
I. O.	−	−	2
D. B.	+	+	14
J. W.	+	+	46
A. K.	−	−	13
G. G.	−	−	13
E. H.	−	−	5
E. S.	−	−	7
E. W.	−	−	30
E. B.	−	−	12
U. C.	−	−	12
Y. F.	−	−	12
Y. W.	−	+	62
G. Z.	−	−	32
E. P.	−	+	6
G. H.	−	−	68
G. B.	+	+	36
E. B.	+	+	32

Total: 17 cases
Agreement: 15/17
Disagreement: 2/17
ER status in primary tumours and metastases

investigated is so far very small as yet (Fig. 7); nevertheless, a very high degree of conformity of the ER status between primary tumours and metastases was found (88%). However, the percentage of ER-positive cancers in this group was remarkably low (4 out of 17 cases), and cannot be explained, unless the well-known high degree of ER-negativity in breast cancers with a bad prognosis plays a role in this phenomenon.

Summary

The estradiol receptor (ER) status and the ER concentration in human breast cancers were investigated in relation to the prognosis of the disease. The percentage of ER-positive breast cancers was found to be higher in postmenopausal than in premenopausal patients. Except for stage I, there was a gradual increase in the percentage of ER-negative cancers from stage II to stage IV of the disease. The existence of metastatic axillary lymph nodes lowers the probability of finding an ER-positive primary tumour. The free interval and survival time were found to be longer in ER-positive than in ER-negative cancers. The ER status of primary tumours and of metastatic axillary lymph nodes determined at the same time as the tumour specimen were very comparable as was the comparison of the ER status of primary tumours and distant metastases, which appeared several months after removal of the primary tumour.

References

1. Steroid Receptors and the Management of Cancer. Eds. E. B. THOMPSON and M. E. LIPPMANN CRC Press, Inc., Boca Ratou, Florida, 1979
2. HEUSON, I. C., LECLERQ, G., LONGEVAL, E., DEBOEL, M. C., MATTHEIEM, W. H. and HEIMANN, R.: Estrogen Receptors: Prognostic Significance in Breast Cancer. In: Estrogen Receptors in Human Breast Cancer. Eds: McGuire, W. L., CARBONE, P. P., VOLLMER, E. P. New York, Raven Press, 1975, pp. 57—72
3. ELSTON, C. W., JOHNSON, J., BISHOP, H. H., MAYNARD, P. V., HAYBITTLE, J. L., GRIFFITHS, K. and BLAMEY, R. W.: Oestradiol Receptor in Primary Breast Cancer: Correlation with Histological Grade. Reported on: Second Breast Cancer Working Conference of E.O.R.T.C. Breast Cancer Cooperative Group, Copenhagen, 1979
4. COOKE, T., MAYNARD, P., GEORGE, D., GRIFFITHS, K. and SHIELDS, R.: Oestrogen Receptors: A Guide to Prognosis in Early Breast Cancer. Reported on: Second Breast Cancer Working Conference of E.O.R.T.C. Breast Cancer Cooperative Group, Copenhagen, 1979
5. E.O.R.T.C. Breast Cancer Cooperative Group: Standards for the Assessment of Oestrogen Receptors in Human Breast Cancer. Europ. J. Cancer 9 (1973), 379—381
6. LOWRY, G. H., ROSEBROUGH, N., FARR, A. L. and RANDALL, R. J.: Protein Measurement with Folin Phenol Reagent. J. Biol. Chem. 193 (1951), 265—270
7. MARTIN, P. M., ROLLAND, P. H., JACQUEMIER, J., ROLLAND, A. M. and TOGA, M.: Multiple Steroid Receptors in Human Breast Cancer. Cancer Chemother. Pharamcol. 2 (1979), 107—113
8. SINGHAKOWINTA, A., POTTER, H. G., BURCKER, T. R., SAMEL, B., BROOKES, S. C. and VAITKEVICIUS, V. K.: Estrogen Receptor and Natural Course of Breast Cancer Surgery. 183 (1976), 84—88
9. TNM-Klassifizierung der malignen Tumoren und allgemeine Regeln zur Anwendung des TNM-Systems Berlin, Heidelberg, New York, Springer-Verlag 1976, S. 51—55
10. HOEHN, J. L., PLOTKA, E. D. and DICKSON, K. B.: Comparison of Estrogen Receptor Levels in Primary and Regional Metastatic Carcinoma of the Breast Ann. Surg. 190 (1979), 69—71

* Istituto di Radiologia — Universita, Ferrara,
and
** Istituto di Ricerche Biomediche 'A. Marxer' RBM, Ivrea, Italy

External Quality Assessment Scheme of Estradiol Receptor Assay: An Italian Survey

A. Piffanelli*, S. Fumero**, D. Pelizzola,* G. Giovannini* and L. Ricci*

Introduction

Quality of performance in pathology laboratories has been discussed by a W.H.O. working group (9).

External quality assessment schemes have been largely accepted as a valuable aid to self-improvement and continuing education, but it has been emphasized that governements have a prime responsibility for obtaining not only a retrospective evaluation of interlaboratory comparability but also an actual control, professionally established (7).

In the field of steroid receptors in breast cancer experience of external quality schemes has been successfully accumulated through a few medical research laboratories. It was time to extend external quality assessment to laboratories in Italy directly involved in the clinical use of steroid receptor assays. The main objective of the quality control programme was to evaluate the methods applied by laboratories that determine estradiol receptor in tumours, in order to achieve both standardized methods and, consequently, more reliable and comparable data.

The programme was based on assays of lyophilized animal uterus cytosol. Estradiol receptor in these preparations proved stable in time (4) (6).

The use of lyophilized supernatant, permits identification of variations due to the final steps of the ER determination method. Future phases of the programme will deal with the homogenization and centrifugation steps.

Since no reference samples of known content are available, a series of lyophilized cytosols were prepared at scalar receptor concentrations in order to cull as much information as possible about the intra- and interlaboratory variability.

Preparation of the lyophilized calf uterus cytosols

The uterus of a young calf was homogenized with phosphate buffer, pH 7.4, 5 mM, containing 0.15 g/l of dithioerythrol, for 30 sec at 4 °C. The homogenate was centrifuged at 28,000 g for 1 h at 0—4 °C. The calf uterus surnatant was diluted 1:2 (Preparation no. 4) with a pool of female human serum diluted 30-fold with physiologic solution. The calf uterus surnatant was further diluted 1:2, 1:4, and 1:8 with the same diluted serum. This diluted serum was also used as negative cytosol (preparation no. 8). 1 ml of each preparation was placed in a lyophilizing vial and lyophilized overnight. The vials were vacuum sealed. The lyophilized samples, stored at 4 °C, were dispatched by normal mail to the collaborating laboratories. Each dispatch was accom-

Table 1.
Features of methods used by laboratories participating in the Italian Quality Control programme (1980).

Laboratory	Date of determ.	Protein assay method	Protein standard	Range $^3H\text{-}E_2$ conc.	Ci/mmole Specific activity of $^3H\text{-}E_2$	DES concent. nM	Dextran percentage in final incubation	Charcoal percentage in final incubation	DCC Contact time	Incubation time/temp.
A	9. 7. 80	Lowry	BSA	1.8 Sc 4.62 S	115	360	0.14	0.0014	10'	18^h —4 °C
B	17. 2. 81	Bio Rad	5% HSA— 3% IgG	0.15—2.3	100	230	0.31	0.031	10'	18^h —4 °C
C	31. 7. 80	Bio Rad	BSA	0.13—4.17	110	834	0.28	0.028	10'	16^h —4 °C
D	29. 8. 80	Bio Rad	KABI	0.13—4.17	101	834	0.31	0.031	15'	16^h —4 °C
E	17. 7. 80	Bio Rad	BSA	n. r.—4.17	108	4170	0.28	0.028	30'	16^h —4 °C
F	14. 7. 80	Bio Rad	BSA	n.r.—3.33	101	666	0.25	0.025	10'	16^h —4 °C
G	15. 7. 80	Lowry	HSA	0.06—0.4	91	40	0.25	0.025	30'	2^h —15 °C
H	9. 9. 80	Bio Rad	BSA	0.09—5.0	85	2500	0.25	0.025	15'	18^h —4 °C
I	29. 9. 80	Lowry	BSA	0.62—20	91	2000	0.5	0.05	10.	18^h —4 °C
L	9. 80	Lowry	BSA	0.065—4.16	91	830	0.31	0.031	10'	18^h —4 °C
M	19. 5. 81	Bio Rad	BSA	0.06—4.17	112	800	0.62	0.031	15'	18^h —4 °C

n.r. = not reported

panied by a form giving indications of how to dissolve the lyophilized powder, and requesting that the laboratory specify the features of the assay method that it used.

Methods

Each laboratory dissolved the lyophilized substance with 5 ml of the recommended solvent (phosphate buffer) and determined the estradiol receptor by the dextran coated charcoal method (DCC) (1, 2, 3). The essential features of the methods followed by the participating laboratories are reported in Table 1.

Generally, the receptor concentration was evaluated by Scatchard analysis without correction.

Since preparations no. 5, 6, and 7 were obtained by scalar dilutions of preparation no. 4, it was possible to make a variance analysis of each laboratory's linear regression and of the mean values of all laboratories.

Results and discussion

Table 2 gives the results that the participating laboratories reported after determining estradiol receptor concentration, expressed as fmoles/ml and as fmoles/mg of protein and after determining protein level in each of the lyophilized preparations.

In the same table are reported the mean values, the standard deviations and the variation coefficients of these results.

One laboratory (F) reported that its determinations on samples no. 6 and 7 were lost. Only one laboratory (D) considered the result obtained on preparation no. 7 (the one with the lowest receptor content) as borderline.

The variation coefficient of the results of estradiol receptor, expressed as fmoles/ml, ranges from 25—46%, while the same expressed as fmoles/mg p, ranges from 36 — 43%.

The highest variation coefficient proved to be for the sample with the lowest receptor content.

Data expression as fmoles/ml markedly lowers the variability of the results, because a factor that increases variability is constituted by protein determination, the variation coefficient of which ranges from 35—42%.

Considerable variability is also evident in the dissociation constant values given in Table 3.

Statistical analysis of the receptor content in these preparations of the scalar concentration permits identification of intramurally variable parameters, identification of the systemic factors among the participating laboratories and, finally, a better estimation of receptor content obtainable by similar methods in different laboratories.

The regression coefficient for each laboratory ranges from 0.9850—0.9994.

The regression of mean values of estradiol receptor expressed as fmoles/ml is in excellent agreement with the theoretical scalar dilutions, with a highly significant coefficient (0.9993).

A first goal of any quality control programme concerns the qualitative, positive or negative response that the assay can provide on a sample and the present programme has amply achieved it. The positive/negative distinction is, for the present, the cardinal factor for selecting the therapy appopriate to each case, and every laboratory in the study defined all samples containing receptor as positive, and the one without receptor as negative.

Table 2.
Estradiol receptor concentration expressed as fmoles/ml and as fmoles/mg protein in the five lyophilized calf uterus cytosols used in the Italian Quality Control programme (1980).

Labo-ratory	Prep. No. 4 (100%)			Prep. No. 5 (50%)			Prep. No. 6 (25%)			Prep. No. 7 (12.5%)			Prep. No. 8		
	a	b	c	a	b	c	a	b	c	a	b	c	a	b	c
A	355	135	2.5	168	55	2.9	72	23	3.1	44	14	3.1	0	0	3.0
B	200	200	1.0	90	72	1.2	43	31	1.4	26	18	1.4	0	0	1.5
C	326	233	1.4	130	86	1.5	46	31	1.5	25	16	1.5	0	0	1.6
D	225	225	1.0	129	129	1.0	63	58	1.1	32	27	1.2	0	0	1.4
E	361	425	0.8	145	145	1.0	63	53	1.2	31	25	1.2	0	0	1.2
F	201	102	1.9	90	41	2.2	lost			lost			0	0	1.0
G	361	230	1.5	132	66	2.0	44	28	1.5	24	14	1.7	0	0	2.0
H	380	344	0.9	180	133	1.2	86	63	1.3	47	28	1.6	0	0	1.9
I	184	205	0.9	70	70	1.0	43	39	1.1	17	17	1.0	0	0	0.5
L	300	250	1.2	137	106	1.3	83	69	1.2	22	11	2.1	0	0	n.m.
M	272	323	0.8	150	113	1.3	64	43	2.4	29	15	1.9	0	0	n.m.
Mean	287	242	1.26	129	92.3	1.50	60.7	43.8	1.58	26.8	16.0	1.67	—	—	1.56
SD	74.5	92.3	0.53	33.7	34.7	0.60	16.3	16.0	0.65	12.5	6.9	0.60	>	>	0.70
VC	25.9	38.1	42.0	26.1	37.5	40.0	26.8	36.5	41.1	46.6	43.6	35.9	>	>	44.8

a = fmoles/ml
b = fmoles/mg p
c = prot. mg/ml
n.m. = not measurable

Table 3.
Dissociation constant values obtained for estradiol receptor in the five lyophilized calf uterus cytosols used in the Italian Quality Control programme (1980)

Laboratory	Prep. No. 4	Prep. No. 5	Prep. No. 6	Prep. No. 7	Prep. No. 8
A	0.19	0.56	1.63	2.04	—
B	1.23	1.63	2.84	2.66	—
C	0.39	1.30	2.41	1.31	—
D	0.17	1.40	1.60	n.d.	—
E	1.08	1.09	1.70	5.16	—
F	1.60	1.60	lost	lost	—
G	2.80	2.90	2.50	4.40	—
H	1.00	3.00	2.90	2.20	—
I	13.00	4.38	3.70	5.80	—
L	1.72	1.57	1.50	2.15	—
M	1.13	2.70	2.70	2.00	—
Mean	2.21	2.01	2.35	3.08	—
SD	3.66	1.10	0.73	1.61	—

A second, qualitative objective dealing with the concentration response obtainable from the assay, met with variability. When the concentration was expressed in fmoles/ml, the variability was acceptable, except for sample 7, which had the lowest concentration. But variability rose markedly when the concentration was expressed as fmoles/mg, due to the high variability in the protein determination.

While other European quality control programmes (5) reported similar variability levels, it is a point of concern that the protein assay represents one of the major sources of variability in receptor determination. The distribution of dissociation constant (Kd) values, also, was rather high. As the receptor concentration decreases, the Kd tends to increase. Further study is needed to ascertain whether this trend is due to the lyophilized preparations themselves or to some other factor, yet to be identified.

The results obtained so far indicated that there was good intramural reproducibility, as the single correlation coefficients demonstrate. From analysis of these regressions, the systematic intramural variables can be identified.

Very probably, quality control conducted on lyophilized tissue including the homogenization and centrifugation phases, which in the initial Italian experience were not required, would produce increased variability of concentrations as assayed. Therefore, before this second phase of the programme is undertaken further efforts are necessary to pin-point the sources of variability and to standardize methods, aiming at a closer uniformity of responses. Only then can the numerous variables in the homogenization and centrifugation phases be appropriately dealt with.

Acknowledgement

The authors wish to thank their colleagues from the following participating laboratories for their scientific collaboration:

1. Istituto di Cancerologia — Università di Bologna
2. Istituto Nazionale Tumori di Milano
3. Servizio Oncologia — Ospedali Riuniti di Padova

4. Clinica Medica Generale V — Università di Roma
5. Divisione Oncologica Fond. Clinica Lavoro — Università di Pavia
6. Clinica Ostetrica — Università di Padova, Sede di Verona
7. Istituto di Patologia Generale — Università di Napoli
8. Istituto per lo Studio e la Cura dei Tumori — Genova

References

1. E.O.R.T.C. Breast Cancer Cooperative Group: Standards for the Assessment of Estrogen Receptors in Human Breast Cancer. I Workshop Europ. J. Cancer 9 (1973), 379—381
2. E.O.R.T.C. Breast Cancer Cooperative Group: Standards for the Assessment of Estrogen Receptors in Human Breast Cancer. II Workshop, Amsterdam 1979. Europ. J. Cancer 16 (1980), 1513—1515
3. E.O.R.T.C. Breast Cancer Cooperative Group: Standards for the Assessment of Estrogen Receptors in Human Breast Cancer. III Workshop, Copenhagen 1980. Europ. J. Cancer (in press)
4. FUMERO, S., BERRUTO, G. P., MONDINO, A. PELIZZOLA, D., GRILLI, S., BUTTAZZI, C., DI FRONZO, G., BERTUZZI, A., BOZZETTI, C., MORI, P., CONCOLINO, G., MAROCCHI, A., ROBUSTELLI della CUNA, G., ZIBERA, C., CERRUTTI, G., Ros, A. and PIFFANELLI, A.: Results of the Italian Interlaboratory Quality Control Program for Estradiol Receptor Assay. Tumori (in press)
5. KING, R. J. B., BAMES, D. N., HAWKINS, R. A., LEAKE, R. E., MAYNARD, P. V. and ROBERTS, M. M.: Measurements of Estradiol Receptors by Five Institutions on Common Tissue Samples. Br. J. Cancer 38 (1978), 428—430
6. KOENDERS, A. J., GEURTS-MAESPOTS, J. KHO, K. H. and BENRAAD, Th. J.: Estradiol and Progesterone Receptor Activities in Stored Lyophilized Target Tissue. Journ. of Steroid Biochemistry 9 (1978), 947—950
7. Quality of performance in pathology laboratories. The Lancet i (1981), 599
8. RAAM, S., GELMAN, R., COHEN, J. L., et al: Estrogen receptor assay: interlaboratory and intralaboratory variations in the measurement of receptors using dextran-coated charcoal technique: a study sponsored by E.C.O.G. Europ. J. Cancer, 17 (1981), 643—649
9. W.H.O. External quality assessment of health laboratories. Euroreports and studies No. 38. Copenhagen, W.H.O. Regional Office for Europe, 1981.

National Institute of Oncology, H-1525 Budapest, Hungary

Methodological and Clinical Studies of the Steroid Receptor Assay in Primary Breast Cancer

I. Szamel, B. Vincze, E. Svastits, J. Tóth, S. Kerpel-Fronius and S. Eckhardt

Introduction

Approximately one-third of breast cancer patients have hormone-dependent tumours (1). Primary breast tumours are treated by combined treatment consisting of surgery, irradiation and chemo- and hormone therapy, depending on the clinical and pathological stage of the disease and the steroid receptor (SR) content of the tumour (2). In choosing the most suitable treatment, the oestradiol receptor (ER) and progesterone receptor (PR) assays are of great importance (3, 4, 5, 6).

This paper describes our determinations of ER and PR, using two different buffer compositions, and presents some clinical results which show the correlation between the receptor content of a tumour and the endocrine therapy to be used.

Material and methods

Principle

Cytoplasmic ER and PR binding capacities were measured as described by the CMEA recommendation (7). This method is based on a charcoal-adsorption (DCC) technique performed essentially according to the standard procedure defined by the E.O.R.T.C. Breast Cancer Cooperative Group, revised in 1979 (8, 9). The DCC assay proved to be the most suitable method for routine clinical purposes. The specificity of each assay was monitored by verifying that by Scatchard analysis (10) the dissociation constant (K_d) was in the range of 10^{-10} M. In order to increase the sensitivity of receptor determination and to minimize the denaturation and loss of receptor protein during the assay procedure we also carried out studies of a new buffer composition. On the basis of data published by Anderson et al (11) and Krozowski et al (12), we used a buffer containing 20 mM sodium molybdate (Na_2MoO_4).

Reagents

2,4,6,7-^{3}H-Oestradiol, specific activity: 3.37 TBq/mmol, radiochemical purity: 97% (RCC, Amersham); ^{3}H-R 5020, 17α-methyl-^{3}H-promegestone, specific activity: 3.219 TBq/mmol, radiochemical purity: 97% (New England Nuclear); Tris/EDTA buffer: 10 mM Tris-HCl, 0.5 mM EDTA, 12 mM thioglycerol, 10% glycerol, pH 7.4; Tris/EDTA buffer containing Na_2MoO_4: 10 mM Tris-HCl, 0.15 mM EDTA, 1 mM dithioerythritol, 10% glycerol, 20 mM Na_2MoO_4, pH 7.4; Dextran-coated charcoal (DCC) suspension: 0.5% Norit A, 0.05% Dextran T70, 0.1% gelatine suspended in Tris/EDTA buffer.

Assay

The technique used is a saturation analysis. Tumour samples were divided for histopathological diagnosis and for receptor assay. The specimens were frozen in liquid N_2, powdered by a Mikrodismembrator (B. Braun Melsungen AG) and homogenized with four volume of buffer. Cytosol was prepared by ultracentrifugation at 100,000 × g for 1 hour. The cytosol was incubated with ^{3}H-oestradiol in five concentrations ($2 \times 10^{-10} - 2.5 \times 10^{-8}$ M) in the case of the ER assay; and ^{3}H-R 5020 was used in seven concentrations ($8 \times 10^{-10} - 2 \times 10^{-8}$ M) for the PR determination. Five-point and seven-point Scatchard plots were applied to the calculation of the number of binding sites and kinetic parameters, respectively. (Recently, a computer program for fitting curves and for calculating the parameters has been developed by G. Ringwald in our Institute.) In both determinations, incubation was carried out at 0—4 °C for 18 hours. Free and protein-bound, labelled ligands were separated by DCC treatment and centrifugation at 1,500 × g for 15 min. The radioactivity of the supernatant was counted in a liquid scintillation counter (LKB-Wallac 81,000). According to the CMEA recommendations, the borderline value of receptor-positivity is 5 fmol/mg protein in the case of ER, and 10 fmol/mg protein for the PR. The protein content of the cytosol was measured according to the method of LOWRY et al. (13).

Results and discussion

The influence of Na_2MoO_4 on the ER and PR content of breast cancer cytosol is shown in a representative case in Figure 1. Calculated ER binding capacities in the absence and presence of Na_2MoO_4 were 66.67 and 113.33 fmol/mg protein, respectively, and in the case of PR, 111.11 and 155.56 fmol/mg protein, respectively. In the presence of Na_2MoO_4, there was a 70% increase in ER binding and a 40% increase in that of PR. The kinetic parameters were within the predicted range; and neither the dissociation constants nor non-specific binding were influenced by molybdate.

ER and PR contents were determined in tumour samples from 10 and six patients, respectively (Fig. 2). The mean ER values $\pm$ SD (n = 10) in the absence and presence of Na_2MoO_4 were 67.46 $\pm$ 39.67 and 121.22 $\pm$ 79.11 fmol/mg protein, respectively; and a significant 80% increase in sensitivity was demonstrated (p < 0.01 calculated by Student's paired statistics). A higher PR content (49% increase) in the presence of molybdate was also observed: 215.62 $\pm$ 273.5 versus 144.61 $\pm$ 193.53 fmol/mg protein in the absence of the salt.

The presence of Na_2MoO_4 during the ER and PR assay increased the absolute concentration of receptors in both cases. This observation is particularly important for

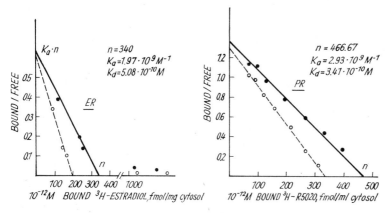

Fig. 1. Scatchard plots of oestradiol receptor (ER) and progesterone receptor (PR) in the presence (●) and absence (○) of Na_2MoO_4. n = number of binding sites; K_a = association constant; K_d = dissociation constant.

100

cases in which the receptor content of the tumour is very low. By increasing the receptor concentration, Na_2MoO_4 contributes to a more accurate evaluation; however, due to increased sensitivity, it might later become necessary to reevaluate the cut off point of receptor-positivity. The mechanism by which Na_2MoO_4 increases the recep-

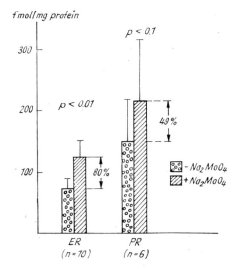

Fig. 2. Effect of Na_2MoO_4 on the estrogen receptor (ER) and progesterone receptor (PR) contents of human breast cancer cytosols. n = number of patients.

tor content has not yet been elucidated, but it is hypothesized that it stabilizes the receptor protein-radioactive ligand complex.

In our clinical studies, because of the small number of samples involved, we continued to use the recommended CMEA technique.

Oestrogen receptor

The presence of ER has been determined in more than 100 patients. Breast cancer cases and the presence of ER are shown as a function of age in Figure 3. Most of the patients were 40—60 years old. In patients over 70 years old, receptor-positivity was 100%; in premenopause, the frequency of ER-positive tumours was 50%, and that in postmenopause, 81%.

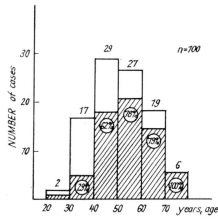

Fig. 3. Distribution of ER-positive tumours (striped areas) among breast cancer cases, in relation to the age of patients (10-year-age groups).

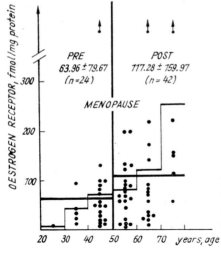

Fig. 4. ER content of breast cancer cases in relation to age of patients (10-year age groups). ER levels over 300 fmol/mg protein values are shown as vertical arrows.

ER content in relation to the age of patients was studied in 66 women with ER-positive tumours (Fig. 4). For this calculation, menopause was arbitrarily set at 50 years. The ER content varied widely, from undetectable levels to over 800 fmol/mg protein. In premenopausal patients, the average ER content was lower than that in postmenopausal ones, but this difference was not significant.

Progesterone receptor

PR was measured in 20 tumour specimens. The PR binding capacity was found to be 380.84 ± 351.66 fmol/mg protein in premenopausal women and 784.99 ± 823.58 fmol per mg protein in postmenopausal cases.

In agreement with other reports (14, 15), it was observed that the presence of PR was correlated with ER-positivity. Primary tumours with high ER levels had a higher PR content than tumours with a low ER concentration. This observation demonstrates that PR synthesis is under oestrogenic control.

ER and PR assays of primary tumours could thus be used to select patients for endocrine or other types of treatments after surgery. Of our group of patients, 49% were UICC stage I and all the others stage II. Hormone therapy was indicated when the axillary nodes were positive and the tumour had an ER content higher than 5 fmol per mg protein. Ovariectomy was carried out in premenopausal patients, in combination with Tamoxifen treatment. In some cases, only chemotherapy was used. Postmenopausal ER-positive patients with massive lymph node metastases were treated with Tamoxifen and irradiation. Hormone therapy was not used for ER-negative patients, for oncological considerations.

Determinations of SR content can also be used as a guide to appropriate endocrine therapy when a patient subsequently develops metastasis. According to DeSombre and Jensen (16), the ER content of primary breast tumours predicts the response to subsequent endocrine therapy in the case of recurrence.

102

Summary

Addition of 20 mM Na_2MoO_4 to buffer resulted in approximately 80% and 49% increases in the sensitivity of ER and PR determinations, respectively. This increased sensitivity is of decisive importance in evaluating tumours with borderline SR content. We hope that use of this modification will assist in the selection of patients for endocrine therapy.

Acknowledgements

We gratefully acknowledge the cooperation of Dr. G. RINGWALD, and the skillful technical assistance of Miss Eva VARGA and Mrs. Marta JANCSIK. The authors wish to acknowledge the collaboration of Mr. Ferenc GÁL.

References

1. DAO, T. L.: Ablation therapy for hormone dependent tumours. Ann. Rev. Med. *23* (1972), 1—18
2. McGUIRE, W. L.: Steroid receptors and clinical breast cancer. In: BRESCIANI, F., ed., Perspectives in Steroid Receptor Research, New York, Raven Press, pp. 239—246
3. McGUIRE, W. L., CARBONE, P. P., SEARS, M. E. and ESCHER, G. C.: Estrogen receptors in human breast cancer; an overview. In: McGUIRE, W. L., CARBONE, P. P. & VOLLMER, E. P., eds. Estrogen Receptor in Human Breast Cancer, New York, Raven Press, 1975, pp. 1—7
4. JENSEN, E. D., SMITH, S. and DeSOMBRE, E. R.: Hormone dependency in breast cancer. J. Steroid Biochem. *7* (1976), 911—917
5. DiCARLO, R., MUCCIOLI, G., CONTI, G., REBOANI, C. and DiCARLO, R.: Estrogen and prolactin receptor concentrations in human breast tumours. In: GENAZZANI, E., DiCARLO, F. and MANWARING, W. I. P., eds. Pharmacological Modulation of Steroid Action, New York, Raven Press, 1980, pp. 261—266
6. VORHERR, H.: Breast Cancer, Baltimore, Munich, Urban & Schwarzenberg, 1980, pp. 247—281
7. CMEA Meeting Problem Nr. 5.3 (1979) Clinical Pharmacology of Antineoplastic Drugs, Experimental Group, Chariman: Dr. E. Heise, Berlin, Dec. 18—19
8. E.O.R.T.C. Breast Cancer Cooperative Group (1973) Standards for the assessment of estrogen receptors in human breast cancer. Eur. J. Cancer *9* (1973), 379—381
9. E.O.R.T.C. Breast Cancer Cooperative Group. Revision of the standards for the assessment of hormone receptors in human breast cancer. Eur. J. Cancer *16* (1980), 1513—1515
10. SCATCHARD, G.: The attraction of proteins for small molecules and ions. Ann. N.Y. Acad. Sci. *51* (1949), 660—672
11. ANDERSON, K. M., MAROGIL, M., BONOMI, P. D., HENDRICKSON, C. and ECONOMU, S.: Stabilization of human breast cancer progesterone (5020) receptor by sodium molybdate. Clin. Chim. Acta *103* (1980), 367—373
12. KOROZOWSKI, Z. and MURPHY, L. C.: Stabilisation of the cytoplasmic oestrogen receptor by molybdate. J. Steroid Biochem. *14* (1981), 363—366
13. LOWRY, O. H., ROSENBROUGH, N. J., FARR, A. R. and RANDALL, R. J.: Protein measurement with folin phenol reagent. J. Biol. Chem. *193* (1951), 265—275
14. KOENDERS, A. J. M., BEEX, L. V. M. and BENRAAD, T. J.: Steroid hormone receptors in human breast cancer. In: BRESCIANI, F. ed. Perspectives in Steroid Receptor Research, New York, Raven Press, 1980, pp. 247—257
15. McGUIRE, W. L., RAYNARD, J. P. and BAULIEU, E. E.: Progesterone receptors. Introduction and overview. In: McGUIRE, W. L., RAYNAUD, J. P. & BAULIEU, E. E., eds., Progesterone Receptors in Normal and Neoplastic Tissues, New York, Raven Press, 1977, pp. 1—8
16. DeSOMBRE, E. R. and JENSEN, E. V.: Hormone dependency in breast cancer. In: MAYER, M., SAEZ, S. & STOLL, B. A., eds., Hormone, Deprivation in Breast Cancer, ICI, (1978) pp. 15—28

Institute of Oncology, Warsaw, Poland

The Value of Hormone Receptor Assays for Prediction of the Effectiveness of Endocrine Therapy in Breast Cancer

Z. Paszko, H. Padzik, F. Pieńkowska, S. Chrapusta, B. Wasowska and E. Kwiatkowska

Jensen et al (5) were the first authors to suggest that the presence of estrogen receptor (ER) in human breast cancers might be an index of their hormone dependence; since this time, the determination of the steroid hormone receptors and their clinical applications are one of the main features of endocrine therapy of breast carcinomas. Many studies performed during the past decade have — despite certain disagreement — generally confirmed the usefulness of the determinations of hormone receptors for diagnostic, prognostic and therapeutic purposes. According to these studies, the tissues of 50—85% of breast tumours contain ER (3, 9, 11, 15). However, only 55—60% of the receptor-positive (ER+) tumours react by a regression to endocrine therapy, the remaining ER+ tumours being non-reactive (3, 11).

Since 1972, studies performed at this laboratory were aimed at: 1. characterization of various receptors in the breast tumour tissues in Polish women, and 2. evaluation of the usefulness of receptor determinations for clinical practice. These studies may — apart from their practical importance for therapy — be of some significance for biology of tumours, since, it is well known that the incidence of breast cancer is much lower in Polish women than in those from West Europe and U.S.A. (7). A part of the studies reported in this paper (111 tumours and 20 patients treated) have been successively published (13—16).

The present communication sums up the whole of our previous investigations (extended by studies of 373 breast tumours and 18 cases treated). Moreover, in addition to the ER determinations, the receptor of: progestin (PR), androgens (AR) and glucocorticosteroids (GR) were assayed.

Materials and methods

Clinical material: In total, 484 cases of primary or metastatic breast cancer were investigated. The distribution of patients according to age was as follows: 10.7% of cases were 19—40 years old; 25.4% — 41—50; 29% — 51—60; 22.9% — 61—70; and 12% — over 70 years old.

This age distribution of patients reflects the morbidity of breast cancer in Warsaw, as described by Koszarowski et al (6). It can be assumed that our cancer material is representative of the Polish population.

Chemicals: Radioactive steroids — 2,4,6,7(N)-^{3}H-estradiol (^{3}H-E$_2$, 90—100 Ci/mmole) was from Amersham, whereas ^{3}H-promegestone (^{3}H-R 5020, 86 Ci/mmole) and ^{3}H-methyltrienolone (^{3}H-R 1881, 87 Ci/mmole) were from NEN. The labelled steroids were purified by TLC and stored in absolute ethanol at −20 °C. The non-labelled compounds R 5020 and R 1881 were gifts from Dr. J. P. Raynaud, Roussel-Uclaf, France, and diethylstilbestrol was from Sigma. Other chemicals were of analytical grade.

Preparation of cytosols: Tumour specimens stored in liquid nitrogen for 1—2 weeks were powdered in liquid N_2, dispersed in 3 vol. of TEDG buffer (10 mM Tris, 1.5 mM EDTA, 0.5 mM dithiothreitol, 10% glycerol, pH 7.4) in a Polytron apparatus (Kinematica GmBH), and centrifuged at 220000 $\times$ g for 30 min. Supernatants (cytosols) were stored at -25 °C for up to 1 week before assay.

Steroid receptor analysis: Estrogen receptor (ER) was assayed as described before (13, 15, 16). Progestin (PR) and androgen (AR) receptors were assayed analogously to ER, using the DCC-competitive-binding assay in the presence or absence of a 100-fold molar excess of non-labelled competitor (without ethylene glycol in the incubation mixture). Some tumours were examined for AR using agar-agarose gel electrophoresis (18). Whenever possible, the amount of each receptor was determined by Scatchard plot analysis; in other cases, a single saturating concentration (10 nM) of the radioactive ligand was used. Tumour tissues were assumed to be ER+, PR+, AR+ and GR+, when the concentrations of the respective receptors were greater than 5 fmoles per mg of tumour cytosol protein. Protein content was assayed according to Lowry (10). Sucrose density gradient centrifugation was performed as described before (2).

Results and discussion

1. Content of steroid hormone receptors in breast cancer tissues

The content of ER in breast cancer tissues (484 cases) varied from barely detectable levels to very high ones (about 1000 fmoles/mg cytosol protein). In normal mammary gland tissue, ER cannot be detected by the present method; thus, the border-line value in the classification into receptor-positive tumours (ER+) and receptor-negative ones (ER—) can only be arbitrary and depends on the sensitivity of the detection methods. For practical clinical purposes, the following arbitrary classification was accepted (Tab. I): range I comprises values of 0—5 fmoles/mg cytosol protein, which indicate a relative lack of receptor (ER—) (our material comprised 36% of ER— cases); range II includes ER levels of 6—20 fmoles/mg cytosol protein, which we regard as border-line positive ones (our material contained 26% of these cases); range III comprises ER levels of 21—1000 fmoles/mg cytosol protein, which we classify as definitely positive, (and which in the present material accounted for 38% of cases).

Therefore, our clinical material included 36% of ER— and 64% of ER+ cases. Although the classification criterion was arbitrarily selected, these percentages remained nearly unchanged throughout 6 series of assays performed during 9 years. It is note-

Table 1.
Frequency and levels of estrogen, progestin, androgen and glucocorticosteroid receptors in human breast cancer

Receptor sites* (fmoles/mg cytoplasmic protein)	% of total number of tumours			
	ER	PR	AR	GR
0	25%	38%	33%	49%
1—5	11%	10%	34%	23%
6—20	26%	17%	20%	28%
21—1000	38%	35%	13%	—
Total number of tumours	484	259	76	43

* ER — ³H-estradiol; PR — ³H-R 5020; AR — ³H-R 1881; GR — ³H-dexamethasone.

worthy that the incidence of tumours in range III (21—1000 fmoles/mg cytosol protein) increased with age of patients from 25% (19—40 years) to 54% (over 70 years). The incidence of tumours in ranges I and II (0—20 fmoles/mg cytosol protein) evidently dropped with age of patients from 75% (19—40 years) to 46% (over 70 years) (Fig. 1). This phenomenon is usually interpreted in terms of changes in the hormonal status of women, particularly after menopause. However, the fact that the incidence of ER+ and ER— tumours persisted at the same level, may suggest the occurrence of two biological types of tumours. One type would — like the normal tissue of the

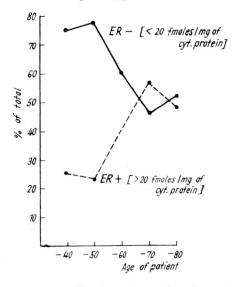

Fig. 1. The frequency of ER+ and ER— in breast cancers as a function of age of patients.

mammary gland — show a low basic level of ER, whereas the second type would be characterized by increased production of ER. In young women, the first type would predominate, and in older women both types would occur in the same proportion. ALLEGRA et al (1) have found an evident correlation between the increase in ER content and age of patients. They claim that this correlation is related to the women's state of menopause, since it is not observed in the pre- and post-menopausal groups. Likewise LECLERCQ et al have observed higher ER values in women after menopause than before (9). The present are similar to other findings in stating that in breast cancer, ER+ values occur in 50—77% of cases (3, 11, 17). Some authors report a much higher incidence of ER+ tumours (e.g. LECLERCQ: 85—87%) (9). This dispersion of the results may be due to differences in the sensitivity of the detection methods and to differences in the criterion of classification into ER+ and ER— tumours.

For the distribution of PR in breast cancer, we accepted the same classification as for ER (Tab. 1); we found that 38% of tumours contained no PR and 10% of them exhibited extremely low levels, these together amounting to 48% of PR— tumours. The percentage of PR+ tumours was 52%, including 17% within the border-line range and 35% being evidently positive. In contrast to the proportion of ER+ and ER— tumours (irrespective of age), which remained constant in our material, the proportion of PR+ and PR— tumours was evidently variable. The variability concerned in particular the definitely PR+ and definitely PR— tumours. On the other hand, the behaviour of the incidence of PR+ and PR— tumours considered in relation to age, was quite different. Between 19—60 years of age, the incidence of PR+ and PR— tumours remained at the same levels (59% and 41%, respectively — Fig. 2).

Above 60 years of age, the incidence of PR+ tumours decreased to 35%, and that of PR— tumours increased to 65%. Thus, the variability of the PR content in breast cancer is different from that of ER.

Compared with the present results for the PR level in tumours, the data from the literature are lower for Japanese women (12), but other authors give results close to ours (4, 9).

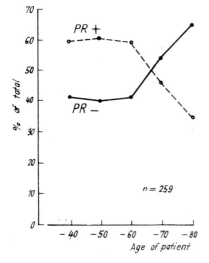

Fig. 2. The frequency of PR+ and PR— in breast cancers as a function of age of patients.

The levels of AR and GR in breast cancer, compared with those of ER and PR, were usually low. In a group of 76 patients, the range of the AR values was only 0—110 fmoles/mg cytosol protein, and the GR values found for 43 tumours were even smaller. Assuming, for AR and GR, the same criteria of classification as for ER and PR, AR+ occurred in only 33%, and GR+, in 28% of cases. However, if — taking account of the very small content of AR and GR in tumours — the level of 1 fmole/mg cytosol protein could be accepted as the criterion of classification into R+ and R— tumours, then the incidence of AR+ and GR+ tumours would be closely similar to that of the ER+ and PR+ tumours. Studies of the frequency of AR and GR in breast cancer are rare. From the few available papers, the frequency of AR in breast cancer is evaluated at 19—36% (1, 12, 17).

On account of the physiological interrelation between ER and PR in cells, much attention is given to studies of the simultaneous occurrence of these receptors. HORWITZ and McGUIRE (4) suggest that the simultaneous presence of ER and PR is a more reliable index of the hormone-dependence of tumours than the occurrence of ER alone. In the present material we evaluated the simultaneous occurrence of: ER and PR (260 cases), ER and AR (76 cases), and ER and GR (43 cases) (Tab. 2). This evaluation indicated that combinations ER+ PR+ occurred most often (39%), ER+ AR+ were present less often (28%) and ER+ GR+ occurred least frequently (14%). Combinations ER+ PR— (26%), ER+ AR— (32%) and ER+ GR— (40%) occurred simultaneously in a reverse order (Tab. 2). It is noteworthy that ER—, PR+, AR+ and GR+ were present in tumours least often, i.e. in 5—14% of cases; ER— tumours and the remaining R— tumours occurred with a nearly equal frequency (22—35%). In 22 tumours, we succeeded in simultaneous assaying ER, PR, AR and GR; this was not always possible, because of the small amount of the specimens.

107

Table 2.
Simultaneous occurrence of estrogen receptor and other steroid receptors* in human breast cancer

Receptor	No. of tumours		Receptor	No. of tumours	
	per total of tumours assayed	percentage		per total of tumours assayed	percentage
ER+ PR+	102/260	39%	ER− PR+	32/260	13%
ER+ AR+	21/76	28%	ER− AR+	4/76	5%
ER+ GR+	6/43	14%	ER− GR+	6/43	14%
ER+ PR−	68/260	26%	ER− PR−	58/260	22%
ER+ AR−	24/76	32%	ER− AR−	27/76	35%
ER+ GR−	17/43	40%	ER− GR−	14/43	32%

* ER, PR, AR and GR levels were assumed to be positive (+) for values > 5 fmoles of specific ligand/mg cytosol protein.

Among ER+ tumours, only one half also contained PR+ and AR+, and a quarter also contained GR+. In contrast, in nearly all ER− tumours, the remaining receptors were also absent.

We found that ER and PR mainly occurred in tumours in two sedimentation forms, i.e. 8S and 4S (60—65% of cases), less often exclusively as 4S (21—34%), and least often, exclusively as 8S (5—13%) (2). Breast tumours with exclusive occurrence of ER in the 4S form often contained PR. In these tumours the average content of ER and PR was rather low (median contents of ER 4S and PR were 21 fmoles/mg cytosol protein). In tumours with ER occurring in both the 8S and 4S form, the simultaneously present PR also appeared in these two forms. In this group, the total receptor contents were greater, as compared with the group of tumours containing only the 4S form of ER (in latter group, the median contents of ER and PR were 63 and 91 fmoles/mg cytosol protein, respectively) (2). The occurrence of exclusively the 4S form of ER in breast cancer is regarded by some authors (8) as a defect of the structure of the receptor, causing inability of cells to respond to estrogen. The simultaneous occurrence, in our material, of ER 4S and PR seems to rule out the presence of a defect in the reactivity of such tumours to estrogen, because PR is produced in cells as an expression of their stimulation by estrogen.

2. Relationship between the presence of ER in breast cancer tissues and the efficiency of endocrine therapy

A total of 38 cases of primary or advanced breat cancer were studied in patients 38—73 years of age. In previous publications (15, 16), 20 of these cases have been reported. Patients were treated by different kinds of endocrine therapy, i.e. castration, treatment with estrogens, androgens, and antiestrogens. The details of the therapeutic procedures and criteria for evaluation of the effectiveness of treatment have previously been reported (15, 16). In this paper, we shall only present the main conclusions.

For a total of 38 patients treated, in 29 cases the tumours contained ER+ > 5 fmoles per mg cytosol protein), whereas in 9 cases the tumours contained very little or no ER (ER− ≤ 5 fmoles/mg cytosol protein, Fig. 3). For a total of 16 patients with ER+

tumours (25—498 fmoles/mg cytosol protein), 13 cases (81.3%) experienced a remission after treatment, whereas 3 cases (18.7%) showed no improvement. Among 13 patients with tumours containing lower levels of ER (6—25 fmoles/mg cytosol protein), remission was found in only 8 cases (61.5%). In the group of ER— patients, only 1 case out of 9 (11.1%) responded by a slight short-term remission. In total, in patients with ER+ tumours, endocrine treatment induced remission in 72% of cases, whereas in 28%

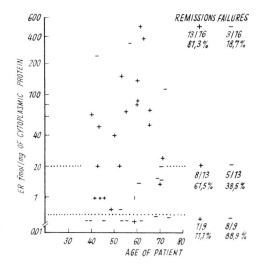

Fig. 3. Relationship between the effectiveness of endocrine therapy of breast cancer and estrogen receptor status of tumours.

of cases this treatment was ineffective. It is noteworthy that in patients with higher ER levels in tumours, the frequency of remission was evidently increased (Fig. 3). The present data, similar to those of other authors (3, 11), indicate that proportion of ER+ tumours do not respond to endocrine therapy. In the present material, compared with the data from the literature, a much higher proportion of ER+ tumours (72%) responded by a regression. This may be due to the small numbers of patients in the present material.

Summary

The frequency of steroid hormone receptors in breast cancer in Polish women, 19—80 years of age, was studied. Estrogen receptor (ER+) occurred in 64% of cases (310/184); progestin receptor (PR+), in 53% (134/200); androgen receptor (AR+); in 33% (25/76); glucocorticosteroid receptor (GR+), in 28% (12/43). The receptor level was assumed to be positive for values exceeding 5 fmoles/mg cytosol protein. The frequency of ER+ and PR+ in breast cancer was evidently age-dependent. ER+ tumours occurred more frequently in older than in younger women. The proportions of PR+ and PR — tumours remained unchanged in women between 19—60 years of age (60 and 40% of cases, respectively). Between 60 and 80 years of age, the incidence of PR+ tumours dropped (from 60% to 35%), and that of PR — tumours increased (from 40% to 65%). There were differences in the coexistence of several receptors in breast tumours. This coexistence was most frequent for ER+ PR+ (39%), less frequent for ER+ AR+ (28%), and least frequent for ER+ GR+ (14%), In ER-tumours, other receptors (i. e. PR+, AR+ and GR+) either occurred very seldom (5—14% of cases), or more often were absent (22—36% of cases). In 60—65% of breast cancer cases, ER and PR were present in two sedimenting forms, 8S and 4S. Exclusive occurrence of ER and PR in only the 4S form was less frequent (21—34% of cases), and that in only the 8S form was still less frequent (5—13%). In breast tumours containing ER in only the 4S form, PR very often coexisted. In these tumours, the total concentrations of ER and PR were less than one third of those in tumours with ER in the 4S and 8S forms.

In a material of 484 patients, 38 cases were treated by various methods of endocrine therapy. In 21 of 29 patients (72%) with ER-positive tumours, endocrine therapy resulted in objective remission. However, the remaining 8 ER+ tumours (28%) failed to regress following endocrine therapy. Endocrine therapy more often induced remissions in patients with higher ER levels in tumours (81%) than in those with lower ER levels (62%). Among 9 patients with ER-tumours, only 1 case showed a remission. It was concluded that the presence of ER in the tumour tissue is a valuable, though not fully reliable, critierion in the selection of patients for endocrine therapy. It seems that ER is most important for evaluation of the hormone-sensitivity of breast cancer, the role of the other steroid receptors being no more than auxiliary.

References

1. ALLEGRA, J. C., LIPPMAN, M. E., THOMPSON, E. B., SIMON, R., BARLOCK, A., GREEN, L., HUFF, K. K., DO, H. M. T. and AITKEN, S. C.: Cancer Res. *39* (1979), 1447—1454
2. CHRAPUSTA, S., KWIATKOWSKA, E., PASZKO, Z. and PADZIK, H.: 1981, in press
3. DESOMBRE, E. R., GREENE, G. L. and JENSEN, E. V.: In: Hormones, Receptors and breast cancer. Ed. W. L. MCGUIRE, Raven Press, New York 1978, p. 1
4. HORWITZ, K. B. and MCGUIRE, W. L.: In: Progesterone receptors in normal and neoplastic tissues. Ed. W. L. MCGUIRE et al. Raven Press, New York, 1977, pp. 103
5. JENSEN, E. V., DESOMBRE, E. R. and JUNGBLUT, P. W.: In: Endogeneous factors influencing host-tumour balance. (WESSLER, R. W.; DAO, T. L.; WOOD, S. Jr. eds.). Chicago Press, 1967, pp. 15—30
6. KOSZAROWSKI, T. et al.: Przeglad Lekarski 1966, XXII-11, 677
7. KOSZAROWSKI, T., GADOMSKA, H. and WRONKOWSKI, Z.: Nowotwory 1973, XXIII, 3
8. KUTE, T. E., HEIDEMANN, P. and WITTLIFF, J. L.: Cancer Research *38* (1978), 4307—4314
9. LECLERCQ, G., HEUSON, J. C., DEBOEL, M. C., LEGROS, N., LONGEVAL, E. and MATTHEIM, W. H.: In: Progesterone receptors in normal and neoplastic tissues. Ed. W. L. MCGUIRE et al. Raven Press, New York, 1977, pp. 141
10. LOWRY, O. H., ROSENBROUGH, N. J., FARR, A. L. and RANDALL, R. J. J.: Biol. Chem. *193* (1951), 265
11. MCGUIRE, W. L.: Cancer *36* (1975), 638
12. OCHI, H., HAYASHI, T., NAKAO, K. YAYOI, E., KAWAHARA, T. and MATSUMOTO, K.: J. Natl. Cancer Inst. *60* (1978), 291
13. PASZKO, Z. and PADZIK, H.: Nowotwory 1973, XXIII, 1—2
14. PASZKO, Z. and PADZIK, H.: Arch. Geschwulstforschung *45*, 5 (1975), 430—443
15. PASZKO, Z., PADZIK, H., DABSKA, M. and PIENKOWSKA, F.: Tumori *64* (1978), 495
16. PIENKOWSKA, F., PASZKO, Z., PADZIK, H. and DZIADEK, T.: Nowotwory 1980, XXX, 1
17. TREMS, G. and MAASS, H.: Cancer Res. *37* (1977), 258—261
18. WAGNER, R. K. Z.: Physiol. Chem. *353* (1972), 1235—1245

Acknowledgements — The authors are grateful to Mrs. Wanda PORZYCKA and Mrs. Teresa KRAUZE for their skilled technical assistance and for typing the manuscript.

This investigation was supported by grant no. 1302 from the Polish Governmental Research and Development Program PR-6 "Control of malignant neoplasms".

110

The Cancer Cell Surface as a Target for Therapy

Laboratory of Histology, Faculty of Medicine, University of Nice, France

Normal and Pathological Cell Communication

B. F. Deys

Mechanisms of cell binding, contact and communication are a wide open question. Current evidence suggest that contact-mediated intercellular communication requires the formation of specialized membrane structures. Obviously the lipid-protein membrane plays an essential role in cell communication, which can be effected by at least three different, but equally important ways:

(I)   by induction during embryogenesis, when an inductive tissue exerts its action on another tissue by diffusible substances

(II) by other biochemical regulation of cellular processes (hormones, enzymes) after embryogenesis and

(III) by intercellular junctions facilitating a direct diffusion of cellular substrates from one cell to the next.

(i) It has long been evident that growth of normal tissues depends largely on some form of interaction between cells. In embryogenesis, cells decending from one single fertilized egg cell, develop along divergent pathways. Firstly, with remarkable precision, decisive factors influence the developing cell from outside. It is therefore essential that every immature cell is able to perceive and interpret signals from its environment. Secondly, cells that act as inducers, not only dictate future structures to embryonic cell populations, but appear also to appreciate the stage of differentiation reached by their target cells. Such mutual recognition is of great importance when embryonic cells migrate to specific parts of the body, where they ultimately will settle down. This "homing" can clearly be observed in germ cells of the developing gonads (8). They migrate from the yolk sac to the genital ridges and settle there to become the ovary or testis.

The phenomena of locomotion and recognition can be also followed *in vitro*. Freshly dissociated cells of embryonic tissues show a tendency to aggregate, and after sorting out, to reconstitute histiotypic structures. Nerve, cartilage, muscle and epithelial cells reaggregate *in vitro* in a three-dimensional ordering (9). It is not clear how homing cells meet each other, nor what is the nature of their communication. The type of signal to different cells seems to be the same, but the interpretation of the message is different. It has been shown that contact properties change during embryonic development and disappear completely in later stages of embryogenesis (1).

Adult forms of homing can be observed in the immune defense mechanism against malignant growth, or bacterial infections. Activated lymphocytes and macrophages can detect, damage, or lyse target cells, which they recognize as abnormal (Fig. 1). Observations with isotopes (13) have shown that certain lymphocytes home to the thymus, stay there for several weeks, and, subsequently; migrate to other organs.

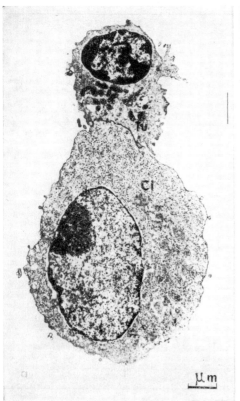

Fig. 1—a. Homing lymphocyte in contact with target cell (E. M. × 8400).

Fig. 1—b. Lymphocyte after lyse of target cell (E. M. × 8400). G. Nocolas, Biol. Cellul., 1980, 33, 231.

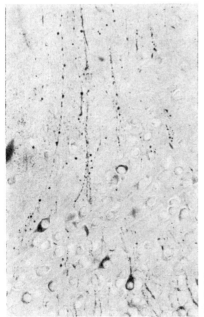

Fig. 2. Cellular communication *via* a transport of neurosecretion. The passage goes through axons of nerve cells. Hypothalamus of a frog (× 500).

(ii) The action of inductive stimuli during embryogenesis, as a means for cell communication, is gradually taken over by hormonal activities in neonates and adults. Even if target cells are far away, effective communication can be achieved by hormones. One of the leading endocrine glands, the hypophysis, plays an important role in the regulation of organs like, for example, thymus, breasts, ovaries, and testis. The hypophysis itself is directed by a hormone, excreted by nerve cells of the hypothalamus. This neurosecretion is transported along preformed pathways and reaches the hypophysis (Fig. 2). Here the communication between different cells is based on the existence of specialized membrane structures.

(iii) Intercellular junctions facilitate a direct diffusion of cellular substrates from one cell to the next. Both in embryonic and in regenerating systems (e.g., in wound healing), where rapid cellular proliferation and morphogenic movements cause frequent disruption of cell contacts, the speed at which de novo junctions may be established is of great importance. It has been observed (11) that formation of gap junctions (i. e. channels between cells facilitating a direct flow of small molecules) can be very rapid. Indeed, time-lapse cinematography shows a brief contact between cells, established in a short time and, depending on tissue type, sometimes of short duration (Personal observation).

Such gap junctions are found in almost every multicellular organism (12). They have also been described in neuroblastoma (9), in macrophages and glia cells (4), in sti-

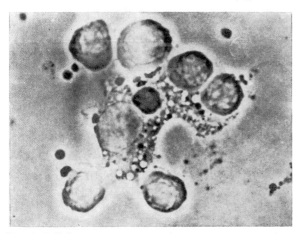

Fig. 3. Cellular communication *via* micropinocytosis. A nursing histiocyte surrounded by maturing erythroblasts (phase contr.)

mulated lymphocytes (5), and synaptic junctions have been observed between neuroblastoma and muscle cells (4). The existence of structures for cellular communication is based on observations with electron-microscopy and freeze-etching techniques. It has been observed that both the passage of an electric current and contact feeding are associated with the presence of gap junctions (10). Such metabolic cooperation is not uncommon. A distinct manifestation of transfer of nutrients, probably by micropinocytosis, is seen in Fig. 3. A nursing histiocyte is surrounded by erythroblasts. These nursing cells are situated in the bone-marrow, where ferritin and erythropoietin are transferred during maturation of the immature erythrocyte (3).

Fig. 4 shows another cellular structure, obviously related to cell communication. Endplates of nerve fibres are closely connected to muscle cells. The communication between two functional units is facilitated by acetylcholine which is secreted at the site of the endplates.

Yet the transfer of the message may be perturbed as a result of changes in cell surface receptors or surface-associated glycoproteins (7). Several compounds have been reported, that influence cellular communication. Curare, for example, is a poison, acting selectively on endplates. Although the message has been passed, its meaning could not be understood.

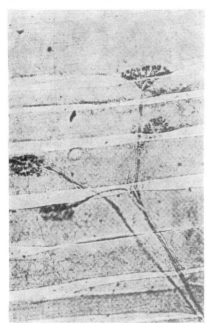

Fig. 4. Communication *via* specialized membrane structure. Endplates of nerve fibres in close contact with muscle syncitiae.

Normal cell growth is also largely dependent on, and influenced by, a distribution of intrinsic membrane proteins, and communication with neighbouring cells passes *via* junctional structures. Growth control (i.e., contact inhibition of proliferation), is largely dependent on cell surface-associated functions. But there is increasing evidence, that under pathological conditions, the number of these functional elements is reduced (14), so that cellular communication becomes perturbed. Malignant cells have an altered proliferation pattern. They show a reduced contact inhibition of movement and of growth, and tend to invade normal tissues indiscriminately. One could consider the invasion of tumour cells in normal tissues and the successive formation of metastases as a manifestation of autonomy of cells, which have partially lost their homing capacity.

Although morpho-kinetic studies cannot reveal the functioning of the specialized structures of which the cell membrane is constituted, time-lapse microcinematography makes it possible to study cellular interactions. Films of cultures of fibroblasts, derived from an osteosarcoma of a mouse, and of normal epithelial cells, derived from a rat ureter, display the individual growth characteristics of these two lines (6) and their behaviour towards each other. Epithelial cells are seeking close contact in order to form a tight sheet of cells. When confluent, these cells derived from a rat ureter display the formation of "holes" in this sheet. A number of cells, ranging from 4 to 9, are apparently obeying at the same time signals of unknown origin. They retract simultaneously to form a "hole", which closes again some hours later. The nature of such

116

a "hole" and the way it develops can only be explained by an intensive communication between the individual cells.

Fibroblasts of malignant origin seem to have lost the regulatory action of contact inhibition. They move in criss-cross fashion and while migrating, may overlap other cells. Yet it appears that there exists a frequent communication between cells, since they are directing pseudopodial extensions towards each other.

One of the most prominent features observed is the visualization of the phenomenon of recognition. When crawling about the bottom of the culture flask, fibroblastic cells may sometimes lose a small part of their cytoplasm. This small part is either abandoned and lost for the cell, or it is selectively reintegrated by the moving cell within its own cytoplasm (Fig. 5). A non-homologous fragment has never been observed being incorporated by one of the cells. Apparently the tumour cell, that has lost the ability to recognise cells of other origin, is still able to recognize itself. Probably the mechanism for communication between tumour cells and normal cells is present, but the message can no longer be understood.

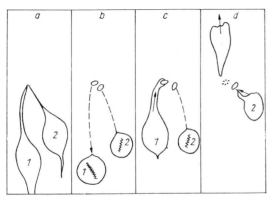

Fig. 5. Communication and recognition.

5—a Two fibroblasts (1) and (2) in close contact with their pseudopodial extensions.

5—b While rounding up for mitosis cells (1) and (2) lose a small part of their cytoplasm.

5—c After mitosis, cell (1) recognizes its lost part, moves towards it and reintegrates only its bit.

5—d After mitosis, cell (2) moves towards its part, reaches out with a pseudopodial extension and reintegrates it.

References

1. ADLER, R.: Cell interactions and histogenesis in embryonic neural aggregates. Exp. Cell Res. 77 (1973), 367—375
2. BELL, P. B.: Locomotory behaviour, contact inhibition and pattern formation of 3T3 and polyoma virus-transformed 3T3 cells in culture. J. Cell. Biol. 74 (1977), 963—982
3. BESSIS, M.: Cellules du sang normal et pathologique. Edit. Masson et Cie., Paris VI, 1972
4. COOPER, A. et al.: The growth of mouse neuroblastoma cells in controlled orientations on thin films of silicon monoxide. Exp. Cell. Res. 103 (1976), 435—438
5. COX, R. P. et al: Absence of metabolic cooperation in PHA stimulated human lymphocyte cultures. Exp. Cell Res. 101 (1976), 411—413
6. DEYS, B. F. et al: Characteristics of primary and serially transplanted tumours and derived cultures. Exc. Med. Congress Series, 375 (1976), 374—378
7. EKBLOM, P. et al: Inhibition of morphogenic cell interactions by 6-diazo-5-oxonorleucine (DON). Exp. Cell Res. 121 (1979), 121—126

8. Gondos, B.: Intercellular bridges and mammalian germ cell differentiation. Differentiation, *1* (1973), 177—182

9. Msocona, A.: Cell suspensions from organ rudiments of chick embryos. Exp. Cell Res. *3* (1952), 535

10. Loewenstein, W. R. et al: Intercellular communication and tissue growth. J. Cell Biol. *33* (1967), 225—234

11. Pederson, D. C. et al: The development of metabolite transfer between reaggregating Novikoff hepatoma cells. Exp. Cell Res. *127* (1980), 159—178

12. Pitts, J. D. et al: Permeability of junctions between animal cells. Exp. Cell Res. *104* (1977), 153—163

13. Röpke, C. et al: Migration of small lmyphocytes in adult mice demonstrated by parabiosis. Cell Tissue Kinet. *7* (1974), 137—150

14. Tremblay, G. et al: Intercellular junctions between Novikoff hepatoma cells and hepatic cells. Exp. Cell Res. *74* (1972), 355—358

Institut für Medizinische Chemie und Biochemie, University of Innsbruck, Innsbruck, Austria

The Cells Surface as Target for Alkylating Agents

H. Grunicke, H. Putzer, F. Scheidl and E. Wolff-Schreiner

Introduction

In previous reports we have demonstrated that alkylating antitumour agents affect several transport systems of the plasma membrane (1—3).

In view of increasing evidence for a role of the plasma membrane in the regulation of cell division (4—8) it seemed worthwhile to investigate the effect of alkylating agents on the cell membrane in greater detail.

Two questions seemed to be of special interest:

(a) Are the alterations of the cell membrane caused by a direct alkylation of membrane constituents or are they due to preceding intracellular events, e.g. inhibition of protein synthesis?

(b) Are the effects of the cell membrane correlated to the antitumour activity of the drug?

The present paper answers these questions for two parameters of the cell membrane which are affected by alkylating agents: The Na^+/K^+-ATPase and the membrane fluidity.

Material and methods

Ehrlich ascites tumour cells were grown intraperitoneally in NMRI/Han mice and harvested at the fourth day after transplantation. Trenimon (2,3,5-trisethyleneiminobenzoquinone) was kindly donated by Farbenfabriken Bayer A.G., Leverkusen, W. Germany. Chlorambucil was a gift from the Wellcome Research Laboratories, Beckenham, Kent, England. Cyclophosphamide, phosphamide mustard, (N,N-bis(2-chloroethyl)-diamido-phosphoric acid), 4-hydroperoxycyclophosphamide and 4-hydroxyurea cyclophosphamide were gifts from ASTA-Werke A.G., Brackwede, W.Germany. Nitrogen mustard (Nor-N-mustard) was obtained from Sigma Chemie, Munich, W.Germany.

Na^+/K^+-ATPase activity of whole cells or of membrane vesicles was determined by the uptake of ^{86}Rb as described previously (3). Membrane fluidity was determined by fluorescence polarization using diphenylhexatriene (DPH) as a probe as described by Shinitzky and Inbar (9).

Lipid extraction of isolated membranes was performed according to van Hoeven and Emmelot (10). Cholesterol was determined by the Liebermann-Burchard reaction. Phospholipids were measured according to Bartlett (11).

Measurement of antitumour activity:

The alkylating agents were dissolved in 0.14 M NaCl and injected i. p. into Ehrlich ascites tumour bearing animals. After the time intervals indicated in the legends to the corresponding tables and figures, the mice were killed, the cells collected and transplanted i. p. into fresh mice.

10 days after tumour transplantation, the animals were killed, the cells harvested and the tumour cell mass determined in hematocrit tubes. For each concentration of the alkylating agent (see corresponding figures and tables) groups of 10 mice were used. The antitumour activity is expressed as "per cent cell multiplication", i. e. the tumour cell mass of the untreated controls was set 100% and the tumour cell mass recovered after treatment with the alkylating agent was given as per cent of the controls.

Results

1. Effect of alkylating agents on Na$^+$/K$^+$-ATPase

As shown previously, (2, 3) treatment of Ehrlich ascites tumour cells with the alkylating agent Trenimon leads to a decrease in Na$^+$/K$^+$-ATPase activity. From the observation that this effect occurs within 30 seconds after administration of the drug (3) it was concluded, that the depression of the enzyme is caused by direct attack of the alkylating agents on the plasma membrane. However, as the turnover of the Na$^+$/K$^+$-ATPase in Ehrlich-ascites tumour cells is unknown, it remains possible that the reduced activity of the enzyme is caused by an inhibition of protein synthesis.

Table 1.
Effect of Trenimon and cycloheximide on the uptake of ^{86}Rb and the incorporation of ^{3}H-lysine by Ehrlich ascites tumour cells

	Rb-uptake		^{3}H-Lysine incorporation	
	ng-atom Rb/mg · min	%	dpm/mg protein	%
Control	2.1 ± 0.12	100	494.610 ± 2.811	100
+ Trenimon 10^{-6} mol/kg	1.06 ± 0.13	50.4	578.694 ± 10.2206	117
+ Cycloheximide 2 × 10^{-4} mol/kg	2.1 ± 0.26	100	20.139 ± 91	4.1

Ehrlich ascites tumour bearing mice were given i. p. injections of 40^{-6} moles/kg of Trenimon. Cycloheximide was administered at the concentration of 40^{-4} moles/kg. The cycloheximide administration was repeated after 60 minutes. Tumour cells were harvested 2.5 hours after the application of Trenimon or the first injection of cycloheximide respectively. The Rb-uptake was measured as described in materials and methods. To measure the effect of cycloheximide on protein synthesis, controls and cycloheximide treated animals were injected with 1 μCi of ^{3}H-lysine per gram body weight 30 minutes before the cells were harvested. The data for lysine incorporation are expressed as dpm/mg acid precipitable protein.

As Table 1 demonstrates, however, this is not the case. An inhibition of protein synthesis by cycloheximide for a total period of 2 hours has no effect on the Na$^+$/K$^+$-ATPase as measured by the uptake of ^{86}Rb. 2 hours after administration of Trenimon, however, the Rb-uptake is decreased to 50% of the control level. Thus, the reduction of the Rb-uptake by Trenimon is not caused by an inhibition of protein synthesis by the alkylating agent. This conclusion is further supported by the observation that ^{3}H-lysine incorporation into total acid precipitable material is not reduced by the drug. Together with the previously reported observation demonstrating that the

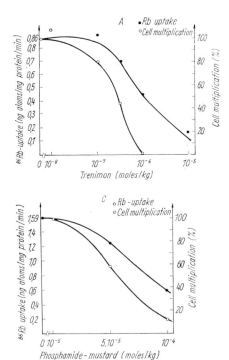

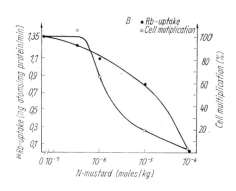

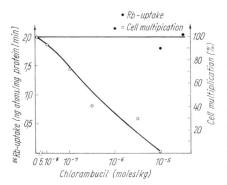

Fig. 1. A, B, C Effects of Trenimon (A), nitrogen mustard (HN2) (B) and phosphamide mustard (N,N-bis(2-chloroethyl)-phosphoricacid) diamide (C) on the uptake of ^{86}Rb and the cell multiplication of Ehrlich ascites tumour cells. Tumour bearing animals were injected i. p. with the alkylating drugs solubilized in 0.14 M NaCl and administered at concentrations indicated in the graphs. Controls received the equivalent volume of NaCl solution. The tumour cells were harvested 2 hours after administration of Trenimon and nitrogen mustard and 5 hours after adminstration of phosphamide mustard and the Rb-uptake measured as described in Methods. For the determination of cell multiplication see material and methods. ●-●-● Rb-uptake; ○-○-○ cell multiplication.

Fig. 2. Effect of chlorambucil on the Rb-uptake and cell multiplication by Ehrlich ascites tumour cells. Chlorambucil was administered i. p. in 0.2 ml 10 mM Na$_2$CO$_3$ solution. Cells were harvested 12 hours after administration of the drug. Rb-uptake and cell multiplication were determined as described under Methods. ●-●-● Rb-uptake; ○-○-○ cell multiplication.

inhibition of the ^{86}Rb-uptake by Trenimon occurs within seconds, the data of table 1 are in accordance with the assumption that the reduction of ^{86}Rb-uptake is caused by direct intercation of the alkylating drug with the plasma membrane.

Is there a correlation between the antitumour activity of the alkylating drug and the inhibition of Na$^+$/K$^+$-ATPase? The data of Fig. 1 suggest that such a correlation exists — although the Rb-uptake seems to be slightly less sensitive to the alkylating agents employed than the multiplication of the tumour cells. By evaluating these curves it should be considered, however, that the determination of cell multiplication is much less precise than the measurement of the Rb-uptake. The graphs demonstrate, however, that all concentrations of the alkylating agents which produce a clear cut reduction of cell multiplication, significantly inhibit Na^+/K^+-activity.

However, this statement cannot be generalized for all alkylating drugs. Chlorambucil is one of those substances which do not affect the Na^+/K^+-ATPase at concentrations which cause a complete block of the transplantability of the ascites tumour cells (Fig. 2).

2. The effect of akylating agents on membrane fluidity.

What is the mechanism for the inhibition of Na^+/K^+-ATPase? One possibility is, of course, a direct alkylation of the enzyme protein. An alternative would be a decrease of the fluidity of the membrane lipids. An increase of the viscosity of the lipid environment of membrane proteins would impede the conformational changes of transport proteins which are assumed to occur during catalyzed transport. An inverse relation between viscosity and the rate constant of membrane bound enzymes has been described (12) (Thus, a decrease in fluidity, i.e. an increase in viscosity, would explain why so many membrane bound transport processes are inhibited by alkylating agents.)

Table 2.

Effect of alkylating agents on membrane fluidity of Ehrlich ascites tumour cells

Drug	Fluorescence polarization	Microviscosity		Cholesterol/ phospholipid ratio
	performed on	Poise (37 °C)	%	mol/mol
None	isolated vesicles	1.60 ± 18^a	100	0.42
Trenimon (10^{-6} moles/kg)	isolated vesicles	2.41 ± 0.20^a	150	0.42
Nitrogen mustard (HN2) (10^{-5} moles/kg)	isolated vesicles	2.64 ± 0.25^a	165	n. d.[b]
Cyclophosphamide (10^{-4} moles/kg)	isolated vesicles	2.02 ± 0.2^a	126	n. d.
Chlorambucil (10^{-5} moles/kg)	isolated vesicles	2.05 ± 0.15^a	128	n. d.
None	whole cells	1.72 ± 0.1^a	100	n. d.
Nitrogen mustard (HN2) (10^{-5} moles/kg)	whole cells	2.34	136	n. d.
4-Hydroperoxycyclo-phosphamide	whole cells	2.34	136	n. d.
4-Hydroxyureacyclo-phosphamide	whole cells	2.44	141	n. d.

[a] means $\pm$ SD
[b] not determined

Ehrlich ascites tumour bearing mice were injected i. p. with the alkylating agent dissolved in 0.2 ml 0.14 M NaCl. Chlorambucil was solubilized in 0.2 ml 10 mM Na_2CO_3. The concentrations administered are listed in the table. Four hours after administration of Trenimon, HN2, cyclophosphamide or 16 hours after 4-Hydroxyperoxycyclophosphamide or 4-Hydroxyureacyclo-phosphamide the tumour cells were harvested and the microviscosity determined. For each alkylating agent as well as for controls, tumour cells from 5 mice were used and pooled. Microviscosity was determined by fluorescence polarization as described under methods. As indicated in the table, fluorescence polarization measurements were either performed on isolated membranes or on whole cells. Plasma membrane vesicles were prepared from the tumour cells according to the procedure of IM and SPECTOR (17). The isolated membrane vesicles were labelled with the fluorescence probe diphenylhexatriene. For labelling a solution of 2×10^{-3} M diphenylhexatriene in tetrahydrofuran was mixed with 300 volumes isotonic phosphate buffered saline (pH 7.4) under rapid stirring. An equal volume of the membrane preparation suspended in phosphate buffered saline was added to the diphenylhexatriene dispersion yielding final concentrations of membrane proteins of 0.5 mg per ml and of diphenylhexatriene of 3×10^{-6} M.

Whole cells were washed 3 times with phosphate buffered saline at $700 \times g$ and diluted to a concentration of 5×10^6 cells/ml. An equal volume of the diphenylhexatriene suspension in phosphate buffered saline described above was added to the cell suspension.

Fluorescence polarization measurements were performed according to SHINITZKY and INBAR (9) using a Perkin-Elmer 650-10S fluorescence photometer equipped with polarization filters. For measurements of intact cells, scattering light below 400 nm was eliminated with lead glass filters containing ceroxide produced by Swarowski & Co., Wattens, Tyrol, Austria.

Membrane fluidity was measured by fluorescence polarization using diphenylhexatriene as a lipophilic probe according to (9). Table 2 demonstrates that numerous alkylating agents increase the viscosity of the lipid phase of the membrane. As a matter of fact, all alkylating drugs which we have studied so far, decrease the fluidity of the plasma membrane.

Is the decrease in membrane fluidity correlated to the antitumour activity? Fig. 3 demonstrates the effect of nitrogen mustard on cell multiplication of Ehrlich ascites tumour cells and on membrane fluiditiy as function of the concentration of the drug. As can be seen, there is a correlation between these parameters. All concentrations of the drug which reduce the multiplication of the tumour cells, increase the viscosity of the membrane lipids.

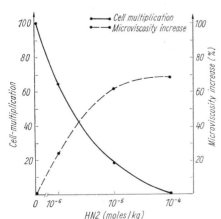

Fig. 3. Effect of nitrogen mustard (HN2) on membrane fluidity and cell multiplication Ehrlich ascites tumour cells. Mustard treatment was performed as described in the legend to Table 2. Microviscosity was measured on isolated membranes as described in the legend to Table 2. Determination of the cell multiplication was performed as described under Methods.

Is the decrease in membrane fluidity caused by a direct interaction of the alkylating agent with the cell membrane? Table 3 demonstrates that the change in membrane fluiditiy can also be produced by treating isolated membrane vesicles with the alkylating agent. It has to be concluded, therefore, that a decrease in membrane fluidity is the result of an alkylation of the membrane. Incubation of liposomes (cholesterol/phospholipid vesicles) with alkylating drugs has no effect. This indicates that the decrease in membrane fluidity is caused by an alkylation of membrane proteins. The detailed mechanism by which an alkylation of membrane proteins affects the fluidity of membrane lipids is still unclear. The cholesterol:phospholipid ratio of the plasma membrane is not changed by the alkylating agent (Table 2).

Table 3.
Viscsoity of membrane vesicles from Ehrlich ascites tumour cells and of liposomes after in vitro treatment with Trenimon

	Microviscosity (poise at 37 °C)
Control membranes	1.60
Trenimon treated membranes	2.05
Control liposomes	1.83
Trenimon treated liposomes	1.79

Membranes were isolated from Ehrlich ascites tumour cells as described in the legend to Table 2. Liposomes (Cholesterol/phospholipid ratio 0.25) were prepared according to SHINITZKY and INBAR (9). The quality of the liposome preparation was controlled by electronmicroscopy indicating more than 90% lipid bilayer vesicles. Membranes and liposomes were incubated in the presence of 10^{-6} M Trenimon at 37 °C for 15 minutes and microviscosity was determined as described in the legend to Table 2.

3. Does the decrease in membrane fluidity affect

As outlined above it could be assumed that the reduced activity of the Na^+/K^+-ATPase activity is the result of an increase in viscosity of the lipid environment of the enzyme. This, however, is not the case. The viscosity of the cell membrane can be increased by incubation of the tumour cells in presence of cholesterol (13). By these means the viscosity is raised to a level above those observed under the influence of the alkylating drugs. The increase in the viscosity, however, had almost no effect on the Na^+/K^+-ATPase (Table 4). From these data it can be concluded that the inhibition of Na^+/K^+-ATPase is caused by an alkylation of the enzyme.

Table 4.
Effect of an increase in membrane viscosity on the ^{86}Rb-uptake of Ehrlich ascites tumour cells

	Microviscosity poise	^{86}Rb-uptake ng atoms/mg protein/min
Control	1.55	1.00
+ Cholesterol	2.35	0.85

Ehrlich ascites tumour cells were suspended in 100 volumes of Krebs-Ringer-tris buffer (pH 7.4) and incubated at 37 °C in the presence of cholesterol hemisuccinate according to LYTE and SHINITZKY (14). Control cells were incubated in the absence of the cholesterol ester but otherwise treated in the same way.
Microviscosity was determined on intact cells as described in the legend to Table 2. Rb-uptake into cells was measured as described under methods.

Discussion

The data presented here support previous reports from our laboratory indicating an interference of alkylating antitumour agents with the plasma membrane of Ehrlich ascites tumour cells (1—3). For the two membrane effects studied here, i.e. inhibition of Na^+/K^+-ATPase and decrease in membrane fluidity, it could be demonstrated that these effects are due to a direct interaction of the alkylating agent with the plasma membrane and that both effects are correlated with the antitumour activity of Trenimon, nitrogen mustard and "phosphamide mustard" (N-mustard phosphoro-diamidic acid). In view of these data one may ask whether the alkylation of the plasma membrane is essential for the antitumour activity of alkylating agents. The use of an alkylating drug which cannot penetrate the cell membrane would answer the question whether an alkylation of the plasma membrane is sufficient to inhibit proliferation of tumour cells. LENSSEN and HOHORST (15) have reported that phosphamide mustard is not taken up by Ehrlich ascites tumour cells. If this is also the case for the condition used in our experiments, the antitumour effect demonstrated in Fig. 1 C should be caused by an alkylation of the cell surface. The same is possibly true for the antitumour activity of polymer-bound chlorambucil (2). However, it still remains to be demonstrated that all alkylating agents exert their antitumour activity by alkylation of the cell membrane. Furthermore, it is still unclear how an alkylation of the cell membrane leads to the inhibition of cell division. It is conceivable that the depression of Na^+/K^+-ATPase is responsible for the cytostatic effect. However, not all alkylating agents produce an inhibition of the Na^+/K^+-ATPase. Chlorambucil for instance does not affect this enzyme at concentrations which completely block the multiplication of tumour cells. Thus, the inhibition of Na^+/K^+-ATPase may be essential in those cases where this inhibition occurs but this is not a general mechanism of all alkylating drugs.

A decrease in membrane fluidity, however, is produced by all alkylating agents we have studied so far. Thus, all alkylating agents studied so far affect the cell membrane, but — with the exception of the decrease in membrane fluidity — the spectra of effects which are expressed at the cell membrane differ and depend on the alkylating agent employed. At present it is unclear how an alkylation of the cell membrane affects the proliferation of the tumour cell. An increase in membrane fluidity seems to be a prerequisite for cell proliferation (8, 16). It is conceivable, therefore, that rigidization of the cell membrane may inhibit tumour growth. Of course, this is just one out of many other possible working hypotheses which can be built to explain the cytostatic activity of alkylating agents by interaction with the cell membrane.

Summary

The alkylating agents Trenimon (2,3,5-trisethyleneiminobenzoquinone), nitrogen mustard and phosphamide mustard (N-bis(2-chloroethyl)-diamidophosphoric acid) inhibit the Na^+/K^+-ATPase of the plasma membrane of Ehrlich ascites tumour cells. The dose effect curves for this inhibition are similar to those of the antitumour activity of the drug. The reduced activity of Na^+/K^+-ATPase is not caused by a depression of protein synthesis. No inhibition of Na^+/K^+-ATPase can be seen after treatment with Chlorambucil (p-N,N-bis(2-chloroethyl)aminophenylbutyric acid).

The influence of the alkylating agents on membrane fluidity was measured by fluorescence polarization with diphenylhexatriene as a probe. All alkylating agents studied so far decrease the fluidity of the plasma membrane. This effect is caused by a direct interaction of the alkylating agent with the plasma membrane and occurs at all concentrations which exhibit an antitumour activity. No effect on membrane fluidity is observed if protein-free lipid vesicles are treated with alkylating agents.

References

1. GRUNICKE, H., HIRSCH, E., WOLF, H., BAUER, U. and KIEFER, G.: Exptl. Cell Res. *90* (1975), 357
2. GRUNICKE, H., GANTNER, G., HOLZWEBER, F., IHLENFELDT, M. and PUSCHENDORF, B.: Adv. in Enzyme Regulation (WEBER, G. ed.) vol. 17, p. 291, Pergamon Press, New York, 1979
3. IHLENFELDT, M., GANTNER, G., HARRER, M., PUSCHENDORF, B., PUTZER, H. and GRUNICKE, H.: Cancer Res. *41* (1981), 289
4. BURGER, M. M.: Fed. Proc. *32* (1973), 91
5. EDELMAN, G. M.: J. Biochem. *79* (1976), 1
6. PRESCOTT, D. M.: in: Reproduction of eukaryotic cells, pp. 47—106, Academic Press, New York, 1976
7. HYNES, R. O. (ed.): Surface of normal and malignant cells. J. Wiely and Sons, Chichester, New York, Toronto, 1979
8. BRUSCALUPI, G., CURATOLA, G., LENAZ, G., LEONI, S., MANGIANTINI, M. T., MAZZANTI, L., SPAGNUOLO, S. und TRENTALANCE, A.: Biochim. Biophys. Acta *597* (1980), 263
9. SHINITZKY, M. and INBAR, M.: Biochim. Biophys. Acta *433* (1979), 133
10. van HOEVEN, R. P. and EMMELOT, P.: J. Membrane Biol. *9* (1972), 105
11. BARTLETT, G. R.: J. Biol. Chem. *234* (1959), 466
12. SHINITZKY, M., BOROCHOV, H. and WILBRANDT, W. (1980) in: Membrane Transport in erythrocytes (Lassen, U. V., Ussing, H. H. Wieth, J. O. eds.) p. 91, Munksgaard, Copenhagen
13. SHINITZKY, M. and BARENHOLZ, Y.: Biochim. Biophys. Acta *515* (1978), 367
14. LYTE, M. and SHINITZKY, M.: Chem. Phys. Lipids *24* (1979), 45
15. LENSSEN, U. and HOHORST, H. J.: J. Cancer Res. Clin. Oncol. *93* (1979), 161
16. CHENG, S. and LEVY, D.: Arch. Biochem. Biophys. *196* (1979), 424
17. IM, W. B. and SPECTOR, A.: J. Biol. Chem. *255* (1980), 764

Acknowledgement

These studies were supported by the Austrian Science Foundation (Fonds zur Förderung der Wissenschaftlichen Forschung in Österreich, Project 3890).

Dept. of Surgery, University of Cambridge
Addenbrooke's Hosp., Cambridge, England

The Synergistic Effect of Drugs and Antibodies

D. A. L. Davies

Introduction

While a cell mediated immune response (CMI) can be mounted by a patient against his own tumour, a humoral antibody response is less frequently demonstrable. This may be due to limitations by the methods available, but also because for the last two decades CMI has attracted nearly all the attention and a vast literature exists covering this topic. Attempts have been made to use the information for clinical application and the stimulation of CMI has been tried in many different forms; the treatment has had benefits but these are not on a scale such as to radically alter a patient's prospects in any form of cancer. This approach is, of course, non-specific because transfer of specifically immune cells is not possible due to immune rejection.

This disappointing outcome became clear by about the time that methods were invented for producing monoclonal antibodies by fusion (KOHLER and MILSTEIN 1975) and this is now attracting increasing attention as a means for obtaining useful amounts of antibody exactly specific for particular tumours. Treatment of animals bearing experimentally induced tumours, using humoral antibody against the tumour cells, has not had an illustrious history, but examples of small successes can be found in model systems (GORER and AMOS 1956; DAVIES 1963). It has not been possible to test this clinically in any clear way. Most reviews of immunotherapy in cancer do not actually mention specific immunotherapy, or they pass it over in a few words.

In the following text data are given to show a substantial synergy between tumour directed antibody and synthetic drugs in experimental animals carrying transplanted tumours. The drugs used in cancer treatment are rather non-specific cell poisons with little difference between therapeutic and toxic doses. The question arises as to whether these drugs work because antibody is present and whether the 'better drugs' are those better able to collaborate with antibody in a synergistic way. Is it possible that chemotherapy in cancer works (to the extent it does) more or less because of such a synergy? Does the point at which chemotherapy is no longer effective in a particular case coincide with the time when, for some reason, free antibody is no longer available in the circulation.

The subject of drug attachment to antibodies for homing has been rejuvenated by the advent of monoclonal antibodies. This topic is not dealt with here. However, it is increasingly important with the renewed effort in that field, to establish a baseline such as to detect a homing effect over and above any synergy between the drug and antibody unattached. Claims have been made for homing effects by complexes which dissociated in vivo after injection and the effect found should correctly have been attributed to synergy between drug and antibody. It is also possible (our own

127

unpublished work) for a drug-antibody complex to behave as a (macromolecular) drug and synergize with free antibody; again an apparent homing effect is correctly attributable to synergy of the kind described below. For such reasons the control experiments needed in studies of homing drugs on tumour cells in vivo need to be specially exacting.

Materials and methods

Animals and tumours

EL4 is a lymphoma originally induced with dimethylbenzanthracene in C57BL mice (GORER and AMOS, 1956) and grows readily as an ascites tumour. EL4 has been extensively studied serologically and has at least 3 distinguishable specificities not possessed by C57BL/6 mice: these are 'X' (GORER and AMOS, 1956), 'E' (AOKI et al, 1970) and 'L' (LECLERC et al, 1970). These cells are TL negative (BOYSE, STOCKERT and OLD, 1968). The lymphoma SB1 arose spontaneously in a Balb/c mouse in our colony; it does not grow as an ascites tumour but enlarges the spleen up to 2 g (wet weight) if cells are injected intraperitoneally or subcutaneously; it does not grow at the site of injection. About 5 cells constitutes a lethal dose in the syngeneic host but 10^7 cells fail to grow even in other H-2^d mice (DBA/2, B10.D2).

Immunization

Antisera were recovered by standard methods but the immunization schedules were varied over a series of experiments. Groups of mice or rabbits were used as recipients for immunization with tumour cells or with normal cells as control.

Cytotoxicity

Cytotoxicity of allo- and xenoantisera was assessed on appropriate target cells (lymph node cells or tumour cells) by release of ^{51}Cr label from the cells in the presence of complement. Generally guinea-pig complement has been used and tubes were incubated for 1 h. However, in cases where it has been difficult to obtain a cytotoxic titre against tumour target cells (when none remained after absorption for lymph node cells), rabbit complement has been used and incubation times were increased up to 3 h.

Absorption

Allo- and xenoantisera were absorbed in vitro, mainly using spleen cells but in some cases using liver or membrane preparations ('eluate') (DAVIES, 1966) from lymphoid tissue. Both liver cell suspensions and eluate were quite difficult to pack down sufficiently by centrifugation in order to avoid substantial losses of absorbed serum volume. In any event, absorption was taken to completion as tested by complement mediated cytotoxicity for normal cells.
The amount of absorption required depended on the number of injections given to raise a particular serum. In all experiments, antisera were submitted to small scale absorption tests to determine likely requirements before committing whole batches. Generally 3 or 4 absorption stages were needed to remove all cytotoxicity for normal cells. Each stage was monitored in order not to add absorbing material in excesss with the prospect of losing tumour specific antibody nonspecifically. When spleens alone were used, 3000—5000 were usually required to absorb fully 100 ml of antiserum. All absorptions included material from mice of the same H-2 genotype as that of the tumour cells used for immunization. Thus, spleens from a variety of mouse strains were

128

used for the bulk absorptions but some H-2^b spleens were always included in absorptions of EL4 antisera and some H-2^d spleens always included in absorptions of SB1 antisera. This was to remove xeno-antibodies having individual recognition discrimination (STAINES et al, 1973). All the sera were centrifuged at 80,000 g for 60 min before use.

Fractionation

Ammonium sulphate (AmSO$_4$) was used and sera precipitated at 40% saturation at 4 °C. The 40% precipitate was recovered, after several hours of equilibrium, re-dissolved and re-precipitated at the same level a second time. The precipitate was then washed with 40% AmSO$_4$, centrifuged out and re-dissolved for dialysis and recovery. The quality of the immunoglobulin and an assessment of loss and recovery were made by checking the rabbit Ig by immunodiffusion with a goat Ig anti-rabbit Ig.

Protection tests

The immunoglobulin fractions were tested for their ability to interfere with the growth of lymphoma in vivo after suitable absorption until non-reactive with normal cells. The severity of the tests was adjusted as necessary by selecting different numbers of cells for challenge, by selecting routes (intraperitoneal or subcutaneous), by adjusting the time-lapse between challenge and treatment and by altering as necessary the number of treatment doses. Groups of mice varied from 5 to 15 (depending on the availability of serum) and the day of death recorded.

Results

In the SB1(Balb/c) and EL4(C57/BL) combinations it is possible, after complete absorption with normal syngeneic tissue to detect a direct cytotoxic effect on tumour cell targets, if not using guinea-pig complement, at least using rabbit complement (DAVIES and O'NEILL, 1974). When absorbed serum is tested against normal lymphoid cells to find if absorption is adequate, it is not easy to decide if there is residual antibody against normal tissue antigens and whether what remains (detectable or not) would constitute a hazard on injection. We have taken an endpoint as referred to above.

In Fig. 1 it can be seen that progression in growth of SB1 was significantly inhibited by absorbed alloantiserum. An immunoglobulin preparation from that alloantiserum was a little less effective in postponing death in these mice, at the amount used.

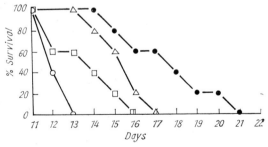

Fig. 1. Protection of Balb/c mice against SB1 cells, challenge dose 10^3, i. p. Treatment, injections i. p. 4 h after challenge and again at 24 h intervals 3 times with: normal mouse serum (0.4ml), O——O; indiluted, absorbed alloantiserum from C3H mice (0.25 ml), □——□; Ig prepared from that antiserum, (2 mg) △——△; the same amplified by 0.2 mg chlorambucil, ●——●.

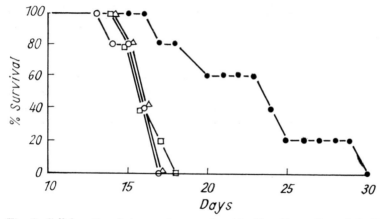

Fig. 2. Collaboration between drugs and antibodies. Protection of C57BL/6 mice against EL4 with cyclophosphamide (500 μg) and tumour specific antiserum (R129/130 0.5 ml, at 1:2 dilution). Treatment started 96 h after challenge. Saline controls, ○—○; antiserum alone, △—△: cyclophosphamide alone, □—□; drug followed 1 h later by antiserum, ●—●.

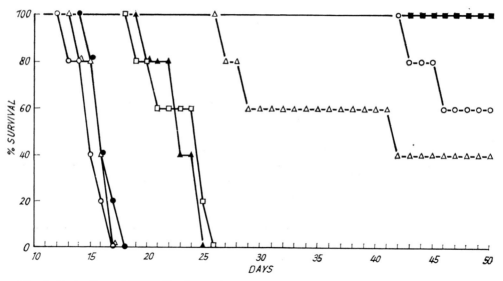

Fig. 3. Protection of C57BL/6 mice against syngeneic EL4 lymphoma (10,000 lethal dose challenge). ○—○, controls, 0.9% NaCl solution injections only; △—△, normal rabbit serum only, with a time lapse of 48 h between challenge and treatment. Treatment with absorbed rabbit anti-EL4 specific serum (0.5 ml, doses at 1:2 dilution): time lapse, 48 h (□) and 96 h (●); with melphalan (20-μg doses), time-lapse, 48 hr (▲). Treatment with melphalan (20-μg doses) followed 1 h later by antiserum (0.5 ml doses at 1:2 dilution): time-lapse 24 h (■); 48 h (○—○); and 96 h (△—△).

In collaboration with a maximum permissible dose of chlorambucil, which was unable to influence the outcome when used alone, a significant prolongation of life is evident.

The experiment shown in Fig. 2 employed EL4 with cyclophosphamide. In this case the time-lapse between tumour challenge and the beginning of treatment was 96 h and it will be noted that no attempt was made to 'save' the animals in that only 4 treatment doses were given and the ensuing life span recorded. In this case no difference can be seen between mice injected with saline, with antiserum, or with drug. However substantial prolongation of life can be seen when antiserum and drug were used (injected within an hour of each other) each at the dose levels used previously.

The experiment shown in Fig. 3 makes the point that an amount of serum able to influence tumour growth when the time-lapse between challenge and the beginning of treatment was 48 h., was insufficient when the time-lapse was increased to 96 h. The largest tolerated dose of melphalan, used alone, gave a modest effect but used with absorbed antitumour xenoantiserum, substantial improvement can be seen with a time lapse of 96 h, over half survival using a 48 h delay, and with a lapse of 24 h, all mice survived indefinitely.

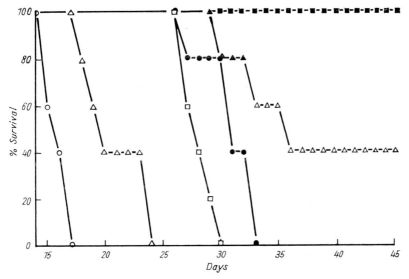

Fig. 4. Protection of C57BL/6 mice against syngeneic EL4 lymphoma. Time-lapse is 96 h throughout. 0, control mice, given injections of normal rabbit serum (0.5 ml); △, treatment with absorbed tumour specific xenoantiserum (0.5 ml doses); □, treatment with cytosine arabinoside (5 mg doses). Treatment with drug followed 1 h later by antiserum (0.5 ml doses at 1:2 dilution), using chlorambucil at 200-μg doses (●); melphalan at 20-μg doses (▲); cytosine arabinoside at 5-mg doses (■).

It will be seen from Fig. 4 that in combination with the same amount of antiserum, and based on a relevant set of controls, cytosine arabinoside was more effective than melphalan (phenylalanine mustard), and melphalan better chlorambucil.

A gross improvement seems to be obtainable by these kinds of combinations between antibody and drug. From the graphs in Figs. 1—4 it cannot be decided whether the effect is e.g. additive or synergistic. By abstracting data from a series of experiments carried out, the figures in Table 1 were obtained, confined to animals which survived permanently (and ignoring those whose lives were only prolonged). Inspection of the figures for drug alone, antibody alone and both together show very clearly that the effect is actually a synergy.

Table 1.
Protection of C57BL mice from EL4 lymphoma by drug, antibody or both

Drug (no. of experiments)	Permanent survivors*		
	Antibody	Drug	Both
Cytosine arabinoside (17)	16/275	5/120	126/260
Adriamycin (2)	0/15	0/15	1/15
Daunomycin (1)	1/5	1/5	4/5
Methotrexate (2)	0/15	0/15	1/15
Chlorambucil (9)	4/76	0/70	32/67
Melphalan (14)	6/195	6/125	187/310
Phenylenediamine mustard (6)	1/55	1/30	16/30
Cyclophosphamide (2)	0/20	0/10	2/10
DTIC (1)	0/10	0/10	7/10

* (over 100 days).

Discussion

The synergy described is a powerful effect; it is not confined to a particular tumour (others than those mentioned here have been used); nor to a particular mouse strain; nor to a particular drug; nor to a particular preparation of antibody; nor to a particular inoculation site. Susceptible tumours may grow as ascites, as a subcutaneous growth or as a spleen enlarging lymphoma (inoculated subcutaneously). The effect was first revealed in control series when putative drug-Ig complexes were being tested for homing. Homing drugs and toxins is not yet a clinical reality so we should take this synergy (ADS = antibody-drug synergy) seriously as having clinical possibilities. Pilot studies, (something less than clinical trials) were carried out, initially in patient's with advanced secondary melanoma (EVERALL et al, 1977) and in view of the problem-free course of that exercise, a series of post lung resection bronchial carcinoma patients were treated (NEWMAN et al, 1977). In both instances goat anti-patient's tumour serum was used, after extensive absorption with normal human tissue. The lung cancer study also ran a trouble-free course, with suggestive results that should be followed up.
It is possible that ADS is a part of chemotherapy and that progression to lack of response to chemotherapy is loss of free antibody, e.g. by binding into antigen-antibody complexes. In any event the same amount of drug can be made more effective in the presence of antibody or alternately a smaller amount of drug might be used in the presence of antibody with undiminished effect and concomitant reduction in general toxicity.
Actual in vivo homing of drugs carried by antibodies has been achieved but not in a spectacular way so far. Positive results were recorded in mice (DAVIES & O'NEILL, 1975) using direct carbodiimide linked drug and also using a carrier system, drug-carrier-Ig (e.g. melphalan-polyglutamic acid-immune Ig) to minimize loss of antibody activity (ROWLAND et al, 1975). This was tested in a single melanoma patient with good results; the patient did not produce an immune response against the goat Ig over a year of intermittent treatment. Other carriers have been used successfully (ROWLAND, 1977), In experimental work it is important to be sure that ADS is not confused with genuine ADC.

The important new development for both these effects is the availability of monoclonal antibodies to replace laboriously prepared and absorbed immune Ig. Purity and reproducibility are features of these new reagents and methodology has advanced such that monoclonal antibodies could be prepared against a particular patient's tumour in time to be made use of for such a patient.

Until such time as linkage of drugs and toxins to monoclonal antibodies is successfully perfected for clinical use, the ADS system should be used, — drug-monoclonal antibody synergy, — it is a likely source of untapped help in clinical cancer.

References

AOKI, T., STÜCK, B., OLD, L. J., HAMMERLING, U. and DEHARVEN, E.: 'E' Antigen: A cell surface antigen of C57BL leukaemias. Cancer Res. *30* (1970), 244

BOYSE, R., STOCKERT, E. and OLD, L. J.: Isoantigens of the H-2 and TLa loci of the mouse. J. Exp. Med. *128* (1968), 85

DAVIES, D. A. L.: Occurrence of X antigenic specificity in histocompatibility antigens prepared from mouse leukaemic cells. Br. J. Exp. Path. *44* (1963), 546

DAVIES, D. A. L.: Mouse histocompatibility isoantigens derived from normal and from tumour cells. Immunology *11* (1966), 115

DAVIES, D. A. L.: The combined effect of Drugs and tumour-specific antibodies in protection against a mouse lymphoma. Cancer Res. *34* (1974), 3040

DAVIES, A. D. L., BUCKHAM, S. and MANSTONE, A. J.: Protection of mice against syngeneic lymphomas. 2. Collaboration between drugs and antibodies. Brit. J. Cancer *30* (1974), 305

DAVIES, A. D. L., MANSTONE, A. J. and BUCKHAM, S.: Protection of mice against syngeneic lymphomas. 1. Use of antibodies. Brit. J. Cancer *30* (1974), 297

DAVIES, D. A. L. and O'NEILL, G. J.: In vivo and in vitro effects of tumour specific antibodies with Chlorambucil. Brit. J. Cancer *28* (Suppl. 1.) (1973), 285

DAVIES, D. A. L. and O'NEILL, G. J.: Methods of cancer immuno-chemotherapy (DRAB and DRAC) using antisera against tumour specific cell-membrane antigens. VII Int. Cancer Congr. 218, Excerpta Medica, Amsterdam, 1975

DAVIES, D. A. L., O'NEILL, G. J., ROWLAND, G. F., NEWMAN, C. E. and FORD, C. H. J.: Tumour antigens and the use of xenoantisera: experimental and clinical applications. In: Tumour-associated antigens and their specific immune response. Serono Symp. Vol. 16. Ed. F. SPREAFICO & R. ARNON. Academic Press, 1974

EVERALL, J. D., DOWD, P., DAVIES, D. A. L., O'NEILL, G. J. and ROWLAND, G. F.: Treatment of melanoma by passive humoral immunotherapy using antibody drug synergism. Lancet *i* (1977), 1105

GORER, P. A. and AMOS, D. B.: Passive immunity in mice against C57BL leucosis EL4 by means of iso-immune serum. Cancer Res. *16* (1956), 338

KOHLER, G. and MILSTEIN, C.: Continuous cultures of fused cells secreting antibody of predefined specificity. Nature, Lond. 256 (1975), 495

LECLERC, J. C., LEVY, J. P., VARET, B., OPPENHEIM, S. and SENIK, A.: Antigenic analysis of L strain cells: a new murine leukemia-associated antigen, "L". Cancer Res. *30* (1970), 2073

NEWMAN, C. E., FORD, C. H. J., DAVIES, D. A. L. and O'NEILL, G. J.: Antibody-drug synergism: an assessment of specific passive immunotherapy in bronchial carcinoma. Lancet *ii* (1977), 163

ROWLAND, G. F.: Effective anti-tumour conjugates of alkylating drug and antibody using dextran as the intermediate carrier. Europ. J. Cancer *13* (1977), 593

ROWLAND, G. F., O'NEILL, G. J. and DAVIES, D. A. L.: Prevention of lymphoma growth in mice by a covalent drug-carrier-antibody complex. In: Chemotherapy Vol 8. Ed. K. HELLMANN & T. A. CONNORS. New York: Plenum Press, 1976

STAINES, N. A., O'NEILL, G. J., GUY, K. and DAVIES, D. A. L.: Xenoantisera against lymphoid cells: specificity and use in monitoring purification of mouse and human histocompatibility antigens. Tissue Antigens *3* (1973), 1

Norsk Hydro's Institute for Cancer Research and The Norwegian Cancer Society,
The Norwegian Radium Hospital, Oslo, Norway

Cancerostatic Lectins

A. Pihl and O. Fodstad

Lectins constitute a large group of sugar binding proteins of non-immune origin. Most lectins are found in plants and have two or more sugar binding sites and are hence able to bind together and agglutinate cells and glucoconjugates (Sharon and Lis, 1972; Lis and Sharon, 1977). Due to their ability to bind to cell surface glycoproteins and glycolipids, lectins like phytoagglutinin, wheat germ agglutinin and concanavalin A have been widely used for the study of the surface properties of cells. There is now considerable evidence that the surface of cancer cells has altered properties and many authors have reported that transformed cells are more easily agglutinated by lectins than are normal cells. However, most lectins have rather low toxicity to cells and only two rather special and highly toxic lectins, abrin and ricin, have been shown to possess cancerostatic properties.

Abrin and ricin which are among the most toxic proteins known, occur, together with powerful agglutinins, in the seeds of *Abrus precatorius* and *Ricinus communis*. Originally, the toxic properties of abrin and ricin preparations were believed to be associated with their agglutinating properties. However, subsequent work demonstrated that the pure toxins virtually lack agglutinating activity, as they possess only a single sugar binding site. We termed these proteins monovalent lectins (Olsnes et al, 1974) since they bind specifically to cell surface receptors and have many features in common with the agglutinins. Koucurek and Hořejši (1981) likewise feel that the term lectin should include also such proteins as abrin and ricin which have a single sugar binding site, whereas Goldstein et al (1980) have proposed that the term lectin should be reserved for substances capable of agglutinating cells and precipitating glycoconjugates.

The cancerostatic properties of abrin, ricin and related proteins, appear to be of considerable interest, as these proteins act by inhibiting cellular protein synthesis, i.e. by a mechanism different from that of most cancerostatic agents in clinical use.

Biochemical properties

Considerable information is now available on the biochemical and biological properties of abrin, ricin and the related protein modeccin (for review, see Olsnes and Pihl, 1976, 1981). Although they occur in widely different plants, they are very similar in structure and mechanism of action. The proteins have molecular weights of about 65,000 and consist of two polypeptide chains, joined by a disulfide bond. The larger chains, the B-chains, have molecular weights of about 35,000 and are glycopeptides that bind to cell surface receptors containing terminal galactose residues. The toxic action is associated exclusively with the A-chains.

The interaction of abrin and ricin with the cell surface has been extensively studied in our laboratory. The surface of animal cell contains a large number of binding sites for abrin and ricin and the binding of the toxins through the B-chain is the first and obligatory step in the uptake of the toxins (or their A-chains). An appreciable fraction of the toxin bound is internalized by endocytosis, but only a small number of A-chains seems able to penetrate the membrane and enter into the cytosol. The entry of the A-chains requires metabolic energy (SANDVIG and OLSNES, 1981). However, the detailed mechanism whereby the hydrophilic A-chains penetrate the lipophilic membranes is not understood.

The A-chains inhibit protein synthesis by inactivating specifically the large ribosomal subunit, as first demonstrated by STIRPE and collaborators (SPERTI et al, 1973). The A-chains act catalytically and inactivate a large number of ribosomes per molecule. They do so by modifying the surface of the 60 S ribosomal subunit in such a way that its affinity for the elongation factor 2 is decreased.

The enzymatic activity of the A-chains accounts for the high toxicity of these proteins and there is evidence that the presence of a single A-chain in the cytosol is sufficient to kill a cell (EIKLID et al, 1980). The A-chains appear to be inactive when they are joined to the B-chains through the disulfide bond. The enzymatic activity is acquired when the A-chains change conformation as they are liberated from the B-chains.

When cells are exposed to abrin or ricin, inhibition of protein synthesis is seen only after a certain lag time which decreases with increasing concentration of the toxins. After the inhibition of protein synthesis is evident, DNA synthesis is also inhibited and still later, RNA synthesis as well is inhibited. These effects are believed to be secondary to the inhibition of protein synthesis. Studies of synchronized HeLa cells indicate that these are equally sensitive to the toxins during the different phases of the cell cycle (OLSNES and REFSNES, 1978).

Pharmacological properties

The LD_{50}-doses of abrin and ricin in animals are of the order 1 to 3 µg/kg of body weight (FODSTAD et al, 1976, 1979). For both toxins the dose-response curves decline steeply after an initial horizontal phase (Fig. 1a). Thus, all animals die within a narrow dose range. The minimum lethal dose which is about 0.7 and 2.7 µg/kg for abrin and ricin, respectively, is a more meaningful parameter than the LD_{50}.

The relationship between dose and survival time is shown in Fig. 1b. Even after supralethal doses no animals die before 10 h and the survival time is strictly related to the dose (FODSTAD et al, 1976, 1979). The curve is highly reproducible and is used in our laboratory for the biological standarization of the toxins.

The main toxic effect observed in mice, rats and dogs were anorexia, weakness, weight loss and a moderate fever. In dogs recovering from non-lethal doses, no delayed abnormalities were observed (FODSTAD et al, 1979).

An important finding is that abrin and ricin, in contrast to most cytostatic agents, have only little effect on myelopoiesis. After sublethal doses a rapid but transient decrease of the peripheral thrombocytes occurred. However, even after doses that eventually led to the death of the animals, abrin and ricin did not depress the number of peripheral leukocytes (FODSTAD et al, 1977, 1979).

In studies where mice were treated with ricin and the survival of the colony-forming bone marrow cells was measured in a spleen colony assay, the effect was not greater on cells that had been induced to proliferate rapidly, than on resting bone marrow cells (FODSTAD and PIHL, 1980). Thus, the effect of ricin on the bone marrow is not proliferation dependent. On this basis ricin and abrin might be expected to be active also on slow-growing tumours with a low growth fraction.

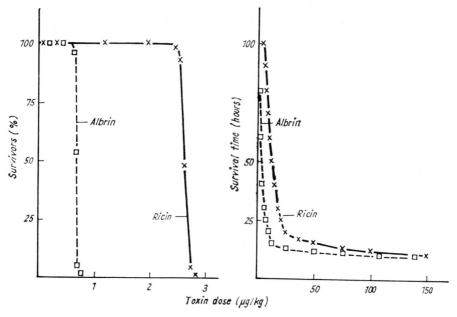

Fig. 1. Effect of abrin and ricin on survival of mice. Groups of mice were given increasing doses of abrin and ricin i. v. and the number of survivors (a) and survival time (b) were observed. Data from FODSTAD et al 1979.

Since abrin and ricin are foreign proteins, they are immunogenic in animals and induce the formation of antibodies. In mice as well as in humans, antibodies to ricin appear somewhat faster than antibodies to abrin. In mice antibody formation can be effectively suppressed by cyclophosphamide and prednisolone treatment (GODAL, unpublished data).

Cancerostatic properties

Effect of murine tumours

The cancerostatic action of abrin and ricin was first clearly demonstrated by LIN et al (1970) who reported that the toxins strongly inhibited the growth of Ehrlich ascites tumour in mice. Later we tested the anticancer activity of abrin and ricin in four murine tumours (FODSTAD et al, 1977; PIHL et al, 1979). It was found that in mice with Ehrlich ascites, abrin given i.p. prolonged the survival of the animals, but the effect was less dramatic than that earlier reported by LIN et al, (1970). The effect of abrin was comparable to that of adriamycin, but less than that of cyclophosphamide. Ricin was less active. In contrast, in L 1210 ascites, ricin gave better results than abrin, but both toxins were inferior to adriamycin and cyclophosphamide. In the more slowly growing B16 melanoma, abrin and ricin were about as efficient as cyclophosphamide and adriamycin. In Lewis lung carcinoma the toxins inhibited the growth of the primary tumour, but they did not enhance the life span of the animals which succumbed to their lung metastases.

The effect of the toxins on systemic L 1210 leukemia was studied in mice given the cells i. v. (FODSTAD and PIHL, 1978). Treatment with abrin and ricin did not enhance the survival of the animals. This is not surprising, as the proteins would not be expected to pass the blood/brain barrier. However, when the effect of the drugs on the survival of the leukemic colony-forming bone marrow cells was measured in a spleen colony assay, it was found that ricin had a strong differential effect on the leukemic bone marrow cells (FODSTAD and PIHL, 1978). The effect was of the same magnitude as that of adriamycin, whereas abrin had a much lower effect.

Effect of human tumours

The effect of abrin and ricin on human tumours growing as xenografts in athymic, nude mice was then studied (FODSTAD et al, 1977). Tumour specimens obtained at surgery were serially transplanted in nude mice and the tumour growth was evaluated by measuring two perpendicular diameters with Vernier callipers. The experimental

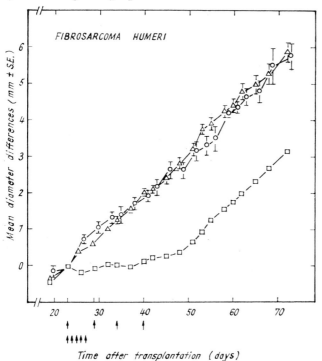

Fig. 2. Effect of abrin on the growth in nude mice of the fibrosarcoma from human humerus. On day 23 after implantation 26 mice were treated i. v. with 7 ng of abrin per 20 g body weight and the injection was repeated on days 29, 34 and 40 (upper row of arrows). In addition 5 mice were treated with 5-fluorouracil (200 µg per 20 g body weight per day for 5 days; lower row of arrows). Twenty mice were used as controls. Bars, S. E. ▲, untreated mice; ○, mice treated with 5-fluorouracil; □, mice treated with abrin. Data taken from FODSTAD et al, (1977).

Table 1.
Effect of abrin and ricin on human tumours in athymic, nude mice

Tumour type	Number	Effect of		
		Abrin	Ricin	Reference drug
Malignant melanoma	40	++	+	++(+) (DTIC)
Colon carcinoma	3	++	++	(+) (5-Fluorouracil)
Breast carcinoma	1	+	+	++++ (Cyclophosphamide)
Ovarian carcinoma	4	++	+(+)	+++(+) (Thiotepa)
Ovarian sarcoma	2	+(+)	+	+ (Cyclophosphamide)
Fibrosarcoma humeri	1	++(+)	++	+ (Cyclophosphamide)
Ewing's sarcoma	1	++	+	+ (Actinomycin D)
Embryonal testicular carcinoma	1	—	++	++++ (Cyclophosphamide)

—	No inhibtion
+	Definite growth inhibition
++	Slope of growth curve reduced by 50% or more
+++	Cessation of tumour growth for more than a week
++++	Disappearance of tumour

animals were treated i. v. with maximum tolerable doses of the toxins. In Fig. 2 a typical example is shown. It is seen that in this fibrosarcoma, abrin induced a pronounced growth inhibition which lasted for about 30 days. Then growth resumed at about the same rate as in the untreated control animals. The results obtained with different xenografts are summarized in Table 1 (PIHL and FODSTAD, 1980). It can be seen that the effect of abrin and ricin was as good as that of some of the standard drugs currently used in the treatment of these tumours. This was the case with several melanomas, colorectal carcinomas and with ovarian sarcomas, a fibrosarcoma and a Ewing's sarcoma. It should be noted that although abrin and ricin are similar in structure and mechanism of action, they showed definite differences in their effect on various tumours.

Mechanism of action

The above data do indicate that both abrin and ricin have definite cytostatic properties. The reason for this selective growth inhibiting effect on malignant tumours is poorly understood. In vitro, all eukaryotic nucleated cells appear to be sensitive to abrin and ricin. It seems unlikely that the ribosomes of cancer cells are more sensitive to the A-chains than are those of normal cells. Possibly the difference is related to altered surface properties in cancer cells, facilitating their uptake of the A-chains into the cytosol.

Combination therapy

The finding that abrin and ricin have little or no bone marrow-suppressive effect and act by a mechanism different from that of most cancerostatic agents, suggested that the toxins might be of value in combination therapy. Data have been obtained in support of this view.

138

In Lewis lung carcinoma a small to moderate dose of abrin which had little or no effect when given alone, potentiated strongly the effect of cyclophosphamide, without increasing the toxicity (GUNDERSEN and FODSTAD, 1979). Furthermore, in a melanoma xenograft where abrin had a modest effect and DTIC a more pronounced effect, the combination of the two (Fig. 3) was clearly more effective than each drug given alone. Thus, in this case the growth curve initially followed that after abrin treatment alone, whereupon the tumour decreased in size to a level beneath that of the start of the treatment (FODSTAD et al, 1980).

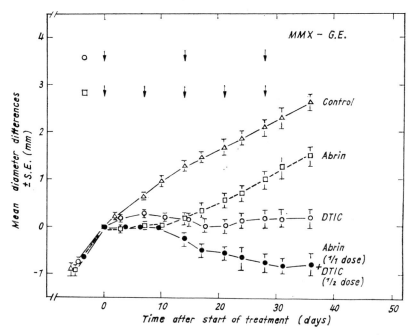

Fig. 3. Effect of abrin and DTIC, given singly and in combination on the growth of a human malignant melanoma xenograft. Each group of mice consisted of 8—12 animals. Abrin was given in single doses i. v. 350 ng/kg every week and DTIC was given i. p. (50 mg/kg) every second week. Bars, S. E. Data taken from FODSTAD et al, 1980).

Particularly interesting results were obtained in mice inoculated with L 1210 cells i.v. and subsequently treated with mixtures of ricin and adriamycin. Spleen colony assays demonstrated that when a small constant dose of ricin (1 µg/kg) was given together with increasing doses of adriamycin, a dramatic, synergistic effect on the leukemic bone marrow cells was observed (PIHL and FODSTAD, 1979, FODSTAD and PIHL, 1980). The effect of the combination on leukemic cells residing in spleen and liver was examined by using end point dilution technique, according to HEWITT (1978). The results showed (FODSTAD and PIHL, 1980) that in liver and spleen the effect of the combination was 5 to 10 times greater than that expected if the drugs had acted additively.

Recently, we have found synergistic effect also with mixtures of abrin and adriamycin, as well as with mixtures of ricin with daunorubicin, a substance closely related to adriamycin (FODSTAD and PIHL, submitted). Also, a fixed dose of ricin enhanced considerably the antileukemic effect of cisplatinum and of vincristine (Fig. 4). The dose of ricin did not enhance the toxicity of the conventional drugs on resting or proliferating normal bone marrow cells or the overall toxicity, as measured by the survival of non-leukemic animals. Since the antileukemic effect was more than additive by all assays used, this implies that a small dose of ricin gave a true potentiation of the effect of daunorubicin, cisplatinum and vincristine in L 1210 leukemia. We feel that these data are rather promising from a clinical point of view and they clearly warrant further studies.

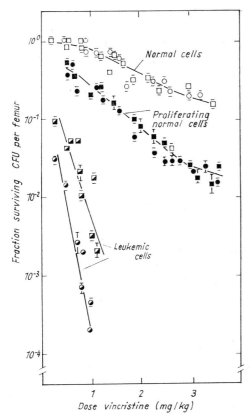

Fig. 4. Effect of increasing doses of vincristine, alone and in combination with a fixed dose of ricin on resting and proliferating normal bone marrow cells and on leukemic bone marrow cells. Groups of mice were treated i. v. with vincristine, as indicated, and a fixed dose of 1 μg/kg of ricin. Then the number of surviving colony-forming bone marrow cells was determined by spleen colony assays. The symbols represent the average for 8 mice: Bars, S. E., CFU, colony forming units; squares, vincristine alone; circles, ricin/vincristine combinations. Open symbols, normal cells; filled symbols, proliferating normal cells; half filled symbols, leukemic cells.

The simplest interpretation of the synergism between the toxic proteins and the conventional drugs is that somehow the presence of the one component facilitates the uptake of the other one. Since binding to cell surface receptors is the first step in the uptake of the toxins, such binding may conceivably alter the permeability of the cell membrane to other drugs. However, in view of the evidence that the presence of a single A-chain in the cytosol is sufficient to kill a cell, the other possibility, i.e. that the conventional drugs somehow increase the uptake of the toxins may perhaps be more probable. In attempts to elucidate the nature of the interaction between the drugs, experiments are in progress to see whether ricin will overcome the resistance of cells to e.g. adriamycin and vice versa.

Potential use in human cancers

A Phase-I clinical trial of abrin was initiated at the Norwegian Radium Hospital several years ago. Therapy-resistant cancers in late stages have been treated with increasing doses of abrin i.v. In most cases the side effects have been moderate and several favourable responses have been seen. However, since the dose-lethality curves are steep in animals and possibly also in man, we have postponed further testing until we are able to monitor the levels of the toxins in the blood. We now have an ELISA method which is sensitive enough to measure picogram levels of toxins in the blood (GODAL, unpublished data).

Although our results with murine tumours and human tumour xenografts show that abrin and ricin do have cancerostatic properties when given in adequate doses, we feel that these agents offer greatest promise as components in combination therapy. The fact that these toxins are immunogenic and that the antibody formation can be rather effectively suppressed by concurrent treatment with alkylating agents and prednisolone, further supports this view.

References

1. BRUCE, W. R. and van der GAAG, H. A.: Nature (Lond.) *199* (1963), 79
2. EIKLID, K., OLSNES, S. and PIHL, A.: Exp. Cell Res. *126* (1980), 321
3. FODSTAD, Ø., OLSNES,S. and PIHL, A.: Br. J. Cancer *34* (1976), 418
4. FODSTAD, Ø., OLSNES, S. and PIHL, A.: Cancer Res. *37* (1977), 4559
5. FODSTAD, Ø., and PIHL, A.: Int. J. Cancer *22* (1978), 558
6. FODSTAD, Ø., JOHANNESSEN, J. V. SCHJERVEN, L. and PIHL, A.: J. Toxicol. Environ. Health *5* (1979), 1073
7. FODSTAD, Ø and PIHL, A.: Cancer Treat. Rep. *64* (1980), 1375
8. FODSTAD, Ø. and PIHL, A.: Cancer Res. *40* (1980), 3735
9. GOLDSTEIN, I. J., HUGHES, R. C., MONSIGNY, M., OSAWA, T. and SHARON, N.: Nature *285* (1980), 66
10. GUNDERSON, S. and FODSTAD, Ø: Int. J. Cancer *23* (1979), 530
11. HEWITT, H. B.: Br. J. Cancer *12* (1958), 378
12. KOUCUREK, J. and HOŘEJŠI, V.: Nature *290* (1981), 188
13. LIN, J.-Y., TSERNG, K.-Y., CHEN, C.-C., LIN, L.-T., and TUNG, T.-C.: Nature *227* (1970), 292
14. LIS, H. and SHARON, N.: In: The Antigens. p. 429. Ed.: M. SELA. Academic Press, New York, 1977
15. OLSNES, S., SALTVEDT, E. and PIHL, A.: J. Biol. Chem. *249* (1974), 803
16. OLSNES, S. and REFSNES, K.: Eur. J. Biochem. *88* (1978), 7
17. OLSNES, S. and PIHL, A.: In: The Specificity and Action of Animal, Bacterial and Plant Toxins, p. 131. Ed.: P. CUATRECASES, London: Chapman and Hall, 1979
18. OLSNES, S. and PIHL, A.: In press. In: The Molecular Actions of Toxins and Viruses. Ed.: P. COHEN and S. van HEYNINGEN, Elsevier/North Holland, Amsterdam
19. PIHL, A., FODSTAD, Ø. and OLSNES, S.: In: Proceedings of XVII Annual Colloquium on Protides of the Biological Fluids. p. 631. Ed. H. PEETERS, Pergamon Press, Oxford and New, York, 1979
20. PIHL, A., FODSTAD, Ø. and OLSNES, S.: In: Biology of the Cancer Cell. p. 261, Ed.: K. LETNANSKY, Kugler Medical Publications, Amsterdam, 1980
21. SANDVIG, K. and OLSNES, S.: In press. J. Biol. Chem.
22. SHARON, N. and LIS, H.: Science *177* (1972), 949
23. SPERTI, S., MONTANARO, L., MATTIOLI, A. and STIRPE, F.: Biochem. J. *136* (1973), 813

Istituto di Patologia generale dell'Universitá di Bologna,
I-40126 Bologna, Italy

Ribosome-inactivating Proteins as Possible Chemotherapeutic Agents

F. Stirpe and L. Barbieri

Some proteins purified from several plant materials have the property of damaging in a still unknown manner the 80S (eukaryotic) ribosomes, rendering them unable to perform protein synthesis. For this reason they have been and still are referred to as "inhibitors of protein synthesis". However, we prefer not to use this definition, which may turn out to be incorrect, once the mechanism of action of these proteins will be known.

Distribution

Ribosome-inactivating proteins have been identified in a variety of plants (1, 2). There is evidence that they may be present in all plants, in some cases in more than one form, although their concentration may vary greatly, in some plants being very high (up to 2 mg/g), whilst in others being so low that detection of their activity in crude extracts may be difficult. These variations occur in an apparently impredictable manner, although we observed a higher frequency of very active materials in plants belonging to some families (for instance, *Cucurbitaceae*). The proteins have been found in seeds, leaves, roots and in a latex, and we can assume they may be present in any part of the plants. The ribosome-inactivating proteins purified so far are listed in Table 1.

Characteristics

The ribosome-inactivating proteins are all single-chain basic proteins, with molecular weight 30,000, approximately, all of them binding to carboxymethyl cellulose. They are glycoproteins, with the only exception of PAP, in which no sugars were detected. This suggests that the carbohydrate component is not essential for their activity, and indeed gelonin, which contains mannose, is equally as active after demannosylation (9). No free sulphydryl groups have been demonstrated in any of the proteins, nor their biological activity is affected by reagents of sulphydryl groups.

Biological activity

The main property of these proteins is the arrest of protein synthesis they bring about in cell-free systems (reticulocyte lysates or purified ribosomes). This effect occurs at very low concentrations, of the order of ng/ml (10^{-10} M, approximately). All proteins

Table 1.
Properties of the purified ribosome-inactivating proteins

Name	Plant source	Molecular weight	Isoelectric point	LD_{50} mouse (mg/kg)	Inhibitory activity ID_{50}* (M)	Reference
Pokeweed antiviral protein	*Phytolacca americana* (pokeweed)					
PAP	Leaves	29,000	8.40		2.4×10^{-10}	3, 4
PAP II	Summer leaves	30,000	8.50		2.5×10^{-10}	5
PAP-S	Seeds	30,000	8.45	3.2	3.7×10^{-11}	+
Tritin	*Triticum aestivum* (wheat germ)	30,000			5.7×10^{-11}	6, 7
Momordica charantia inhibitor (MCI)	*Momordica charantia* Seeds	31,000	8.60	4.3	5.5×10^{-11}	8
Gelonin	*Gelonium multiflorum* Seeds	28,000	8.15	40	4.2×10^{-10}	9
Dianthin 30	*Dianthus caryophyllus* (Carnation)	29,500	8.65		3.1×10^{-10}	10
Dianthin 32	Leaves	32,000	8.55	30	1.1×10^{-10}	
Agrostin A	*Agrostemma githago* (corn cockle)	30,000	7.70		5.9×10^{-10}	+
Agrostin B		29,500	8.70		4.7×10^{-10}	+
Agrostin C	Seeds	29,600	8.75		5.7×10^{-10}	+
Hura crepitans inhibitor (MCI)	*Hura crepitans* Latex	28,000			1.2×10^{-10}	+

* Concentration giving 50% inhibition of protein synthesis by a rabbit reticulocyte lysate
+ Unpublished experiments
Abbreviations:
MCI: *Momordica charantica* inhibitor
PAP: Pokeweed antiviral protein

isolated in our or in other laboratories, with the exception of the inhibitor from *Hura crepitans*, have been tested on purified ribosomes, which were subsequently washed and assayed, and found inactive in performing protein synthesis. This demonstrates that the proteins act on ribosomes and not on any of the soluble components of the protein-synthesizing system. The effect of PAP and gelonin on ribosomal subunits was studied, and it was ascertained that they inactivate the larger (60 S) subunit (3, 9). No cofactors are required for the activity of the proteins, which seems to be catalytic (i.e. enzymatic) since all proteins inactivate a molar excess of ribosomes. The alteration of ribosomes seems to be irreversible, although it was reported that ribosomes treated with PAP show protein-synthetic activity in the presence of high concentrations of Mg^{2+} (11). Experiments performed with PAP and tritin showed that they reduce the ability of ribosomes to bind the elongation factor 2 (3, 7).

Thus the action of the ribosome-inactivating proteins in cell-free systems strongly resembles that of the A-chains of the plant toxins ricin, abrin (12), modeccin (13, 14) and of the more recently identified toxin from *Viscum album* (mistletoe) (15). Like the A-chains of the toxins, the ribosome-inactivating proteins are relatively non-toxic to intact cells, in most cases the ID_{50} being much higher as compared with the complete toxins, and of the order of 1 mg/ml (10^{-5} M, approximately). However, the sensitivity of cells to these proteins varies greatly, depending on the type or on the conditions of the cells, as it will be discussed below. This scarce effect on cells presumably is due to the lack of a B-chain, and consequently to poor penetration of the proteins into cells: indeed, it was observed that gelonin does not bind to HeLa cells (9). As a consequence, the toxicity of the ribosome-inactivating proteins to animals is relatively low, the LD_{50} for the mouse, when determined, ranging from 3—4 (PAP, MCI) to 30—40 mg/kg (dianthin 32, gelonin).

Possible applications

The similarities between the ribosome-inactivating proteins and the A-chains of the toxins suggested that the former could be used instead of the A-chains to prepare conjugates with suitable carriers (antibodies, hormones, lectins). These "A-chain-like" proteins should have several advantages over the A-chains, such as (1) the easier preparation and the better yield, (2) the greater stability, (3) the absence of contaminating toxin traces, and (4) the fact that they are numerous, and this may allow circumventing the problem of a possible immune reaction.

The first attempt to prepare a conjugate with one of these proteins was performed by binding gelonin to concanavalin. A through an artificial disulphide bond: the resulting complex was more toxic cells to than the mixture of the components (9). Another conjugate was prepared by linking gelonin to an anti-$Thy_{1.1}$ monoclonal antibody, and resulted specifically toxic to cells bearing the $Thy_{1.1}$ antigen. More recently, mannose-6-phosphate was linked to gelonin, which became toxic to K-562λ and F-265 cells (17). Other results revealed other properties of these proteins which could possibly be exploited. It should be recalled here that PAP was purified initially as an inhibitor of tobacco-mosaic virus replication, and that subsequently it was found to reduce protein synthesis and viral yield in virus-infected mammalian cells (18—20). With experiments performed with some of these proteins we observed that all those tested, like PAP, reduced lesions by tobacco-mosaic virus (MCI, gelonin, dianthins, agrostins) (10, 21), and impaired protein synthesis in cells infected with Herpes simplex virus (type 1) or with poliovirus, more than in uninfected cells; viral yield was also reduced (22).

Further, various types of cells show considerable differences in their sensitivity to the ribosome-damaging proteins: thus SV40-transformed cells and mouse peritoneal macrophages were more sensitive, by some 10-fold and 1000-fold, respectively, as compared with non-transformed or other cells tested (Table 2). While the effect on other transformed cells is currently being investigated, the high sensitivity of macrophages led us to study the effect of the proteins on the immune response. The results obtained so far showed that at least PAP and MCI, at doses well below the LD_{50}, suppress antibody formation in the mouse (as determined by the Jerne's test) (F. SPREAFICO, S. FILIPPESCHI, L. BARBIERI and F. STIRPE, unpublished results). We do not know yet whether this effect is due to the action of the substances on macrophages or occurs through a different mechanism.

Table 2.
Effect of ribosome-inactivating proteins on protein synthesis by various types of cells

Cells	PAP-S	MCI LD_{50}* (M)	Gelonin	Dianthin 30
EUE	1.7×10^{-5}	1.6×10^{-5}	1.7×10^{-5}	
HeLa	3.3×10^{-5}	3.2×10^{-5}	3.4×10^{-5}	
Mouse fibroblasts	3.3×10^{-5}	3.2×10^{-5}	3.4×10^{-5}	
SV40-transformed mouse fibroblasts	1.4×10^{-6}	3.5×10^{-6}	3.1×10^{-6}	
Mouse peritoneal marcophages	$1.6 + 10^{-8}$	3×10^{-8}	4.8×10^{-8}	1.4×40^{-8}

* Concentration giving 50% inhibition

At the beginning of our research on ribosome-inactivating proteins we hoped they could be useful to prepare conjugates. The results obtained along this line are encouraging, but the effects of the proteins on cells suggest that they could be used also as such, at least for experimental purposes.

The research performed in Bologna was supported by the Consiglio Nazionale delle Richerche, Rome, through the Progetto finalizzato "Controllo della crescita neoplastica", and by the Pallotti's legacy for cancer research. F. S. acknowledges support also from EMBO and from the Medical Research Council, London.

References

1. GASPERI-CAMPANI, A., BARBIERI, L., LORENZONI, E. and STIRPE, F.: FEBS Lett. *76* (1977), 173—176
2. GASPERI-CAMPANI, A., BARBIERI, L., MORELLI, P. and STIRPE, F.: Biochem. J. *186* (1980), 439—441
3. OBRIG, T. L., IRVIN, J. D. and HARDESTY, B.: Arch. Biochem. Biophys. *155* (1973), 278—289
4. IRVIN, J. D.: Arch. Biochem. Biophys. *169* (1975), 522—528
5. IRVIN, J. D., KELLY, T. and ROBERTUS, J. D.: Arch. Biochem. Biophys. *200* (1980), 418—425
6. ROBERTS, W. K. and STEWART, T. S.: Biochemistry *18* (1979), 2615—2621
7. COLEMAN, W. H. and ROBERTS, W. K.: Biochim. Biophys. Acta *654* (1981), 57—66
8. BARBIERI, L., ZAMBONI, M., LORENZONI, E., MONTANARO, L., SPERTI, S. and STIRPE, F.: Biochem. J. *185* (1950), 203—210
9. STIRPE, F., OLSNES, S. and PIHL, A.: J. Biol. Chem. *255* (1980), 6947—6955

10. Stirpe, F., Williams, D. G., Onyon, L. J., Legg, R. F. and Stevens, W. A.: Biochem. J. *195* (1981), 399—405

11. Rodes, T. L. III and Irvin, J. D.: Biochim. Biophys. Acta *652* (1981), 160—167

12. Olsnes, S. and Pihl, A.: In: Receptors and Recognition, series B, vol. 1 (Cuatrecasas, P., ed.), pp. 129—173, Chapman and Hall, London 1977

13. Olsnes, S., Haylett, T. and Refsnes, K.: J. Biol. Chem. *253* (1978), 5069—5073

14. Gasperi-Campani, A., Barbieri, L., Lorenzoni, E., Montanaro, L., Sperti, S., Bonetti, E. and Stirpe, F.: Biochem. J. *174* (1978), 191—196

15. Stirpe, F., Legg, R. F., Onyon, L. J., Ziska, P. and Franz, H.: Biochem. J. *190* (1980), 843—845

16. Thorpe, P. E., Brown, A. N. F., Ross, W. C. I., Cumber, A. J., Detre, S. I., Edwards, D. C., Davies, A. J. S. and Stirpe, F.: Eur. J. Biochem. *116* (1981), 447—454

17. Forbes, J. T., Bretthauer, R. K. and Oeltmann, T. N.: Proc. Natl. Acad. Sci. U.S.A.

18. Tomlinson, J. A., Walker, V. M., Flewett, T. H. and Barclay, G. R.: J. gen. Virol. *22* (1974), 225—232

19. Ussery, M. A., Irvin, J. D. and Hardesty, B.: Ann. N.Y. Acad. Sci. *284* (1977), 431—440

20. Fernandez-Puentes, C. and Carrasco, L.: Cell *20* (1980), 769—775

21. Stevens, W. A., Spurdon, C., Onyon, L. J. and Stirpe, F.: Experientia *37* (1981), 257—259

22. Foá-Tomasi, L., Campadelli-Fiume, G., Barbieri, L. and Stirpe, F.: Arch. Virol.

Department of Microbiology
University of Texas Health Science Center
Dallas, Texas 75235, USA

Selective Targeting of Ricin A Chain to a Murine B Cell Tumour by Anti-Immunoglobulin Antibodies

K. A. Krolick, J. W. Uhr and E. S. Vitetta

The targeting of toxic agents to tumour cells in vivo has been a goal of immunological research since the studies of Ehrlich (1). Successful application of this technique requires tumour-specific antibody whose activity remains unaltered following its covalent conjugation to a toxic agent. Moreover, the toxic portion of the conjugate should remain inactive until bound to the tumour cell via its antibody portion. In the studies described in this report, we have used an antibody against the cell surface immunoglobulin idiotype (Id) of a B cell tumour as our model system. B cell tumours are virtually always monoclonal in origin; hence each tumour cell that bears surface immunoglobulin expresses a particular Id (2—4). Since the Id is present on only a very small number of normal B cells (approximately $1/10^6$), the Id is operationally a tumour-specific antigen. Other advantages for using B cell tumours as model systems for antibody targeting studies include the availability of antibodies against other determinants on the cell surface immunoglobulin molecule (isotype, allotype, etc.) and a large body of information concerning the role of particular organs (e. g., spleen), cell types (T cells, macrophages) and lymphokines on the replication and differentiation of both normal and neoplastic B cells. In addition, a large number of humans with B cell tumours do not respond well to conventional chemo/radiotherapy (5) and there is, therefore, a need to improve treatment.

In our studies, as well as those of others (Table 1), the enzymatically active component of various biological toxins have been tested as covalent conjugates with specific anti-tumour antibodies. The polypeptide toxins are particularly attractive for tumour therapy because their primary action is to inhibit protein synthesis and they are, therefore, capable of killing non-dividing tumour cells which are refractory to anti-mitotic agents and can be clinically silent for long periods of time.

The toxic agent we have employed in our studies is the A chain of the plant lectin, ricin. In this report, we describe the capacity of antibody-ricin A chain conjugates (we will use the term "immunotoxins" for simplicity) to selectively kill tumour cells from the murine B cell tumour, BCl_1. Our studies first determined the extent to which BCl_1 cells could be selectively killed in vitro. We next investigated whether BCL_1 cells present in tumour-infiltrated bone marrow could be killed in vitro without harming hemapoietic stem cells. This maneuver has important clinical implications for the management of disseminated cancer by autologous bone marrow rescue after supralethal irradiation and/or chemotherapy. Finally, we discuss experiments in progress design to determine the effectiveness of the anti-Ig immunotoxins in vivo using mice bearing advanced BCL_1 tumours.

10*

147

Table 1.
Toxins or toxic peptides coupled to antibodies

Toxin	Tumour	Antibody	Reference
Diphtheria	TRD14 (SV40-induced hamster lymphoma)	Antibody-SV40 induced tumour antigens	Moolten, et al. 1975 (25)
	Human lymphoblastoid	F(ab')$_2$ ALG	Ross, et al. (1980) (26)
Diphtheria Fragment A	L1210 (mouse leukemia)	F(ab')$_2$ anti-L1210	Musuho, et al. 1979 (27)
Abrin	Daudi	ALG	Thorpe, et al. 1981 (28)
Ricin	EL4 (mouse thymoma)	Anti-Thy 1.2	Youle and Neville 1980 (29)
Ricin A Chain	WEHI-7	IgM hybridoma Anti-Thy 1.2	Blythman, et al. 1981 (30)
	L1210 (mouse leukemia)	F(ab)-anti-L1210	Musuho and Hara 1980 (31)
	Human colon carcinoma	Hybridoma anticolon carcinoma	Gilliland, et al. 1980 (32)
	ZR75 (human breast carcinoma	IgM hybridoma anti-ZR75	Krolick, et al. 1981 (33)
	Daudi, EBV Human lymphoblastoid line	F(ab)-anti-Ig	Raso and Griffin 1980 (34)
	Mouse BCL$_1$	AP R-anti-Id	Krolick, et al. 1980 (17)

The BCL$_1$ tumour model

The transplantable BCL$_1$ tumour which arose spontaneously in an elderly BALB/c mouse (6) is in many respects similar to the prolymphocytic variant of human chronic lymphocytic leukemia (PL-CLL) (7). The malignant cells are of B cell origin, bear λ-containing immunoglobulins, IgM and IgD, which have the same Id (8, 9). The neoplastic BCL$_1$ cells resemble immature B cells as determined by their surface phenotype and their in vitro behaviour (10, 11). The tumour grows primarily in the spleen and blood of recipient BALB/c mice or their F$_1$ hybrids (9, 12) and invades the bone marrow only late in the course of the disease (13). Tumour cells are absent from the lymph nodes and thoracic duct lymph (7, 13). Between 1 and 10 cells are sufficient to induce the tumour in normal BALB/c recipients (12). Depending on the number of tumour cells injected, recipient mice survive for 3—5 months after injection with tumour cells. The tumour-bearing mice are profoundly immunosuppressed due primarily to the development of suppressor monocytes in the lymphoid tissues (14). In vivo, the BCL$_1$ tumour cells do not secrete Ig. In vitro, the cells can be stimulated by mitogens (15), anti-immunoglobulins (10), or T cell factors (11, 16) to proliferate and/or differentiate into IgM-secreting cells.

In vitro inhibition of protein synthesis in BCL₁ tumour cells by anti-idiotype coupled to A chain (17)

To evaluate the immunotherapeutic potential of a tumour specific antibody conjugate, an affinity-purified rabbit anti-Id specific for the Ig on BCL₁ tumour cells (18) was coupled to ricin A chain. The antibodies were first derivitized with the disulfide-containing crosslinker, SPDP and then attached to the A chain of ricin by disulfide exchange (17). The anti-Id immunotoxin was then cultured with BCL₁ tumour cells or control cells as previously reported (17). Following 15 minutes of culture at 4 °C, the cells were washed and cultured for 2 days in the presence of the B cell mitogen, LPS. Protein synthesis was evaluated by ³H-leucine incorporation. Treatment of splenic BCL₁ cells (70—80% Id-positive) with anti-Id immunotoxin caused 70% inhibition of protein synthesis in LPS-stimulated spleen cells from mice bearing the BCL₁ tumour, suggesting that virtually all BCL₁ cells were killed. The same conjugate caused only 5% inhibition of protein synthesis in LPS-stimulated normal BALB/c splenocytes. Neither normal rabbit Ig-A chain (Figure 1), A-chain alone nor antibody alone (not shown), had a detectable effect on either normal cells or the tumor cells. Furthermore, as shown in Figure 1, the anti-Id-A chain immunotoxin did not inhibit protein synthesis in a T cell tumour (ASL-1) and had no effect on cells from another

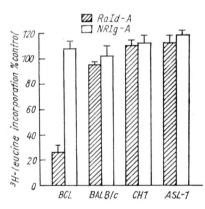

Fig. 1. Inhibition of protein synthesis in BCL₁ tumour cells by anti-Id immunotoxin. Spleen cells from BCL₁-bearing mice or control cells were pulsed for 15—30 min with 0.2 µg/ml of anti-Id immunotoxin at 4 °C, washed, and then cultured in triplicate for 2 days in the presence of LPS at 50 µg/ml. Cultures then received 1 µCi of (³H)-leucine, and were incubated for an additional 14—16 h. Labeled cells were then harvested and analyzed for incorporation of ³H-leucine into protein. ASL-1 is a T cell tumour and CH1 is a B cell tumour that bears IgMλ but lacks the BCL₁ idiotype. Hatched bars, anti-Id-A chain; empty bars, normal rabbit Ig-A chain.

B cell tumour (CH-1). The CH-1 cells express surface IgMλ lacking the BCL₁ Id. These results demonstrate the potential usefulness of the anti-Id immunotoxin as a B cell tumour-specific agent. The results do not, however, exclude the presence of a small number of surviving tumour cells in the treated cell population since the assay used to demonstrate inhibition of protein synthesis can give only an approximation of the number of tumour cells killed.

Adoptive transfer of BCL₁ cells treated with antibody A-chain immunotoxin

Since the injection of 1-10 BCL₁ cells into normal BALB/c mice will cause tumour (6, KROLICK, et al, this communication), the adoptive transfer assay represents an ex-

149

tremely sensitive measurement of the number of residual viable tumour cells in a treated cell population. In order to assess the effectiveness of specific immunotoxins in eliminating tumour cells from a treated cell population, rabbit anti-mouse Ig (RAMIg)-immunotoxin (which binds to both the BCL_1 tumour cells and to normal B cells) was employed. $1-10 \times 10^5$ spleen cells from the BCL_1-bearing mice (of which approximately 80% were tumour cells) were treated with optimal concentrations of the specific (RAMIg) or control (R-anti-ovalbumin) immunotoxin. After treatment, 10^4 cells were injected into normal BALB/c mice. A group of mice also received untreated cells. At 6 and 12 weeks after adoptive transfer, recipient mice were sacrificed and examined for tumour cells in their spleens and for leukemia. As shown in Figure 2, untreated cells, or cells treated with the control immunotoxin caused significant tumour in adoptive recipients. Animals receiving the cells treated with RAMIg-immunotoxin had background concentrations of Id-positive cells and the numbers did not increase between 6 and 12 weeks. Furthermore, the WBC in the blood of mice treated with RAMIg-immunotoxin never exceeded levels observed in normal mice ($\sim 5 \times 10^6$ per ml).

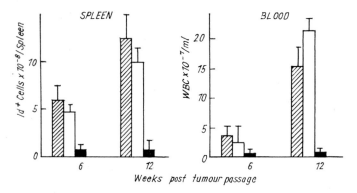

Fig. 2. Adoptive transfer of splenic BCL_1 cells treated with RAMIg-immunotoxin. 10^7 spleen cells from BCL_1-bearing mice containing 8×10^6 tumour cells were treated for 15 min at 4 °C with 1 µg/ml/10^7 cells with either RAMIg-A chain (solid bars) or R-anti-OVA-A chain (open bars). The treated cells, as well as untreated cells (hatched bars), were washed and injected i. v. into groups of 5 normal BALB/c mice (10^4 cells/mouse). At 6 and 12 weeks following adoptive transfer, recipient mice were sacrificed and examined for Id+ (tumour) cells in the spleen and for leukemia.

In order to determine how many transferred viable tumour cells in the above experiment would have been necessary to cause tumour at 12 weeks, additional experiments were performed using untreated tumour cells. In these experiments, groups of 15 mice received 1, 10, or 100 BCL_1 tumour cells and the time at which hepatosplenomegaly became apparent was noted. As seen in Table 2, at 12 weeks after transfer of tumour cells, all the animals receiving 100 or 10 tumour cells and 20% of the animals receiving 1 tumour cell had overt tumour.

There are two interpretations consistent with the above data: 1) animals injected with BCL_1 spleen cells treated with RAMIg-immunotoxin received fewer than 10 viable tumour cells. Thus, using an inoculum of 10^4 tumour cells, at least 99.9% of the cells were eliminated; 2) more than 10 viable tumour cells were injected but their growth was inhibited by an immune response transferred with the treated splenocytes. At present, we cannot distinguish between these two alternatives.

150

Table 2.

The time required for small doses of tumour cells to cause hepatosplenomegaly in BALB/c recipients

Number of BCL$_1$ cells injected	Weeks after transfer	Tumour-positive mice*
100	9	15/15
10	9	12/15
	12	15/15
1	9	0/15
	12	3/15

* positive mice/total mice injected.

The elimination of BCL$_1$ tumour cells from bone marrow: Implications for autologous bone marrow transplantation in the treatment of malignancy

One approach to management of patients with disseminated neoplasia involves supra-lethal chemotherapy/radiotherapy followed by autologous bone marrow rescue (19). Current clinical strategy is to remove bone marrow during remission. Following relap-se, the patient is treated with supralethal doses of chemotherapy and/or radiotherapy. The autologous marrow is then injected in order to reconstitute the hemopoietic system. This approach eliminates the problem of GVH disease but not the risk of reintroducing tumour cells with the marrow graft. To surmount the problem of reintro-ducing tumour cells, we have applied the immunotoxin technique to treat marrow cells from BCL$_1$-bearing mice. The marrow from animals with advanced tumours con-tains approximately 10—20% tumour cells. As shown in Figure 3, the transfer of untreated marrow cells or marrow cells treated with control-immunotoxin into normal mice caused tumour at 6 weeks. Marrow treated with RAMIg-immunotoxin did not cause detectable tumour at this time. Thus, RAMIg-A chain is very effective in killing BCL$_1$ tumour cells present in bone marrow as well as in spleen cell suspensions. The potent effect of the immuntoxin is contrasted with the results of similar experiments

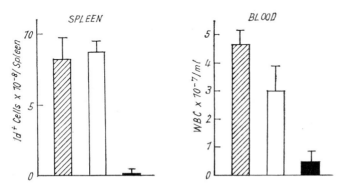

Fig. 3. Adoptive transfer of bone marrow BCL$_1$ cells treated with RAMIg-A chain into normal recipients. 10^6 bone marrow cells from BCL$_1$-bearing mice containing $1-2 \times 10^5$ tumour cells were treated as described in Fig. 7. Groups of 5 mice received 10^6 marrow cells/mouse. At 6 weeks following adoptive transfer, mice were sacrificed and examined for Id$^+$ (tumour) cells in the spleen and for leukemia.

151

using RAMIg and complement to kill BCL$_1$ cells in bone marrow in which hepatospleno-megaly was racdily detectable by 3—4 weeks after adoptive transfer of treated cells and the spleens and blood of the recipient mice contained large numbers of tumour cells (not shown). The above results emphasize the advantage of using immunotoxin compared to the more conventional approach of using antibody and complement.

In order to demonstrate that marrow cells treated with immunotoxin contain functional hemopoietic stem cells, treated cells were transferred into lethally irradiated mice. Preliminary experiments had established that a dose of 750r was 100% lethal for normal BALB/c mice, but that all of these mice could be rescued with an intravenous injection of 10^6 (but not 10^5) bone marrow cells. Thus, mice given 750r were injected with 10^6 untreated or RAMIg-A chain treated marrow cells from BCL$_1$-bearing mice. As seen in Table 3, although both groups of mice were rescued by this dose of marrow cells, the mice given untreated marrow cells had tumour cells in their spleens 6 weeks later. In contrast, the mice given bone marrow cells treated with RAMIg-A chain had no detectable tumour cells and exhibited normal numbers of T and B cells in their spleens.

Table 3.
The ability of RAMIg-A chain conjugates to eliminate tumour cells but not stem cells from the bone marrow of BCL$_1$-bearing mice

Source of BALB/c (donor) BM*		Treatment of donor BM cells	% of lethally irradiated mice which survived[+]	% of spleen cells in recipient mice that were[++]		
Normal	BCL$_1$-bearing			Tumour cells	B-cells	T-cells
None	None	None	0	—	—	—
10^6	None	None	100	0	37	55
None	10^6	None	100	54	8	14
None	10^6	RAMIg-A Chain	100	1	40	42

* 10^6 cells injected.

+ Prior to marrow reconstitution, mice were irradiated with 750r. Id+, Ig+ or Thy-l+ cells in spleen were determined by indirect immunofluorescence assay 6 weeks later. 5—10 mice/group

++ As dected by indirect IF on the FACS:
Tumour cells = Id+
B cells = Ig+ minus Id+
T cells = Thy 1.2+

These results indicate that: 1) virtually all BCL$_1$ tumour cells bear surface immuno-globulin, i.e., the BCL$_1$ tumour does not have a major pre-B cell component; 2) treatment with RAMIg-A-chain eliminates more than 99% of tumour cells from the marrow but leaves sufficient number of stem cells intact for reconstitution of hemopoietic function; 3) neoplastic B cells can be destroyed by an immunotoxin containing an antibody that is not tumour-specific. Thus, for the above approach to be applicable to autologous bone marrow transplantation, a *tumour reactive, stem cell non-reactive* antibody is all that is required.

Inhibition of BCL₁ tumour growth in vivo by immunotoxin

In the case of the BCL_1 tumour, the enormous tumour mass present in mice with advanced disease, precludes the use of small amounts of immunotoxins. Thus, at the peak of disease, the tumour mass is approximately $5 \times 10^9 - 1 \times 10^{10}$ cells and this probably represents $10-25\%$ of body weight. Our strategy, therefore, was to reduce the tumour burden by non-specific therapy and subsequently to use immunotoxins to eliminate residual tumour cells from the animal. Our choice of cytoreductive therapy, total lymphoid irradiation (TLI), has been used effectively in treating Hodgkin's disease in humans (20) and has the additional advantage of directing the irradiation solely to tumour infiltrated tissues. In the experiments described here, animals bearing advanced tumours were first treated with 9 doses of TLI (200 rads per dose). Larger or more numerous doses of TLI were not found to be significantly more effective. During such treatment, the vital organs and a portion of the long bones were shielded and X-irradiation was delivered primarily to the lymphoid tissues. Following 9 doses of TLI, it was shown that approximately 95% of the tumour cells had been eliminated from the spleen and blood (Figure 4). Such animals were then injected with a Rabbit-anti-δ (Rα-δ) immunotoxin. We chose to use Rα-δ rather than anti-Id immunotoxin for these first series of experiments. BCL_1 cells freshly harvested from tumour-bearing animals display small amounts of surface IgD (8, 9). Anti-δ immunotoxin offers the potential advantage of a reagent that could be effective against any IgD-bearing tumour. Furthermore, serum levels of IgD in mice are low (21, 22) and following TLI, the few remaining normal B cells are IgD⁻ (MAY, R. and E. VITETTA, unpublished results). The doses od immunotoxin were determined by preliminary experiments using NRIg-A chain. The dose chosen (1 dose of 20 μg) caused *reversible* damage to liver, spleen and lymph nodes as determined by gross morphology and

Effect of TLI on Tumour Cells in Vivo

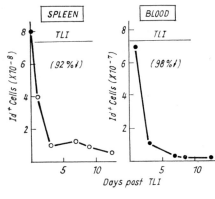

Fig. 4. Effect of total lymphoid irradiation (TLI) on the number of tumour cells in the spleens and blood of BCL_1-bearing mice. Nine doses of 200 R each were administered on consecutive days beginning on day 0. Indirect staining was performed using R-anti-Id and FITC-GARIg and the cells were analyzed on the FACS.

microscopic examination. This non-specific toxicity was not abolished by using $F(ab')_2$ fragments coupled to A chain. In preliminary experiments using Rα-δ immunotoxin or R-anti-Id immunotoxin, it could be shown that there was a slight delay in the reappearance of leukemia. However, approximately 2 weeks following immunotoxin injection, tumour cells had returned to levels observed in the control mice. Since tumour cells did reappear, further cytoreductive therapy was performed prior to administration of immunotoxin. Thus, in additional experiments, animals were splenectomized following the 9 doses of TLI since the majority of remaining tumour cells were present in the spleen. Following such treatment, the animals were injected with 3 to 4 weekly doses of Rα-δ immunotoxin and the appearance of leukemia was monitored. Controls included animals splenectomized but not injected with immunotoxin or splenectomized animals injected with the control (R-anti-OVA) immunotoxin. It should be mentioned that splenectomy per se delays the onset of leukemia, and leukemia is less severe (7. 23, 24). As seen in Figure 5, leukemia was evident 3—5 weeks after the completion of TLI in all the control mice and approximately 2—7 weeks later,

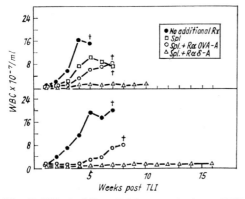

Fig. 5. Effect of R-anti-δ immunotoxin on BCL_1-bearing mice following combined cytoreductive therapy by TLI and splenectomy. Groups of 4—6 mice received TLI. One control group received no further therapy. Other groups were splenectomized one day following the last TLI treatment and rested two days before immunotoxin adminstration. Spl = splenectomy. + indicates death. Top panel: Mice received 3 intravenous injections of 5 μg R-anti-δ immunotoxin or control immunotoxin. One injection was given before splenectomy and 2 after splenectomy. Bottom panel: Mice received 4 weekly intravenous injections of 5μg R-anti-δ or control immunotoxin.

all control mice had died. In contrast, all the animals treated with the Rα-δ immunotoxin have survived and thus far remained leukemia-free for a period of $2^1/_2$—4 months. Recent experiments using *unconjugated* α-δ in BCL_1-bearing mice previously treated with TLI and splenectomy showed no effect on tumour growth.

The major finding to emerge from the present studies is that anti-Ig immunotoxins directed against the BCL_1 cell surface Id, isotype or L chain are highly effective in killing BCL_1 cells (in vitro and in vivo). The results presented in this report suggest that remission can be achieved in mice with far-advanced BCL_1 disease by a combination of cytoreduction and administration of anti-Ig-ricin-A chain immunotoxins.

Acknowledgements

We would like to thank Drs. S. ANDERSON, P. ISAKSON, M. MUIRHEAD, E. PURÉ, S. SLAVIN, C. VILLEMEZ, and A. van der HOVEN who have collaborated with us on portions of these studies. The technical assistance of Mr. Y. CHINN, Ms. M. BAGBY-WYATT, Ms. B. HUBER, Ms. L. TRAHAN, Ms. R. HIMMEL and Ms. S. SHEIKH is gratefully acknowledged. We are grateful to Drs. S. STROBER and S. SLAVIN for providing us with the BCL_1 tumour. We thank Ms. G. A. CHEEK for secretarial assistance. These studies were supported by NIH grants AI-11851, AI-12789 and CA-23115.

References

1. HIMMELWEIT, F.: In: The Collected Papers of Paul Ehrlich, ed. F. HIMMELWEIT (Pergamon Press, Elmsford, N.Y.), Vol. 3, 1960
2. FU, S. M., WINCHESTER, R. J. and KUNKEL, H. G.: J. Immunol. *114* (1975), 250

3. SALSANO, F., FROLAND, S. S., NATVIG, J. B. and MICHAELSON, T. E.: Scan. J. Immunol. *3* (1974), 841
4. SCHROER, K. R., BRILES, D. E., van BOXEL, J. A. and DAVIE, J. M.: J. Exp. Med. *140* (1974), 1416
5. LENNERT, K. and MOHRI, N.: In: Malignant Lymphomas, K. LENNERT, ed., pp. 111—136, 1978
6. SLAVIN, S. and STROBER, S.: Nature *272* (1977), 624
7. MUIRHEAD, M. J., ISAKSON, P. C., KROLICK, K. A., UHR, J. W. and VITETTA, E. S.: Amer. J. Pathol., In press, 1981
8. KNAPP, M. R., JONES, P. P., BLACK, S. J. VITETTA, E. S., SLAVIN, S. and STROBER, S.: J. Immunol. *123* (1979), 992
9. KROLICK, K. A., ISAKSON, P. C., UHR, J. W. and VITETTA, E. S.: Immunol. Rev. *48* (1979), 81
10. ISAKSON, P. C., KROLICK, D. A., UHR, J. W. and VITETTA, E. S.: J. Immunol. *125* (1980), 886
11. ISAKSON, P. C., PURE, E., UHR, J. W. and VITETTA, E. S.: Proc. Natl. Acad. Sci. U.S.A. *78* (1981), 2507
12. STROBER, S., GRONOWICZ, E. S., KNAPP, M. R., SLAVIN, S., VITETTA, E. S., WARNKE, R. A., KOTZIN, B. and SCHRODER, J.: Immunol. Rev. *48* (1979), 169
13. KROLICK, K. A., ISAKSON, P. C., UHR, J. W. and VITETTA, E. S.: J. Immunol. *123* (1979), 1928
14. ANDERSON, S. A., ISAKSON, P. C., PURE, E., MUIRHEAD, M., UHR, J. W. and VITETTA, E. S.: J. Immunol. *126* (1981), 1603
15. KNAPP, M. R., SEVRINSON-GRONOWICZ, E., SCHROEDER, J. and STROBER, S.: J. Immunol. *123* (1979), 1000
16. PURE, E., ISAKSON, P., TAKATSU, K., HAMAOKA, T., SWAIN, S. L., DUTTON, R., DENNERT, G., UHR, J. and VITETTA, E. S.: J. Immunol. 1981, in press
17. KROLICK, K. A., VILLEMEZ, C., ISAKSON, P. C. UHR, J. W. and VITETTA, E. S.: Proc. Natl. Acad. Sci. U.S.A. *77* (1980), 5419
18. VITETTA, R. S., YUAN, D., KROLICK, K., ISAKSON, P., KNAPP, M., SLAVIN, S. and STROBER, S.: J. Immunol. *122* (1979), 1649
19. GALE, R. P.: J. Amer. Med. Assoc. *243* (1980), 540
20. KAPLAN, H. S.: Hodgkin's Disease. Harvard University Press, Cambridge, Mass., 1972
21. VITETTA, E. S., MELCHER, U., McWILLIAMS, M., PHILLIPS-QUAGLIATA, L., LAMM, M. and UHR, J. W.: J. Exp. Med. *141* (1975), 206
22. ABNEY, E., HUNTER, I. R. and PARKHOUSE, R. M. E.: Nature *259* (1976), 404
23. SLAVIN, S., MORECKI, S. and WEISS, L.: J. Immunol. *124* (1980), 586
24. KOTZIN, B. L. and STROBER, S.: Science *208* (1980), 59
25. MOOLTEN, F. L., CAPPARELL, N. J., ZAJDEL, S. H. and COOPERBAND, S. R.: J. Natl. Cancer Inst. *55* (1975), 473
26. ROSS, W. C. J., THORPE, P. E., CUMBER, A. J., EDWARDS, D. C., HINSON, C. A. and DAVIES, A. J. S.: Eur. J. Biochem. *104* (1980), 381
27. MUSUHO, Y., HARA, T. and NOGUCHI, R.: Biochem. Biophys. Res. Commun. *90* (1979), 320
28. THORPE, P. E., CUMBER, A. J., WILLIAMS, N., EDWARDS, D. C., ROSS, W. C. J. and DAVIES, A. J. S.: Clin. Exp. Immunol. *43* (1981), 195
29. YOULE, R. J. and NEVILLE, D. M.: Proc. Natl. Acad. Sci. U.S.A. *77* (1980), 5483
30. BLYTHMAN, H. E., CASELLAS, P., GROS, O., GROS, P., JANSEN, F. K., PAOLUCCI, F., PAU, B. and VIDAL, H.: Nature *290* (1981), 145
31. MUSUHO, Y. and HARA, T.: Gann *71* (1980), 759
32. GILLILAND, D. G., STEPLEWSKI, Z., COLLIER, R. J., MITCHELL, K. F., CHANG, T. H. and KoPROWSKI, H.: Proc. Natl. Acad. Sci. U.S.A. *77* (1980), 4539
33. KROLICK, K. A., YUAN, D. and VITETTA, E. S.: Cancer Immunol. and Immunother. 1981 in press.
34. RASO, V. and GRIFFIN, T.: J. Immunol. *125* (1980), 2610

Development of New Drugs

* Laboratoire de Biochimie Enzymologie, INSERM U140, CNRS LA 147, Institut Gustave Roussy, 94800 VILLEJUIF, France

and

** Laboratoire de Pharmacologie et Toxicologie Fondamentales du CNRS, 31078 TOULOUSE, France

The Generation of Reactive Molecular Species during the Oxidation of 9-Hydroxyellipticine Derivatives. Interest of Prooxidant Compounds in the Design of Anti-Cancer Drugs.

C. AUCLAIR*, B. MEUNIER* and C. PAOLETTI**

Introduction

Ellipticine, 5,11-dimethyl-(6H)-pyrido(4-3,b)carbazole, is an alkaloid occurring in plants of the Apocynaceae family, which are found in several countries near the Indian Ocean. The antitumoural properties of ellipticine and related compounds were discovered in 1967 by DALTON et al (1) and further confirmed in 1968 by SVOBODA et al (2). The relatively simple structure of ellipticine prompted chemists to devise ways of synthesizing congeners, in order to improve the antitumoural activities of the natural compounds. It was found that the substitution in ellipticine of an OH group at the C-9 position resulted in a strong increase in both cytotoxic and antitumoural activities (3); whereas the addition of a methyl group to hydroxyellipticine at the N-2 position

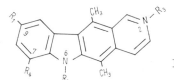

Fig. 1. Structure of ellipticine derivatives.

Table 1.
Structure of ellipticine derivatives (See also Fig. 1)

Radical				Name	Abbreviations	
R_1	R_2	R_3	R_4			
H	H		H	ellipticine	E	
H	H	CH$_3$	H	ellipticinium	2 N-CH$_3$, E	NME
OH	H		H	9-hydroxyellipticine	9-OH-E	HE
OH	H	CH$_3$	H	9-hydroxyellipticinium	2 N-CH$_3$, 9-OH-E	NMHE
O			H	9-oxoellipticine	9-Oxo-E	OE
O		CH$_3$	H	9-oxoellipticinium	2 N-CH$_3$, 9-Oxo-E	NMOE

yielding the quaternary drug 2N-CH$_3$, 9-OH-E (see Fig. 1 and Table 1), resulted in a marked increase in antitumoural efficiency in vivo. The latter drug has shown preliminary favourable results in an ongoing phase II clinical trial and appears to be especially active against osteolytic metastases of breast cancer (4, 5). For the development

159

of new, active drugs in the series of ellipticines, it is of interest to determine why modifications of their structure increase their cytotoxic and antitumoral activities. Up to now, two hypothesis have been put forward. The first is based on the increase in affinity for DNA following hydroxylation (3), and the second takes into account possible oxidation of the hydroxylated ellipticines to reactive products endowed with potential toxicity (6). The present report summarizes some experimental data that support the second hypothesis. These data are discussed in terms of the selective toxicity of antitumoural drugs for cancerous cells.

Effects of structural modifications on the cytotoxic and antitumoural activities of ellipticine

Results presented in Table 2 summarize the effects of both hydroxylation and quaternarization of ellipticines on their cytotoxic and antitumoral activities. Hydroxylation of E and NME, yielding, respectively, HE and NMHE, results in a strong increase in the cytotoxic properties of these compounds of L1210 cells in vitro, as evidenced from the values for the ID_{50}, which indicates the concentration of drug which reduces

Table 2.
Effect of hydroxylation of ellipticine (E) and of ellipticinium (NME) on their cytotoxic and antitumoural activies (after LE PECQ et al. (3) and PAOLETTI et al (13)).

Ellipticine derivative	ID_{50} $(\mu M)^a$	LD_0 $(mg/kg)^b$	ILS $(\%)^c$
E	0.99	50	68
HE	0.015	50	53
NME	1.68	12.5	18
NMHE	0.050	5	62

[a] Dose which reduces L1210 cell growth in vitro by 50% after 48 hours as compared with controls
[b] Highest non-lethal intraperitoneal dose in DBA/2 mice
[c] Increase in lifespan (ILS) over that in controls after a single intraperitoneal injection of drug 24 hours after grafting of 10^5 L1210 cells/mouse

the rate of L1210 cell multiplication by 50%. The second interresting feature is that NME does not display significant antitumoural activity against L1210 leukaemia in mice (ILS < 25%), whereas the corresponding hydroxylated compound NMHE exhibits a high antitumoural efficiency. As for hydroxylation, the quaternarization of E and HE to NME and NMHE significantly affects some of the pharmacological properties of the parent compounds. One of the most striking features is that the, quaternarization of E and HE results in a strong increase in their toxicity in mice, as indicated by the values of LD_0 (Table 2). In the case of NMHE, the increase in toxicity is associated with an increase in antitumoural activity, since an ILS of 62% is obtained with doses ten-fold lower than those required with the parent compound HE. In contrast, it must be noted that the quaternarization of E to NME results in a loss of antitumoural activity.
These results indicate that the association of hydroxylation and quaternarization yields structures suitable for optimal antitumoural activity.

Oxidation of the hydroxyellipticines HE and NMHE
to reactive species

Results shown in Table 3 indicate that hydroxylation of E and NHE to HE and NMHE, respectively, results in possible further oxidation of the hydroxylated compound to quinone-imine products, OE and NMOE (see Table 1 and Fig. 1). This oxidation may occur in vitro either through autoxidation (using molecular oxygen as electron acceptor) or through a peroxidase-catalysed reaction (using hydrogen peroxide as electron acceptor). In both cases, the oxidation reactions involve a one-electron transfer process generating free radicals as intermediates. Electron Paramagnetic Resonance (E.P.R.) experiments have effectively indicated that the phenoxy-free radical of the

Table 3.
Effect of hydroxylation and quaternarization of ellipticine derivatives on their oxidative activation to oxidizing species (after AUCLAIR et al (6, 7))

Ellipticine derivative	Reactive species generated during the oxidation of ellipticines[a]	
	Autoxidation	Peroxidase-catalysed oxidation
E	no oxidation	
HE	$O_2^{\cdot-}$, 9-O$\cdot$-E	9-O$\cdot$-E
	9-Oxo-E	9-Oxo-E
NME	no oxidation	
NMHE	$O_2^{\cdot-}$	2 N-CH$_3$, 9-O$\cdot$-E
	2 N-CH$_3$, 9-O$\cdot$-E	2 N-CH$_3$, 9-Oxo-E

[a] Free radicals ($O_2^{\cdot-}$, 9-O$\cdot$-E and 2 N-CH$_3$, 9-O$\cdot$-E) were identified by electron spin resonance spectrometry, as described in references 6 and 7; and quinone products were identified by mass spectrometry and nuclear magnetic resonance, as described in reference 6.

drugs was generated as an intermediate in the enzyme-catalysed oxidation of HE and NMHE, whereas both superoxide anion ($O_2^{\cdot-}$) and phenoxy radicals were generated during the autoxidation reaction (6, 7). It is clear that the presence of an OH group at position 9 of the ellipticine ring may result in further transformation of the drugs, generating at least three potentially toxic products, namely superoxide anion, the free radical of the drugs and the quinone-imine derivative.

Chemical reactivity of the oxidized products of HE and NMHE

The chemical reactivity of $O_2^{\cdot-}$ has been studied extensively, and this compound has been found to be involved in various cytotoxic processess (for a general review see ref. 8). In the case of the drugs HE and NMHE, a polarographic study has shown that the standard redox potential of the couple 9-OH-E/9-O$\cdot$-E is $E_0 = +0.50$ V (9). Therefore, the oxidized products obtained from HE and NMHE should be strong oxidizing species. In order to obtain information about the oxidizing power of free radicals and quinone products obtained from HE and NMHE, NADH oxidation has been measured in the presence of peroxidase-H_2O_2-drug (6). This system may be considered a mean of evaluating quantitatively the oxidizing properties of these compounds; it follows the sequences of reactions indicated in Figures 2 and 3. In both cases, the reaction occurs in a cyclic process in which the drugs are regenerated under their initial reduced forms. When the free radical of a drug is involved in the NADH oxidation, the reaction occurs through a one-electron transfer process, and oxygen acts as terminal electron acceptor (Fig. 2). In contrast, when the quinone is directly involved in NADH oxidation through a two-electron transfer, oxygen is not consumed (Fig. 3). Results obtained using this system (Table 4) indicate that the hydroxylated compounds, HE and NMHE, promote NADH oxidation at quite similar rates, whereas no NADH oxidation occurs in the absence of drug or in the presence of E or NME. The absence of oxygen uptake suggests that free radicals are not involved in the system and that reactions proceed according to the sequence shown in Figure 3.

Fig. 2

Fig. 3

Fig. 2. NADH oxidation in the presence of peroxidase-H_2O_2-drug, involving a free radical, HRP-horseradish peroxidase.

Fig. 3. NADH oxidation in the presense of peroxidase-H_2O_2-drug, involving a quinone. HRP-horseradish peroxidase.

Table 4.
Effect of ellipticine derivatives on NADH oxidation in the presence of myeloperoxidase-H_2O_2 (after AUCLAIR et al. (9)).
All experiments were performed at 25 °C in 0.05 M phosphate buffer (pH 7.4) containing 10^{-4} M NADH, 2×10^{-8} M myeloperoxidase, 10^{-4} M H_2O_2 and 2×10^{-8} M ellipticines.

Ellipticine derivative	NADH oxidized (nmol/min)	Oxygen consumed (nmol/min)
E	0	0
HE	10.50	0
NME	0	0
NMHE	12.20	0

An interesting phenomenon is that the peroxidase-hydroxyellipticines system exhibits a Michaelis kinetics for NADH oxidation (Fig. 4). This observation suggests that the drugs HE and NMHE act as coenzymes of the peroxidase. Consequently, it is possible to determine the Km of the peroxidase-drug complex for NADH; and the values so obtained indicate the apparent affinity of the peroxidase-drug for NADH and should reflect the oxidizing efficiency of the quinones OE and NMOE. Results shown in Table 5 give the Km values of horseradish peroxidase (HRP) for HE and NMHE, and of HRP-HE and HRP-NMHE for NADH. These values indicate a similar affinity of HRP for HE and NMHE, whereas HRP-HE exhibits a lower affinity for NADH than does HRP-NMHE. These results indicate

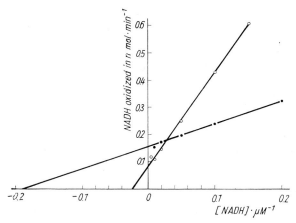

Fig. 4. Double reciprocal plots of NADH oxidation rate as a function of HE and NMHE concentrations. Experiments were performed at 25 °C in 0.05 M phosphate buffer (pH 7.4) containing 10^{-4} M H_2O_2, 10^{-10} M horseradish peroxidase and 10^{-5} M HE (o---o) or NMHE (●---●).

Table 5.
Effect of quaternarization of HE on the affinity of horseradish peroxidase (HRP) for the drugs and on the affinity of HRP-drug for NADH. Experiments were carried out as indicated in the legend to Table 4, except that 10^{-10} M HRP was used.

	Km of HRP-H_2O_2 for the drugs (μM)	Km of HRP-H_2O_2-drug for NADH (μM)
HE	6.5	42
NMHE	5.5	5.3

Table 6.
Reactivity of oxoellipticines towards various nucleophilic groups

Nucleophilic group	NMOE	OE
R—NH$_2$	+	
R—SH	+	+
R—CH$_2$OH	+	
Ar—OH	+	
Ar—NH$_2$	+	
Ar—NH	+	
>N :	+	

that the quinone products of both HE and NMHE are potent oxidizing compounds. In addition, the quaternarization of HE to NMHE strongly increases the oxidizing efficiency of the corresponding quinone-imine. Since OE and NMOE are powerful oxidants, they can be considered as electrophilic molecules which concequently may undergo nucleophilic attack, resulting in covalent binding with the nucleophilic molecules.

It has been effectively demonstrated that NHME activated to NMOE by peroxidase-H_2O_2 readily undergoes irreversible binding with biological nucleophiles such as bovine serum albumin (6) and DNA (unpublished data). The functional nucleophilic groups possibly involved in such binding have been investigated and the information obtained is summarized in Table 6. It is evident that the quinones OE and NMOE can form a covalent adduct with any molecule that contains one of the nucleophilic groups indicated. It can also be seen that the chemical reactivities of OE and NMOE are very different: NMOE can react with even the weakest nucleophiles, while OE reacts only with the reduced thiol group.

The high reactivity of NMOE is related to the presence in the pyridinium ion, of the electrophilic nitrogen which may result in the formation of a resonance hybrid structure (Fig. 5). According to this scheme, electron deficiency may take place either at the C-8 or at the C-10 position, possibly resulting in the formation of a highly reactive carbonium ion which could bind covalently to a nucleophile through a Michael addition reaction.

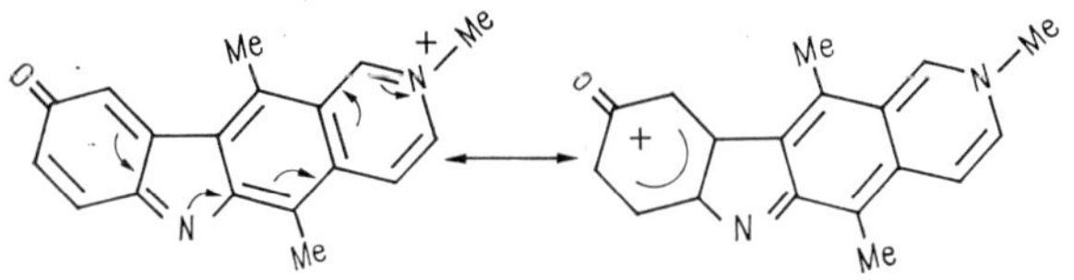

Fig. 5. Resonance hybrid structure of NMOE.

Discussion

The working hypothesis for the studies summarized in this paper has been that the effect of increasing hydroxylation of ellipticines on their cytotoxic and antitumoural activities may be due to the transformation of the hydroxylated drugs to chemically reactive compounds. Experimental data have indicated that 9-hydroxyderivatives, in the series of ellipticines may undergo one- and two-electron oxidation, yielding, respectively, free radicals and quinone-imine products. Quinones, especially NMOE, were found to be strong electrophilic molecules which react readily with both strong and weak nucleophiles to form covalent adducts.

The high reactivity of quinone-imines is related to the ready formation of a carbocation. It is thus of interest to consider that a carbocation is the structure responsible for the alkylation of DNA and proteins that occurs with nitrogen mustards and nitrosoureas and for the formation of interstrand cross-links with DNA that occurs with mitomycin and related compounds. Moreover, it has been pointed out that anthracyclines and related compounds (another major class of drugs that show marked antitumour activity) may undergo bioactivation to electrophilic quinone methides which could function as potent alkylating agents (10). A number of antineoplastic drugs thus owe their cytotoxicity to their ability to form potent electrophilic molecules, and it would appear that hydroxyellipticines can be put into this category.

Another interesting point is that compounds of this class exhibit a satisfying toxic selectivity towards malignant cells: For example, the cytotoxic compound bischlorethyl nitrosourea can divide the number of malignant cells (L1210) in mice by a factor of $10^6 - 10^7$ without affecting the animal host. Among the possible explanations for this impressive selectivity is that cancer cells have modified or new metabolic reactions or require cell components that are not necessary for the normal cell (and

164

conversely). Thus, it has been shown recently that most malignant cells demonstrate superoxide dismutase (SOD) deficiency (11): Lower levels of manganese-containing SOD have been found in all tumours examined to date and lower levels of copper-zinc-containing SOD in the majority. SOD, whose function is to destroy superoxide anion (O_2^-) inside cells, is considered to be the key enzyme in protecting aerobic cells against oxidation (12). Thus, SOD-deficient cells are potentially sensitive to various oxidant stresses. In the same lines of evidence, tumour cells are especially sensitive to ionizing radiation, the toxicity of which involves oxidizing agents such as the free hydroxyl radical (OH·). The selective toxicity of drugs which generate electrophilic species may therefore be due to the inability of tumour cells to exhibit efficient protection against oxidation. This difference between normal and malignant cells might be used to therapeutic advantage, and the synthesis of prooxidant drugs that can be activated to oxidizing species could be an attractive approach in the development of selectively toxic drugs against tumour cells.

Acknowledgement

This work was supported by Research Grant ATP CNRS No. 9764.

References

1. DALTON, L. K., DEMERAC, S., ELMES, B. C., LODER, J. W., SWAN, J. M. and TEITEI, T.: Synthesis of the tumour inhibitory alkaloids ellipticine 9-methoxy ellipticine and related pyrido (4,3-b) carbazoles. Aust. J. Chem. 20 (1967), 2715—2727

2. SVOBODA, G. H., POORE, G. A. and MONTFORT, M.: Alkaloids of ochrosia maculate (*Ochrosia borbonica* G. mel). Isolation of the alkaloids and study of the antitumour properties of 9-metoxy ellipticine. J. Pharm Sci. 57 (1968), 1720—1725

3. LE PECQ, J.-B., DAT-XUONG, N., GOSSE, C. and PAOLETTI, C.: A new antitumoral agent: 9-hydroxy ellipticine. Possibility of a rational design of anticancerous drugs in the series of DNA intercalating drugs. Proc. Natl. Acad. Sci. USA 71 (1974), 5078—5082

4. JURET, P., TANGUY, A., LE TALAER, J. Y., ABBATUCCI, J. S., DAT-XUONG, N., LE PECQ, J.-B. and PAOLETTI, C.: Preliminary trial of 9-hydroxy 2-methyl ellipticinium (NSC 264137) in advanced human cancers. Eur. J. Cancer 14 (1978), 205—206

5. PAOLETTI, C., LE PECQ, J.-B., DAT-XUONG, N., JURET, P., GARNIER, H., AMIEL; J.-L., and ROUSSE, J.: In: G. MATHÉ and MUGGIA, F. M., eds., Recent Results in Cancer Research, Springer Verlag Berlin, 74 (1980), 107—123

6. AUCLAIR, C. and PAOLETTI, C.: Bioactivation of the antitumour drugs 9-hydroxyellipticine and derivatives by a peroxidase hydrogen peroxide system. J. Med. Chem. 24 (1981), 289—295

7. AUCLAIR, C.: In: BANNISTER, J. V., HILL, H. A. O., eds., Chemical and Biochemical Aspects of Superoxide and Superoxide Dismutase 11A, Elsevier North-Holland, 318—327 (1980)

8. FRIDOVICH, I.: The Biology of Oxygen Radicals. Science 201 (1978), 875—880

9. MOIROUX, J. and ARMBRUSTER, A. M.: Electrochemical behaviour of ellipticine derivatives. Part I Oxidation of 9-hydroxy ellipticine. J. Electroanal. Chem. 114 (1980), 139—146

10. MOORE, H. W.: Bioactivation as a model for drug design bioreductive alkylation. Science. 197 (1977), 527—532

11. OBERLEY, L. W and BUETTNER, G. R.: Role of superoxide dismutase in cancer: a review. Cancer Research 39 (1980), 1141—1149

12. MCCORD, J. M., KEELE, B. B. and FRIDOVICH, I.: An enzyme based theory of obligate anaero-biosis: the physiological function of superoxide dismutase. Proc. Natl. Acad. Sci. USA 68 (1971), 1024—1027

13. PAOLETTI, C., CROS, S., DAT-XUONG, N., LECOINTE, P. and MOISAND, A.: Comparative cyto-toxic and antitumoral effects of ellipticine derivatives on mouse L1210 leukemia. Chem. Biol. Interact 25 (1979), 45—58

MRC Clinical Oncology and Radiotherapeutics Unit
Hills Road, Cambridge, England

Development of Nitroimidazoles

P. WORKMAN

Introduction

It is thought by many that the effectiveness of radiation and cytotoxic drug therapy against solid tumours may be limited by the presence of hypoxic tumour cells (21, 22). These have reduced oxygen concentrations because of their distance from blood vessels, and as a result are comparatively resistant to treatment. Oxygen itself has limited value as a sensitizer because its rapid metabolism prevents it from reaching all the hypoxic cells.

In addition to their established roles as antimicrobial agents, nitroimidazoles are of considerable current interest in oncology because of their selective activity against hypoxic cells. This includes preferential cytotoxicity and selective sensitization to radiation and cytotoxic drugs. For an introduction to the nitroimidazoles, the proceedings of three recent conferences can be recommended (4, 11, 12). In this paper the development of nitroimidazoles as anticancer agents is briefly reviewed, with emphasis on more recent progress.

Mechanisms of cytotoxicity and radiosensitization

Radiosensitization and cytotoxicity are both a function of the one-electron reduction potential (E_7^1) (2, 5). This is a measure of the electron affinity of the nitro group. Fig. 1 shows the structures and E_7^1 values for metronidazole (METRO, MAY and BAKER) and misonidazole (MISO, ROCHE). The 2-nitroimidazole MISO is more electron affinic and shows radiosensitization and cytotoxicity at about ten-fold lower concentrations than the 5-nitroimidazole METRO (e.g. Fig. 2). Other oxidising agents, including for example quinones and oxygen itself, show the same dependence of radiosensitization on electron affinity (Fig. 2).

The mechanism of hypoxic radiosensitization is complex and probably involves several factors (13, 38). One involves reaction with free radicals produced in biological

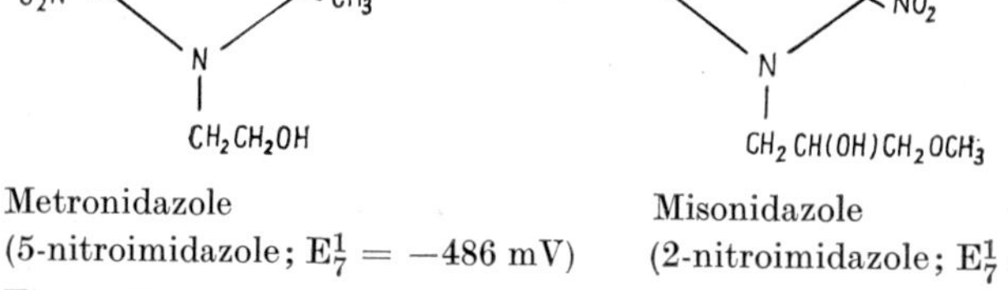

Metronidazole
(5-nitroimidazole; $E_7^1 = -486$ mV)

Misonidazole
(2-nitroimidazole; $E_7^1 = -389$ mV)

Fig. 1. Metronidazole and misonidazole.

166

molecules, including DNA, resulting in 'fixation' of the damage in an unreparable form. This can involve the formation of DNA-sensitizer adducts. Another is reaction with radioprotective SH groups.

Hypoxic cell cytotoxicity is thought to be due to enzymatic reduction to toxic species such as the nitro radical anion, nitroso and hydroxylamine, metabolism to which predominates under hypoxic conditions (31). These metabolites then react with cellu-

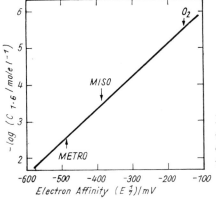

Fig. 2. Relationship between electron affinity and radiosensitization of hypoxic V79 cells in vitro. E_7^1 is the one-electron reduction potential and $C_{1\cdot6}$ the concentration to give an enhancement ratio of 1.6.

lar macromolecules. In contrast to radiosensitization, cytotoxicity is metabolism-dependent and requires prolonged hypoxic contact with the drug. Similar prolonged incubation also gives enhanced radiosensitization (13, 39).

Radiosensitization in vivo

The nitroimidazoles have so far proved to be the most effective sensitizers in vivo, in that radiosensitization of tumours can be demonstrated at doses non-toxic to the host. METRO and MISO have been the most extensively studied: agents more electron-affinic than MISO tend to be too toxic, whereas those less electron-affinic than METRO tend to be inactive. Good radiosensitization has been obtained with large doses of MISO in a wide range of experimental animal tumours (16).

METRO and MISO in man

Both METRO and MISO are currently undergoing clinical trial as radiosensitizers (e.g. see Ref. 11). In one early trial METRO improved survival of glioma patients compared to radiotherapy alone (33) but this study has been critizeied on several grounds (see Ref. 21). MISO is now more popular than METRO because of the lower dose required. Improved tumour growth delay responses suggested radiosensitization may occur with MISO in man (7). A recent small study showed no improvement in survival for radiotherapy of glioma, and several reasons for this were discussed (9).

Many trials are now in progress throughout the world, and in the UK these include the Medical Research Council's glioma, cervix and head and neck studies with MISO. The possible contribution of hypoxic cell cytotoxicity to tumour response in the clinic is unknown.

167

Neurotoxicity: the need for improved sensitizers

Although nausea and vomiting are also troublesome, the dose-limiting toxicity of MISO and METRO in man is peripheral neuropathy (18, 34). With MISO neurotoxicity is reduced, but not eliminated, by restricting the total dose to 12 g/m². Unfortunately this means that in conventional multifraction radiotherapy the amount given with each radiation dose will not be sufficient for maximal radiosensitization, although a significant and valuable improvement might still be obtained.

Patients with prolonged exposure to MISO (i. e. high values for the area under the curve, AUC, of plasma drug concentration versus time) have a greater risk of developing neurotoxicity (18). AUC is significantly diminished by inducing rapid metabolism using phenobarbitone or phenytoin (35, 40, 43), and this may result in a reduction of neurotoxicity (9, 35). The steroid dexamethasone may reduce neurotoxicity (35), possibly by reducing brain penetration by MISO (42). However, dexamethasone also has radioprotective properties (24).

Development of improved sensitizers

Structure-activity relationships with hypoxic mammalian cells in vitro have shown that radiosensitization and acute cytotoxicity are both primarily dependent on electron affinity (2, 5). Unfortunately, this is also true for chronic aerobic cytotoxicity in vitro, used to predict potential toxicity to oxic tissues (3). However despite the general tendency for increased toxicity to go hand-in-hand with improved radiosensitization efficiency this is not always true for individual compounds, some of which exhibit better in vitro 'therapeutic ratios' than MISO. This is particularly true of 2-nitroimidazoles with basic substituents in the side-chains. Compared to MISO which has similar electron affinity, these show an order of magnitude increase in sensitization efficiency with no increase in aerobic cytotoxicity (1, 27). Lipophilicity, pKa and alkyl chain length may each contribute to improved in vitro therapeutic ratio, but no simple explanation is apparent at this time. Analogues such as Ro 03-8799, developed by Roche and the Gray Laboratory, and RSU 1047, developed at Sutton, exhibit in vivo radiosensitization and toxicological properties sufficiently promising to warrant further investigation (Ref. 27 and ADAMS et al, personal communication).

Another class of nitroimidazoles exhibiting more efficient in vitro radiosensitization than would be predicted from their electron affinities are the 5-substituted 4-nitroimidazoles, such as the NCI compound NSC 38087 (25). Unfortunately this compound is rapidly metabolised and highly toxic in vivo, and no radiosensitization is seen (SHELDON et al, personal communication). NSC 38087 is also interesting in that it shows preferential cytotoxicity towards *oxic* cells, and a different mechanism appears to be involved (25).

Earlier structure-activity relationships with neutral nitroimidazoles suggested that lipophilicity was not important for in vitro radiosensitization (2, 5). However, more recent studies with bacteria have shown improved radiosensitization for highly lipophilic analogues (6), possibly due to association with a hydrophobic target site. Conversely, very hydrophilic analogues show reduced radiosensitization of mammalian cells in vitro because they fail to penetrate the cell membrane (BROWN, D. M. et al, personal communication).

Lipophilicity is even more important for radiosensitization, principally because of its effect on pharmacokinetics.

Lipophilicity and pharmacokinetics in the development of improved sensitizers

The approach to radiosensitizer development used by the Cambridge and Stanford groups has concentrated on the relationship between structure and pharmacokinetic behaviour for neutral analogues of MISO with similar electron affinity but widely different lipophilicity (for review see Ref. 41). In particular, it was felt that the unusually broad structural specificity for hypoxic radiosensitization in vitro facilitates the rational manipulation of structure to produce the required pharmacokinetic behaviour. High-performance liquid chromatography (HPLC) techniques have been developed for nitroimidazoles (45) and have now become the methods of choice.

The lipophilicity approach to nitroimidazole development is based on the concept that toxicity is related to AUC in critical normal tissues (18), whereas radiosensitization is a function of the concentration in the hypoxic cells only during the irradiation period (23) (Fig. 3). Improvement in therapeutic ratio might therefore be obtained by maintaining or increasing peak tumour levels while minimising the AUC in normal tissues.

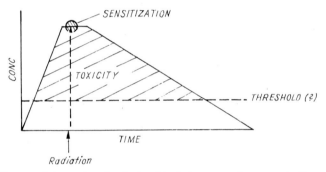

Fig. 3. Schematic of relationship between peak concentration and radiosensitization, and area under the curve and neurotoxicity.

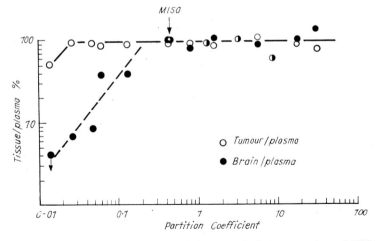

Fig. 4. Relationship between lipophilicity and the penetration of MISO into brain and EMT6 mammary tumours in BALB/c mice (Data from ref. 10 and WORKMAN, unpublished).

With hydrophilic analogues of MISO, synthesized at Roche and at Stanford Research International, reduced AUCs are obtained through rapid renal clearance and peak tumour levels and radiosensitization are maintained with intravenous administration (10, 36, 37, 44). In addition, they are progressively excluded from brain and peripheral nerve but not from tumour (e. g. Fig. 4) (10, 35).

The demethylated metabolite of MISO Ro 05-9963 (Roche) has entered Phase 1 clinical trial (17, 19). Although it has a shorter half-life than MISO (6 h compared to 10 h) (17) its neurotoxicity was comparable to MISO (19) possibly due to similar nervous tissue penetration (BLEEHEN et al, unpublished). This may be overcome with the much more hydrophilic SR-2508 (SRI) which is excluded from nerves more effectively (1p, 37). SR-2508 is now undergoing preclinical toxicology in the U.S.A.

Reduced AUCs can also be achieved with neutral analogues more lipophilic than MISO as a result of very fast metabolism (WORKMAN et al, unpublished). These analogues have tumour/plasma and nervous tissue/plasma ratios similar to MISO (Fig. 4). Rapid metabolic clearance is also seen with some basic 2-nitroimidazoles, such as Ro 03-8799; in addition, some of these are excluded from the brain to varying extents, but show some tendency to concentrate in tumours (30). Human studies are now underway with Ro 03-8799.

Various methods are available for determining the neurotoxicity of nitroimidazoles in experimental animals, e.g. histochemical (14) and rotarod performance (15). These have indicated reduced neurotoxicity for hydrophilic and basic MISO analogues, but remain to be validated clinically.

Chemosensitization

Since 1980 a number of studies have shown that the response of experimental tumours to cytotoxic drugs can be enhanced by MISO both in vitro (28) and in vivo (25, 26, 32). This is seen particularly with alkylating agents and nitrosoureas. In some cases there is evidence that the enhancement is greater in tumour than in critical normal tissues, for example with melphalan (25) and CCNU (26, 32). However, there is greater variation between tumours than is seen with radiosensitization.

We have recently demonstrated that several lipophilic analogues, e.g. benznidazole (Ro 07-1051, Roche) exhibit enhancement of CCNU response considerably superior to MISO (46). Dose-modification factors >2 can be obtained.

The mechanism of action for chemosensitization, if indeed there is a common mechanism, is not certain at this time. Possibilities include selective sensitization of hypoxic tumour cells (possibly through SH depletion and similar to the in vitro hypoxic pre-incubation sensitization to drugs and radiation), inhibition of repair of potentially lethal damage, and modification of pharmacokinetics. Our studies favour the latter.

Nitroimidazoles also increase the response of hypoxic cells to hyperthermia (8).

Prospects

Many clinical trials are now in progress throughout the world to assess the value of MISO as a radiosensitizer, and some will be completed in the near future. The problem is the dose-limitation imposed by its neurotoxic effects. Several analogues are now under investigation as potentially superior to MISO, and it is hoped that this problem may be overcome and the therapeutic ratio improved. Enhancement of the antitumour effects of cytotoxic agents shows considerable promise and is currently under intensive investigation, in both laboratory and clinic.

References

1. ADAMS, G. E., AHMED, I., CLARKE, E. D., O'NEILL, P., PARRICK, J., STRATFORD, I. J., WALLACE, R. G., WARDMAN, P. and WATTS, M. E.: Int. J. Radiat. Biol. *38* (1980), 613
2. ADAMS, G. E., CLARKE, E. D., FLOCKHART, I. R., JACOBS, R. S., SEHMI, D. S., STRATFORD, I. J., WARDMAN, P., WATTS, M. E., PARRICK, J., WALLACE, R. G. and SMITHEN, C. E.: Int. J. Radiat. Biol. *35* (1979), 133
3. ADAMS, G. E., CLARKE, E. D., GRAY, P., JACOBS, R. S., STRATFORD, I. J., WARDMAN, P., WATTS, M. E., PARRICK, J., WALLACE, R. G. and SMITHEN, C. E.: Int. J. Radiat. Biol. *35* (1979), 151
4. ADAMS, G. E., FOWLER, J. F. and WARDMAN, P. (Eds.): Br. J. Cancer *37*, Suppl III, (1978)
5. ADAMS, G. E., STRATFORD, I. J., WALLACE, R. G., WARDMAN, P. and WATTS, M. E.: J. Natl. Cancer Inst. *3* (1980), 555
6. ANDERSON, R. F. and PATEL, K. B.: Br. J. Cancer *39* (1979), 705
7. ASH, D. V., PECKHAM, M. J. and STEEL, G. G.: Br. J. Cancr *40* (1979), 883
8. BLEEHEN, N. M., HONESS, D. J. and MORGAN, J. E.: Br. J. Cancer *35* (1977), 299
9. BLEEHEN, N. M., WILTSHIRE, C. R., PLOWMAN, P. N., WATSON, J. V., GLEAVE, J. R. W., HOLMES, A. E., LEWIN, W. S., TREIP, C. S. and HAWKINS, T. D.: Br. J. Cancer *43* (1981), 436
10. BROWN, J. M. and WORKMAN, P.: Radiat. Res. *82* (1980), 171
11. BRADY, L. W. (Ed): Radiation Sensitizers, Masson, New York (1980)
12. BRECCIA, A., RIMONDI, C. ADAMS, G. E. (Eds): Radiosensitizers of Hypoxic Cells, Elsevier, Amsterdam, (1979)
13. CHAPMAN, J. D., NGAN-LEE, J. and MEEKER, B. E.: Proc. 2nd Annual Bristol-Meyers Cancer Conference, Academic Press (1980)
14. CLARKE, C., DAWSON, K. B., SHELDON, P. W., CHAPLIN, D. W., STRATFORD, I. J. and ADAMS, G. E.: In: Radiation Sensitizers, (Brady, L. W. Ed.). Masson, New York, p. 245. (1980)
15. CONROY, P. J., SHAW, A. B., McNEILL, T. H., PASSALACQUA, W. and SUTHERLAND, R. M.: In: Radiation Sensitizers (BRADY, L. W., Ed.), Masson, New York, p. 397 (1980)
16. DENEKAMP, J.: In: Radiation Sensitizers (BRADY, L. W., Ed.), Masson, New York, p. 215 (1980).
17. DISCHE, S. D., FOWLER, F. J., SAUNDERS, M. I., STRATFORD, M. R. L., ANDERSON, P., MINCHINTON, A. I. and LEE, M. E.: Br. J. Cancer *42* (1980), 153
18. DISCHE, S., SANDERS, M. I., FLOCKHARDT, I. R., LEE, M. E. and ANDERSON, P.: Int. J. Radiat. Oncol. Biol. Phys. *5* (1979), 851
19. DISCHE, S., SAUNDERS, M. I., and STRATFORD, M. R. L.: Br. J. Radiol. *54* (1981), 1561
20. GANGJI, D., SCHWADE, J. G. and STRONG, J. M.: Cancer Treatment Rep. *64* (1980), 155
21. HALL, E. J.: Radiobiology for the radiologist, Harper and Row, Maryland, 2nd ED. (1978).
22. HILL, R. P. and STANLEY, J. A.: Cancer Res. *35* (1975), 1147
23. McNALLY, N. J., DENEKAMP, J., SHELDON, P., FLOCKHART, I. R. and STEWART, F. A.: Radiat. Res. *73* (1978), 568
24. MILLAR, B. C. and JINKS, S.: Br. J. Radiol. *54* (1981), 505
25. ROSE, C. M., MILLAR, J. L., PEACOCK, J. H., STEPHENS, T. C.: In: Radiation Sensitizers (BRADY, L. W., Ed.), Masson, New York, p. 250 (1980)
26. SIEMANN, D. W.: Br. J. Cancer *43* (1981), 367
27. SMITHEN, C. E., CLARKE E. D., DALE, J. A., JACOBS, R. S., WARDMAN, P., WATTS, M. E. and WOODCOCK, M. In: Radiation Sensitizers, (BRADY, L. W., Ed.), Masson, New York, p. 22 (1980)

28. STRATFORD, I. J., ADAMS, G. E., HORSMAN, M. R., KANDAIYA, S., RAJARATNAM, S., SMITH, E. and WILLIAMSON, C. In: Radiation Sensitizers (BRADY, L. W., Ed.), Masson, New York, p. 276 (1980)
29. STRATFORD, I. J., WILLIAMSON, C. and HARDY, C.: Br. J. Cancer *44* (1981), 109
30. STRATFORD, M. R. L., MINCHINTON, A. I., STEWART, F. A. and RANDHAWA, V. S. In: Radio-sensitizers of Hypoxic Cells, Plenum, Nato ASI Series (in press)
31. TAYLOR, Y. C. and RAUTH, A. M.: Cancer Res. *38* (1978), 2745
32. TWENTYMAN, P. E. and WORKMAN, P.: Br. J. Cancer (in press)
33. URTASUN, R., BAND, P., CHAPMAN, J. D., FELDSTEIN, M. L., MIELKE, B. and FRYER, C.: New Engl. J. Med. *294* (1976), 1364
34. WASSERMAN, T. H., PHILLIPS, T. L., JOHNSON, R. J., GOMER, C. J., LAWRENCE, G. A., SADEE, W., MARQUES, R. A., LEVIN, V. A. and van RAALTE, G.: Int. J. Radiat. Oncol. Biol. Phys. *5* (1979), 775
35. WASSERMAN, T. H. PHILLIPS, T. L., JOHNSON, R. J., van RAALTE, G., URTASUN, R., PAR-TINGTON, J., KOZIOL, D., SCHWADE, J. G., GANGJI, D. and STRONG, J. M.: Br. J. Radiol. *53* (1980), 172
36. WHITE, R. A. S. and WORKMAN, P.: Br. J. Cancer *41* (1980), 268
37. WHITE, R. A. S., WORKMAN, P. and BROWN, J. M.: Radiat. Res. *84* (1980), 542
38. WILLSON, R. L. In: Metronidazole (FINEGOLD, S. M., Ed.), Excerpta Medica, Amsterdam, p. 147 (1977)
39. WONG, T. W., WHITMORE, G. F. .and GULYAS, S.: Radiat. Res. *75* (1978), 541
40. WORKMAN, P.: Br. J. Cancer *40* (1979), 335
41. WORKMAN, P.: Cancer Clinical Trials *3* (1980), 237
42. WORKMAN, P.: Biochem. Pharmac. *29* (1980), 2709
43. WORKMAN, P., BLEEHEN, N. M. and WILTSHIRE, C. R.: Br. J. Cancer *41* (1980), 302
44. WORKMAN, P. and BROWN, J. M.: Cancer Chemother. Pharmacol. *6* (1981), 39
45. WORKMAN, P., LITTLE, C. J., MARTEN, T. R., DALE, A. D., RUANE, R. J., FLOCKHART, I. R. and BLEEHEN, N. M.: J. Chromatog. *145* (1978), 507
46. WORKMAN, P. and TWENTYMAN, P. R.: Int. J. Radiat. Oncol. Biol. Phys. (in press)

[1] Institute for Cancer Research, University of Vienna and
[2] I. Surg. Department, University of Vienna and
[3] II. Department of Dermatology, University of Vienna and
[4] Clinic for Chemotherapy, University of Vienna and
[5] V. Intern. Department and L. Boltzmann Research Institute, Wilhelminenspital, Vienna, Austria

Development of New Drugs — Immunomodulating Agents

M. Micksche[1], M. Colot[1], A. Fritsch[2], E. M. Kokoschka[3], R. Kolb[2], R. Lenzhofer[4], Th. Luger[3], K. Moser[4], H. Rainer[4], P. Sagaster[5] and A. Uchida[1]

I. Introduction

Since the first clinical attempts to improve chemotherapy-induced remissions in leukemia by additional immunotherapy with bacille Calmette-Guérin (BCG) in 1967, intensive efforts have been made to define agents which can improve the immune response in tumour bearers (1). Early clinical studies were performed mainly with microbial adjuvants such as BCG, *Corynebacterium parvum* and methanol-extractable residue (MER), and also with the synthetic immune modulating agent Levamisole. Immunomodulation in both animals and in cancer patients has been achieved by all these agents (2, 3, 4). Moreover, it has recently been demonstrated that immunotherapy with these products has an effect on the clinical outcome of the disease. It has achieved increases of response rate to chemotherapy, induction of remission and prolongation of remission-free interval and survival rate, when given alone, or in combination with chemo- or radiotherapy, for palliation or adjuvant therapy (5, 6, 7, 8).

Beside these suggestive results, there are also many studies, in which the efficacy of immunotherapy was not demonstrated, independent of whether its application was together with conventional therapy, or as sole treatment (9).

The development is necessary of more standardized preparations. Such as non-viable bacterial organisms or defined synthetic agents. Broader investigations into their immunopharmacology, prior to their introduction in randomized clinical trials should be an aim for the future, in order to give clearer evidence, whether or not immunomodulation in cancer patients has some influence on their clinical outcome. In recent years, some candidate drugs for broad clinical application have been developed.

This report deals with our approaches to defining the immunopharmacology and clinical efficiency of newly developed immunomodulating agents, such as OK-432, a streptococcal preparation (10), 2-cyanaziridine derivatives (Imexon, Azimexon) (11),

Table 1
Development of new immunomodulating agents: immunopharmacologic study parameters

T-, B-lymphoyte differentiation
T-lymphocyte subsets (monoclonal antibodies)
Lymphocyte blastogenic response to mitogens
Natural killer (NK)-cell activity
Suppressor cells to NK
Macrophage maturation
DCHR — delayed cutaneous hypersensitivity reaction (dinitrochlorobenzene, recall antigens)

NPT 15392, an Isoprenosine-related compound (12), and synthetic polynucleotides Poly A:U (19).

Methods used to investigate the immunopharmacology of these agents are given in Table 1.

Our own approaches are, first, to test the drug or agent in vitro, measuring in-vitro parameters. The second step is to investigate the in-vitro reactivity of patients' lymphocytes, after in-vivo application of the drug, and, furthermore, to investigate skin test response in vivo after therapy. Side effects of each agent investigated are summarized in Table 2.

Imexon led to vomiting in 20% of the patients, Azimexon, NPT 15392 and poly A:U had no side effects. OK-432 was applied via several routes; intravenous application produced fever and chills in 100% of the patients, whereas systemic routes, intradermal or intramuscular, were well tolerated.

Table 2.
Phase I—II trials with immunomodulating agents

Agent	Route[a]	Dose	Toxicity	Immune[b] modulation
Imexon	i.v.	5—200 mg	20% vomiting!	yes
Azimexon	i.v.	100—400 mg	no	yes
NPT 15392	p.o.	0.4, 0.7 mg	no	yes
Poly A:U	i.m., i.v.	10, 30, 150 mg	no	no
OK-432	i.m., i.v., i.t., i.p.	0.2 KE-25 KE	100% fever!	yes

[a] i.v. = intravenous; p.o. = oral, i.m. = intramuscular; i.t. = intramuroal;
 i.p. = intraperitoneal
[b] yes = immune restoration
    immune potentiation

II. Characteristics of agents and clinical applications

Imexon:

With Levamisole, a new era of synthetic immune modulating agents, which have the advantage of an exact dose regimen, was initiated.

A further step was the synthesis of the group of 2-cyanaziridines by BICKER (11), especially of BM 06 002 (4-imino-1,3-diazabicyclo-(3,1.0)-hexan-2-on) which is an isomer of 1-carboxamido-2-cyanaziridine. In animal studies, this substance has been found to potentiate cell-mediated immune reactions, and to inhibit both primary tumour growth and metastatic spread in several tumour systems (13).

Here, we summarize the clinical and immunological data obtained so far in the phase I study with Imexon. The last patient to be included in this investigation was at the end of 1977 (14).

Acute toxicity studies were followed by an investigation of chronic toxicity, the drug being administered for 4—8 weeks, in one study and by administering Imexon, at intervals, for more than 3 months up to 3 years in another. At the time of Imexon therapy patients did not receive any other tumour therapy.

Sixty patients with high risk of recurrence or with advanced malignant disease, with no therapy except surgery for 3 months prior to time of investigation, were included in this study. Conventional therapy had either been considered ineffective or not indicated.

BM 06 002 was supplied by Boehringer Mannheim (FRG) in ampoules of 20 and 100 mg. Patients received a single or several doses of this drug once, twice or three times a week over a period of 1 week, up to 39 months. In some patients anti-emetic drugs were given before therapy in order to reduce side effects.

Imexon therapy induced two complete remissions — one in a case of metastatic lung cancer and one in a case of malignant melanoma metastasizing to the lung. Neither patient shows evidence of disease after observation periods of 33 and 42 months, respectively. One remission from pleural effusion of breast cancer with lung involvement has also been obtained after therapy.

Stabilization of disease was achieved in 3 of 11 patients with breast cancer (mean duration, 4.5 months), in 3/7 patients with lung cancer (mean duration, 4.3 months), and in 1 case of melanoma and 1 of liver cancer, the latter lasting for at least 24 months. Stabilization of disease was maintained by additional therapy with Imexon in 14 patients (4 breast, 3 lung, 3 melanoma, 4 other solid tumours).

Azimexon:

A similar compound — Azimexon — has been developed recently. It has been demonstrated in animal experiments that this substance has an immunomodulating and tumour growth-inhibiting capacity comparable to that of Imexon. Studies in man, including our own, revealed that this compound has no side effects (15, 16).

In a clinical trial in progress (initiated in 1977), Azimexon is included in adjuvant therapy for breast cancer. After surgery, patients are randomized to three treatment arms: (A) no further therapy; (B) chemotherapy; and (C) chemo-immunotherapy (Azimexon, 1×400 mg, after each chemotherapy cycle). So far, 180 patients have taken part in this trial. In group A, the relapse rate is 29%; in group B 17%; and in group C, 12%. These preliminary observations require confirmation by further follow up.

NPT 15392

Isoprenosine and NPT 15392 are synthetic compounds wich have been introduced recently into clinical trials after extensive investigations for toxicity and immunopharmacology in animals (17). Neither substance is toxic, and both can be considered potent modulators of immune functions in both animals and man (18).

NPT has not yet been subjected intensive experimental and clinical studies; therefore, several aspects of its effects on immunomodulation have not yet been investigated. The present study, as part of a cooperative trial with the EORTC Cancer Immunology and Immunotherapy Project Group, was performed in order to investigate the effect of two fixed dose regimens of NPT on several immune parameters.

A total of 10 patients (7 females, 3 males), 5 with diagnoses of malignant melanoma and 5 with gastrointestinal cancer (3 stomach, 1 colon, 1 pancreatic cancer) were studied. All of these patients were considered to be at high risk of recurrence or had locally advanced disease (observed at surgery) which had not been radically operated.

NPT 15392 was kindly supplied by Newport Pharmaceutical Company, USA, in ampoules containing 0.4 mg in 4 ml or 0.7 mg in 7 ml, and was given orally, in the same dose, to each patient. Therapy was well tolerated, with no evidence of subjective or objective side effects.

The influence of therapy on the outcome of disease was not evaluated because of the limited number of patients and the short observation period.

Polyadenylic: polyuridylic acids (poly A: U):

Poly A:U, a weak interferon (IFN) inducer, has been reported recently to prolong significantly the survival of patients with breast cancer when given as adjuvant therapy subsequent to surgery and conventional therapy (18). In that randomized clinical trial, immunological tests gave no evidence for immunomodulation by poly A:U. Furthermore, the authors could demonstrate no immune stimulation by poly A:U therapy in cancer patients (19). The effect of poly A:U on immune response in cancer patients thus appear still undefined.

The purpose of our investigation was to determine whether poly A:U can induce endogenous IFN in cancer patients, and, furthermore, whether it modulates the immune response.

After obtaining verbal consent, 13 patients with locally advanced but not widespread disease (breast, colorectal, and prostatic cancer, and one malignant melanoma) were included in this investigation. Eight patients received 10 mg of poly A:U (Boehringer, Mannheim, FRG) intramuscularly (i. m.); three received 30 mg intravenously (i.v.) (same dose as used by Lacour (18)); and another three patients were given 150 mg i.v.

No negative side effects of poly A:U were observed in these patients. Furthermore, no interferon was detected in serum after 2, 4, 8, 12 and 24 hours after i.v. and i.m. injection. Patients could not be evaluated for clinical response, since they had received only a single injection of poly A:U. The results of immune monitoring (see below) do not allow the conclusion that poly A:U is a potent immunomodulator.

OK-432:

A pharmaceutical preparation known as OK-432 (non-viable *Streptococcus pyogenes* SU strain, lyophilized and sealed in ampoules) has recently been developed in Japan (Chugai Co., Japan); it has been investigated intensively in clinical studies as an anticancer agent which stimulates host defense mechanisms (20).

In cancer patients, OK-432 has also been shown to bring about immunomodulation: it enhances delayed cutaneous hypersensitivity reactions, increases circulating lymphocyte counts anb regulates the levels of lymphocyte subpopulations, enhances proliferative responses of lymphocytes to mitogens; and, as shown recently, reduces suppressor cells for mitogen response (21, 22, 23).

A phase I trial was initiated to study the acute and chronic toxicity and immunomodulating activity of OK-432 (24). A single dose of 0.1 mg lyophilized bacterial preparation (1 Klinische Einheit) was given to 15 patients (12 malignant melanomas, 2 gastrointestinal and 1 breast cancer) by i.v., i.m., intradermal, intratumoural and intraperitoneal routes; patients were not evaluated for response of disease (24).

Two of six patients with metastatic malignant melanoma which had not responded to chemotherapy but who received OK-432 i.v. several times might be considered to have responded, since in one of the patients no progression of the disease was observed after three months, and the other, who had hemiparetic symptoms (due to brain metastases) could move again due to cessation of symptoms after OK-432 therapy. All the other patients still had progressive disease.

The combination of local and systemic OK-432 therapy appears to be the most effective, since five of eight patients with metastatic malignant melanoma responded to such therapy. This streptococcal preparation appears to be effective as an anti-tumour agent, since several patients with advanced malignant melanoma were maintained without tumour progression for some months.

III. Immunopharmacology of Imexon, Azimexon, NPT 15 392, Poly A: U and OK-432

All of these compounds influence several immune parameters after either in-vivo and in-vitro applications (Fig. 1). Their mechanisms of action, however, appear to be different and have not yet been fully characterized.

Lymphocyte blastogenic response (LyBl) to phytohaemagglutinin was significantly increased when Azimexon was added to lymphocytes from patients (26). Poly A:U had a significant suppressive effect (27).

Immunopharmacologic investigations

Appl-testing	Parameter	Imexon	Azimexon	NPT 15392	Poly AU	OK 432
in vitro-in vitro	LyBl		↑		↓	
	aTRFC		↑			
	NK			↔	↔	↑
in vivo-in vitro	LyBl	↑	↔		↓	↑
	T-subsets			↔		
	NK				↓	↓
	Suppressor (NK)					↓
in vivo-in vivo	Recall Ag	↔	↔			↔
	DNCB	↑	↑	(↑)		↑

Fig. 1. Immunopharmacology of the agents investigated.
Symbols: ↑ enhanced response; ↓ suppressed response; ↔ unchanged response
Abbreviations: LyBl — lymphocyte blastogenic response
        aTRFC — active T-rosette forming cells
        NK — natural killer cells
        Ag — antigen
        DCNB — dinitrochlorobenzene

The percentage of active T-rosette forming cells (aTRFC) was also found to be increased after in-vitro incubation of lymphocytes with Azimexon (28).

In-vitro incubation of lymphocytes with Poly A:U (27) or with NPT 15392 (29) had no effect on the activity of natural killer cells (NK), whereas OK-432 significantly enhanced their reactivity (30).

Upon administration of these agents to patients, the following change swere observed: Imexon significantly stimulated LyBl in about 50% of patients (14), whereas Azimexon appeared to have no influence on this parameter, when tested in a randomized trial (unpublished data).

Poly A:U, injected i.v., had a significant depressive effect on this in-vitro reactivity (27), whereas OK-432 therapy enhanced it significantly (23). Cells that suppress NK cells, recently observed by us (31), have been found to be functionally reduced in peripheral blood after OK-432 therapy (unpublished data).

Imexon (14), Azimexon and OK-432 induced no significant changes in skin reactivity to microbial recall atigen (25). The response to dinitrochlorobenzene (DNCB) was significantly augmented (or anergic patients were immunorestored) by Imexon (14), Azimexon, NPT 15392 (29) and OK-432 (25).

It can be concluded from these studies that all of the agents tested, except for poly A:U, have a restorative and/or potentiating effect on several immune functions after either in-vivo or in-vitro application.

Some clinical effectiveness has already been documented for Imexon and OK-432 in phase II studies. Azimexon seems to be effective when combined with chemotherapy, for example in adjuvant therapy of breast cancer. The role of NPT 15392 in cancer treatment is not yet established. All of these agents appear to be useful for the study of immunomodulation in cancer patients and should be investigated further.

References

1. MATHÉ, G., SCHWARZENBERG, L. and AMIEL, J. L.: The role of immunology in the treatment of leukaemias and haematosarcomas. Cancer Res. 27 (1967), 2542—2546
2. McKNEALLY, M. F., MAVER, C. and KAUSEL, H. W.: Regional immunotherapy of lung cancer with intrapleural BCG. Lancet I (1976), 377—381
3. ISREAL, L. and HALPERN, B.: Le *Corynebacterium parvum* dans les cancers avancés. Nouv. Presse Med. 1 (1972), 19—23
4. AMERY, W. K.: Double blind levamisole trial in resectable lung cancer. Ann. N.Y. Acad. Sci. 277 (1976), 260—268
5. STEWART, T. H. M., HOLLINSHEAD, A. C., HARRIS, J. E., RAMAN, S., BELANGER, R., CREPEAU, A., CROOK, A. F., HIRTE, N. E., HOOPER, D., KLAASEN, D. J., RAPP, E. F. and SACHS, H. J. (1978): Survival study of immunotherapy of lung cancer. In: TERRY, W. D. & WINDHORST, D., eds., Immunotherapy of Cancer: Present Status of Trials in Man, New York, Raven Press, pp. 203—216
6. WANEBO, H. J., HILAL, E. Y., PINSKY, C. M., STRONG, E. W., MIKE, V. HIRSHAUT, Y. and OETTGEN, H. F.: Randomized trial of levamisole in patients with squamous cancer of the head and neck. Cancer Treatment Rep. 62 (1978), 1663—1670
7. GALL, St. A., BLESSING, J. A., DISAIA, P. J. and CREASMEN, W. T. (1980): The effect of chemo-immunotherapy in the treatment of primary stage III epithelial ovarian cancer. In: TERRY, W. D., ed. Immunotherapy of Cancer: Present Status of Trials in Man, New York, Elsevier/North Holland (in press)
8. ALBERTS, D. S., SALMON, S. E. and MOON, T. E.: Chemo-immunotherapy for advanced ovarian carcinoma with adriamycin + cyclophosphamide ± BCG. Rec. Results Cancer Res. 68 (1980), 160—166
9. TERRY, W. D. and WINDHORST, D., eds. (1978): Immunotherapy of Cancer: Present Status of Trials in Man, New York, Raven Press
10. OKAMOTO, H., SHOIN, S., KOSHIMURA, S. and SHIMIZU, R.: Studies on the anticancer and streptolysin S-forming abilities of hemolytic streptococci. A review. Jpn. J. Microbiol. 11 (1967), 323—334
11. BICKER, U.: Biochemische und pharmakologische Eigenschaften neuer 2-substituierter Aziridine. Fortschr. Med. 96 (1978), 661—664
12. HADDEN, J. W. and GINER-SOROLLA, A. (1981): Isoprenosine and NPT 15392: modulators of lymphocyte and macrophage development and function. In: Chirigos, M., HERSH, E. & MASTRANGELO, M., eds., Biologic Response Modifiers, New York, Raven Press (in press)

13. Bicker, U. (1978): BM 06 002: a new immune stimulating drug. In: Chirigos, M., ed., Immune Modulation and Control of Neoplasia by Adjuvant Therapy, Basel, Karger, p. 389

14. Micksche, M., Kokoschka, E. M., Sagaster, P. and Bicker, U. (1978): Phase I study for a new immunostimulating drug, BM 06 002, in man. In: Chirigos, M. A., ed., Immune Modulation and Control of Neoplasia by Adjuvant Therapy, New York, Raven Press, pp. 403—413

15. Bicker, U.: Immune modulating effects of BM 12 531 in animals and tolerance in man. Cancer Treat Rep. *62* (1978), 1987—1995

16. Micksche, M., Colot, M., Kokoschka, E. M., Sagaster, P., Bicker, U. and Müller, L.: Immune modulation by 2-cyanaziridine analogs — studies in animals and man. Int. J. Immunopharm. *2* (1980), 202—203

17. Hadden, J. W. and Wybran, J. (1981): Isoprenosine, NPT 15 392 and Azimexon: modulators of lymphocyte and macrophage development and function. In: Müller, P. N. & Hadden, J. W., eds., Advances in Immunopharmacology, New York, Pergamon Press

18. Florentin, I., Bruley-Rosset, M., Schulz, J., Davigny, M., Kiger, N. and Mathé, G. (1981): Attempt at functional classification of chemically defined immunomodulators. In Müller, P. N. & Hadden, J. W., eds., Advances in Immunopharmacology, New York, Pergamon Press

19. Lacour, J., Spira, A., Petit, J.-Y., Sarrazin, D., Lacour, F., Michelson, M., Delage, M., Contesso, G. and Viguier, J.: Adjuvant treatment with polyadenylic-polyuridylic acid (polyA-polyU) in operable breast cancer. Lancet I (1980), 161—166

20. Wanebo, H. J., Kenemy, M., Pinsky, C. M., Hirshaut, Y. and Oettgen, H.: Influence of poly(A)-poly(U) on immune response in cancer patients. Ann. N.Y. Acad. Sci. *277* (1976), 288—298

21. Chugai Pharmaceutical Co. (1977): Host defense stimulator: antitumor Str. pyogenes preparation: picibanil (OK-432). Compendium

22. Uchida, A. and Hoshino, T.: Clinical studies on cell-mediated immunity in patients with malignant disease. I. Effects of immunotherapy with OK-432 on lymphocyte subpopulation and phytomitogen responsiveness in vitro. Cancer *45* (1980), 476—483

23. Uchida, A. and Hoshino, T.: Reduction of suppressor cells in cancer patients treated with OK-432 immunotherapy. Int. J. Cancer *26* (1980), 401—404

24. Micksche, M., Kokoschka, E. M., Sagaster, P. and Kofler, A.: Klinische und immunologische Untersuchungen mit OK-432 (*Streptococcus pyogenes*) zur Immuntherapy bei Krebspatienten. Onkologie *1* (1978), 106—111

25. Micksche, M., Kokoschka, E. M., Jakesz, R., Luger, Th., Rainer, H., Sagaster, P. und Uchida, A. (1980): Phase I study with *Streptococcus* preparation OK-432. In: Terry, W., ed., Immunotherapy of Cancer: Present Status of Trials in Man, New York, Elsevier/North Holland (in press)

26. Colot, M., Micksche, M. and Bicker, U.: Enhanced PHA stimulation of cancer patients lymphocytes by addition of BM 12 531 (Azimexon) in vitro. Cancer Immunol. Immunother. *6* (1979), 110—114

27. Lenzhofer, R., Graninger, W., Uchida, A. and Micksche, M. (1980): Lack of interferon induction by poly(A:U) in cancer patients. In: Current Chemotherapy and Immunotherapy, Waverly Press Inc., (in press)

28. Colot, M., Müller, L., Yamagata, Sh. and Micksche, M. (1980): Immune modulation by BM 12 531 in vitro and in vivo. In: Biology of the Cancer Cell, Proceedings of the 5th Meeting of the European Association for Cancer Research, Vienna, September 9—12, 1979, Amsterdam, Kugler Publications, pp. 149—155

29. Micksche, M., Kokoschka, E. M., Rainer, H. and Uchida, A. (1982): Immunopharmacological studies in patients receiving NPT 15 392. (Submitted for publication)

30. Uchida, A. and Micksche, M. (1982): In vitro augmentation of natural killing activity by OK-432. Int. J. Immunopharmacol. (In press)

31. Uchida, A. and Micksche, M.: Suppressor cells for natural killer activity in carcinomatous pleural effusions of cancer patients. Cancer Immunol. Immunother. *11* (1981), 255—263

Department of Biochemical Pharmacology,
Institute of Cancer Research,
Belmont, Sutton, Surrey,
England

Development of Potential Clinical Alternatives to Hexamethylmelamine

C. J. RUTTY, D. R. NEWELL, J. R. F. MUINDI and K. R. HARRAP

Introduction

Hexamethylmelamine (HMM) [Structure I] is an active agent in the treatment of human cancer, but its usefulness is limited by severe gastrointestinal toxicity. Because of the poor aqueous solubility of HMM the drug must be administered orally, and it was reasoned that such administration led to local irritation of the gastrointestinal tract. Therefore, in search for a water soluble derivative which could be administered intravenously, a large series of analogues of HMM were synthesized by Prof. W. C. J. Ross and his colleagues at the Chester Beatty Research Institute (1). Pentamethyl-melamine (PMM) [Structure II] was found to be 24 times more water soluble than HMM and was not significantly more toxic in terms of mouse LD_{50} values (Fig. 1). In addition, PMM showed comparable activity to HMM against a mouse ADJ/PC6 plasma-cytoma (2) and a human lung tumour xenograft (P246) growing in immune-deprived mice (3).

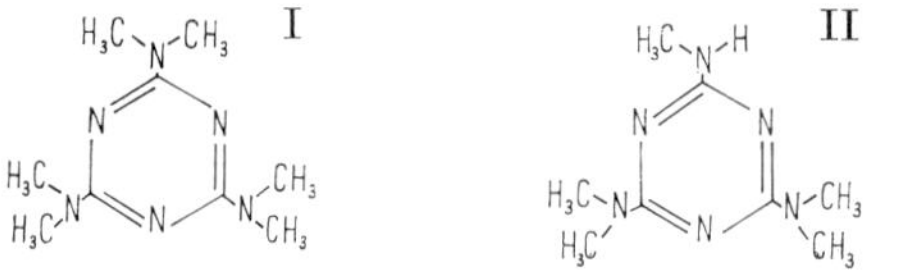

Fig. 1.

	I	II
Aq solubility	0.09 mg/ml	2.16 mg/ml
LD_{50} (mouse)	113 mg/ml	95 mg/ml
PC6 TI*	3.2	2.3
P246 T/C %**	1.0	0.1

* Therapeutic index

** $\dfrac{\text{vol. of treated tumour (mm}^3)}{\text{vol. of control tumour (mm}^3)} \times 100$

Structure-activity and N-demethylation relationships

As well as testing a number of HMM analogues for antitumour activity (and Table 1 shows but a few of the compounds which have been synthesized and tested) the ability of these compounds to undergo N-demethylation by mouse liver microsomes in vitro has also been examined as described previously (2). As the number of methyl groups decreases from HMM, through PMM to N^2, N^2, N^4, N^6-tetramethylmelamine the extent of N-demethylation decreases, but initially the antitumour activity is little affected. However, when three methyl groups have been lost N-demethylation is

180

Table 1

N-demethylation vs. antitumour activity in the melamine series

General formula

$$\begin{array}{c}
\text{H}_3\text{C} \quad \text{R}_1 \\
\text{N} \\
\text{N} \qquad \text{N} \\
\text{H}_3\text{C} \quad \text{N} \qquad \text{N} \qquad \text{CH}_3 \\
\text{R}_3 \qquad \text{N} \qquad \text{R}_2
\end{array}$$

R_1	R_2	R_3	% N-demethylation in vitro (mouse microsomes)	% inhibition of tumour growth at M.T.D. PC6	P246
$-CH_3$	$-CH_3$	$-CH_3$	113	93	100
$-H$	$-CH_3$	$-CH_3$	99	89	91
$-H$	$-H$	$-CH_3$	54	90	83
$-H$	$-H$	$-H$	19	15	0
$-CH_2COOH$	$-CH_3$	$-CH_3$	2.7	7.4	0
$-CH_2CH_3$	$-CH_2CH_3$	$-CH_2CH_3$	74	92	99
$-CH_2OH$	$-CH_3$	$-CH_3$	>100	95	91
$-CH_2OH$	$-CH_2OH$	$-CH_2OH$	>100	95	99

slight and antitumour activity is lost. The highly water soluble carboxymethyl derivative does not undergo significant N-demethylation and is inactive as an antitumour agent. In contrast, the highly lipid soluble triethyl derivative is well demethylated and is active in vivo. Of particular interest are the two N-methylol derivatives, i.e. the mono- and tri-substituted compounds, which have also shown antitumour activity. These data clearly indicate that N-demethylation is necessary for antitumour activity in the melamine series, and that N-methylols may be responsible for the activity.

In vitro cytotoxicity

To further examine the requirement for metabolic activation and the possibility that N-methylolmelamines may represent the active intermediates, we have studied the effects of these compounds on tumour cells in vitro. Using firstly a bioassay system in which TLX/6 lymphoma cells are treated in vitro and then re-injected back into the animal and increase in survival time recorded (4), HMM alone at very high concentrations is totally non-toxic. However, it can be activated by liver microsomes to cytotoxic products (Table 2). Pentamethylmonomethylolmelamine, however, is toxic per se on a 2 hr exposure to these cells. Using PC6 cells in culture (5) followins a 72 hr exposure both HMM and PMM do exhibit toxicity, but N-methylolmelamines are significantly more toxic. N^2,N^4,N^6-trimethylmelamine is relatively non-toxic, HMM does show some activity versus the Walker carcinosarcoma 256 tumour in vivo (6) but is quite non-toxic to these cells in vitro. PMM is also relatively non-toxic, but the two N-methylols do exhibit cytotoxicity. The formation of such intermediary metabolites might therefore be responsible for the antitumour activity in vivo. Furthermore, N-methylolmelamines are chemically unstable and break down to formaldehyde which is itself highly cytotoxic.

Table 2.
In vitro cytotoxicity of N-methyl and N-methylolmelamines

Compound	PC6 ID$_{50}$ (µg/ml) 72 hr	TLX/5 bioassay (µg/ml)* 2 hr	Walker ID$_{50}$ (µg/ml) 72 hr
HMM	39	>2000	Non toxic
HMM + microsomes	—	500	—
PMM	53	—	181
N^2, N^4, N^6-TriMM	370	—	—
PMM-methylol	12.5	200	12.4
Trimethyltrimethylol	4.3	—	3.9
HCHO	1.4	25	1.8

* Concentration to give 99.9% cell kill

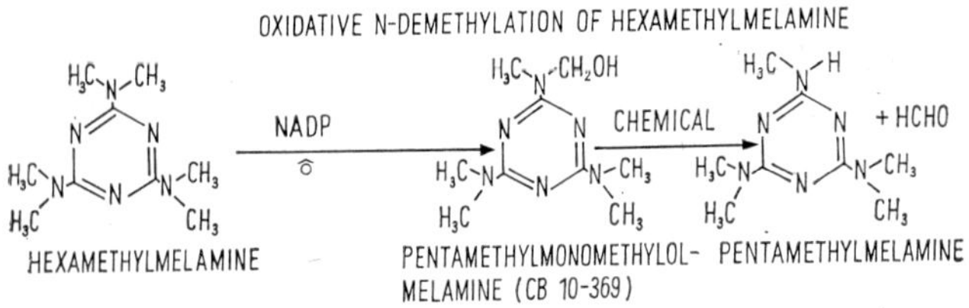

OXIDATIVE N-DEMETHYLATION OF HEXAMETHYLMELAMINE

Fig. 2.

PMM is the primary product of oxidative N-demethylation of HMM. The formation of PMM from HMM requires NADPH and oxygen and occurs via the formation of PMM-methylol as intermediate, i.e. CB 10-369 (Fig. 2) (7).

The toxicity of N-methylolmelamines and formaldehyde to two cell lines in vitro has been examined, i.e. the L1210 leukaemia which is inherently resistant to melamines in vivo (8) and the PC6 plasmacytoma which is sensitive (2). PMM-methylol is toxic to L1210 cells and formaldehyde is similarly toxic. Toxicity to PC6 cells is somewhat greater and again quantitatively formaldehyde toxicity is similar. An important difference between these two cell lines shown in Table 3 is the lack of ability of semicarbazide, a formaldehyde trapping agent, to reverse the toxicity of CB 10-369 to PC6 cells whereas the toxicity of formaldehyde to both cell lines is readily reversed. This suggests that in the sensitive cell line free formaldehyde never exists, but that the N-hydroxymethyl moiety may be transferred to some other carrier within the cell.

Table 3.
In vitro cytotoxicity of CB 10-369 and formaldehyde

Drug	Cell line	ID$_{50}^*$ (µm)	Effect of semicarbazide
CB 10-369	L1210	93	reversal
HCHO	L1210	73	reversal
CB 10-369	PC6	55	no reversal
HCHO	PC6	66	reversal

* Concentration to inhibit growth of cells by 50% (72 h exposure)

182

Effects of melamines on macromolecular synthesis

Under the bioassay conditions described earlier, HMM (500 µg/ml) inhibits both
³H-thymidine and ³H-uridine incorporation into TLX/5 lymphoma cells in vitro
(20 mins flash label). PMM is a somewhat more effective inhibitor, probably by
virtue of its greater water solubility (Fig. 3). CB 10-369 markedly inhibits thymidine
and uridine incorporation at a lower drug concentration (200 µg/ml) than for HMM
or PMM, and there is an increase in inhibition with time which is probably a result
of formaldehyde release.

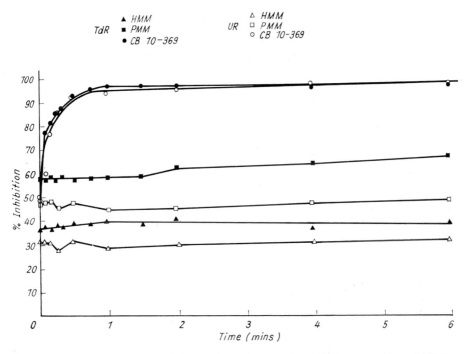

Fig. 3. Progressive effect of HMM, PMM and CB 10-369 on the incorporation of H-Thymidine
and H-uridine by the TLX/5 lymphoma

The inhibition of incorporation of both thymidine and uridine by PMM following a
30 min initial exposure is rapidly and completely reversed following removal of the
drug from the medium (Fig. 4). In marked contrast the effects of the N-methylolmelamine, CB 10-369, are totally irreversible, suggesting quite a different mechanism
of action for the two drugs. The latter finding suggests that CB 10-369 is capable of
covalently binding to the DNA and RNA of tumour cells, and that this may be the
mechanism by which these compounds exert their antitumour activity.

Phase I clinical trial of PMM

A number of recent Phase I clinical trials have been carried out with PMM, including
our own study at the Royal Marsden Hospital (9). In our study PMM was given as an
intravenous infusion over 1—4 h over the dose range 100—1300 mg/m² (Table 4).

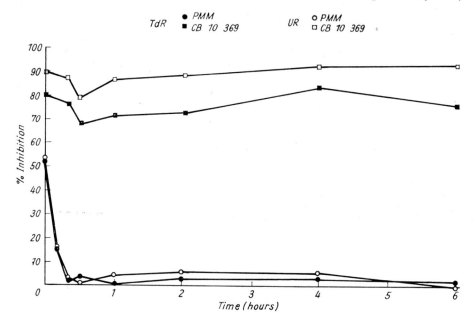

Fig. 4. Reversibility of effects of PMM and CB 10-369 on TdR UR incorporation by TLX/5 cells

Table 4.
Phase I clinical trial of PMM
PMM administered as an i.v. infusion

Dose (mg/m²)	Infusion time (hr)	Gastrointestinal toxicity (nausea and vomiting)
100	1	
200	1	mild
300	1	
500	2	moderate
800	3	severe and prolonged
1300	4	

No myelosuppression or neurological side effects were observed.

The major toxic side effect observed for PMM in this and in other studies reported (10—12) was gastrointestinal, i.e. nausea and vomiting and this effect was dose related. These findings are disappointing in view of the early surmise that by giving a melamine parenterally it should be possible to overcome the gastrointestinal toxicity. It would therefore now appear that this toxicity is central nervous system mediated rather than due to local irritation of the gastrointestinal tract as thought previously. PMM undergoes N-demethylation to give N^2,N^2,N^4,N^6-tetramethylmelamine and N^2,N^4,N^6-trimethylmelamine (Fig. 5). We have measured PMM and its N-demethylated metabolites in human plasma by gas chromatography and by high performance liquid chromatography during the Phase I clinical study (13). From Table 5 it would appear that, unlike for HMM (14), there is a definite relationship between the dose

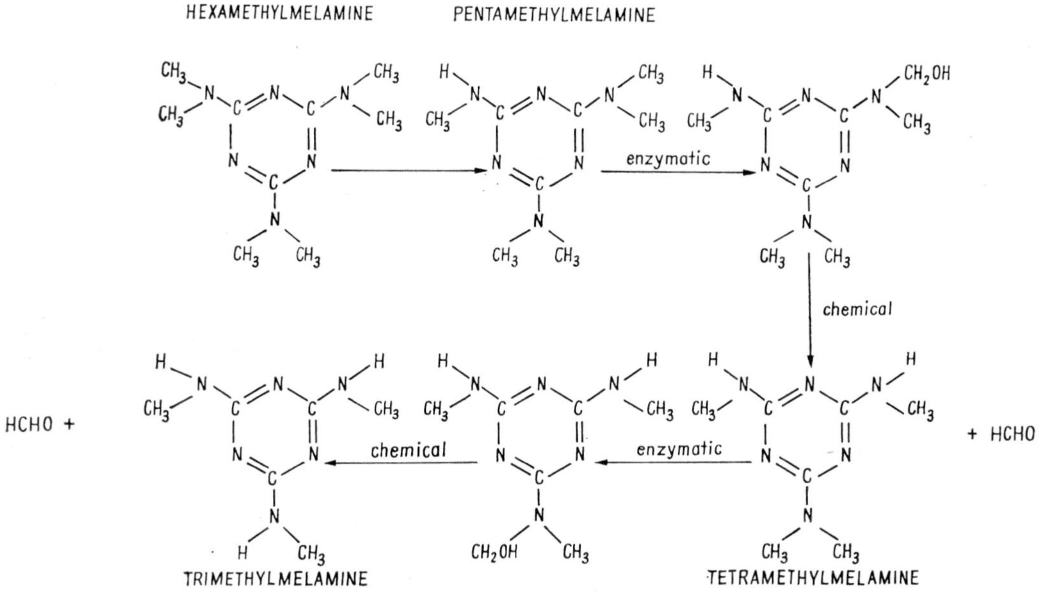

HEXAMETHYLMELAMINE   PENTAMETHYLMELAMINE

enzymatic

chemical

HCHO +   chemical   enzymatic   + HCHO

TRIMETHYLMELAMINE   TETRAMETHYLMELAMINE

Fig. 5.

of PMM administered and circulating levels of parent drug and its metabolites. The average plasma half life ($t^1/_2\beta$) for PMM in patients with normal liver function is approximately 65 min, but is significantly longer for those with poor liver function. The pharmacokinetic data shown here further suggested that much higher circulating levels of N-methylmelamines were obtained following intravenous administration of PMM than for HMM given orally, as compared with published data (14).

A comparative trial of oral HMM versus intravenous PMM in two patients was therefore carried out. PMM was given at 500 mg/m² as a 24 hr infusion, whilst HMM was

Table 5.

Patient	PMM dose (mg/m²)	Hepatic function	PMM plasma $t^1/_2\beta$ (min ± SEM)	Area under the plasma conc. v time curve (μm × min)			
				PMM	N^2, N^2, N^4, N_6-TMM	N^2, N^4, N_6- TriMM	Total Methyl-malamines
M. S	100	Good	N.D.*	317	151	189	657
A. K	100	Good	54.1 ± 3.5	734	204	573	1511
M. M	200	Good	N.D.	1694	397	1070	3161
A. O	300	Good	72.8 ± 6.0	6232	3697	4091	14020
A. C	500	Good	68.6 ± 3.6	3940	2693	3710	10343
E. H	200	Poor	135.0 ± 14.1	7175	1804	1438	10417
J. B	300	Poor	152.6 ± 9.0	6019	2121	627	8767
P. P	500	Poor	127.0 ± 11.1	7179	6206	7995	21380

* N.D. = PMM pharmacokinetics did not follow a one compartment open model in the disposition phase

given orally for 5 days at a dose of 100 mg/m², such that patients received the same total dose of each drug. In both patients studied the total methylmelamine area under the concentration versus time curve for PMM far exceeds that obtained for HMM (Table 6). Despite these findings PMM has proved to be very disappointing clinically with no complete or partial responses being reported (9—12, 15).

Metabolism of PMM occurs via the formation of N-methylolmelamines (Fig. 5) and data presented earlier strongly suggest that these intermediary metabolites, rather than N-methylmelamines, are responsible for the in vivo antitumour action. In a comparative pharmacokinetic study in mouse, rat an man we have therefore measured the levels of N-methylolmelamines in plasma in an attempt to explain the antitumour activity of PMM in experimental tumour systems as opposed to the lack of clinical response to this agent. PMM was measured by HPLC and N-methylolmelamines by a micro-Nash technique (13). In two strains of mouse studied PMM rapidly disappears from the plasma with a half-life of about 15 min. This gives rise to high levels of Nash-positive metabolites (N-methylolmelamines) which are readily cytotoxic (5)

Table 6.
Comparative pharmacology of HMM and PMM

Treatment	Total methylmelamine area under curve (μm × hr)	
PMM 500 mg/m² × 1 24 hour infusion	372	73
HMM 100 mg/m² orally daily × 5	18	17

Table 7.
Pharmacokinetics of pentamethylmelamine

Species	strain	PMM dose	PMM plasma $t^{1/2}$	Nash + Ve metabolites		
				peak plasma concentration	time of peak level	A.U.C. μm × hr
Mouse	Balb/c⁻	90 mg/kg	~10 min	575 μm	30 min	757
	CBA/LAC	90 mg/kg	17 min	700 μm	30 min	1157
Rat	Wistar	90 mg/kg	41 min	225 μm	60 min	715
Man	—	2—35 mg/kg	108 (70—156) min	<50 μm	—	—

(Table 7). In the rat the PMM half-life is significantly longer (approx. 40 min) and the peak levels of N-methylolmelamines achieved are correspondingly lower. The reduced levels of N-methylolmelamines in the rat may explain the relatively low activity of PMM versus the Walker tumour grown in the rat (unpublished data). PMM metabolism in man is even slower than in the rat, and very much slower than in the mouse. More importantly no Nash positive metabolites were detectable in plasma of patients given up to 1.3 g/m² PMM, i.e. the levels of N-methylolmelamines achieved were below the limit of cytotoxicity. It is therefore concluded that the inability to produce sufficiently high levels of cytotoxic N-methylolmelamines in man is responsible for the poor clinical activity of PMM.

Assuming this hypothesis to be correct the direct administration of an N-methylolmelamine would circumvent the need for metabolic activation and might thereby lead to a therapeutic effect in man. N^2,N^4,N^6-trimethylol, N^2,N^4,N^6-trimethylmelamine (CB 10-375) is a compound synthesized in this Institute. Unfortunately, like all N-methylolmelamines, CB 10-375 is unstable breaking down to give N^2,N^4,N^6-trimethylmelamine and formaldehyde (Fig. 6). This would obviously make clinical administration difficult. However, the synthesis of a suitable stabilised derivative would overcome this problem.

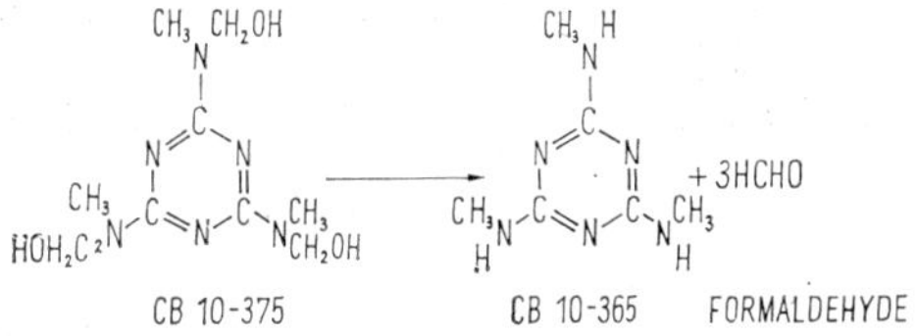

Fig. 6. Trimethyltrimethylolmelamine (CB 10-375) decomposition

Nevertheless, CB 10-375 has several advantages over PMM which suggests this may be a useful approach (Table 8). For example, it is approximately 10-times more cytotoxic in vitro, and shows comparable activity to PMM versus mouse tumours and some human tumour xenografts (2, 3, 8, 16). It is also more water soluble than PMM and may therefore be administered more quickly as an infusion thus minimising breakdown. CB 10-375 is much less acutely neurotoxic than PMM as estimated by hypokinesia and loss of righting reflex. More importantly, the direct administration of CB 10-375 in the rat gives rise to much higher circulating levels of N-methylolmelamines than are achieved using PMM where metabolism of the latter is relatively slow, Correspondingly, CB 10-375 has significantly better antitumour activity versus the Walker tumour grown in the rat.

Further antitumour and toxicological evaluation of CB 10-375 is currently being undertaken with a view to using this compound as an alternative to PMM in the clinic.

Table 8.
Advantages of CB 10-375 over PMM

	PMM	CB 10-375
In vitro cytotoxicity ID_{50} PC6 (µg/ml)	53	5.0
In vivo a.t. activity PC6/P246	++	++
Aq. solubility (mg/ml)	2.2	9.0
Acute neurotoxicity	++++	+
Peak N-methylol levels in rat (µm)	105	608
A.t. activity vs. rat tumour	+	++

187

References

1. CUMBER, A. J. and ROSS, W. C. J.: Chem.-Biol. Interactions *17* (1977), 349
2. RUTTY, C. J. ynd CONNORS, T. A.: Biochem. Pharmacol. *26* (1977), 2385
3. CONNORS, T. A., CUMBER, A. J., ROSS, W. C. J. CLARKE, S. A. and MITCHLEY, B. C. V.: Cancer Treat. Rep. *61* (1977), 927
4. CONNORS, T. A., MANDEL, H. G. and MELZACK, D. H.: Int. J. Cancer *8* (1972), 126
5. RUTTY, C. J. and ABEL, G.: Chem.-Biol. Interactions *29* (1980), 235
6. MIICHLEY, B. C. V., CLARKE, S. A., CONNORS, T. A. and NEVILLE, A. M.: Cancer Res. *35* (1975), 1099
7. GESCHER, A., D'INCALCI, M., FANELLI, R. and FARINA, P.: Life Sciences *26* (1980), 147
8. Data on file with Drug Evaluation Branch, National Cancer Institute
9. SMITH, I. E., MUINDI, J. F. R., NEWELL, D. R., MERAI, K., RUTTY, C. J., WILMAN, D. E. V. and TAYLOR, R. E.: Proc. Am. Ass. Cancer Res. *21* (1980), 136
10. IHDE, D. C., DUTCHER, J. S., YOUNG, R. C., CORDES, R. S., BARLOCK, A. L., HUBBARD, S. M., JONES, R. B. and BOYD, M. R.: Cancer Treat. Rep. *65* (1981), 755
11. GOLDBERG, R. S., GRIFFEN, J. P., McSHERRY, J. W. and KRAKOFF, I. H.: Cancer Treat. Rep. *64* (1980), 1319
12. CASPER, E. S., GRALLA, R. J., LYNCH, G. R., JONES, B. R., WOODCOCK, T. M., GORDON, C., KELSEN, D. P. and YOUNG, C. W.: Cancer Res. *41* (1981), 1402
13. RUTTY, C. J., NEWELL, D. R., MUINDI, J. F. R. and HARRAP, K. R.: Cancer Chemother. Pharmacol. (in press)
14. D'INCALCI, M., BOLIS, G., MANGIONIE, C., MORASCA, L. and GARATTINI, S.: Cancer Treat. Rep. *62* (1978), 2117
15. ECHO, D. A., CHIUTEN, D. F., WHITACRE, M., AISNER, J., LICHTENFIELD. J. L. and WIERNIK, P. H.: Cancer Treat. Rep. *64* (1980), 1335
16. GOLDIN, A., VENDITTI, J. M., MacDONALD, J. S., MUGGIA, F. M., HENNEY, J. E. and DeVITA, V.: Europ. J. Cancer *17* (1981), 129

Central Institute for Tumours and Allied Diseases, Ilica 197, 41000 Zagreb, Yugoslavia[a]
and
Laboratory for Experimental Oncology, Indiana University School of Medicine, 1100 W. Michigan Street, Indianapolis, IN 46223[b], USA

Synergistic Interaction of an Alkylating Agent (Lycurim) and an Antimetabolite (Pyrazofurin) on Hepatoma 3924A Cells in Culture

J. Ban[a], E. Olah[b] and G. Weber[b,*]

Introduction

The purpose of this study was to test for a possible synergism in the antitumour action of the antimetabolite Pyrazofurin (PF) and the alkylating agent, Lycurim (LY) (1,4-di-(2'-mesyloxy-ethylamine)-1,4-dideoxy-m-erythritol dimethylsulfonate), on proliferating and resting rat hepatoma 3924A cells in tissue culture.

PF inhibited the growth of some rodent tumours (7, 15) and showed potential chemotherapeutic action in human tumours (3, 6). It was suggested that PF might be used in combination chemotherapy (2, 3). It was recently demonstrated that in combination with galactosamine a synergistic decrease of uridine- and cytidine-5'-triposphate pools of hepatoma cells in vivo and in vitro was obtained (10, 18, 19). In active form, PF is an inhibitor of orotidylate (OMP) decarboxylase (2, 3, 6, 7). In cell culture PF was a phase-specific agent (11, 18, 19), while LY showed cycle specificity (1). In some solid tumours, LY was found to be a potential chemotherapeutic agent (8, 13). When used sequentially with cyclophosphamide a synergistic response was detected in leukemia L1210 cells in mice (14). LY, which is an alkylating agent (5, 12, 13) also inhibited transaldolase activity in extracts of solid hepatoma 3924A (1).

Materials and methods

Cell culture. Hepatoma 3924A cell line was grown in monolayer cultures in McCoy's 5A medium with 10% fetal calf serum (Grand Island Biological Co., Grand Island, N.Y.) and incubated in 5% CO_2: 95% air atmosphere. Cells were subcultured 3 times a week. For experiments on exponentially growing populations hepatoma 3924A cells were seeded (5×10^5) into plastic flasks (25 cm²), and incubated for 48 hrs. For studies on plateau phase cells, cultures were incubated for 96 hrs without changing the medium.

Survival studies. Cellular survival was measured by the colony formation technique. The experimental details of this technique and also induction of the plateau phase cultures with definitions and cytogenetic characteristics of plateau and exponential phases were reported elsewhere (1, 11).

Drugs. LY (NSC-122402) was obtained through courtesy of the G. Richter Company, Budapest, Hungary. PF (NSC-143095) was donated by Eli Lilly and Co., Indianapolis, IN. Both lyophilized drugs were stored at 4 °C.

Results and discussion

Survival studies. Exponentially growing or plateau phase cells were treated with different concentrations of drugs. LY and PF were dissolved in sterile phosphate

* Supported by grant no. CA-05034 from the USPHS, National Cancer Institute, to whom correspondence and requests for reprints should be addressed.

189

buffered saline (PBS) just before use and were immediately added to the cell culture. Cells were exposed to the individual drug or both drugs together for 1 or 2 hrs. LY and PF were then removed and flasks were rinsed 3 times with PBS. The cells were trypsinized and seeded into culture flasks (500 cells/25 cm²). The pH of the medium was adjusted with 5% CO_2 in air. After an incubation period of 6 days, the medium was removed and the cells were stained with crystal violet. Colonies were counted and the surviving fraction was calculated as percent of untreated cells. In combination experiments, control survival curves were performed for each individual drug.

Lethal effects of PF. The survival curves of exponentially growing cells treated with different doses of PF for 1 or 2 hr, respectively, were of a biphasic type, yielding an LD_{50} of 20 µM. The same or even 10 times higher drug concentrations in the plateau phase had no inhibitory effect on the growth of tumour cells. Thus, PF inhibited proliferating cells only (11, 18, 19).

Lethal effects of LY. The survival curves of both exponential and plateau phase cells exposed to increasing concentrations of LY or 1 or 2 hr, respectively, were the threshold exponential type. Curves indicated similar lethal effects on both cell cultures, yielding an LD_{50} of 5 and 1 µM after one- or two-h treatment, respectively (1). This points to the possible usefulness of this drug in combination with a phase-specific agent, e.g. PF.

Lethal effects of a combination of PF and LY. To test the hypothesis that a combination of LY and PF might potentiate the killing of hepatoma 3924 A cells, proliferating and resting cells were exposed to the action of both drugs for 1 and 2 hr and 7 days. Both drugs were given in combination of their respective LD_{50} concentrations. The predicted survival and possible synergism were calculated according to WEBB (17) (see Fig. 1). Details were described elsewhere (1).
Exponentially growing cells were simultaneously treated with LD_{50} concentrations of LY and PF for different lengths of incubation (Fig. 1). Predicted survival was in all cases 25%. After 1 hr treatment only summation was observed. Synergistic po-

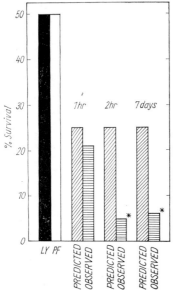

Fig. 1. Survival of proliferating hepatoma 3924A cells exposed to LD_{50} concentrations of LY and PF alone and both drugs given simultaneously. The cells were treated for 1 and 2 hrs, and 7 days with the drug. Colonies were then counted.

Predicted survival (PS) =

$$\frac{\text{Mean \% of LY survival} \times \text{Mean \% of PF survival}}{100}$$

* Significantly lower survival than the predicted one ($p < 0.05$). Means of triplicate determinations are given.

190

tentiation was noted when hepatoma cells were treated for 2 hr with both drugs (LY of 1 μM and PF of 20 μM). Observed survival was 4.6%. It was also detected that lower concentrations of LY (0.1 μM) together with PF (10 μM) gave only summation. When cells were treated for 7 days, very low concentrations of LY (0.016 μM) and PF (0.085 μM) were needed to obtain the synergistic killing action. Observed survival was 5.9%.

It was of interest to test whether even lower concentrations of drugs would be effective after long-term treatment. The survival curves of proliferating cells treated for 7 days with different doses of PF and LY alone and in combination are shown in Fig. 2. Dose-response curve of cells treated with PF was of a threshold exponential type with a broad shoulder region ($D_q = 0.025$ μM; $D_0 = 0.065$ μM; where D_q is a quasi-threshold dose equal to the intercept with the abscissa of the exponential part of survival curve, and D_0 is the mean lethal dose equal to the concentration required to reduce survival by 63% on the exponential part of survival curve). The survival curve of hepatoma cells treated with LY alone was also threshold exponential with a small shoulder and a steep exponential part ($D_q = 0.012$ μM; $D_0 = 0.014$ μM). When

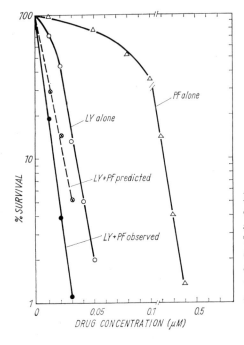

Fig. 2. Survival of proliferating hepatoma 3924 A cells exposed to increasing concentrations of LY and PF alone and both drugs given simultaneously. The cells were treated for 7 days. Cells were seeded (500/flask) and supplemented with the drug for 7 days. Colonies were counted and predicted survivals were calculated as in Fig. 1. Each point is the average of triplicate samples of 3 experiments.

two drugs were given together, cells were exposed to increasing concentrations of LY, as indicated in Fig. 2, while PF was always added in the concentration of 0.1 μM. Obtained dose-response curve was exponential, with no shoulder region ($D_0 = 0.0092$ μM). The increase in killing activity by PF was reflected in the reduction or the elimination of shoulder region and in the magnitude of the slope of the survival curve of LY.

These results suggested that the synergistic activity of LY and PF was primarily time-dependent and secondarily concentration-dependent.

The survival of the plateau phase cells treated with LY and PF simultaneously is shown in Fig. 3. As PF did not inhibit the growth of plateau phase cells, LD_{50} concentrations were not obtained. After 1 and 2 hr treatment only very high concentration of LY (5 μM) together with PF (50 or 100 μM) resulted in synergistic action. Observed survivals were 14.4% and 7.2% after 1- and 2- hr treatment, respectively. PF was selected for drug combination with LY because their mechanisms of action are different and increased activities of certain tumour enzymes could be targets for the action of these drugs. In hepatomas adenosine kinase activity was retained (9), and OMP decarboxylase activity, the target of PF inhibitory action of de novo uridine-5′-monophosphate synthesis (7) was increased (18, 19, 20). LY, as an alkylating agent, would damage DNA molecule (4). As an inhibitor of transaldolase activity, LY might inhibit the biosynthesis of purines (1).

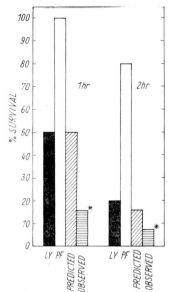

Fig. 3. Survival of plateau phase hepatoma 3924 A cells exposed to different concentrations of LY and PF alone and both drugs given simultaneously. The cells were treated for 1 and 2 hrs with the drug. Colonies were counted, and predicted survivals were calculated as in Fig. 1.
* Significantly lower survival than the predicted one (p < 0.05). Means of triplicate determinations are given.

The decreased effectiveness of synergistic action in plateau phase cells is important because of the presence of such low growth fractions in the most common human neoplasms, e. g., colon, breast and others. It has been suggested that the DNA in plateau phase might be less sensitive to alkylating agents than in proliferating cells (16). If this is so, the decreased synergistic action in plateau cells may be accounted for, in part at least, by the fact that the activity of OMP decarboxylase was 3.3-fold lower than in the proliferative phase (11, 20). Thus, there should be less sensitivity to pyrazofurin which has indeed been demonstrated (11). Further studies should provide other drug combinations effective against plateau phase cells.

References

1. BAN, J., OLAH, E. and WEBER, G.: Cancer Treat. Rep. *66* (1982), (in press)
2. BROCKMAN, R. W., SHADDIX, S. C. and ROSE, L. M.: Cancer *40* (1977), 2681
3. CADMAN, E. C., DIX, D. E. and HANDSCHUMACHER, R. E.: Cancer Res. *38* (1978), 682
4. CALABRESI, P. and PARKS, R. E., Jr.: (1980) In: The Pharmacological Basis of Therapeutics. p. 1256 (GILMAN, G. A., GOODMAN, L. S., GILMAN, A., eds.), Macmillan, N.Y.
5. CSANY, E. and ELEKES, I.: Neoplasma *19* (1972), 189
6. GRALLA, R. J., CURRIE, V. E., WITTES, R. E., GOLBEY, R. B. and YOUNG, C. W.: Cancer Treat. Rep. *62* (1978), 451

7. GUTOWSKI, G. E., SWEENEY, M. J., DeLONG, D. C., HAMILL, R. L., GERZON, K. and DYKE' R. W.: Ann. N.Y. Acad. Sci. *255* (1975), 544

8. HINDY, I., SELLEI, C., ECKHARDT, S., SZENTKLARAY, J. and HARTAI, F.: Neoplasma *18* (1971), 277

9. JACKSON, R. C., MORRIS, H. P. and WEBER, G.: Br. J. Cancer *37* (1978), 701

10. LUI, M. S., JACKSON, R. C. and WEBER, G.: Biochem. Pharmacol. *28* (1979), 1189

11. OLAH, E., LUI, M. S., TZENG, D. Y. and WEBER, G.: Cancer Res. *40* (1980), 2869

12. SANDBERG, J. and GOLDIN, A.: Cancer Chem. Rep. *53* (1969), 367

13. SELLEI, C., ECKHARDT, S. and NEMETH, L. (1970): In: Chemotherapy of Neoplastic Disease. p. 164. Publishing House of the Hungarian Academy of Sciences, Budapest.

14. STOYCHKOV, J. N., MILUSHEV, A. S. and TODOROV, D. K.: Neoplasma *27* (1980), 33

15. SWEENEY, M. J., DAVIS, F. A., GUTOWSKI, G. E., HAMILL, R. L., HOFFMAN, D. H. and POORE, G. A.: Cancer Res. *33* (1973), 2619

16. VALERIOTE, F. and PUTTEN, L.: Cancer Res. *35* (1975), 2619

17. WEBB, J. L.: (1963) In: Enzyme and Metabolic Inhibitors. Vol. 1, 487. Academic Press, N.Y.

18. WEBER, G., OLAH, E., LUI, M. S. and TZENG, D. Y.: (1979) In: Advances in Medical Oncology, Research and Education. p. 151, (Fox, B. W., ed.), Pergamon Press, Oxford and N.Y.

19. WEBER, G., OLAH, E., LUI, M. S. and TZENG, D. Y.: Adv. Enzyme Regul. *17* (1979), 1

20. WEBER, G., OLAH, E., LUI, M. S., KIZAKI, H., TZENG, D. Y. and TAKEDA, E.: Adv. Enzyme Regul. *18* (1980), 3

Istituto Scientifico per lo Studio e la Cura dei Tumori, Genova,
and
* Divisone Otorinolaringoiatrica, Ospedale S. Martino, Genova, Italy

Phase II Evaluation of 4-Thiazolidine-Carboxylic Acid (Thioproline) in Advanced Epidermoid Head and Neck Tumours

F. Boccardo, R. Rosso, A. Barbieri*, L. Canobbio, D. Guarneri and M. Merlano

Introduction

Thioproline (thiazolidine-4-carboxylic acid) has recently been reported to be effective against epidermoid tumours in humans. In particular, a 100% response rate was achieved in 10 patients with head and neck cancer and in one patient with lung cancer, without side effects (11).

The results of a phase II trial with thioproline in advanced epidermoid head and neck tumours form the subject of the present report.

Material and methods

Between November 1980 and February 1981, 20 patients with histologically proven epidermoid head and neck cancer entered the trial. The main characteristics of the study patients are summarized in Table 1. Bevofe treatment, all patients underwent a complete assessment, including full blood counts, electrocardiogram, chest roentgenogram and scintiscan, when indicated. In addition, measurements and colour photographs were taken of tumour lesions. Full, informed consent was obtained in all cases.

Thioproline was supplied in ampoules containing 750 mg of the sodium salt of thiazolidine-4-carboxylic acid and administered according to one of the schedules described by Brugarolas and Gosalvez (7). Therapy was started with a dose of 40—60 mg/kg daily, given by continuous intravenous infusion on five consecutive days, after appropriate dilution in 2 litres of normal saline, and was repeated every three weeks for a total of three therapy cycles. Therapy was discontinued when clear progression of disease was observed. Infusion was performed through a central or peripheral venous catheter, using millipore filters to decrease the risk of febrile and septic complications. Fluid and saline balance were monitored closely during infusion.

Responses were assessed and toxicity recorded at the end of each therapeutic cycle. Patients were considered to be fully evaluable for response after three therapy cycles. Complete response (CR) was defined as disappearance of all measurable diseases for at least one month. Partial response (PR) was defined as a decrease of at least 50% in all measurable lesions during one month. An objective improvement of at least 25% was considered to be a minor response (MR). Progressive disease (PD) was defined as an increase of at least 25% in all lesions or the appearance of new lesions. All cathegories between MR and PD were considered to be stationary disease (SD).

Results

Two patients died of PD after completion of the first therapy cycle; one patient died of congestive heart failure; and one patient was lost to follow-up after two therapy

Table 1.
Main characteristics of study patients (n = 20)

Median age in years (range)	58 (36—73)
Sex	
Males	18
Females	2
Median initial performance status (range)	1 (0—3)
Distribution of primary tumour sites	
Oropharynx	7
Hypopharynx	1
Larynx	2
Nasal sinus	2
Oral cavity	6
Lower lip	1
Primary tumour size	
T_0-T_2	9
T_3-T_4	11
Nodal status	
N_0-N_1	11
N_2-N_3	9
Previous treatment	
None	6
Radio- + chemotherapy	6
Surgery + radio- + chemotherapy	8

cycles. In all of these cases, disease appeared to be unchanged. One patient showed acute neurologic toxicity during the first therapy cycle, and treatment was discontinued. Therefore, 15 patients were fully evaluable for response.

Five out of six patients with no prior treatment showed SD, while one showed PD. Of nine patients who had had previous radio- and/or chemotherapy, one showed a MR lasting four weeks, three had SD and five had PD. The patient who showed a MR had completed radiotherapy 25 days before commencing the treatment with thioproline; thus, it cannot be excluded that radiotherapy rather than thioproline produced the improvement.

Fifty therapy cycles were considered for toxicity. In general, therapy was well tolerated: most patients had a feeling of well-being and no nausea, vomiting, myelosuppression or major disturbances of fluid or saline balance were noted. However, serious neurotoxicity was encountered in four cases. One patient, aged 73, developed seizures and coma during the first therapy cycle, which disappeared after discontinuation of therapy; two patients developed confusion and frank psychosis with paranoid delusions in the course of the third therapy cycle; and a fourth patient showed a neurological syndrome similar but less intense than the above one month after completing the last therapeutic cycle. In three cases tumour biopsies were repeated, and two patients underwent major surgery at the end of the third cycle; in all of these, the disease appeared to be clinically unchanged, and in no case could significant changes in the histological picture be demonstrated.

Discussion

Thioproline derives from the reaction of cysteine with formaldehyde and is a physiological metabolite which occurs in the liver of mammals. Due to its ability to transfer

SH groups, it has been employed since the 1960s as a liver-protective drug (2). More recently, it has been shown to produce a morphological change in HeLa cells similar to that obtained with dibutyryl cyclic AMP in CHO-K1 cells, probably by restoring membrane functions such as contact inhibition (3). Thus, the drug has been described as one of the first of a new series of non-cytotoxic anticancer agents, capable of inducing reverse transformation of tumour cells rather than killing them. In support of this possible mechanism of action, significant changes have been reported, in the histological pictures of tumours that regressed after treatment with thioproline (1). In particular, differentiation of epidermoid tumours with horn pearl formation, involution and regression of previously invasive tumours and healing with production of scar tissue were noted.

The results of our study seem to indicate that thioproline is not effective in epidermoid head and neck tumours. These findings do not confirm those reported by BRUGAROLAS and GOSALVEZ (1), despite the fact that a similar dosage and schedule were employed; and, on the contrary serious neurological toxicity was encountered.

Pharmacokinetic studies showed that after intravenous administration thioproline occurs as such in the urine (4): when the drug is administered orally, it is rapidly hydrolysed to cysteine and formaldehyde in the stomach and liver. It is possible that, at least in some cases, intravenously administered thioproline may follow the same metabolic pathway as orally administered drug.

With the high dosage employed in this clinical trial, an accumulation of formaldehyde may have occurred, leading to the observed neurotoxicity. Formaldehyde accumulation was responsible for severe convulsions, accompanied by status epilepticus, in chilbren who had accidentally ingested toxic amounts of thioproline (5).

SAPPINO and SMITH (6), reporting on five patients with squamous malignancies of the lung and tongue treated with 40 mg/kg daily delivered intramuscularly in four divided doses, found a similar lack of effectiveness and neurological toxicity. NASCA et al (7), who treated 48 patients with different epidermoid tumours (lung, head and neck, oesophagus, skin and cervix) with daily doses of 20 mg/kg orally or 40 mg/kg intramuscularly, also obtained no effect of the drug but noted neurotoxicity and renal function abnormalities.

NEWMAN and coworkers (8) tested thioproline in vitro on transformed HeLa and other cell lines (W1-38VA13, C1300 neuroblasma and CHO-K1) and showed that it had no effect in producing a reversal of the transformed state. Thioproline also produced severe, life-threatening central nervous system toxicity in both mice and rats after intraperitoneal administration at levels far below those previously reported to be without toxic effects (8).

In summary, a number of clinical and experimental studies have failed to confirm the biological and, in particular, the antineoplastic effects of thioproline that were described earlier. Disagreement concerning the efficacy of this drug and the possible existence of severe neurotoxic effects contraindicate further investigation of thioproline in humans.

References

1. BRUGAROLAS, A. and GOSALVEZ, M.: Treatment of cancer by an inducer of reverse transformation. Lancet *I* (1980), 68—70
2. BURBERI, S.: Ricerche farmacologiche sull'acido thiazolidin-carbossilico. Boll. Chim. Farm. *114* (1975), 659—662

3. Gosalvez, M., Viveiro, C. and Alvarez, I.: Restoration of contact inhibition of tumour cells in tissue culture by treatment with thiazolidin-4-carboxylic acid. Biochem. Soc. Trans. 7 (1979), 191—192

4. Gosalvez, M.: Thioproline. Lancet I (1980), 597—598

5. Garnier, R., Conso, F., Eftymion, M. L. and Fournier, E.: Thioproline. Lancet I (1980), 417

6. Sappino, A. P. and Smith, S. E.: Thioproline in squamous cell cancer. Lancet I (1980), 417

7. Nasca, S., Galichet, V., Jardillier, S. C., Garee, E. and Conox, P.: Thioproline toxicity. Lancet I (1980), 778

8. Newmann, R., Hacter, M. P., McCormack, J. J. and Krakoff, I. H.: Pharmacologic and toxicologic evaluation of thioproline: a proposed non-toxic inducer of reverse transformation. Cancer Treat. Rep. 64 (1980), 837—844

Institute for Drug Research, Budapest, Hungary

The Effect of a Bifunctional N-Nitrosoureido Derivative (GYKI-13324) on Experimental Metastasis Models

E. Csányi, Z. Hargittay, E. Király, T. Horváth, L. Bogdány and K. Tory

GYKI-13324 is a new N-nitrosoureido sugar alcohol derivative (Fig. 1) that produces a curative effect on a broad scale of transplantable and induced rodent tumours as well as on human tumour xenografts. Such an effect has also been shown on various leukaemia models (1). In the present study its inhibitory effect on experimental metastasis was demonstrated.

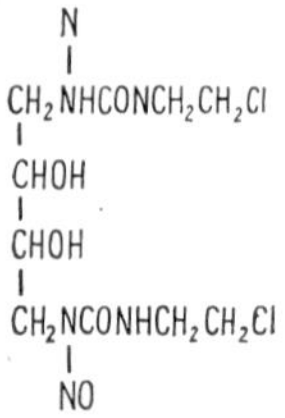

```
        N
        |
CH₂NHCONCH₂CH₂Cl
 |
CHOH
 |
CHOH
 |
CH₂NCONHCH₂CH₂Cl
 |
 NO
```

Fig. 1. Chemical structure of 1-(3-(2-chloroethyl)-3-nitrosocarbamoyl)-4-(3-(2-chloroethyl)-1-ni-trosocarbamoyl)-1,4-dideoxy-D,L-threitol (GYKI-13324).

Lewis lung cancer is known to be a good but relatively resistant model for testing compounds that affect the steps of formation and development of metastases. To study the effect of GYKI-13324 on this model, 5×10^5 cells in a volume of 50 µl were implanted into the right hind legs of BDF_1 mice. In most experiments, the primary tumour was removed under pentobarbital anaesthesia by amputation of the leg. Increase in survival time and 90-day tumour-free survival were considered to be positive responses.

The effect of chemotherapy alone was studied first (Table 1). Early therapy of this type had first to depress the primary tumour, then to prevent dissemination of tumour cells and finally to prevent the development of metastases in the lung. Thus,

Table 1.
Effects of GYKI-13324 given alone, orally, on Lewis lung carcinoma

Dose (mg/kg)	Treatment[a]	Increase in lifespan (%)	Cures[b]
30	Once, on day 2	36	0/8
60	Once, on day 2	54	1/8
100	Once, on day 2	70	6/8
100	Twice, on days 2 and 8	—	8/8
Control		0	0/8

[a] Day of implantation was regarded as day 1
[b] Number of 90-day tumour-free survivors

a well-tolerated oral dose of GYKI-13324 produced a 100% cure rate. The approximate DC_{50} value was calculated to be 85 mg/kg; the $LD_{50}:DC_{50}$ ratio was 1.59. Under the same conditions, bischloroethylnitrosourea (BCNU) produced a maximum cure rate of 2/8 at a dose close to the maximum tolerated dose (25 mg/kg).

Lower doses of GYKI-13 324 were required to produce a high cure rate when they were combined with surgical removal of the primary tumour. Surgery was performed on days 8, 10 or 12 after implantation, and a single oral dose of GYKI-13 324 was given simultaneously, one day before or one day after surgery.

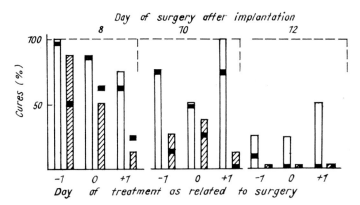

Fig. 2. Curative effect on Lewis lung carcinoma of GYKI-13 324, given orally before or after surgical removal of the primary tumour.

▨, 30 mg/kg; □, 60 mg/kg; ■, bischloroethylnitrosourea at 12.5 mg/kg corresponding to ▨ and 25 mg/kg corresponding to □.

As can be seen in Figure 2, the compound had a curative effect on the lung metastases. This effect was most pronounced in the case of treatment before surgery on day 8: a single 30 mg/kg dose produced 7/8 cures, and 60 mg/kg resulted in a 100% cure rate. When surgery was performed on day 10 or 12, postoperative chemotherapy was more effective, the low and high doses producing 50% and 100% cure rates, respectively. BCNU, tested as a positive control, was less effective: when given after late day 12 surgery, only 1/24 animal was cured, while administration of GYKI-13324 under the same conditions produced a 50% cure rate. Mayo et al (2) found weaker effects of 1-(2-chloroethyl)-3-(4-methyl-cyclohexyl)-1-nitrosourea (me-CCNU) and BCNU given around early day 7 surgery, obtaining a maximum 40% cure rate in contrast to our results of 90—100%.

Since a potentiating synergism had previously been found between GYKI-13324 and 5-fluorouracil (5-FU) on the L-1210 leukaemia system, we tested the two compounds in the Lewis lung cancer system, in combination with surgery on day 8. Pretreatment with 40 mg/kg 5-FU intraperitoneally on days 9—12, followed by a single dose of 40 mg/kg GYKI-13324 on day 12 was found to be the most effective. Treatment with GYKI-13324 or 5-FU alone resulted in 2/8 or 3/8 cures, respectively, while the combination produced 6/8 cures.

The intravenous implantation of ascites cells may simulate haematogenic dissemination; intravenous administration of Walker ascites cells results in the development of lung metastases that kill the animals within two weeks. The effect of GYKI-13 324 was tested on this metastasis model (Table 2). When administered as early, single-dose

Table 2.
Effect of GYKI-13 324 on the Walker carcinosarcoma

Compound	Treatment[a]		Increase in life span	Cures[c]
	Dose (mg/kg)	Day[b]	(%)	
GYKI-13 324	12 (1 × i.p.)	2	156	1/7
	12 (2 × i.p.)	2, 3	270	6/7
	30 (1 × p.o.)	2	95	1/6
	60 (1 × p.o.)		44	4/6
BCNU	20 (1 × i.p.)	2	106	1/6
	25 (1 × p.o.)	2	107	1/6
Control[d]	— —		0	0/7

[a] i. p., intraperitoneal; p.o., oral
[b] After intravenous implantation of Walker ascites cells
[c] Number of 90-day tumour-free survivors
[d] Lifespan of controls, 13.6 days

therapy, it produced a high percentage of long-term survivors after either intravenous or oral treatment. In parallel experiments on this model, BCNU was found to be much less effective.

In conclusion, GYKI-13 324 has a very strong antimetastatic action, as seen in the Lewis lung cancer model, both with and without surgery. In comparative studies, its effect was superior to that of BCNU.

References

1. Csányi, E., Horváth, T., Király, E., Lapis, K. and Kopper, L.: Oncology 37 Suppl. 1 (1980), 59—66
2. Mayo, J. G., Laster, W. R., Jr. Andrews, C. M. and Schabel, F. M., Jr.: Cancer Chemother. Rep. 56 (1972), 183—195

Institute of Toxicology and Chemotherapy,
German Cancer Research Center, Heidelberg, FRG

Long-term Toxic and Carcinogenic Effects
of Cytostatic Drugs

M. Habs and D. Schmähl*

Today more than ever, drug-induced effects and diseases are gaining in significance:
Two factors seem to be largely responsible for this development:
1. The number of drugs and their use are increasing constantly.
2. More and more drugs are being developed, which have far-reaching effects on physiologic and pathologic biochemical reactions.

The physician administering drugs has been trained to take acute and subacute toxic side effects into consideration. Nowadays he also ought to expand this caution to possible chronic toxicity, including carcinogenicity.

It is necessary to undertake a risk-benefit analysis in each invididual case, making sure that therapeutic effects are not outweighed by risk. A carcinogenic effect of a drug, which may possibly manifest itself many years or even decades after the therapeutic treatment, will hardly be of significance if the case has a poor prognosis or there is no alternative to this therapy. If, however, this is not so, then the physician has to consider whether the potentially hazardous drug should be administered or whether alternatives are at hand.

From the point of view of overall cancer incidence, drug-induced malignant tumours do not play a very important role. However, it is not known how many drugs carrying a carcinogenic risk are being used at present. These circumstances should not obscure the fact that certain groups of patients who are subjected to a particularly intensive treatment with carcinogenic drugs run a considerably higher risk.

The statistical methods of analytic epidemiology have definite limits in detecting slight increases in the frequency of diseases. If a drug increases the risk of developing a relatively frequent tumour type, its detection will consequently be more difficult than the detection of an increased risk of forming a tumour which seldom occurs in the general public.

It is not easy to identify a drug exerting a carcinogenic activity in man. This is primarily due to the fact that a disease is only seldom treated with one drug. Thus it is very difficult to detect the suspect carcinogen in combination therapy, particularly since several drugs may produce mutually modifying effects (Habs and Schmähl 1980). Furthermore, the often long induction times of iatrogenic tumours are frequently a hindrance to an epidemiologic approach.

Seen historically, the carcinogenic activity of cancer chemotherapeutic agents, including most of the alkylating agents, has been known from experimental investigations for many years. In the late 60s, Japanese investigators indicated that following exposure to mustard gas, neoplasms may occur in the respiratory tract of man. It

* Dedicated to John H.Weisburger, Ph. D., M. D. h. c. on the occasion of his 60th birthday

was found that among workers, who had been employed in the production of mustard gas in the years between 1929 and 1945, the rate of malignant tumours of the respiratory tract was 33-fold higher than in the general population. Beside a statistically proven increased occurrence of bronchus carcinomas, in former mustard gas-exposed workers carcinomas of the urinary bladder and leukemias were observed to a three-fold higher extent than expected. Also, the occurrence of glioblastomas and neurofibromas in association with exposure to N-mustard has been discussed (SCHMÄHL and HABS 1980).

These observations in occupational medicine as well as the large amount of experimental data on carcinogenic effects of corresponding drugs caused us to test alkylating agents in particular and, in addition, antimetabolites, antineoplastic natural substances, and antibiotics in comparative and quantitative dose-response investigations (SCHMÄHL and HABS 1980). Our earlier studies can be summarized as follows: At a dose corresponding to that administered clinically to patients, alkylating compounds induced significant carcinogenic effects in rats. Compared with untreated controls, we observed a four- to six-fold increase in tumour yield. The antimetabolites investigated by us (methotrexate, 6-mercaptopurine, 5-fluorouracil) as well as the alkaloids vinblastine and demecolcine (Colcemide) (desacetyl-methylcolchicine) did not prove to be carcinogenic. Regarding tumour localizations, no preselection for certain organ sites could be seen in our experiments; however, an increase in leukemias and hemangiosarcomas was recorded by WEISBURGER (1977).

Using cyclophosphamide as a model, since it is one of the most frequently used chemotherapeutic alkylating agents, we undertook some quantitative experiments. Our primary objective was to determine whether small doses, lower than those presently administered in clinical chemotherapy, are carcinogenic or not. Rats were given various doses orally, the lowest dose being only 25% of the dose used in man in maintenance therapy.

In our experiment, we found the same types of malignant tumours as those described following treatment with cyclophosphamide and other alkylating agents used in the therapy of human cancer diseases, namely carcinomas of the urinary bladder and leukemias (Table 1). After elimination of mortality influences in the different groups, a linear dose-response relationship of the tumour frequency was obtained by logarithmic transformation of the dose and pro bit transformation of the response (Fig. 1).

At present we are investigating the influence of mesna (sodium 2-mercaptoethane sulfonate) on the carcinogenicity of cyclophosphamide. BROCK and coworkers have submitted evidence that the highly water-soluble and virtually non-toxic mesna is

Table 1.
Carcinogenic action of low-dose cyclophosphamide given orally to rats in a lifetime experiment (according to SCHMÄHL, D., HABS, M. 1979)

| Group | Number of evaluable animals | | Individual dose | Median total dose | Animals with tumours in: | | |
	m	f	(mg/kg)	(g/m^2)	Urinary bladder	Lymphoid and hematopoietic tissue	Others
I	31	27	2.50	10.2	8	4	12
II	35	33	1.25	5.8	5	6	23
III	36	37	0.63	4.0	2	6	23
IV	34	37	0.31	2.0	2	3	21
V	38	34	0	0	0	0	9

capable of reducing acute hemorrhagic cystitis following cyclophosphamide treatment without interfering with the cytostatic activity of this oxazaphosphorine. It seems possible to lower the bladder cancer risk after cyclophosphamide treatment by additional administration of mesna (BROCK 1980, HABS and SCHMÄHL 1981).

In 1976, BONADONNA et al were among the first to report favourable results obtained in adjuvant chemotherapy of carcinomas of the breast. The empirically selected therapy scheme consisted of the drug combination cyclophosphamide-methotrexate-

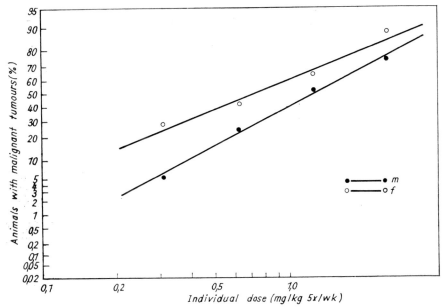

Fig. 1. Carcinogenic action of low-dose cyclophosphamide given orally to Sprague-Dawley rats in a lifetime experiment. Dose response of tumour frequencies after elimination of mortality influences.

5-fluorouracil (CMF). Postoperative adjuvant chemotherapy is increasingly being introduced into clinical cancer treatment programs. The time which has elapsed since the onset of a broader use of adjuvant chemotherapy is still inadequate in comparison with known tumour induction periods in man. Clinical findings are therefore limited, and no reliable risk assessment of secondary tumours related to drug treatment in patients can be made so far. To describe the carcinogenic effect in a limited number of animals in relation to the number of patients at risk, a lifetime experiment was carried out using doses comparable to the human situation (Table 2).

Among the three drugs combined in the investigated regimen, only cyclophosphamide is known to be carcinogenic. In October 1980, an IARC working group (IARC 1981) concluded that there is sufficient evidence for the carcinogenicity of cyclophosphamide in mice and rats, and in humans. There is, however no evidence to suggest carcinogenicity of methotrexate in rats, the available data from studies in humans being inadequate for evaluations. There is also no evidence showing carcinogenic activity of 5-fluorouracil in the limited number of studies carried out with experimental animals, the data from studies in humans being insufficient to arrive at a conclusion. The results of this bioassay are summarized in Table 3 (HABS et al 1981).

It is not possible to decide whether the carcinogenic response observed in the present experiment was due to a combined effect of the three drugs used or should be

Table 2.
Scheme of combined treatment with cyclophosphamide (C), methotrexate (M), and 5-fluorouracil (F) in Sprague-Dawley rats (according to HABS, M. et al 1981)

Group*	Mode of treatment	Individual dose (mg/m²)	Number of monthly cycles	Maximum total dose (g/m²)	Median total dose (g/m²)	95% Confidence limits
0	untreated control	0	0	0.00	0.00	0.00
1	C day 1—14 p.o.	50		4.20	4.20	4.20
	M day 1+8 i.p.	20	6	0.24	0.24	0.24
	F day 1+8 i.v.	300		3.60	3.60	3.60
2	C day 1—14 p.o.	25		5.25	5.25	5.25
	M day 1+8 i.p.	10	15	0.30	0.30	0.30
	F day 1+8 i.v.	150		4.50	4.50	4.50
3	C day 1—14 p.o.	50		10.50	6.30	6.15
	M day 1+8 i.p.	20	15	0.60	0.36	0.34
	F day 1+8 i.v.	300		9.00	6.00	5.70
Administration to humans (according to BONADONNA et al 1976)						
	C day 1—14 p.o.	100			1,200	
	M day 1+8 i.v.	40	12		480	
	F day 1+8 i.v.	600			7,200	

* Initial number of animals: 40 male and 40 female rats per group, total number: 320 rats

Table 3.
Organs in which an increased tumour risk was diagnosed after repeated CMF treatment in Sprague-Dawley rats (according to HABS, M. et al 1981)

Organ	Males*	Females*
Nervous tissue	++	++
Urinary bladder	(+)	(+)
Hematopoietic and lymphatic tissue	(+)	+
Suprarenal gland	+	±
Mammary gland	0	(+)
Uterus		±

*
++ $p < 0.001$
 + $p < 0.01$
(+) $p < 0.05$
 ± $p < 0.1$

attributed to the alkylating agent cyclophosphamide alone. The organs in which an increased tumour risk manifested itself in this study were also found as target organs after administration of cyclophosphamide alone to rats. However, the main target organ affected by CMF treatment was the nervous tissue, which to our knowledge has seldom been described in single-drug studies with cyclophosphamide (SCHMÄHL and HABS 1980). Irrespective of whether or not a shift in the organotropism of the carcinogenic effects of cyclophosphamide is assumed or a combined carcinogenic action of the three-drug combination is suggested, the results demonstrate that the carcinogenic activity of a combination of xenobiotic agents cannot simply be predicted from the known effects of the individual compounds of this combination.

A large number of nitrosoureas have recently been introduced into cytostatic therapy. Among the nitrosoureas, there are many substances, which exert a strong carcinogenic effect in animals. Chlorozotocin, for instance, has been shown to be highly carcinogenic (HABS et al 1979). There have also been first reports on the carcinogenic activities of N-nitrosoureas in man (COHEN et al 1976, JOCHIMSEN et al 1976). In an experimental study on inoculated leukemia ZELLER and SCHMÄHL (1979) stated that after curative treatment with BCNU, secondary tumours occurred in 11% of the treated animals, which were caused by the BCNU administration.

In addition or as an alternative to an evaluation of acute toxicity, chronic toxicity is an obvious criterion for these selection among analogues. A reduced or absent carcinogenic activity might thus be an important parameter in the choice of novel nitrosourea analogues. Following the above rationale, nitrosourea analogues were compared with clinically used nitrosoureas in rats as to their influence on life span and induction of neoplasms. CCNU and methyl-CCNU were the least toxic among the substances

Table 4.
Chemical structure of N-nitroso-(2-chloroethyl)-urea derivatives tested

Cl—CH₂—CH₂

CNU-derivatives	—R
CCNU	
MeCCNU	—CH₃
Morpholino-CNU	—NO
Chlorozotocin	D-Glucopyranose
BCNU	—CH₂—CH₂Cl
HECNU	—CH₂—CH₂OH
HECNU-MS	—CH₂—CH₂—OSO₂CH₃

tested (Tables 4, 5). Qualitatively, the toxicity was similar for all compounds (Table 6). The most prominent manifestations were loss of weight and death following terminal infections. Histologic examination almost invariably revealed signs of liver damage, chlorozotocin showing additionally a high degree of dose-dependent renal toxicity, observable to a lesser extent and severity in CCNU-treated animals. Morpholino-CNU was much more toxic than CCNU and methyl-CCNU, the median survival times being significantly reduced even at the lowest dose of 9.5 mg/m². In the case of chlorozotocin, doses exceeding 38 mg/m² could not be administered, because 7 of 30 rats died within 14 days after a single injection of 75 mg/m². BCNU was the most toxic in this series of substances. The water-soluble HECNU and HECNU-MS were clearly less toxic than BCNU.

Table 5.

Scheme of repeated intravenous administration of N-nitroso(2-chloroethyl)urea derivatives in male Wistar rats (Total number of animals: 990)

Compound tested	Initial number of animals per group	Individual dose (mg/m²) administered every 6 weeks (max: 10 applications)					Clinically used individual dose* (mg/m²)
		150	75	38	19	9.5	
CCNU	30	+	+	+	+	−	70−150
Methyl-CCNU	30	+	+	+	+	−	70−160
Morpholino-CNU	30	+	+	+	+	+	−
Chlorozotocin	30	−	+⃞	+	+	+	100−130
BCNU	30	−	+	+	+	+	70−130
HECNU	30	−	+	+	+	+	−
HECNU-MS	30	−	+	+	+	+	−
Control	120						r

* according to MACDONALD et al 1980, CARTER 1980.
+   = investigated
−   = not investigated
⃞+⃞ = toxic (median survival time < 200 days)

Table 6.

Qualitative comparison of the organ-specific toxic effect of N-nitroso(2-chloroethyl)-urea derivatives in male Wistar rats

Compound	Organ affected:			
	Brain	Liver	Kidneys	Heart
Solvent	?	∅	∅	∅
CCNU	?	+	+	(+)
MeCCNU	?	+	∅	(+)
Morpholino-CNU	?	+	+	∅
Chlorozotocin	?	+	+	+
BCNU	?	∅	∅	∅
HECNU	?	+	∅	∅
HECNU-MS	(+)	∅	∅	

+   = probable
(+) = indications in the dissection material
?   = questionable
∅   = no toxicity observed

The carcinogenicity data are summarized in Tables 7 and 8. These findings demonstrate clear differences in the long-term toxic and carcinogenic effects of the four clinically employed nitrosoureas in rats. Under the conditions of this experiment, BCNU emerged as the most toxic of these substances with regard to life span reduction upon repeated administration and to carcinogenic potential. In the absence of undisputed evidence for a clinical superiority of BCNU over CCNU, chlorozotocin, and methyl-CCNU, these results may have a direct clinical impact to select less empirically among available drugs. They also support the assumption that chemotherapeutic effective-

Table 7

Qualitative comparison of the neoplastic effect observed after repeated intravenous administration of N-nitroso(2-chloroethyl)urea derivatives in male Wistar rats

Compound	Organotropism of the neoplastic activity*:					Decrease in the incidence of spontaneous tumours
	Nervous tissue	Lung	Hematopoietic and lymphatic tissue	Foresto-mach	Pituitary gland	
CCNU	(+)	+	(+)	Ø	Ø	?
MeCCNU	Ø	+	Ø	Ø	(+)	Ø
Morpholino-CNU	Ø	+	Ø	Ø	Ø	Ø
Chlorozotocin	(+)	+	Ø	Ø	Ø	Ø
BCNU	+	+	Ø	Ø	Ø	(+)
HECNU	+	Ø	Ø	(+)	Ø	(+)
HECNU-MS	+	Ø	Ø	Ø	Ø	(+)

* + = proven evidence
(+) = clear indications
? = questionable
Ø = no evidence

Table 8.

Lowest dose (mg/m²) of the tested N-nitroso(2-chloroethyl)urea derivatives, which evidently increased the cancer risk in male Wistar rats (two-tailed $p < 0.05$)

compound	Individual dose (mg/m²)	Median total dose (mg/m²)
CCNU	38	380
MeCCNU	150	1200
Morpholino-CNU	38	380
Chlorozotocin	38	380
BCNU	38	266
HECNU	38	380
HECNU-MS	(75)	(380)

( ) = not proven

ness is not necessarily linked with certain types of toxicity, since even minor chemical modifications produce analogues of enhanced cell-killing ability, but with reduced toxicity, as in the case of HECNU-MS.

There are a number of examples, in which carcinogenicity data of animal experiments predicted an elevated tumour risk in man (Table 9). In the case of carcinogenesis induced by alkylating cytostatic agents, animal experiments also predicted results seen several years later in humans. It is hard to understand, why cytostatic agents with structural formulae suggesting a carcinogenic activity have been put on the market. A typical example is chlornaphazine. It contains a mustard group at the basic molecule of β-naphthylamine. During metabolism the chloroethyl function is

Table 9
Examples of compounds, which proved to be carcinogenic in animal experiments, predicting thus a later on confirmed, elevated cancer risk in man (according to HABS 1980)

Compound	Carcinogenic activity in experimental animals proven in:	Confirmation of experimental results in man in:
Diethylstilbestrol	1947	1971
4-Aminobiphenyl	1952	1955
Vinylchloride	1970	1974
Polychlorinated biphenyls (e. g. Arochlor 1254)	1972	1976
Cyclophosphamide	1967	1970
S-Lost (mustard gas)	1950	1960
Aflatoxin	1961	1971
Dichloromethylether	1969	1973

probably cleaved off so that β-naphthylamine is formed, the carcinogenic effect of which has been known for many decades. Chlornaphazine has been administered in the treatment of polycythemia, predominantly in Scandinavian countries, and has induced carcinomas of the urinary bladder in many cases after surprisingly short induction times (2—10 years) (THIEDE and CHRISTENSEN 1969, VIDEBAEK 1964).

The drugs used in cytostatic chemotherapy — alkylating drugs as well as antimetabolites or antibiotics of the adriamycin type — represent highly reactive substances, which should be employed only in cases with a correspondingly poor prognosis. We consider this all the more necessary if these antineoplastic substances are recommended for use in diseases without a fatal prognosis.

The existing experimental and clinical data on carcinogenesis induced by cytostatic drugs permit to draw the following conclusions:

1. Cytostatic agents should be used only in cases with a poor prognosis. This includes all those cancers, which occur systemically or can no longer be treated by "classical" therapy. It is important, however, to know whether the tumour in question is chemosensitive as far as one can tell with existing knowledge.

2. Non-malignant diseases should be treated with cytostatic drugs only if no alternative is available.

3. Particular restraint should be exercised in using potentially carcinogenic cytostatic agents in "experimental adjuvant" chemotherapy, because by randomizing the patients, potentially healthy people who have already been cured by classical treatment might be subjected to potential hazards. Special caution is required if young patients are affected. This warning seems to be particularly justified, since some cases of leukemia in man have been described after adjuvant chemotherapy of breast cancer (LERNER 1977). If the adjuvant chemotherapy with carcinogenic alkylating compounds is applied indiscriminately, it is to be expected that a large number of patients who have been subjected to this treatment will later on develop a secondary tumour induced by the adjuvant chemotherapy.

4. The implementation of cytostatic therapy should be carried out by clinicians who have special training in this field of chemotherapy. Inexperienced physicians should never employ this form of treatment in cancer patients.

The development of our knowledge of carcinogenesis induced by cytostatic agents in experimental animals and in man during the last two decades has precisely predicted the "late effects" observed in man. The detection of these late effects has initiated more restrictive practices in chemotherapy. These more restrictive practices will hopefully protect patients against possible late effects in the future. In the case of otherwise incurable diseases, such as Hodgkin's disease and plasmocytomas, these late effects will have to be accepted in order to prevent acute danger to life.

References

1. BONADONNA, G., BRUSAMOLINO, E., VALAGUSSA, P., ROSSI, A., BRUGNATELLI, L., BRAMBILLA, C., DELENA, M., TANCINI, L., BAJETTA, E., MUSUMECI, R. and VERONESI, U.: Combination chemotherapy as an adjuvant treatment in operable breast cancer. New Eng. J. Med. *294* (1976), 405—410

2. BROCK, N. (1980): Konzeption und Wirkmechanismus von Uromitexan (Mesna). In: BURKERT, H., NAGEL, G. A. (eds) Neue Erfahrungen mit Oxazaphosphorinen unter besonderer Berücksichtigung des Uroprotektors Uromitexan. pp 1—11. Karger Basel—München—New York

3. COHEN, R. J., WIERNIK, P. H. and WALKER, M. D.: Acute nonlymphocytic leukemia associated with nitrosourea chemotherapy: Report of two cases. Cancer Treat. Rep. *60* (1976), 1257—1261

4. HABS, M.: Was uns Kanzerogenitätsstudien lehren. Ärztl. Praxis *99* (1980), 3399

5. HABS, M., EISENBRAND, G. and SCHMÄHL, D.: Carcinogenic activity in Sprague-Dawley rats of 2-[3-(2-chloroethyl)-3-nitrosoureido]-D-glucopyranose (chlorozotoxin). Cancer Letters *8* (1979), 133—137

6. HABS, M. and SCHMÄHL, D.: Synergistic effects of N-nitroso compounds in experimental long-term carcinogenesis studies. Oncology *37* (1980), 259—265

7. HABS, M., SCHMÄHL, D. and LIN, P. Z.: Carcinogenic activity in rats of combined treatment with cyclophosphamide, methotrexate and 5-fluorouracil. Int. J. Cancer *28* (1981), 91—96

8. HABS, M. and SCHMÄHL, D. (1981): Prevention of urinary bladder tumours in cyclophosphamide-treated rats by additional medication with the uroprotectors sodium 2-mercaptoethane sulfonate (mesna) and disodium 2,2'-dithio-bis-ethane sulfonate (dimesna). Cancer, submitted for publication

9. IARC (1981) IARC Monographs on the evaluation of the carcinogenic risk of chemicals to humans. Vol 26: Some antineoplastic and immunosuppressive agents. IARC, Lyon

10. JOCHIMSEN, P. R., PEARLMAN, N. W. and LAWTON, R. L.: Pancreatic carcinoma as a sequel to therapy of lymphoma. J. Surg. Oncol. *8* (1976), 461—464

11. LERNER, H.: Second malignancies diagnosed in breast cancer patients while receiving adjuvant chemotherapy at the Pennsylvania Hospital. Proc. Amer. Assoc. Cancer Res. *18* (1977), 340

12. SCHMÄHL, D. and HABS, M.: Carcinogenic action of low-dose cyclophosphamide given orally to Sprague-Dawley rats in a lifetime experiment. Int. J. Cancer *23* (1979), 706—712

13. SCHMÄHL, D. and HABS, M. (1980): Drug-induced cancer. In: GRUNDMANN, E. (ed) Current topics in pathology. Vol. 69 Drug-induced pathology. pp 333—369. Springer Berlin-Heidelberg-New York

14. THIEDE, T. and CHRISTENSEN, B. C.: Bladder tumours induced by chlornaphazine. Acta Med. Scand. *185* (1969), 133—137

15. VIDEBAEK, A.: Chlornaphazine (Erysan) may induce cancer of the urinary bladder. Acta Med. Scand. *176* (1964), 45—50

16. WEISBURGER, E. K.: Bioassay program for carcinogenic hazards of cancer chemotherapeutic agents. Cancer *40* (1977), 1935—1949

17. ZELLER, W. J. and SCHMÄHL, D.: Development of second malignancies in rats after cure of acute leukemia L5222 by single doses of 2-chloroethylnitrosoureas. J. Cancer. Res. Clin. Oncol. *95* (1979), 83—86

Dept. of Med. Oncology, Charing Cross Hospital, London, England

VP 16-213 (Etoposide; NSC-141540; Vepesid): A Review

E. S. Newlands

The history of the development of podophyllotoxins in human therapy is a long one since the root of the American mandrake (podophyllin peltatum) was used traditionally by the North American Indians as a cathartic and anti-helminthic agent. An extract of podophyllin was also in the USA pharmacopoeia from 1820 to 1942 as an emetic. In 1942 Kaplan (1) first used podophyllotoxin to treat anal warts and in 1947 experiments by Sullivan and Wechsler (2) demonstrated the anti-mitotic activity of podophyllin extracts. Between 1964 and 1967 early clinical trials with the podophyllin derivatives SP1 and SPG were conducted but these compounds were found to be fairly toxic (3). In 1971 Keller-Juslin et al (4) described the synthesis of VP 16-213. This was followed in 1972 by Nissen et al (5) who published the Phase I trial using VP 16-213. Since this time there have been extensive clinical studies using VP 16-213 in a wide range of human as well as experimental tumours. However, many questions remain to be answered about the exact mechanism of action of this compound and how it should be given clinically to obtain the maximum therapeutic effect. There has been little work done during the last decade in attempting to identify further derivatives of podophyllotoxin which might have different clinical patterns of activity from the two compounds that are currently available (VP 16-213 and VM 26).

Although podophyllotoxin itself binds avidly to tubulin and disrupts microtubular function, the semi-synthetic derivates VP 16-213 and VM 26 have little affinity for tubulin but can be shown to disrupt DNA in intact cells (6, 7). At present the evidence is in favour of the anti-tumour activity of VP 16-213 being more related to its ability to induce strand breaks in DNA than to any effect on microtubular function.

In experimental models, VP 16-213 has been shown to be active in some tumours and also to have schedule dependency in L.1210 leukaemia (8). In man, the clinical schedules that have been used differ considerably (Table 1). VP 16-213 can also be given orally and the absorption of the oral capsules is approximately 50 per cent, but the bioavailability of the oral ampoules is probably higher and closer to 80 per cent of the drug absorbed. Newer formulations for oral administration of VP 16-213 will be available in the near future.

Creaven and Allen (9) described a study using tritiated VP 16-213 in a dose of 220 to 290 mg/m² given by an i.v. infusion over one hour. The principal findings from this study showed that approximately 44 per cent of the labelled VP 16-213 appeared in the urine within the first 72 hours. Sixty-seven per cent of this was apparently unchanged drug. Only 2—16 per cent. of the label was recovered in the faeces in the first 72 hours. The CSF concentration varied between 1 and 10 per cent of the plasma levels. Only 50—60 per cent of the total radioactivity administered was recovered.

Table 1.
Schedules used clinically with VP 16-213

Schedule	Route	Dose (mg/m²)	No. Patients
Days 1—5 every 2—4 weeks	i.v. p.o.	50—60 120—130	271 96
Days 1—5 every 2—4 weeks	i.v.	100	100 plus
Weekly	i.v.	290	40
Twice weekly	i.v.	69—86	25
Days 1, 3, 5 every 4 weeks	i.v.	125	15

More recently, using high pressure liquid chromatography assays, the $T^1/_2$ beta is just over five hours and the renal clearance in adults is approximately 25 ml/minute. CSF concentrations were still undetectable at the end of a 24-hour infusion of VP 16-213 at a dose of 100 mg/m². In the circulation, approximately 93 per cent of VP 16-213 is protein-bound (10, 11).

The clinical toxicity of VP 16-213 has shown that the main dose-limiting toxicity is reversible myelosuppression. This is related both to the dose given and also increases with the number of consecutive days over which it is administered. Nausea and vomiting is rarely a problem with VP 16-213 but some degree of alopecia occurs in approximately half the patients receiving the drug. Mucositis is extremely rare. Occasional cases of chest or abdominal pain associated with hypotension can occur with VP 16-213 and VM 26. In both cases that we have seen (one patient received VP 16-213 and the other VM 26) recovery occurred within 30—60 minutes. It is possible that the hypotension is related to the formulation of VP 16-213 and VM 26 which includes Tween-80, polyethylene glycol and ethyl alcohol.

In the initial clinical studies, NISSEN et al (5) detected some anti-tumour activity in patients with malignant lymphomas. In most reports the activity of VP 16-213 in patients with malignant lymphomas has been modest but recently TAYLOR et al (12) reported results in resistant Hodgkin's disease using VP 16-213 in a dose of 120 mg/m² for five consecutive days. There were 3 (25 per cent) complete responses and 5 (42 per cent) partial responses in 12 patients. The dose of VP 16-213 in this series was higher than that reported in most studies and suggests that there may be a dose-response effect in terms of antitumour activity. There are now a number of studies reporting single agent activity of VP 16-213 in small cell carcinoma of the bronchus, and it is probably the most active single drug against this tumour (13). VP 16-213 is currently being integrated into a number of Phase III studies in small cell carcinoma of the lung, with certainly a high initial response rate, but unfortunately in many series the disease progresses after a period of months on chemotherapy. However, a small fraction of patients with small cell carcinoma of the bronchus remain in remission for several years, and it is possible that some of these patients have had their tumour eliminated with a combination of chemotherapy and radiotherapy (either to the primary site and, in some cases, including prophylactic skull irradiation).

Our experience in using VP 16-213 has been principally in two rare tumours, malignant teratomas and gestational choriocarcinoma. In a combined study with the Royal

Marsden Hospital the complete and partial response rate in heavily pretreated patients with malignant teratomas was 11 (46 per cent) out of 24 patients (14). A number of other investigators have subsequently confirmed the activity of VP 16-213 in patients with malignant teratomas. Since our initial recognition (15) that VP 16-213 was an active agent in malignant teratomas, we have integrated VP 16-213 into a Phase III study in patients with metastatic malignant teratomas, using sequential combination chemotherapy (16). The results indicate that even patients with very large volumes of tumour can obtain complete remissions with chemotherapy combined in selected cases with surgery. At the last analysis to 1st May 1981, 74 per cent of the 64 male patients with malignant teratomas and 71 per cent of the 18 female patients with ovarian teratomas are currently alive, with the majority of patients off treatment.

We have previously reported our initial experience using VP 16-213 in patients with drug-resistant gestational choriocarcinoma (17). Subsequently we have integrated VP 16-213 as one of the first line agents in patients with gestational trophoblastic tumours who present with adverse prognostic factors (18).

CAVALLI et al (19) originally reported 3 responses out of 6 patients with malignant hepatomas. Subsequent studies indicate that the activity of VP 16-213 is fairly modest in this disease and the cumulative results show that only 11 (19 per cent) out of 56 patients responded. Originally the results in breast cancer were very disappointing and only 5 (5 per cent) out of 99 patients showed any clinical response. However, recently some responses have been reported by SCHELL et al (20) in heavily pretreated patients with breast cancer. At present their results indicate that 9 (14 per cent) out of 66 patients have had a complete or partial response. It should be noted that the dose that they have used is relatively modest ($50-70$ mg/m² intravenously daily fo- 5 days). It is possible that with dose escalation to at least 100 mg/m² for five consecutive days intravenously, there might be a higher response rate in patients with rer fractory breast cancer. Paediatric tumours are fairly rare but some activity has been seen in patients with leukaemias and occasional responses have been seen in some solid paediatric malignancies (21). Tumours in which VP 16-213 appears to be inactive include adult acute lymphoblastic leukaemia, non-small cell carcinoma of the bronchus, colon carcinoma, malignant melanoma and ovarian carcinoma. In the case of ovarian carcinoma, we have treated a number of patients who had highly resistant tumours, having failed on multiple prior therapy. Although no objective tumour regressions have been seen, there have been brief tumour stabilisations in some cases. This may indicate that VP 16-213 should be explored further in ovarian adenocarcinomas, either at an earlier stage of the disease or in a higher dose (i.e. greater than 100 mg/m² intravenously for days 1 to 5).

In summary, VP 16-213 is clearly a clinically useful drug which is well tolerated and has activity in a range of human tumours. We do not know the optimum schedule for using this drug and it is possible that either by a change in schedule or by using it in a higher dose responses may be seen in tumour types which have been refractory to the lower doses which have been used in some studies. Now that the antitumour activity of some podophyllin derivatives has been clearly demonstrated in man, it will be very interesting to see whether further chemical modifications can produce either agents with a different spectrum of activity or compounds with greater antitumour activity than either VP 16-213 or VM 26.

References

1. KAPLAN, I. W.: Condyloma acuminata. New Orleans Med. Surg. J. *94* (1942), 388
2. SULLIVAN, B. J. and WECHSLER, H. L.: The cytological effects of podophyllin. Science *105* (1947), 433
3. CHAKRAVORTY, R. C., SARKER, S. K., SEN, S. and MUKERJI, B.: Human anticancer effect of podophyllum derivatives (SPG and SPl). Br. J. Cancer *21* (1967), 33
4. KELLER-JUSLIN, C., KUHN, M., Von WARTBURG, A. and STAHELIN, H.: Synthesis and anti-mitotic activity of glycosidic lignan derivatives related to podophyllotoxin. J. Med. Chem. *14*, (1971), 936
5. NISSEN, N. L., HANSEN, H. H., PEDERSEN, H., STRYER, L., DOMBERNOWSKY, P. and HESSEL-LUND, M.: Clinical trial of the oral form of a new podophyllotoxin derivative, VP 16-213 (NSC 141 540) in patients with advanced neoplastic disease. Cancer Chemother. Rep. *59* (1975), 1627
6. LOIKE, J. D. and HORWITZ, S. B.: Effects of podophyllotoxin and VP 16-213 on microtubule assembly in vitro and nucleoside transport in HeLa cells. Biochemistry *15* (1976), 5435
7. LOIKE, J. D. and HORWITZ, S. B.: Effect of VP 16-213 on the intracellular degradation of DNA in HeLa cells. Biochemistry *15* (1976), 5443
8. DOMBERNOWSKY, P. and NISSEN, N. I.: Schedule dependency of the anti-leukaemic activity of the podophyllotoxin derixative VP 16-213 (NSC 141540) in L 1210 leukaemia. Acta. Path. Microbiol. Scand (A) *81* (1973), 715
9. ALLEN, L. M. and CREAVAN, P. J.: Comparison of the human pharmacokinetics of VM 26 and VP 16-213, two antineoplastic epipodophyllotoxin glucopyranoside derivatives. Eur. J. Cancer *11* (1975), 697
10. EVANS, W. E., SINKULE, J. A., CROM, W. R., Dow, L., LOOK, T. and RIVERA, G.: Pharmaco-kinetics of VM 26 and VP 16-213 in children with cancer. Proc. First Int. Symp. on Podophyllo-toxins in Cancer Therapy, Abstract 8, 1981
11. D'INCALCI, M., FARINA, P., SESSA, C., MANGIONE, C., JANKOVIC, M., MASERA, G., BRAMBILLA M., PIAZZA, E., BEER, M. and CAVALLI, F.: VP 16-213. Pharmacokinetics in Man. Proc. First Int. Symp. on Podophyllotoxins in Cancer Therapy, Abstract 10, 1981
12. TAYLOR, R. E., McELWAIN, T. J., BARRETT, A. and PECKHAM, M. J.: Phase II Trial of VP 16-213 in relapsed Hodgkin's disease and non-Hodgkin's lymphomas. Proc. First Int. Symp. on Podo-phyllotoxins in Cancer Therapy, Abstract 27, 1981
13. ARNOLD, A. M.: Podophyllotoxin derivative VP 16-213. Cancer. Chemother. Pharmacol. *3* (1979), 71
14. FITZHARRIS, B. M., KAYE, S. B., SAVERYMUTTU, S., NEWLANDS, E. S. and McELWAIN, T. J.: VP 16-213 as a single agent in advanced testicular tumours. Europ. J. Cancer *16* (1980), 1193
15. NEWLANDS, E. S. and BAGSHAWE, K. D.: Epipodophyllin derivative (VP 16-213) in malig-nant teratomas and choriocarcinomas. Lancet *2* (1977), 87
16. NEWLANDS, E. S., BEGENT, R. H. J., KAYE, S. B., RUSTIN, J. G. S. and BAGSHAWE, K. D.: Chemotherapy of advanced malignant teratomas. Brit. J. Cancer *42* (1980), 378
17. NEWLANDS, E. S. and BAGSHAWE, K. D.: Anti-tumour activity of the epipodophyllin deri-vative VP 16-213 (Etoposide; NSC 141 540) in gestational choriocarcinoma. Europ. J. Cancer *16* (1980), 401
18. NEWLANDS, E. S. and BAGSHAWE, K. D.: Role of VP 16-213 (Etoposide; NSC 141540) in gestational choriocarcinoma. Proc. First Int. Symp. on Podophyllotoxins in Cancer Therapy, Abstract 18. Full paper submitted to Cancer Chemother. and Pharmacol.
19. CAVALLI, F., SONNTAG, R. W. and BRUNNER, K. W.: Epipodophyllin derivative (VP 16-213) in the treatment of solid tumours. Lancet *2* (1977), 362
20. SCHELL, F. C., YAP, H. Y., BLUMENSCHEIN, G. R., ESPARZA, L. and ISSELL, B.: Phase II study of VP 16-213 (Etoposide) in refractory metastatic breast carcinoma. Proc. First Int. Symp. on Podophyllotoxins in Cancer Therapy. Abstract 23. 1981
21. GUTIERREZ, M. L. and CROOKE, J. T.: Paediatric cancer chemotherapy: an updated review. Cancer Treat. Rev. *6* (1979), 153

Johnson Matthey Research Centre,
Sonning common reading, U.K.

New Platinum Anti-Cancer Drugs

M. J. Cleare, P. C. Hydes and C. F. J. Barnard

1. Introduction

Cis-dichlorodiammineplatinum(II) is now an established member in the armamentarium of antineoplastic agents. It is variously known as Cisplatin (which it will be referred to for the purposes of this paper) and Neoplatin depending on the country in which it is being sold, and has the structure shown in Figure 1 a. It is unique amongst the anticancer drugs in that it is based on a heavy metal namely platinum.

Cis-platinum was first shown to have anti-tumour activity by Rosenberg et al (1) and has since been shown to be clinically active either as a single agent or, more usually, in combination therapy, against several human tumours particularly those of the genito-urinary origin. In general, the addition of cis-platinum to the armamentarium of the chemotherapist has increased the therapeutic responsiveness of a number of solid tumours. This has been summarised by Durant (2) using the definition of chemotherapeutic sensitivity shown in Table 1. Thus, although cis-platinum has

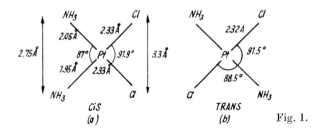

Fig. 1.

Table 1.
Classification of chemotherapeutic sensitivity

Chemotherapy sensitivity	Usual cell kill (log$_{10}$)	Response rate	Complete remissions (%)	Duration response	Cures (%)	Example
Unresponsive	0— 2	< 15%	None	—	None	Kidney
Resistant	2 — 3	15—30%	None	Weeks	None	Colon
Responsive	3 — 4	30—60%	≅ 5%	Months	0-rare	Breast
Sensitive	4 — 8	50—80%	≅ 50%	Months	5—20%	AML
Curable	8—12	≅ 100%	≈ 100%	Years	> 75%	Gestational choriocarcinoma

Table 2.
Contributions of *cis*-platinum

1. Unresponsive	→	Resistant	—	Cervix, bladder and prostate
2. Resistant	→	Responsive	—	Head and neck
3. Responsive	→	Sensitive	—	Ovary
4. Sensitive	→	Curable	—	Testicle

improved responses in cervix, bladder, prostate and head and neck cancer, it has presently only made a major impact on long term survival for ovarian and, particularly, testicular tumours (Table 2).

Although it exhibits activity as discussed above, cis-platin's therapeutic efficacy is somewhat compromised by the occurrence of severe dose limiting side effects. Predominant among these are nephrotoxicity, severe nausea and vomiting, myelotoxicity and ototoxicity. Although hydration techniques have reduced nephrotoxicity, the major dose limiting factor, higher doses have resulted, in some cases, in the appearance of peripheral neuropathy symptoms after several doses (3). Also nausea and vomiting is so severe as to limit the number of courses that some patients will tolerate. There is thus a strong requirement for a less toxic platinum drug with an equivalent or improved spectrum of activity to that of cis-platinum.

Many analogues have been screened since the discovery of cis-platinum. For example, by 1979 the US National Cancer Institute had screened 1055 platinum compounds of which 185 (18%) showed at least minimal activity (4). Indeed, our group at Johnson MATTHEY, in conjunction with a variety of other researchers in the UK (Appendix 1) have tested nearly 500 such compounds. These were eventually narrowed down to a short list of nine from which a candidate for clinical trial was chosen (5). Other compounds have been chosen for clinical trial using various screening criteria (see section 4). However, before discussing preclinical studies on some new platinum analogues, the results of structure-activity relationship studies will be briefly summarised.

2. Structure-activity studies

The chemistry of complexes of the type $[PtA_2X_2]$ (where A_2 is one bidentate or two monodentate amine groups and X_2 is one bidentate or two monodentate anionic groups) is dominated by the strength of the Pt-N bond. Thus, for both cis and trans isomers (Figure 1) the X groups are reactive while the A groups are relatively inert. Screening studies on transplanted animal tumours have clearly established that only cis isomers are active. Many different isomers have been tested and some examples are given in Table 3 (6). Only neutral $cis[PtA_2X_2]$ species show appreciable activity. Although inert, the A groups can have a primary effect on the anti-tumour property. Heterocyclic, alicyclic and straight and branched chain alkyl amines all give compounds with appreciable activity against a range of tumours (6, 7, 8) (see Table 5). Much of the early screening was against the ADJ/PC6A plasmacytoma which is particularly sensitive to platinum compounds. Most of the changes in selectivity (therapeutic index) were associated with toxicity rather than potency which at least indicated that less toxic drugs might be possible. This was confirmed by studies on alkylamine complexes in mice bearing the L1210 system where microtoxicological measurement of blood urea nitrogen (BUN) and total white blood cell count (WBC) indicated much lower nephrotoxicity and marginally lower myelotoxicity than cis-platinum (Table 6) (9).

Table 3.
Comparison of activities for *cis*- and *trans*- isomers

ADJ/PC6 plasma cell tumour complex	Solvent		Dose range mg/kg	Dose response	LD_{50}	ID_{90}	TI
H_3N–Pt(Cl)(Cl)–NH_3 (cis)	cis	A	0.1–40	+	13.0	1.6	8.1
H_3N–Pt(Cl)(Cl)–NH_3 (trans)	trans A			–	27.0	>27.0	<1.0
aziridine–Pt(Cl)(Cl)–aziridine (cis)	cis	A	2.5–160	+	56.5	2.6	21.7
aziridine–Pt(Cl)(Cl)–aziridine (trans)	trans A			–	18.0	>18.0	<1.0
pyrrolidine–Pt(Cl)(Cl)–pyrrolidine (cis)	cis	A	6 –800	+	240	17.5	13.7
pyrrolidine–Pt(Cl)(Cl)–pyrrolidine (trans)	trans A			–	72	>72	<1.0

[a] Only 66 % survivors
[b] Slurry a t higher concentrations.
[c] Sporadic toxicity over this range.

Amines which generally give rise to active $[PtA_2Cl_2]$ complexes are summarized in Table 7. Some of these amines have been incorporated into active Pt(IV) complexes of the type *cis*-$[PtA_2Cl_4]$ and *trans*-$[PtA_2(OH)_2Cl_2]$ dihydroxo derivatives where the latter sometimes have the advantage of activity coupled with higher aqueous solubility (8).

The order of reactivity of X groups in complexes such as PtA_2X_2 has been well established (10) and antitumour active complexes have been identified with widely differing kinetic properties. The X groups that can give rise to active are summarized in Table 8. Physicochemical studies, such as the change in molar conductivity with time in aqueous solution, confirm three groups of active complexes on a kinetic basis (Fiure 2) (9).

1. Reactive species that are rapidly hydrolysed and would be quickly converted to chloro complexes in the presence of physiological concentrations of saline (e.g. X = $= SO_4^{2-}$, NO_3^-).

Table 4.
Changes in activity on varying A in cis-[PtA$_2$Cl$_2$]

ADJ/PC6 plasma cell tumour A	Solvent	Dose range (mg/kg)	Dose response	LD$_{50}$	ID$_{90}$	TI
NH$_3$	A^b	0.1—40	+	13.0	1.6	8.1
CH$_3$NH$_2$	A		−	18.5	18.5	1.0
ClC$_2$H$_4$NH$_2$	A		+	45.0	17.5	2.6
▷NH (cyclopropyl)	A	2.5—160	+	56.5	2.6	21.7
⬠NH (ring)	A	3—200	+	141	10.8	13.1
C$_2$H$_4$OH / ▷N	A		−	90	>90	<1.0
O(⬡)NH (morpholine)	A		−	18	>18	<1.0
▷—NH$_2$	A	1—80	+	56.5	2.3	24.6
◇—NH$_2$	A	6—750	+	67	<6	>11.1
⬠—NH$_2$	A	1—3200	+	80	2.4	200
⬡—NH$_2$	A	1—3200	+	>3200	12	>267
(7-ring)—NH$_2$	A	5—625	+	>625	18	>35

Table 5.
Changes in activity on varying A in cis-[PtA$_2$Cl$_2$]
A   = straight and branched chain alkylamines
Tumour = ADJ/PC6A in BALB/c mice

A^a	ID$_{50}$	LD$_{90}$	TI
i-propylamine	0.9	33.5	37
i-butylamine	6.2	83	13
i-pentylamine	5.8	1150	198
2-aminohexane	27.5	730	26.5
ethylamine	<12	26.5	>2.2
n-propylamine	12	26.5	2.2
n-butylamine	<10	110	>11
n-pentylamine	37	92	2.5

^{a} Compounds given i.p. as a suspension in arachis oil

Table 6.

L1210 tumour - BDF$_1$ Mice; 10^6 cells

Complex	Optimum dose (mg/kg)	Schedule (d)	Median survival (%T/C)	Therapeutic ratio (MTD/MED)	Toxicity (BUN)	(WBC)
Cis-PtCl$_2$(CH$_3$NH$_2$)$_2$	16	1	129	1	+	±
	2	1-9	121	1		
Cis-PtCl$_2$(n-C$_3$H$_7$NH$_2$)$_2$	8	1	157	2	+	+
	8	1-9	157	2		
Cis-PtCl$_2$(i-C$_3$H$_7$NH$_2$)$_2$	32	1	171	1	+	±
	8	1-9	179	2		
Cis-PtCl$_2$(C$_3$H$_5$NH$_2$)$_2$	16	1	157	4	+	+
	8	1-9	164	2		
Cis-PtCl$_2$(OH)$_2$(i-C$_3$H$_7$NH$_2$)$_2$(a)	32	1	171	2	+	±
	16	1-9	207	2		
Cis-PtCl$_2$(i-C$_4$H$_9$NH$_2$)$_2$	64	1	171	4	+	±
	16	1-9	193	8		
Cis-PtCl$_2$(t-C$_4$H$_9$NH$_2$)$_2$	64	1	inactive			
	32	1-9	inactive			
Cis-PtCl$_2$(C$_4$H$_7$NH$_2$)$_2$	32	1	157	4	+	±
	16	1-9	221	4		

Table 7.

Structure-activity studies on cis-[PtA$_2$X$_2$] species

Effective A groups A	Examples
n-alkylamines	C$_2$-C$_4$
i-alkylamines	C$_3$-C$_5$ [a]
Alicyclic amines	C$_3$-C$_5$ [a]
Diamino alkanes	Ethylenediamines (also alkyl substituted) propylenediamine
Diamino cycloalkane	1,2 diaminocyclohexane
Heterocyclic amines	Ethyleneimines, pyrolidine
Aromatic diamines	o-phenylenediamine

[a] Aqueous solubility very low with long carbon chain.

Table 8.

Structure-activity studies on cis-[PtA$_2$X$_2$] species

Effective X groups X	Examples
Halide	chloro, bromo
Oxanions	sulphate nitrate
Carboxylates	halogeno-acetates
Dicarboxylates	oxalate, malonate substituted malonates, phthalates

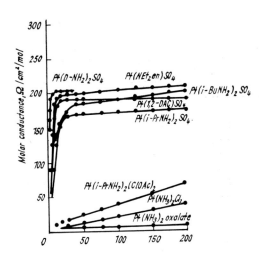

Fig. 2.

Molar conductance in water at 25 °C.

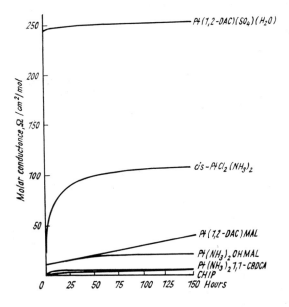

Variation in molar conductivity with time for aqueous solutions of active Pt compounds.

2. Species with intermediate reactivity toward water and chloride and half lives of, say, 1—3 hours (e.g. Cl⁻, Br⁻, chloroacetate — note that reactions of chloro complexes are suppressed in the presence of chloride ion which protects them in the serum.

3. Inert species which presently comprise dicarboxylate complexes. These are very inert in comparison with the other active species and we have previously postulated the involvement of an in vivo activation mechanism. The most common example of these groups are where X is malonate or a substituted malonate and these complexes are usually particularly effective and often show lower nephro- and myelotoxicity than cis-platin in the mouse (Table 9).

The existence of this wide range of reactivity amongst active species has led us to suggest that the initial period of uptake from the blood may be of prime importance.

Table 9.

L1210 tumour - BDF$_1$ mice, 10^6 cells

Complex	Optimum dose (mg/kg)	Schedule (d)	Median survival (per cent T/C)	Therapeutic ratio (MTD/MED)	Toxicity (BUN)	(WBC)
Pt(mal)(1,2-DAC)	32	1	154	—		
	16	1-9	254	4		
Pt(mal)(C$_5$H$_9$NH$_2$)$_2$	128	1	—	—		
	128	1-9	—	—		
Pt(OHmal)(NH$_3$)$_2$	64	1	150	1	±	+
	32	1-9	200	2	+	+
Pt(OHmal)(i-C$_5$H$_{11}$NH$_2$)$_2$	128	1	—	—		
	128	1-9	—	—		
Pt(Etmal)(NH$_3$)$_2$	128	1	171	2	+	±
	64	1-9	186	4	+	+
Pt(1,1-CBDCA)(NH$_3$)$_2$	128	1	150	2	+	±
	64	1-9	157	2	+	+

Key:
+ Denotes toxicity lower than for *cis*-Pt(II).
± Denotes toxicity comparable with *cis*-Pt(II).

By the nature of some of the very reactive species this would mean around the first 10 minutes. As might be expected, reactivity does seem to correlate with side effects with less reactive compounds generally showing lower toxicities.

3. Preclinical studies

In our own collaborative group we selected some eight compounds on the basis of initial screening results for more detailed toxicological and anti-tumour evaluation, with a view to identifying a prime candidate for a Phase 1 clinial trial (5). Compounds were selected not only from our own synthetic programme but included promising compounds reported in the literature (Table 10). A wide range of aqueous solubilities was deliberately included.

The only anti-tumour tests which satisfactorily split the compounds were against a xenografted human bronchogenic carcinoma where only the cyclobutanedicarboxylate derivative (CBDCA) exhibited curative activity without incurring prohibitive host toxicity. Studies on blood urea changes indicated that several of the compounds were less nephrotoxic than cis-platin (Figure 3) and this was confirmed by histopathological studies on the kidney (Table 11). Several of the compounds caused no loss of body weight on treatment with the maximum tolerated dose in complete contrast to cis-platin (11).

The overall conclusion from these studies was that some of the complexes, particularly the malonates, not only exhibited less toxicity overall compared to cis-platin but were strikingly less nephrotoxic in animals. Evidence for superior activity was not convincing although CBDCA showed some evidence for enhanced selectivity on xenograft testing. The latter was chosen for Phase 1 clinical trial on this basis coupled with a low toxicity rating in tests. One of the other compounds (CHIP) was to be the subject of a separate clinical trial elsewhere — see section 4.

Table 10.
Selected platinum complexes (Reference 11)

A	X	Aqueous solubility (MM)
	$[Pt\,A_2\,X]$	
NH_3	Hydroxymalonate	6.4
NH_3	1,1-Cyclobutane dicarboxylate	50
NH_3	Ethylmalonate	160
	$[Pt\,A_2\,X_2\,(OH)_2]$	
Isopropylamine	Cl	44
	$cis\text{-}[Pt\,A_2\,X_2]$	
Isopropylamine	Chloroacetate	16.0
Cyclopropylamine	Cl	1.6
Isobutylamine	Cl	0.1
	$[Pt\,A\,X\,Y]$	

A	X	Y	
1,2-Diaminocyclohexane	SO_4	H_2O	30

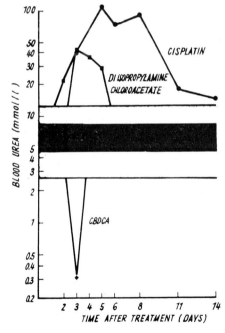

Fig. 3. Circulating blood urea levels in rats receiving maximum tolerated doses of various platinum complexes. ■: range of maximum and minimum individual blood urea levels seen in untreated rats. □: range of maximum and minimum individual blood urea levels seen in rats receiving diisobutylamine, hydroxymalonate, CHIP, ethylmalonate, dicyclopropylamine, or DAC-sulphate.

4. Phase 1 — clinical trials

Three Phase 1 clinical trials are underway where early indications are known to the author. Structures of the compounds involved are shown in Figure 4. Results to date confirm that all three compounds are less toxic than cisplatin particularly in

Table 11.
Summary of Histopathology

JM No.	Compound	Liver	Kidney	Ileum
—	Cisplatin	Capsular thickening	Necrosis pct[a]	—
2	Diisobutylamine	Capsular thickening	Capsular thickening	
5	Hydroxymalonate	—	Necrosis dct[a]	—
8	CBDCA	—	Capsular thickening	Erosion
9	CHIP	Capsular thickening	—	—
10	Ethylmalonate	Mitotic rate 0.5%	—	Erosion
11	Dicyclopropylamine	Capsular thickening	—	Erosion
16	Diisopropylamine chloroacetate	Capsular thickening	Necrosis dct[b]	Erosion
20	DAC-sulphate	Capsular thickening	—	Erosion

[a] pct = proximal convoluted tubule.
[b] dct = distal convuluted tubule.

$$\left[Pt(1,2\text{-}dac)(TMA) \right] \ 4\text{-}carboxyphthalate$$

$$\left[Pt(NH_3)_2(CBDCA) \right]$$

$$\left[Pt(isopropylamine)_2(OH)_2Cl_2 \right]$$

(CHIP) Fig. 4.

Table 12.
Phase 1 — Study on CBDCA (JM-8)

No. of patients	30
Doses:	20—520 mg/m² i.v. infusion over 1 hour on a 3 weekly basis. No diuresis.
Dose limiting toxicity:	Haematological thrombocytopenia, leucopenia — nadirs at 20 days
Side effects:	No renal toxicity (urinary enzymes). Vomiting > 120 mg/m² — less severe than cisplatin.
Responses:	Ovarian carcinoma

CALVERT, HARLAND et al, Royal Marsden Hospital, Sutton, U.K.

222

Table 13.
Effect of structure on activity against DDP resistant leukemia 1210 (L1210/DDP).

PtA_2X_2

A	X	Dose*	Mean	I.L.S.
Control		—	12.0	—
Diammino	Cl_2	6.75	12.3	2.5
Diammino	Cl_2	4.5	13.9	15.8
Diammino	Cl_2	3.0	12.3	2.5
Diaminocyclohexane	Cl_2	7.5	22.9	90.8
Diaminocyclohexane	Carboxyphthalate	20.0	30.9	157.5
Diaminocycloheptane	Cl_2	5.0	18.9	57.5
Diaminocyclopentane	Cl_2	15.0	18.6	55
Orthophenylenediamine	Cl_2	15.0	14.2	18.3
Ethylenediamine	Cl_2	13.0	13.7	14.2
Cytoxan	—	200, D1 only	23.7	97.2
L-PAM	—	10, D1 only	16.9	40.8

* Dose in mg/kg Q4DX4.

Table 14.
Other Phase 1 trials

[Pt(isopropylamine)$_2$Cl$_2$(OH)$_2$] (CHIP)	Roswell Park Memorial Hospital Buffalo, New York, M. D. Anserson Hospital, Houston, Texas, Suny, Upstate Medical Centre, Syracuse, New York.
[Pt(1,1-diaminomethylcyclohexane) (TNO-6) (SO$_4$)(H$_2$O)]	Amsterdam
[Pt(1,2-diaminocyclohexane) (malonate)]	Paris (Prof. Matthé)
[Pt(1,2-diaminocyclohexane) (phic) (isocitrate)]	Paris, Toulouse.

terms of nephrotoxicity. Early results on CBDCA (JM-8) at the Royal Marsden Hospital (Sutton, UK) show that the dose limiting toxicity is haematological rather than renal and some interesting responses have been observed (Table 12). [Pt(1,2 dac) TMA] (Figure 4) entered clinical trial at the Memorial Sloan Kettering Hospital (New York) as a result of its activity against a cisplatin resistant L1210 tumour in mice (Table 13). To date, it has shown much lower toxicity than cisplatin at doses up to 640 mg/m² (12). CHIP (Figure 4) has just commenced a trial at Roswell Park Memorial Hospital (Buffalo) and again initial results show lowered toxicity compared to cisplatin. Other trials either underway or in preparation are shown in Table 14.

5. Summary

Preclinical studies on animals clearly indicate that several of the new platinum drugs are less toxic than cisplatin particularly in terms of nephrotoxicity. Initial results from Phase 1 studies appear to be confirming this and also hold out the possibility of improved selectivity. Although it now seems likely that a second generation drug will emerge on toxicity grounds alone, the successful candidate will be determined by therapeutic performance in the clinic.

Appendix I

Johnson Matthey and Lustenburg Platinum Mines have sponsored a collaborative research programme in the UK on platinum cancer chemotherapy since 1971. The large contributions to our programme of the following and their coworkers are gratefully acknowledged.
Drs. K. HARRAP, T. A. CONNORS and J. J. ROBERTS — Chester Beatty Institute
Professor M. L. TOKE — University College
Dr A. J. THOMSON — University of East Anglia
Dr E. WILTSHAW — Royal Marsden Hospital
Professor T. F. SLATER — Brunel University
Dr P. SLATER — London University
Dr C. A. Mc ANLIFFE — University of Manchester, Institute of Science and Technology

References

1. ROSENBERG, B., VAN CAMP, L., TROSKO, J. E. and MANSOUR, V. H.: Nature (London) *222* (1969), 385—386
2. DURANT, J. R. in: Cisplatin: Current status and new developments (eds. A. W. PRESTAYKO, S. T. CROOKE and S. K. CARTER), p. 317 Academic Press, 1980.
3. WILTSHAW, E. — personal communication
4. WOLPERT-DEFILIPPES, M. K. in: Cisplatin: Current Status and New Developments (eds. A. W. PRESTAYKO, S. T. CROOKE and S. K. CARTER), p. 183 Academic Press, 1980
5. WILKINSON, C. R., COX, P. J., JONES, M. and HARRAP, K. R.: Biochimie *60* (1978), 851—857
6. CONNORS, T. A., JONES, M., ROSS, W. C. J., BRADDOCK, P. D., KHOKAR, A. R. and TOBE, M. L.: Chem-Biol Interactions *5* (1972), 415
7. CLEARE, M. J., HYDES, P. C., MALERBI, B. W. and WATKINS, D. M.: Biochimie *60* (1978), 835
8. CONNORS, T. A., JONES, M., ROSS, W. C. J., BRADDOCKS, P. D., KHOKAR, A. R. and TOBE, M. L.: Chem-Biol Interactions *11* (1975), 145
9. CLEARE, M. J., HYDES, P. C., HEPBURN, D. R. and MALERBI, B. W.: in Cisplatin: Current status and new developments (eds. A. W. PRESTAYKO, S. T. CROOKE and S. K. CARTER), p. 149, Academic Press, 1980
10. BASOLO, F. and PEARSON, R. G.: in 'Mechanisms of Inorganic Recations' (2nd ed.), p. 359, Wiley, New York
11. HARRAP, K. R., JONES, M., WILKINSON, C. P., CLINK, H., McD., SPARROW, S., MITCHLEY, B. C. V., CLARKE, S. and VEASEK, A. in: Cisplatin: Current Status and New Deveopments (eds. A. W. PRESTAYKO, S. T. CROOKE and S. K. CARTER) p. 193, Academic Press, 1980
12. BURCHENAL, J. and PHILLIPS, F. — personal communication

Lucille Reid Cancer Foundation, Bakersfield, California, USA

The Status of Proteolytic Enzymes in Oncology

O. Wildermuth

It is doubtful whether the ancients, observing the rapid healing resulting from their use of herbs as wound dressings, appreciated that they had induced proteolytic debridement. One herb, comfrey or *Symphytum officinale*, was described in Turner's Herbal in 1586 as '. . . good to glue together freshe wounds'. In 1719, Tournefort wrote in his Complete Herbal of curing a rodent ulcer with poultices of ground comfrey root (1). In the 1896 Lancet, Professor William Thompson, president of the Royal College of Surgeons in Ireland, described complete healing of a post-surgical recurrence of a malignant tumour of the antrum with comfrey poultices. With the interruption of the supersonic aircraft project in Seattle in the early 1970s, an unemployed aeronautical engineer and a herbal hobbyist furnished us with sterile, fresh, crushed comfrey leaves three times weekly to tre atnecrotic wound dressings. We found it to be as good as papain or streptokinase-streptodornase (Varidase) solutions from the pharmacy. However, I was unimpressed by any cancerocidal effects. Whether the cell-free liquefaction of tumour masses injected with proteolytic enzymes (PE) as described by Scheef and others was the result of the action of PE on living tumour cells or only on necrotic masses is unknown (2).

John Beard, a professional embryologist, published Enzyme Therapy of Cancer in 1911. His thesis rested on Louis Pasteur's levo- and dextro-rotary states of molecules, then but recently accepted. Beard argued that cancer cells, like germinal cells, were derived from the trophoblast and were made up of levo-rotary moelcules, and that somatic cells were dextro-rotary. His PE attached to the levo-rotary isomer selectively. He felt that the quality of his enzymes explained his unduplicated success in treating cancer. While the rotary state of molecules continues to be important in chemistry, its application to cancer therapy seems more complex. In the world of medical practice, while dextrose is a component of the aerobic energy cycle, *levulose* is inert. Yet *L-dopa* is active in parkinsonism and *L-dromoran* is an active narcotic. Again, *dexadrine* is an active stimulant, and, to complicate things further, *racemephedrine*, a mixture of D- and L-ephedrine, is as effective as the pure levophedrine as a decongestant. The process of racemization of amino acids in proteins is proposed by DeLong and Poplin to be a cause of senescence and cancer: 'normal terminal phases of life (3). Cancer, then, has a much' broader biological connotation than merely a disease state: 'it represents a last effort of the organism to restore the vanishing capacity of mitosis due to shifts in concentration ratios of a few compounds' (4, 5). One example of such a ratio brings us back to racemization, which is said to proceed from a predominantly levo- to dextro-rotary isomeric state at the rate of about 0.1% per year — almost the same as the rate of loss of physiological function with age (3).

Perhaps then, BEARD's simplistic thesis should not be totally forgotten, as a variable ratio of levo-/dextro-rotary cells could relate to the variable effects reported.

PE in the laboratory

In the investigative laboratory, many interesting applications of PE are to be found. As a method of disaggregating cancer cells in preparation for cell culture or for intravenous bolus studies of metastatic potential, PE have been found superior to mechanical techniques (28, 29). In reports from several laboratories, HANKA found eleven amino acids that cancer cells produced poorly or not at all, that could be further reduced with specific PE (6). Since normal cells produce these amino acids adequately, the toxic analogue then administered would be selectively accumulated by the neoplastic cells to their detriment. He also pointed out that the historic road block to chemotherapy of cancer was the lack of biochemical differences between cancer cells and their normal counterparts. The amino acid differences he described may be exploitable to help discover a therapy for cancers with a favourable therapeutic ratio. One attempt at such therapy was the asparagine *versus* L-asparaginase system, which had some success against leukaemia in children, even without the addition of a toxic analogue. However, it failed due to its antigenicity and consequent problems. With the finding that the antigenic property of bovine serum can be altered by the covalent attachment of methoxypolyethylene glycol, reevaluation may be in order (7).

PE in chemotherapy

In cytotoxic drug pharmacology, PE form the target for a number of agents. Many of the vast array of enzymes involved in the regulation of cell metabolism, protein synthesis and effects on the endocrine systems have been studied (8, 9, 10). For example, BAKER's antifol, TZT, acts by inhibiting dehydrofolate reductase (DHFR). The effects of both TZT and methotrexate on DHFR are reversible. A new BAKER's antifol, DTB, now being studied, is non-reversible and attached covalently to serine transhydroxymethylase; this should prove more effective than TZT or methotrexate when it comes to clinical trial. Other systems are as follows: 6-mercaptopurine is inactivated by xanthine oxidase; arabinosyl C (Ara C) is rapidly deaminated by tetrahydro uridinease; Ara C i.p. inhibits ribonucleotide reductase; allopurinal inhibits xanthine oxidase. The anabolism of fluorouracil drugs involves the intermediary of fluorouracil-ribonucleotide *via* uridine phosphorylase, followed by uridinecytidine kinase. (11) The list goes on, but none of these drugs has been specific for cancer cells.

PE in metastases

Many studies support the idea that PE, such as heparin and plasmin, prevent metastases through eliminating the formation of the protective fibrin-platelet coagulum that surrounds the clump of tumour cells adherent to the small ramifications of the vascular tree. The 'cocoon', a popularization of the concept by DVORAK, is necessary to allow leucocytic degradation of the endothelium, leading to invasion of the proliferating cancer cells through the wall of the blood vessel. It provides protection from antibodies and cancerocidal lymphocytes (12, 13). Further, there is evidence that

226

neoplasms produce 'thromboplastic materials' which block the fibrinolytic mechanisms of these PE (14). Several investigators postulated an imbalance between thromboxane-A, released by platelets, and prostacyclin (PGI_2), released by the vascular endothelium (15, 16, 17, 18, 19). Both substances affect the level of cyclic AMP and free calcium, the former preventing and the latter promoting platelet aggregation. HONN further postulated that the lysosomal PE, cathepsin-B, was produced by cancer cells (15).

Cancer cells are also described as glycogen traps (16). ARDENNE and RIEGERS proposed to stimulate the high potential for glycolysis with very high doses of glucose. (20, 21). This would produce an excess of intracellular lactic acid; whereas normal cells, which do not respond to hyperglycaemia with increased glycolysis, would remain unchanged. The low pH created by the accumulation of lactic acid in the cancer cells renders them increasingly vulnerable to damage. This was thought to result in increased permeability of the lysosomal membrane and the release of autolytic enzymes. In the laboratory, vitamin A strongly promotes release of cathepsin-B from lymphocytic lysosomes. The composite effect, then, of hyperglycaemia and vitamin A could further promote selective destruction of cancer cells.

CLIFTON's data seem to indicate that fibrinolytic enzymes not only prevent metastases but also destroy existing fibrin coagula, since repeated doses of PE continue to decrease the rate of metastasis. (22) Of further interest, since he noted a small, early decrease in the number of injected tumour cells in circulation, he postulated a direct cytocidal effect. PE administration suspended growth of measurable tumour masses due to lysis of the 'cocoon' and thus prevented the neovascularization necessary for size increase. The modern western diet produces hyperlipaemia, which has been found to inhibit fibrinolytic effects and thus to promote successful tumour cell implant on the vascular walls (23, 24). This may be relieved in part with consequent respite to coffee lovers, who were publicly advised by MACMAHON, the Harvard epidemiologist of world renown, that coffee was carcinogenic; HONN (15) recently reported that the theophyllins increase PGI_2 clot prevention four-fold, so at least their cancer should stay localized and curable.

PE in radiation therapy

The hallmarks of radiation therapy are post-arterial vascular dilation, erythema and oedema, which convert to late findings of endarteritis, endothelial rosettes and fibrosis. In an ingenious experiment, mice were injected with tagged serum proteins (25), fibrinogen and small molecules being tagged with one radioactivity and the larger molecules with another. After one ear had been irradiated, both ears were exposed by rotation to counters specific to each radiation, and the accumulated activity was plotted. The larger molecules were found to leak out into the tissues of the irradiated ear and to peak at about 12 hours, largely returning into the circulation within 20 hours. The smaller molecule tag appeared later and did not fall for more than 24 hours. Daily irradiation would then have an additive effect on perivascular fibronogen accumulation. Urokinase prevented the fibrinogen-fibrin-fibrosis sequence in the experimental situation. Thus, the pathogenesis of radiation histology is fibrosis constricting vascular spaces with rosette formation, rather than endothelial cell proliferation — a long-standing enigma in radiobiology.

While PE have been advocated for use in radiation oedema and prevention of post-radiation fibrosis in Europe, I know of no randomized prospective study that gives unequivocal laboratory or clinical evidence of successful exploitation of this observations (26). More than two decades ago, at the Tumour Institute of the Swedish Hospital in Seattle, we embarked on a clinical exploratory study on the use of Varidase for prevention of pulmonary oedema in lung irradiation concomitant to mediastinal, hilar nodal or solitary metastasis irradiation. Benefits were equivocal. End-point determination by subjective symptoms, pulmonary ventilation studies or radiographic determinations were unsatisfactory; and, with no area of agreed effectiveness seen in random testing, the project was discontinued.

Discussion

Proteolytic enzymes, directly or through various aspects of their metabolic affects, present a subject for renewed interest and for a reevaluation of their use in systemic cancer therapy. 'Although the use of modern experimental techniques such as mass spectrometry or analogue computers established a lot of new facts, the center of importance lies probably in the new ways of thinking in the evaluation of already known facts from unexpected points of view' (24). A number of facts concerning PE should be listed: (1) There is a direct effect of PE on a small percentage of cancer cells; (2) there is direct effect of PE on the cancer matrix; (3) PE and their target amino-acids are both targets of chemotherapeutic agents; (4) specific PE may eliminate certain amino-acids that are produced inefficiently by tumour cells to make them more ready to take up toxic analogues; (5) PE counteract disseminated intravascular coagulation induced by cancer cells or chemotherapy; (6) PE may prevent metastases from circulating cancer cells; (7) PE may eliminate the complications of radiation therapy of oedema and resultant fibrosis; (8) vitamin A and hyperglycaemia may promote autogenic production of PE, especially cathepsin-B; (9) prevention of hyperlipaemia may allow for more effective action of fibrinolysins; (10) coffee-lovers may drink their beverage so that the theophyllins can aid PGI_2 to inhibit platelet aggregation and resultant metastases.

If, indeed, a certain number of cancer are destroyed directly by PE, and if the result of racemization is to approach equivalency in the levo-/dextro-rotary populations of cells as a result of age, then there may be a justification for the early contention that some PE attack only the levo-optical isomer of a critical protein molecule and result in cancer kill.

Rethinking the facts listed above may result in the formulation of acceptable protocols to interest cooperative chemotherapy test groups. At present, the newer classes of chemotherapy drugs seem to result in greater toxicity. One researcher advised, 'It is important to reemphasize that morbidity of the therapeutic approach and its compromise of the patient's quality of life cannot and should not outweigh the therapeutic benefits for this or any other diseases in oncology' (27). The end of pure toxicity and an increasing interest in research into the development of attacks on unique characteristics of cancer cells is possibly in sight. Our patients may realize their hope that their cancers regress without the universally dreaded agonies of chemotherapy.

A word about where we began: non-specific PE therapy. Aside from anecdotal case reports, there exists no firm evidence of actual selective cancer cell destruction by PE used topically, injected into masses, or injected intravenously or per rectum for systemic effect. Obviously, non-specific PE must be adequately explored in laboratory animals before any serious, combined clinical trial directed toward cancer control, regional or systemic, can be considered. If such preliminaries, required of all new drugs in the US, are carried out and prove successful, there is no doubt in my mind, as a former participant in combined clinical studies, that such studies would be eagerly launched. I hope it will be done with better foundation and less wishful enthusiasm than was involved in the beginning of the immunotherapy of cancer, now largely returned to the laboratory.

Conclusion

In our continuing search for new methods and drugs for cancer therapy, it may be time to look back at some of the accumulated facts from a new point of view. A therapeutic ratio in favour of the patient should be restructed into our thinking, especially when response rates rather than cure rates seem to be the attainable goals in systemic cancer treatment. The identification of actual biochemical differences between cancer cells and their host counterparts should be the target of investigations. Specific proteolytic enzymes must play an important role in widening the differences between cancer and normal cells before the administration of the toxic analogue. Prevention of metastasis seems within our grasp, with the use of heparin and similar fibrinolytic agents. Diet considerations seem more rational. The place of non-specific PE in systemic cancer is, however, still primary. They should be better studied and tested clinically according to the methods developed for chemotherapy agents that have received general acceptance.

References

1. HILLS, L. D: Comfrey Universal Books, N.Y. 1976
2. SCHEEF, W.: Enzymes and vitamine A in cancer therapy. 10th International Cancer Congress, Houston, Texas, 1970
3. DeLONG, R. and POPLIN, L.: On the etiology of ageing. Jour. Theor. Biol. 67 (1977), 111—120
4. DUCHESNE, J.: A unifying biochemical theory of cancer, senescence and maximal life. Span. Jour. Theor. Biol. 67 (1977), 137—145
5. THEOLOGIDES, A.: Cancer cachexia. Cancer 43 (1969), 200402012
6. HANKA, L. J.: Introduction: Possibilities for Biochemically Rational Chemotherapy for some Malignancies with Depleting Enzymes and Unknown Metabolites of Special Amino Acids. Cancer Treat. Repts. 63 (1979), 1009—1011
7. ABUCHOWSKI, A., VAN ES, T., PALCZUK, N. C. and DAVIS, F. F.: Alterations of Immunological Properties of Bovine Serum Albumin by Covalent Attachment of Polyethylene Glycol. Jour. Biol. Chem. 252 (1977), 3578—3581
8. BROADSKY, I.: In: Oncologic Medicine. Clinical Topics and Practical Management. STUTNISK, A. I. & ENGSTROM, P. F. eds. Balto. Univ. Park Press, pp. 247—259, 1976
9. OLSON, R. E.: Introductory Remarks: Nutrients, Hormones & Enzymes Interactions. Am. Jour. Clin. Nutrition 28 (1975), 626—637
10. MANGUM, J. A. and BRAMAN, J. C.: The Antitumour and Biochemical Characterization of an Active-Site-Directed Irreversible Inhibitor of Folate-Dependent Enzymes. 71st Ann. AACR, 1980
11. HAMRELL, M., SEDWICH, D. and LAZZLO, J.: Interrelationship of Drug Transport and Target Enzyme Levels as Determinants of Methotrexate Resistance. 71st Ann. AACR, 1980

12. AHMED, N., HAGGITT, R. C. and WELCH, A. D.: Enzymes of Salvage and de novo Pathways in Human Colorectal Cancer. 71st Ann. AACR. 1980
13. DVORAK, H.: "Cocoon" may Protect Tumours from Immunological Attack. Oncologic Times. p. 1, July 1981
14. THORNES, R. D.: Anticoagulant Therapy in Patients with Cancer. Jour. Irish Med. Assn. *62* (1969), 426—429
15. HONN, K. V.: Prostacyclin: Potential Antimetastatic Agent. Oncologic Times, p. 1, July, 1981
16. SHAPOT, V. S.: On the Multiform Relationships between the Tumour and the Host. Adv. in Cancer Research. *30* (1979), 89—150, Acad. Press, Inc.
17. MONCADA, D., BUNTING, S. and MULLANE, K.: Imidazole: A Selective Inhibitor of Thromboxane Synthetase. Prostaglandins *13* (4) 611—618, Apr. 1977
18. DEMBINSKA, S., KIEC, A., ZMUDA, A. and KRUPINSKA, J.: Inhibition of prostaglandin synthetase by aspirine-like drugs in different microsomal preparations. Adv. Prostaglandin Thromboxane Res. *1* (1976), 93—103
19. ZMUDA, A., DEMBINSKA, A., KIEC, A., CHYTKOWSKI, A. and GRYGLEWSKI R. J., Experimental Atherosclerosis in Rabbits: Platelet Aggregation, Thromboxane A2 Generation and Antiaggregatory Potency of Prostacyclin. Prostaglandins, *14*(C) (1977), 1035—1042
20. ARDENNE, V. and RIEGERS, F.: Arch. Geschwulstforsch. 40; 51—79, 1972. As cited by: SHAPOT, V. S., On the multiform relationships between the tumour and the host., Adv. in Cancer Research, *30* (1979), 137—138
21. CHAN, S. and HIGGINS, E. Jr.: Uncoupling Activity of Endogeneous Free Fatty Acids in Rat Liver Mitochondria. Canad. J. Biochem. (1978), 111—116
22. CLIFTON, E. F.: Effect of fibrinolysin on the spread of cancer. Federation Proceed. *25* (1966), 89—93
23. GJESDAL, K. and ABRAHAMSEN, F. A.: Platelet Consumption and Plasma Concentration of Platelet Factor 4 (PF—J). Scand. Jour. Haematol. *17* (1976), 205
24. HOCMAN, G.: Biochemistry of Ageing. Int. J. Biochem. *10* (1979), 67—76
25. Personal communication, unpublished
26. HOEFER-JANKER, H.: The Importance of Vitamine A and Proteolytic Enzymes in Cancer Therapy. Arztl. Praxis. *23* (1971), 2805
27. SALAZAR, O. M. and CRUSH, R. H.: The State of the Art: Toward Defining the Role of Radiation Therapy in the Management of Small Cell Bronchiogenic Cancer. Rad. Oncol., Biol. & Physics. *6*; 8 (1980), 1103—1117
28. SLOCUM, H. K., RUSTUM, P. J., CREAVEN, Z. P., PAVELIC, F. A., SIDDEQUI, F. a., KARAKOUSIS, H., TAKITA, H. and VINCENT, R. G.: Enzymatic Disaggregation and Mechanical Dissaggregation of Human Melanoma, Sarcoma & Lung Cancer. 71st Ann. AACR, 1980
29. PAVELIC, Z. P., RUSKIM, P. J., CREAVEN, Z. P., KARAKOUSIA, C. and TAKITA, H.: Colony Growth in Soft Agar of Melanomas, Sarcomas & Lung Carcinoma Cells Disaggregated by Mechanical & Enzymatic Methods. 71st Ann. AACR, 1980

Bristol-Myers Company, International Division, USA, Belgium

Marcellomycin: A New Class II Anthracycline

L. Lenaz, R. Canetta and P. Hilgard

Introduction

The mechanism of action of anthracyclines appears to be related to a variety of biochemical effects and sites of action. A number of authors have reported on the interaction of these agents with DNA, thereby interfering with normal nucleic acid synthesis (1—11). Other studies have demonstrated that anthracyclines may induce significant alterations in membranes, characterized by altered ability in cellular agglutination and mitotic arrest, even at concentrations lower than those required to induce inhibition of nucleic acid synthesis (3—8, 12—14).

The two anthracyclines of current major clinical importance, doxorubicin and daunorubicin have been shown to interact with DNA by intercalating between adjacent base pairs (2, 3, 4, 12, 15). They have also been shown to inhibit the synthesis of DNA and RNA at approximately equivalent concentrations, and nucleolar preribosomal RNA (No-RNA) synthesis at concentrations 2—5 fold lower than those required to inhibit DNA synthesis (5, 8, 10, 16).

It has been shown, however, that other anthracyclines have a greater selectivity for No-RNA synthesis, and recently Crooke et al (11) proposed a classification of anthracyclines on the basis of their effects on nucleic acid synthesis. Class I anthracyclines such as doxorubicin and daunorubicin were defined as those shown to inhibit No-RNA synthesis at concentrations comparable to those required to inhibit DNA synthesis. Class II anthracyclines such as marcellomycin and aclacinomycin A, were shown to inhibit No-RNA synthesis at concentrations 200—1500 fold lower than those required to inhibit DNA synthesis. From structure-activity relationship studies, it was also suggested that the presence of a di- or tri-saccharide glycosidic side chain conferred No-RNA synthesis inhibitory selectivity (11).

We have focused the internal anthracycline development program at Bristol-Myers Company on Class II anthracycline oligosaccharides. This paper reviews the results obtained with marcellomycin, the compound selected for clinical trials.

Chemistry

Marcellomycin (NSC-265211) was isolated from a mixture of anthracyclines called bohemic acid complex extracted from fermentations of *Actinosporangium* sp. (17, 18). Structural analysis revealed that the molecule was a trisaccharide anthracycline, with pyrromycinone as aglycone, and a glycosidic side chain containing one rhodosamine and two deoxyfucose residues.

231

Mechanism of action

While doxorubicin and pyrromycin inhibited DNA and RNA synthesis in Novikoff hepatoma ascites cells at approximately equivalent concentrations, marcellomycin was effective in inhibiting RNA synthesis at 6—7 fold lower concentration than that required to inhibit DNA synthesis (19) (Table 1). Table 2 shows that the ratios of the IC_{50} for DNA and No-RNA was about 1 for doxorubicin and pyrromycin, and 1256 for marcellomycin. In comparison, another Class II anthracycline currently in clinical development, aclacinomycin A, had ratio of 170. Thus, marcellomycin appears to

Table 1.
50% Inhibitory concentrations (IC_{50} values) for DNA and whole cell RNA synthesis

Compound	DNA	RNA	DNA/RNA
Doxorubicin	6.1	3.2	1.89
Pyrromycin	5.7	4.5	1.26
Carminomycin	14.7	8.9	1.64
Marcellomycin	11.3	1.7	6.53
Aclacinomycin	6.3	0.8	7.65
10-descarbomethoxy marcellomycin	18.4	7.2	2.54

Table 2.
Inhibition of nucleolar RNA (No-RNA) synthesis, and its ratio to whole cellular DNA synthesis

	IC_{50} No-RNA (μM)	DNA/No-RNA
Doxorubicin	6.0	1.02
Carminomycin	13.1	1.12
Pirromycin	6.1	0.93
Marcellomycin	0.009	1256.00
Aclacinomycin	0.037	170.00
10-descarbomethoxy marcellomycin	2.56	7.42

have the greatest selectivity for inhibiting nucleolar DNA. The difference between the aglycones of marcellomycin and doxorubicin does not appear to contribute significantly to the observed nucleolar selectivity. In fact, pyrromycin has the same aglycone as marcellomycin, but is comparable to doxorubicin in its effects on nucleic acids.

It appears that the critical structural difference is the presence of the trisaccharide side chain, and that the terminal deoxyfucose sugar residue imparts enhanced specificity for inhibition of No-RNA synthesis. The results of studies comparing marcellomycin to its 10-descarbomethoxy derivative provide further support for the concept that No-RNA inhibition may be responsible for the mechanism of anti-tumour action of marcellomycin (20). The removal of the carbomethoxy group in fact resulted in markedly decreased No-RNA selectivity, which was paralleled by a decrease in cytotoxic activity against Novikoff hepatoma cells in vitro, and L-1210 leukemia in vivo (Table 3). However, the effects on DNA and whole cell RNA synthesis were not affected.

Further studies comparing a number of anthracyclines were done in order to evaluate drug localization into the cell by cytofluorescence (21). Marcellomycin and aclacinomycin, unlike doxorubicin and daunorubicin, were found to be localized mainly in the cytoplasm of L-1210 cells and marcellomycin was accumulated both in the whole L-1210 cells and in isolated nuclei to a greater extent than the other drugs.

Table 3.
IC_{50} values of marcellomycin and its 10-descarbomethoxy-derivative for DNA, RNA and No-RNA synthesis, and cell viability in Novikoff hepatoma cells in vitro, in comparison with in vivo antitumour data

	Marcellomycin	10-Descarbomethoxy marcellomycin
IC_{50} (µM) DNA	13.52	18.99
IC_{50} (µM) RNA	3.03	4.07
IC_{50} (µM) No-RNA	0.014	2.56
IC_{50} (µM) Novikoff	0.75	3.80
MED*- L-1210	0.20	4.00

*MED = Minimum effective dose (schedule QD 1 → 5)

Experimental antitumour activity

Marcellomycin was evaluated for its antitumour activity in a broad spectrum of tumours (22). Table 4 summarizes the optimal doses and maximal increases in median survival time (MST) obtained in these studies: marcellomycin shows good activity in murine leukemias, B-16 melanoma, and Lewis lung carcinoma, while activity in colon 26 and Madison 109 lung carcinoma is low. Marcellomycin was compared with doxorubicin in L-1210 leukemia and B-16 melanoma, and, although less effective than doxorubicin, it retained clear effectiveness in these tumours.

Table 4.
Antitumour activity of marcellomycin

Schedule	Optimal dose (mg/kg/day i. p.)	P-388	Maximal % T/C[1] vs. I.p. Tumour				
			L-1210	LL	B-16	C-26	M-109
Day 1	0.8—6.4	144—156	136—157		144—170		120
Days 1 + 4	3—4						126—128
Days 1 + 5	0.18—0.75					104—129	
Days 1, 5 + 9	0.37—1.5					120—139	
QD 1—5	0.4—1.6	150—167	129—150				
QD 1—9	0.5—2				308 (8/10)[2]	138—216	

[1] %T/C = (MST treated/MST control) × 100
[2] 8/10 cures

233

Toxicology studies

The determination of lethal doses in laboratory animals evidenced the existence of a steep slope in the dose response curve of marcellomycin, and, as commonly seen for anthracyclines, and increased toxicity after intraperitoneal administration, reflecting local irritation (Table 5).

Death in laboratory animals after single and multiple dose appeared to be related mainly to gastrointestinal toxicity while bone marrow toxicity was moderate or absent.

Table 5.
Toxicological parameters of marcellomycin in mice and dogs

BDF, mice LD_{50} i.p.	6 mg/kg
BDF, mice LD_{50} i.v.	13 mg/kg
Suiss-Webster mice LD_{50} i.v.	19.9 mg/kg
Dog LD_{100}	3.7 mg/kg
Dog toxic dose high	2.9 mg/kg

Marcellomycin was found to have no leukopenic effects in mice and rats even at lethal doses (22, 23). In rats, two WBC increases, both followed by return to pretreatment levels, were seen at one day and one week after administration.

At the end of the first week mild to moderately decreased platelet counts were observed with prompt recovery within 4—5 days after nadir. Marcellomycin affected the red series, causing an evident reduction of reticulocyte counts during the first week, followed by "reticulocyte crisis" and very mild anemia during the second week, and complete recovery in the third week. Although bone marrow hypocellularity was seen at one week after dosing, increased myeloid activity at all dose levels was seen after 4 weeks. In dogs mild leukopenia was seen after sublethal doses, and was reversible. Only at lethal doses persistent and severe hypocellularity of the bone marrow and lymphoid organs was reported. A multiple dose study in dogs confirmed the results of the single dose study, with dose related leukopenia, clearly evident only in the lethal dose range.

The major site of toxicity of marcellomycin in dogs and mice appears to be the gastrointestinal tract. At supralethal doses massive bleeding was observed both clinically and pathologically. Lower, but lethal, doses led to diffuse hyperplasia and hyperemia of the mucosa with isolated areas of necrosis. Sublethal doses, however, did not produce any remarkable change on G. I. tissue.

No significant myocardial changes indicative of doxorubicin-like cardiomyopathy were seen during the toxicology studies. The potential for cardiotoxicity of marcellomycin was investigated also by examination of the values of creatinine phosphokinase MB isoenzyme, an enzyme released when cardiac muscle is damaged. Elevations of CPK-MB were seen, but lower than after comparable doses of adriamycin (23). Also, marcellomycin did not cause in dogs any significant effect on heart rate, PR interval, QRS duration and voltage (24). In a comparative study vs. doxorubicin, marcellomycin did not cause any significant change in QRS voltage, while doxorubicin induced reduction of QRS voltage approaching 50% (24).

All other toxic effects described with marcellomycin in laboratory animals appear to be similar to those previously reported with other anthracyclines. Particular mention should be made about the drug effects at injection site, leading to severe irritation and/or vesication.

Clinical studies

Marcellomycin has recently entered clinical studies and Phase I studies are currently ongoing according to a single dose intermittent, or a weekly schedule.

Preliminary data indicate that the weekly schedule may be less toxic, allowing administration of higher total doses of the drug per unit of time. Broad Phase II studies are planned to evaluate the clinical spectrum of activity of this new anthracycline.

References

1. WARING, M.: J. Mol. Biol. *54* (1970), 247—279
2. DiMARCO, A., ARCAMONE, F. and ZUNINO, F.: in: Antibiotics III — Mechanism of Action of Antimicrobial and Anti-tumour Agents (CORCORAN, J. W. & HAHN, F. E. — eds.) pp. 101—128, Springer-Verlag, Berlin, (1975).
3. GABBAY, E. J., GRIER, D., FINGELE, R., REINER, R., PEARCE, S. W. and WILSON, W. D.: Biochemistry *15* (1976), 2062—2069
4. TSOU, K. C. and YIP, K. F.: Cancer Res. *36* (1976), 3367—3374
5. THEOLOGIDES, A., YARBRO, J. W. and KENNEDY, B. J.: Cancer *21* (1968), 16—21
6. RUSCONI, A. and DiMARCO, A.: Cancer Res. *29* (1969), 1507—1511
7. MERIWETHER, W. D. and BACHUR, N. R.: Cancer Res. *32* (1972), 1137—1142
8. DANO, K., FREDERIKSEN, S. and HELLUNG-LARSEN, P.: Cancer Res. *32* (1972), 1307—1314
9. HENRY, D. W.: in: Cancer Chemotherapy (SARTORELLI, A. C. — ed.), pp. 15—57, 169th Meeting Amer. Chem. Soc. Div. Med. Chem. Symp., April 7, 1975, Philadelphia, Penna. (1975)
10. DiMARCO, A., SILVESTRINI, R., DiMARCO, S. and DASDIA, T.: J. Cell Biol. *27* (1965), 545—550
11. CROOKE, S. T., DuVERNAY, V. H., GALVAN, L. and PRETAYKO, A. W.: Molecular Pharmacol. *14* (1978), 65—73
12. PIGRAM, W. J., FULLER, W. and HAMILTON, L. O.: Nature New Biol. *235* (1972), 17—19
13. MURPHREE, S. E., CUNNINGHAM, L. S., HWANG, K. M. and SARTORELLI, A. C.: Biochem. Pharmacol. *25* (1976), 1227
14. MURPHREE, S. A., TRITTON, T. R. and SARTORELLI, A. C.: Fed. Proc. *36* (1977), 303
15. ZUNINO, F., GAMBETTA, R., DiMARCO, A., VELCICH, A., ZACCARA, A., QUADRIFOGLIO, F. and CRESCENZI, V.: Biochim. Biophys. Acta *476* (1977), 38—46
16. TONG, G., LEE, W. W., BLACK, D. R. and HENRY, D. W.: J. Med. Chem. *19* (1976), 395—398
17. BRADNER, W. T. and MISIEK, M.: J. Antibiot. *30* (1977), 519—522
18. NETTLETON, D. E., Jr., BRADNER, W. T., BUSCH, J. A., COON, A. B., MOSELEY, J. E., MYLLY-MACKI, R W., O'HERRON, F. A., SCHREIBER, R. H. and VULCANO, A. L.: J. Antibiot. *30* (1977), 525—529
19. CROOKE, S. R., DuVERNAY, U. H., GALVAN, L. and PRESTAYKO, A. W.: Mol. Pharmacol. *14* (1978), 290—298
20. DuVERNAY, U. H., ESSERY, J. M., DOYLE, T. W., BRADNER, W. T. and CROOKE, S. R.: Mol. Pharmacol. *15* (1978), 341—356
21. EGORIN, M. J., CLAWSON, R. E., COHEN, J. L., ROSS, L. A. and BACHUR, N. R.: Cancer Res. *40* (1980), 4669—4676
22. REICH, S. D., BRADNER, W. T., ROSE, W. C., SCHURIG, J. E., MADISSOO, H., JOHNSON, D. F., DuVERNAY, V. H. and CROOKE, S. T.: Marcellomycin. In: Antracyclines: Current Status and New Developments. S. T. CROOKE and S. D. REICH (Editors), Academic Press, New York 1980. Chapt. 20, pp. 343—364
23. SCHURIG, J. E., BRADNER, W. T., HUFTALEN, J. B. and DOYLE, G. J.: In: Antracyclines: Current Status and New Developments. S. T. CROOKE and S. D. REICH (Editors), Academic Press, New York 1980. Chap. 8, pp. 141—149
24. BUYNISKI, J. P. and HIRTH, R. S.: Antracycline cardiotoxicity in the rat. In: Antracyclines: Current Status and New Developments. S. T. CROOKE and S. D. REICH (Editors), Academic Press, New York 1980. Chapt. 10, pp. 157—170

Biological Response Modifiers

Ludwig Institute for Cancer Research, MRC Centre, The Medical School, Cambridge, England

Interferon

K. Sikora

Since its discovery in 1957, interferon has seemed to hover on the brink of a break-through. Its successful clinical exploitation has so far remained elusive. Over the last five years there has been tremendous interest in the drug, mainly because of its potential anticancer action.

Interferon is a glycoprotein produced by mammalian cells in response to viral infection. It can also be produced by certain subpopulations of lymphocytes when exposed to antigens to which they have previously been sensitised. Biologically, it is clearly involved in the prevention, or at least the containment, of viral infection. Its function within the complex interactive network of the immune system is as yet unclear. It may well have a role similar to other lymphokines which act as a communication system amongst the immunocompetent cells. Work performed over the last 20 years has demonstrated that interferon has an antitumour effect in a variety of in vivo and in vitro systems. A major problem has been its species specificity, human interferon being only effective in human cells. In the last few years enough evidence has been gathered to suggest that interferon may have a tumour reducing effect in several human cancers. This evidence has heralded a new wave of research interest amongst oncologists, molecular biologists and biotechnologists.

Sources

The major source of interferon for clinical use so far has been buffy coat leucocytes (1). Dr. Kari Cantell of the National Blood Transfusion Centre in Helsinki in Finland has devoted the last 20 years to the proceeding of human leucocyte interferon. Buffy coat cells are pooled from many donors and stimulated to produce interferon by the addition of Sendai virus. The supernatants are collected and purified using a potassium thiocyanate precipitation technique. Initially the interferon produced activity of 10^5 international units of interferon per mg of protein; current preparations are 20 times more pure, with an activity of 2×10^7 units/mg. However, pure interferon has an estimated activity of 4×10^8 per mg, which is impossible to achieve in large amounts using simple chemical procedures (2).

The logistic problems in producing large quantities of interferon from human leuco-cytes have turned investigators to other sources. Tissue culture cells, either human fibroblast or lymphoblastoid lines, have been used. Fibroblast cells grow as mono-layers and until now have required considerable work to maintain. New techniques involving the use of microspheres which form a substrate for fibroblasts growth pro-mise to revolutionize the growing of large quantities of these monolayer cells. Interferon production by lymphoblastoid cells has yielded sufficient interferon at a con-centration of 2×10^7 units/mg protein for fairly extensive clinical trial (3).

In the last two years remarkable competition amongst new biotechnology groups has resulted in the simultaneous cloning of the structural genes for a variety of inter-ferons (4, 5). Fibroblast, lymphoblastoid and leucocyte interferons have all been cloned, inserted into plasmids and expressed in *E. coli*. In this way large amounts of interferon has been produced relatively cheaply. A further development has been the production of an interferon specific monoclonal antibody (6). By the use of a sui-table affinity column this antibody can purify large amounts of interferon from a com-plex mixture of proteins in a simple single step.

Structure

Surprisingly little is known about the structure of the molecule. One problem is its heterogeneity mainly due to the carbohydrate component. Table 1 lists the basic properties of the three types of human interferon. Recent work on the nucleic acid sequence of various interferon clones suggests that each type of interferon is represent-ed by a family of homologous genes, rather than by a single defined sequence (7).

Table 1.
Human interferon

Name	Alternative names	MW	Source
Hu IFN α	Leucocyte, (Le) Type I	17,000	Leucocyte, lymphoblastoid cells
Hu IFN β	Fibroblast (F)	21,000	Fibroblasts
Hu IFN γ	Immune, Type II	43,000	Antigen stimulated lymphocyte

Mechanism of action

There is good evidence that interferon binds to a cell surface receptor consisting of gangliosides and protein and subsequently triggers a second messenger system, resul-ting in mRNA synthesis and subsequently protein synthesis. The exact nature of this effect is not clear but three separate enzyme systems (Table 2) have been suggested as mediating both the antiviral and growth inhibitory effects of interferon. It is known that interferon can stop the replication of DNA and RNA tumour viruses. For example, in SV-40 virus infected cells, the accumulation of early messenger RNA is inhibited, whilst for the murine leukaemia virus defective viruses with a reduced infectivity is produced by cells in the presence of interferon. Although there are hints that viruses may be implicated in aetiology of human cancer there are no assay systems available in which to determine the effects of interferon on putative tumour viruses.

A direct growth inhibitory effect of interferon has been observed in a wide range of cell lines. Interferon binds to surface receptors in tumour cells and triggers signals that seem to alter the kinetics of the cell cycle. The intracellular mediators may well

240

Table 2.
Interferon enzyme induction

1. PKi	→ Phosphorylation of eiF-2	→ Inhibition of met-tRNA binding
2. Oligoadenylate synthetase	→ (2′—5′) pppApApA	→ Activation of ribonuclease F
3. Phosphodiesterase	→ -CCA removal from tRNA	→ Protein synthesis blocked

be small cyclic nucleotides. Whether the growth inhibitory effect works through the same enzyme system as the viral inhibition is unclear.

Interferon also has a profound effect on the immune system. We know so little about which modes of effector systems are responsible for tumour cell destruction that it is difficult to analyse any potentially immuno-stimulating effect of interferon in cancer. Treated patients do, however, show a fall in the circulating B-lymphocyte level and an increase in natural killer cell activity, together with a post-treatment stimulation of lymphocyte blastogenesis exposure to specific antigens or non-specific mitogens. It is, however, clear that interferon will reduce the growth of tumour cells in vitro in the absence of any immune component, and also in xenograft systems where by definition there can only be minimal residual immunity in the animal bearing the tumour.

Clinical results

The first serious study of the use of interferon against cancer in man was performed by Dr. Hans STRANDER at the Karolinska Institute in Sweden (8). He gave 3×10^6 IU of interferon for thirty days to children who had a recent amputation for osteogenic sarcoma. This was followed by twice weekly injections of the same dose for 18 months. The incidence of pulmonary metastases was found to be 50% in his interferon treated group and 86% in the control group. The survival was 71% in the interferon group and 17% in the control. These apparently dramatic results are overshadowed by the fact that he used a historical control group. Subsequent analysis shows that this group has fared worse than any other group of osteosarcoma patients ever collected. This emphasises the need for concurrent randomization in clinical studies of this nature. STRANDER, however, has now collected data showing responses in multiple myeloma, Hodgkin's disease, non-Hodgkin's lymphoma, advanced osteosarcoma and perhaps most dramatically juvenile laryngeal papilloma. This last disease is rare, occurring in children and adolescents. It presents with tracheal obstruction due to a fleshy papillomatous tumour around the larynx. Treatment of this is difficult but eight complete responses using interferon as above have now been obtained.

The STANFORD group have produced good evidence for a tumour reducing effect of leucocyte interferon in non-Hodgkin's lymphoma (9). Three patients with nodular poorly differentiated lymphoma (NLPD) have entered into complete remission following the administration of interferon 10^7 units daily for thirty days. Three patients with diffuse histiocytic lymphoma (undifferentiated lymphoma) have shown no response. Clearly NLPD is an easy disease in which to obtain responses either by radiation or by chemotherapy, but these results encourage the further investigation of interferon. A randomised clinical trial is now in progress at STANFORD to look at the effects of

Table 3.
Clinical trials of human interferon

	Response Total	NR	LPR	PR	CR	CR + PR
Nodular lymphoma (9, 10)	14	6	2	3	3	42%
Diffuse histocytic lymphoma (9, 10)	7	6	1	0	0	0%
Myeloma (10)	30	16	3	8	3	37%
Breast cacer (10, 11)	38	24	3	11	0	29%
Lung cancer (12)	12	12	0	0	0	0%
Melanoma (13, 14)	4	2	0	1	0	25%

NR, no response; LPR, less than 50% tumour regression; PR, > 50% tumour regression; CR, complete response.

interferon in addition to conventional therapy in patients with "good prognosis" non-Hodgkin's lymphoma.

There is now good evidence of a tumour reducing effect in metastatic breast cancer, myeloma, as well as lymphoma (Table 3). Anecdotal evidence for an effect of interferon in a wide variety of tumour types including bladder papilloma, cervical carcinoma, prostatic cancer, melanoma, chronic lymphocytic leukaemia and childhood A.L.L. also exists.

The future

The evidence so far has been encouraging. A major problem has been the purification and characterization of interferon. The dose limiting side effects of fever, malaise and fatigue are almost certainly caused by impurities. We clearly need to know more about the structure and mode of action of this fascinating substance. Trials of interferon prepared using recombinant DNA techniques are now beginning. With better preparations its true role as an anticancer agent can be determined in the clinic.

References

1. CANTELL, K., HIRVONEN, S., MOGENSEN, K. E. and PHYHALA, L.: Human leucocyte interferon: production purification and animal experiments, In Vitro (Monogr.) 3 (1973), 35—47
2. SIKORA, K.: Does interferon cure cancer ?, Brit. Med. J., 281 (1980), 855—858
3. FINTE, N. B. and FONTES, K. H.: The purity and safety of interferons prepared for clinical use. Interferon 2, p. 65—79. Ed. GRESSER, I. Academic Press London, 1980
4. GOEDDEL, D. V., LEUNG, D. W., DULL, T. J. et al.: The structure of eight distinct cloned human leucocyte interferon cDNA's. Nature 290 (1981), 20—26
5. GOEDDEL, D. V., YELVERTON, E., ULLRICH, A. et al.: Human leucocyte interferon produced by E. coli is biologically active. Nature 287 (1980), 411—415
6. SECHER, D. S.: Immunoradiometric assay of human leucocyte interferon using monoclonal antibody. Nature 290 (1981), 501—503
7. NAGATA, S., MANTEI, N. and WEISSMANN, C.: The structure of one of the eight or more distinct genes for human interferon α. Nature 287 (1980), 401—408
8. STRANDER, H.: Interferons: antineoplastic drugs ?. Blut 35 (1977), 288—299

9. MERIGAN, T. C., SIKORA, K., BREEDEN, J. G., LEVY, R. and ROSENBERG, S. A.: Preliminary observations on the effect of human leucocyte interferon in non-Hodgkin's lymphoma. N. Engl. J. Med. *229* (1978), 1449—1453

10. GUTTERMAN, J. U., BLUMENSCHEIN, G. R., ALEXANIAN, R. et al: Leucocyte interferon induced tumour regression in human breast cancer, multiple myeloma, and malignant lymphoma. Ann. Intern. Med. *93* (1980), 399—406

11. BORDEN, E., DAO, T., HOLLAND, J., GUTTERMAN, J. and MERIGAN, T.: Interferon in recurrent breast cancer. Proc. Am. Assoc. Cancer Res., Abstr. 750 (1980)

12. KROWN, S. E., STOOPLER, M. B., CUNNINGHAM RUNDLES, S. and OETTGEN, H. F.: Phase II trial of human leucocyte interferon in non-small cell lung cancer. Proc. Am. Assoc. Can. Res., Abstr. 715 (1980)

13. HILL, N. O., LOEB, E., KHAN, A. et al: Phase I human leucocyte interferon trials in leukaemia and cancer. Proc. Am. Soc. Clin. Onc., Abstr. C-167 (1980)

14. PRIESTMAN, T. J.: An initial evaluation of human lymphoblastoid interferon in patients with advanced malignant disease. The Lancet *2* (1980), 113—117

Experimental Biology Research, The Upjohn Company, Kalamazoo, MI 49001, USA

Comparative Interferon-Inducing and Anti-Tumour Activity of Substituted Pyrimidinones

D. A. STRINGFELLOW and G. L. NEIL

Introduction

In 1957, while studying the phenomenon of virus interference, ISAACS and LINDEN-MANN (1) discovered that a soluble mediator could transfer this interference from one cell to another; they named this substance interferon. Subsequent research was aimed toward evaluation and development of this substance as a possible treatment of human virus diseases. This, therefore, remained primarily a research area for virologists and individuals interested in antiviral chemotherapy until the 1970's. Then it was discovered by Ion GRESSER et al (2) that interferons could also inhibit tumour cells division in culture and exert antitumour effects in experimental animal models. Since that time, interest in interferons has expanded to include the possibility that these materials might have potential for chemotherapy of human neoplasia.

Essentially two approaches have been taken in the development of interferon as a chemotherapeutic agent. The first has involved developing methods for producing interferon which could be administered for therapeutic purposes, so-called "exogenous" interferon. During the past several years, most of this research has centered upon developing methodology for including human cells in culture to produce interferon which is isolated and purified for exogenous transfer to the exposed or infected individual. The processes developed have generally been very costly, and the amount of interferon that could be produced by them was very small compared to the amount needed to supprt even preliminary clinical trials. During the past two years, however, the human interferon genes have been successfully cloned into bacteria. These bacteria can be grown in large fermentors and produce "interferoids", representing the polypeptide portion of interferons, which then can be isolated and purified for human use. This approach, although not without problems, seems promising since at least the human leukocyte (alpha)-interferoids produced by bacteria have similar biologic activities to the corresponding natural human interferon. Two of these recombinant DNA interferoids are now undergoing clinical trials.

The second approach to development of the interferon system has consisted of identifying and evaluating agents which can be administered to the host and will induce the host's own cells to produce interferon. This approach could, if successful, enlist the participation of the host cells of the treated animal (or patient) in producing interferon endogenously to mediate the desired biologic activity and might have several advantages over the exogenous approach. Several agents are now known which induce interferon production in vivo. Among these are a series of substituted pyrimidinones first reported on in 1980 by STRINGFELLOW et al (3) and WIERENGA et al (4). Agents in this series can induce high levels of interferon in a variety of animal species.

This manuscript will review the comparative abilities of these agents to induce interferon, to modulate the immune system, and to mediate antitumour activity in a variety of animal models.

Interferon induction

Initial research on the pyrimidinone series centered on characterization of the interferon response induced and evaluation of structure-activity relationships. Figure 1 illustrates the chemical structure of three of these agents. ABMP (2-amino-5-bromo-6-methyl-4(3H)-pyrimidinone) was the first lead identified in this series based on its ability to induce an interferon response in mice (ref. 5). Subsequently, a new series of compounds, in which a phenyl group was substitued for the methyl at the 6 position, was synthesized by W. WIERENGA and H. I. SKULNICK. These 5-bromo, 6-phenyl compounds (e.g., ABPP, 5-bromo-6-phenyl-4(3H)-pyrimidinone) turned out to be

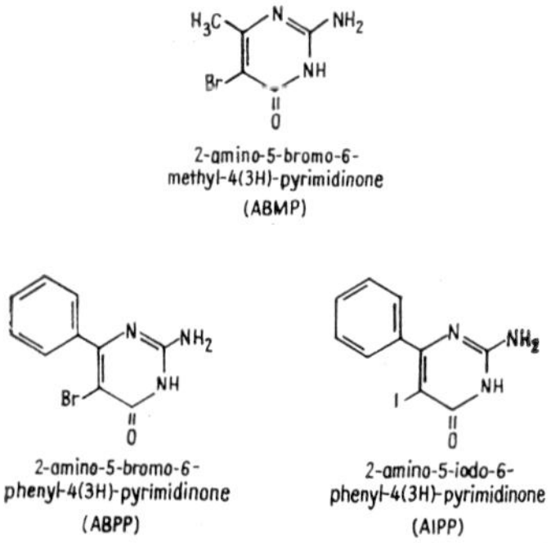

2-amino-5-bromo-6-
methyl-4(3H)-pyrimidinone
(ABMP)

2-amino-5-bromo-6-
phenyl-4(3H)-pyrimidinone
(ABPP)

2-amino-5-iodo-6-
phenyl-4(3H)-pyrimidinone
(AIPP)

Fig. 1.

Table 1.
Maximal tolerated dose (MTD), minimal protective dose (MPD), and minimal interferon-inducing dose (MIID) of pyrimidinones[a] in mice

Compound	MTD (mg/kg)			MPD (mg/kg)			MIID (mg/kg)			Therapeutic Index[b]		
	i.p.	p.o.	s.c.	i.p.	p.o.	s.c.	i.p.	p.o.	s.c.	i.p.	p.o.	s.c.
ABMP	1,000	1,000	2,000	500	250	500	250	250	500	2	4	4
ABPP	1,000	2,000	2,000	100	100	40	50	100	25	10	20	40
AIPP	2,000	2,000	2,000	50	800	25	800	800	800	40	0	80

[a] ABMP = 2-amino-5-bromo-6-methyl-4(3H)-pyrimidinone; ABPP= 2-amino-5-bromo-6-phenyl-4(3H)-pyrimidinone; and AIPP = 2-amino-5-iodo-6-phenyl-4(3H)-pyrimidinone. Drugs were administered intraperitoneally (i.p.), orally (p.o.), and subcutaneously (s.c.)
[b] MTD/MPD.

much more active than ABMP in inducing interferon and were much more effective antiviral agents (see Table 1). ABPP and ABMP induced high levels of interferon when administered intraperitoneally, orally, subcutaneously, intramuscularly, or intranasally to mice, with ABPP being consistently more potent than ABMP. However, a related 5-iodo compound, AIPP (2-amino-5-iodo-6-phenyl-4(3H)-pyrimidinone) was not a very active interferon inducer.

With many of the other agents which have been identified as active interferon inducers, limitation in the range of host species has been observed. Although several agents could induce interferon in one species, e.g. mice, they were unable to elicit an interferon response in other animal species, e.g. cats, dogs, rabbits, or humans. Indeed, one of the first agents identified as being an orally active inducer in mice, tilorone hydrochloride, (6) proved to be totally inactive when administered to rabbits and then humans. Therefore, studies of the host range of the interferon-inducing activity of the pyrimidinone compounds were carried out. Results are summarized in Table 2. ABMP and ABPP were able to induce interferon when administered to a variety of animal species including cats, dogs, cattle, mice, and monkeys. In addition, interferon was produced by certain human tissues when exposed to ABMP and ABPP in vitro. AIPP, on the other hand, was inactive and no circulating interferon could be detected after administration of a single dose of this compound to any of the species or by any of the routes tested.

These results indicated that ABMP and ABPP were active interferon inducers with a broad species range whereas AIPP under comparable conditions, was a very poor inducer.

Table 2.
Induction of interferon in various species

		Maximum IFN response[a]					
	Route	Feline	Bovine	Murine	Canine	Simian	Human tissue (in vitro)
ABPP	p.o.	8,000	2,500	7,500	150	250	
	i.p.	6,500	(IN 1,500)	8,000	ND	ND	150
AIPP	p.o.	<10	30	<10	<10	<10	<10
	i.p.	100	(IN 25)	150	ND	ND	
ABMP	p.o.	6,800	75	6,000	<10	>10	25
	i.p.	7,100	(IN 150)	7,500	ND	ND	

[a] Units/ml of serum.

Spectrum of antiviral activity

The spectrum of antiviral activity of ABPP, AIPP, and ABMP was examined. By definition, an interferon inducer would be expected to have broad spectrum antiviral activity, and consequently it was expected that ABPP and ABMP would have greater antiviral activity than AIPP, a poor inducer (Table 1). For these studies, mice were infected with encephalomyocarditis (EMC), Semliki forest (SFV), West Nile (WNV). vesicular stomatitis (VSV), Friend leukemia (FLV), or type I herpes simplex viruses, One hour after infection, mice were treated intraperitoneally with ABPP, AIPP, or ABMP at a dose of 500 mg/kg/day. Therapy was continued for three days after infection. The virus inoculum employed was such that 90—100% of the control animals died. Increased long-term survival (cure) was evidence of antiviral activity

Table 3.
Spectrum of antiviral activity of pyrimidinones in vivo[a]

Virus	Route	Percent mortality[b]			
		PBS	ABPP	AIPP	ABMP
EMC	i.n.	95	10	10	20
SFV	i.p.	95	15	10	15
WNF	i.p.	100	20	10	40
VSV	i.n.	90	10	0	20
FLV	i.p.	100	20	30	50
HSV-1	i.p.	100	45	30	70

[a] ABPP, AIPP, and ABMP (500 mg/kg, i.p.) were administered 18 hr prior to infection
[b] 30 mice/group.

Table 4.
Duration of antiviral effect

Compound	Route	Dose (mg/kg)	Time of treatment (days)[a]													
			−16	−14	−12	−10	−8	−7	−6	−5	−4	−3	−2	−1	0	+1
AImFPP	i.p.	500	12[b]	50	50	75	83	83	78	79	83	75	88	96	46	33
ABPP	i.p.	500	—	—	—	—	—	—	4	17	15	24	42	92	82	15
AIPP	i.p.	500	30	62	57	67	65	64	75	77	80	83	89	94	42	4
Tilorone	p.o.	250	—	—	—	—	—	19	25	25	56	88	94	100	100	25
Poly (I:C)	i.p.	5	—	—	—	—	—	19	38	31	50	75	88	100	100	19
Pyran	i.p.	20	—	—	—	—	—	53	88	69	81	81	100	81	25	6
CP-20961	i.p.	100	—	—	—	—	—	38	44	88	75	81	88	81	6	12
BL-20803	p.o.	250	—	—	—	—	—	12	12	19	25	12	56	86	50	12

[a] SFV (10 LD50, a 100% lethal dose) was injected i.p. at 0 hr; a single dose of drug was administered between 16 days before to 1 day after infection
[b] Values are % survivors (30 mice/group).

(Table 3). As expected, ABPP, the most active interferon inducer, also had the overall broadest spectrum of antiviral activity. However, AIPP, a poor inducer (Table 1) proved to have good, broad antiviral activity, superior to that observed with ABMP, a better inducer.

The duration of the antiviral effect confered by these agents was also evaluated by determining the length of time, after a single dose of the test compound, over which mice were resistant to subsequent infection with a particular virus. Interestingly, as illustrated in Table 4, AIPP, the poorest interferon inducer, was capable of confering on mice infected with a normally lethal dose of SFV, an antiviral state that persisted for as long as 14 days. A single injection of AIPP protected 60% of the mice who were infected 15 days previously with a uniformly lethal dose of the virus. ABPP and ABMP, although better interferon inducers, had a shorter duration of antiviral activity and, in fact, were active in significantly protecting mice only when the interval between injection of the agent and infection was less than two days.

Immune modulation

Although other explanations related to pharmacokinetics may be involved, the data presented here suggest that the antiviral activity of the pyrimidinones might be unrelated to their ability to induce interferon or at least involve both interferon-dependent and -independent mechanisms. Consequently, several investigations were initiated to determine if the pyrimidinone compounds stimulated or enhanced other host defense systems. Results from these studies are summarized in Table 5. When administered to mice, the pyrimidinones were found to increase natural killer cell and macrophage activities and to stimulate the antibody response to a variety of immunogens. They also increased bone marrow colony-forming units (7—10).

Table 5.
Summary of immune modulating activity of AIPP and ABPP

			Reference
1.	Increased:	Murine natural killer cells invivo.	9, 10
2.	Increased:	Murine macrophage mediated cytotoxicity increased after in vivo or in vitro addition.	10
3.	Increased:	In vivo antibody formation in unimmunized and immunized mice.	7
4.	Decreased:	In vitro spleen cell response to SRBCs.	8
5.	Decreased:	T killer cell cytotoxicity inhibited in vitro.	8
6.	Increased:	Bone marrow colony-forming units.	8
7.	No effect:	In vitro compounds not mitogenic nor did they affect mitogen response.	8

H. E. RENIS et al further demonstrated (11) that coadministration of antithymocyte serum along ABPP or AIPP completely antagonized the anti-herpesvirus activity of these agents. Antithymocyte serum administration did not affect the ability of ABPP or AIPP to induce interferon or reverse their anti-Semliki forest virus activities. These results suggest that an antithymus serumsensitive phenomenon mediated by T-lmyphocytes or possibly macrophages is activated in mice treated with the pyrimidinones and protects them from herpes simplex, but not Semliki forest virus infection.

Antitumour activity

Based on the reported antitumour effect of interferon itself and knowlege of the immunostimulatory properties of the pyrimidinones, these compounds were studied for activity against experimental transplantable tumours in mice. In one series of studies, 2×10^6, 2×10^5, or 2×10^4 B16 malignant melanoma cells, obtained from the U.S. National Cancer Institute, were inoculated intraperitoneally into C-57 black mice. Mice were then treated i.p., beginning 24 hr after tumour inoculation, once daily for nine days with pyrimidinones at doses of 400, 200, or 100 mg/kg. As

Table 6.
Antitumour activity of pyrimidinones in BDF_1 mice injected i.p.[a] with B16 malignant melanoma cells

Tumour load (cells injected i.p.)	Drug (mg/kg/day)	% Survivors (30 mice/group)		
		ABMP	ABPP	AIPP
2×10^6	400	0	0	0
	200	0	0	0
	100	0	0	0
	Placebo		0	
2×10^5	400	10	33	0
	200	0	13	20
	100	0	0	0
	Placebo		0	
2×10^4	400	40	70	20
	200	33	60	13
	100	20	36	47
	Placebo		15	

[a] Mice dosed once daily for 9 days beginning 24 hr after B16 cell injection.

summarized in Table 6, the antitumour activity of each of the compounds proved to be quite tumour-load dependent. With inocula of 2×10^6 or 2×10^5 cells/mouse, animals were not significantly protected by the pyrimidinones. With a lower inoculum of 2×10^4 cells/mouse, however, a significant proportion of mice treated with ABPP, and, to a lesser degree, with ABMP and AIPP survived. In separate studies, the ability of the pyrimidinones to inhibit blood-borne metastasis of B16 cells was evaluated. Metastasis to the lung of mice inoculated intravenously with 2×10 B16 malignant melanoma cells could be significantly reduced when ABPP was administered as much as 2 hr after injection of the tumour cells. In fact, in many situations, the metastatic nodules were reduced on average by over 90% (Table 7).
Similar results have been reported recently by MILAS et al (12) who demonstrated that mice injected with fibrosarcoma cells were significantly protected from metastasis and development of disease if therapy with ABPP or AIPP was initiated before or soon after injection of tumour cells. They further demonstrated, in a system where

Table 7.
Effect of pyrimidinones on B16 pulmonary metastasis[a]

Mouse No.	F_1				F_{10}			
	ABPP	AIPP	ABMP	Placebo	ABPP	AIPP	ABMP	Placebo
1	4[b]	12	50	0	20	21	9	80
2	3	0	1	15	6	44	95	87
3	35	44	9	90	15	7	43	61
4	29	2	0	56	26	48	85	60
5	0	0	53	26	6	21	5	27
6	10	22	3	84	8	19	41	72
7	0	4	9	51	31	32	64	82
8	0	0	48	22	3	1	—[c]	—[c]
9	4	5	2	5	—[c]	14	—[c]	—[c]
10	2	—[c]	—[c]	5	—[c]	—[c]	—[c]	—[c]
Average	8.7	9.9	19	36	14	23	49	67

[a] 2×10^4 melanoma cells injected i.v. 3 weeks prior to sacrifice of mice.
[b] Pulmonary nodules per animal.
[c] Died before 3 weeks.

these tumour cells were implanted intramuscularly followed 2 weeks later by amputating the limb containing the primary tumour, that the number of lung metastasis was greatly decreased by treatment with the pyrimidinones soon after surgery.

Summary

In conclusion, the data presented indicate that a number of substituted pyrimidinone compounds, of interest initially because of their interferon-inducing activity, have antiviral and antitumour activity. Some of the agents in this series, as illustrated by AIPP, effectively protected mice from lethal virus infections, prevented metastasis, and displayed antitumour activity and yet did not induce detectable levels of circulating interferon. Other pyrimidinones, exemplifed by ABPP, which induced high levels of interferon had higher antitumour but lower antiviral activity than AIPP. Each of the agents was an active immune modulator stimulating macrophages, natural killer cells, and antibody response in experimental animals. These data taken together suggest that the pyrimidinones enhance host defenses independent of interferon. The data of RENIS et al. (11) support this concept since antithymocyte serum eliminated the antiherpes virus activity of these agents showing that anti-herpes simplex activity was a T-cell mediated phenomena. These results may be particularly important in considering parameters for use in selecting immune modulators of clinical evaluation. With certain diseases, enhancement of a limited number of specific defenses may be preferable over non-specific stimulation of most host defense components. For example, stimulation of macrophage tumourcidal activity without induction of interferon may, in specific instances, be preferable over stimulation of both. Molecules like the pyrimidinones may provide such a selective stimulation worthy of further evaluation.

References

1. ISAACS, A. and LINDENMANN, J.: Virus interference. I. The interferon. Proc. Roy. Soc., Ser. B 147 (1957)

251

2. GRESSER, I., BOURALI, C., LEVY, J. P., FONTAINE-BROUTY-BOYE, D. and THOMAS, M. T.: Increased survival of mice inoculated with tumour cells and treated with interferon preparations. Proc. Natl. Acad. Sci. U.S.A. *63* (1969), 51

3. STRINGFELLOW, D. A., VANDERBERG, H. C. and WEED, S. D.: Interferon induction by 5-halo-6-phenyl-pyrimidinones. J. Inf. Res. *1* (1980), 1

4. WIERENGA, W., SKULNICK, H. I., STRINGFELLOW, D. A., WEED, S. D., RENIS, H. E. and EIDSON, E.: 5-Substituted 2-amino-6-phenyl-4(3H)-pyrimidinones. Antiviral and interferon inducing agents. J. Med. Chem. *23* (1960), 237

5. STRINGFELLOW, D. A.: Comparative interferon inducing and antiviral properties of 2-amino-5-bromo-6-phenyl-4-pyrimidinone, poly I:C and tilorone. Antimicrob. Agents Chemother. *11* (1977), 984

6. MAYER, G. D. and KRUEGER, R. F.: Tilorone hydrochloride: mode of action. Science *169* (1970), 1214

7. FAST, P. E. and STRINGFELLOW, D. A.: Immune modulation by two antiviral isocytosines with different abilities to induce interferon. Curr. Chemother. Inf. Dis. 1396—1398 (1980)

8. TAGGART, M. T., LOUGHMAN, B. E., GIBBONS, A. J. and STRINGFELLOW, D. A.: Immunomodulatory effects of 2-amino-5-bromo-6-methyl-4-pyrimidinol and its isocytosine analogues. Curr. Chemother. Inf. Dis. 1400—1401 (1980)

9. LOUGHMAN, B. L., GIBBONS, A. J., TAGGART, M. T. and RENIS, H. E.: Modulation of mouse natural killer cell activity by interferon and two antiviral isocytosines. Curr. Chemother. Inf. Dis. 1402—1403 (1980)

10. LOTZOVA, C., SAVARY, C. A., HERSH, E. M., KHANN, A. A. and STRINGFELLOW, D. A.: Potentiation of murine natural killer cell-mediated tumour killing by antiviral pyrimidinone molecules. Annual Meeting, Am. Assoc., Cancer Res., Abstract 1108 (1981)

11. RENIS, H. E. and EIDSON, E. E.: Protection of mice from herpes simplex virus infection by 5-halo-6-aryl-isocytosines. Curr. Chemother. Inf. Dis., 1411—1413 (1980)

12. MILAS, L., HERSH, E. M., STRINGFELLOW, D. A. and HUNTER, N.: Studies on the antitumour activity of pyrimidinone-interferon inducers. I. Effects against artificial and spontaneous lung metastasis of murine tumours. J. Natl. Cancer Inst. (in press, 1981).

Central Institute for Tumours and Allied Diseases, Department of Pathology, Clinical Hospita "Dr. M. Stojanovic"
and
Institute of Immunology, Zagreb, Yugoslavia

Influence of Human Leucocyte Interferon on Squamous-Cell Carcinoma of Uterine Cervix: Clinical, Histological and Histochemical Observations

J. Krušić, Ž. Maričić, V. Chylak, B. Rode, D. Jušić and E. Šooš

Introduction

Clinical testing of leucocyte interferon (HLI) began in 1971 when Strander gave a purified HLI preparation to osteosarcoma patients (Strander, 1973). Numerous studies have since been done in which HLI was used to treat various human malignant and benign tumours. Our studies, begun in 1972, were designed to explore the influence of HLI on cervical carcinoma cells in vitro (Brdar et al, 1975) and in vivo (Krušić et al, 1974).

We present here the results of a controlled clinical trial in which HLI was tested in 37 patients with squamous-cell carcinoma of the uterine cervix, to investigate whether such treatment would alter the results of the Papanicolaou (PAP) test and to study its effects on the tumour tissue itself.

Patients and methods

Native HLI was obtained from the Institute of Immunology, Zagreb, Yugoslavia and was given to three groups of patients, as follows: The first group (1) consisting of 10 patients (six with carcinoma in situ and four with invasive squamous-cell carcinoma), received HLI as daily infiltrating injections (3×10^4 IU) and directly on the cervix as an ointment (5×10^3 IU per gram). The second group (2) comprised 12 patients (10 with stage Ib and IIa squamous-cell carcinoma and two with stage Ia and II adenocarcinoma) who received HLI topically, in the form of powder, which was applied by means of a pessary in a daily dose of 1.25×10^6 IU for 54—80 days. In the third group (3) of 15 patients (two with stage Ia, 10 with stage Ib and three with stage IIb squamous-cell carcinoma), six received HLI topically in the form of powder containing 2×10^6 IU daily, and the other nine received it both topically (as above) and intramuscularly at a dose of 10^6 IU over three weeks. After treatment was completed all patients underwent surgery and irradiation. All patients were examined clinically prior to and during HLI treatment at regular two-week intervals.

The control group consisted of 37 patients with the same type of malignancy who were treated only by surgery and irradiation. The effects of HLI were evaluated according to the microscope criteria described previously by Knežević et al (1979).

Results

The results of the microscope studies show that in the first group, HLI caused regression of the PAP test in four patients, a cure (in terms of disappearance of malignant cells) in three, no change in two, and a deterioration of the PAP test in one patient. The activity of β-glucuronidase before HLI administration was high, 0.37 to 1660 IU, and dropped by the end of administration to 0.05—0.7 IU. According to our studies, β-glucuronidase activity in vaginal secretions of the healthy population does not exceed 0.3 IU. Tumour stromal response was estimated in the second and third groups of patients and compared with biopsy specimens taken prior to HLI application. It was found to be higher in 16 patients, an unchanged in eight; in three, the test was not done. Strong lymph node responses were observed in 17 patients; the nodes did not respond in five; and in two patients there were metastases. The lymph nodes were not examined in five cases. The therapeutic effects of HLI are summarized in Table 1. There was complete disappearance of tumour in 21.6%, regressions in 27.03%, and stable disease in 35.13% of cases. In 16.22% of patients the disease progressed under the treatment.

Table 1.
Therapeutic effects of human leucocyte interferon

	Stage In situ	Ia	Ib	II	Total	(%)
Cured	3	3	2	0	8	21.62
Regression	0	3	2	5	10	27.03
Unchanged	2	0	7	4	13	35.13
Progressions	1	0	2	3	6	16.22
Total	6	6	13	12	37	100%

Finally we analysed the results obtained with HLI and with conventional treatment (surgery and irradiation) on the basis of five-year survival. All patients with carcinoma in situ and stage Ia carcinoma survived more than five years, both with HLI and conventional treatment. Of the patients with stage Ib cancer, 12 survived more than five years, and one died of pulmonary embolism; in the group treated with conventional therapy there were nine survivors and the other four died. Of the patients with more advanced disease (stages IIa and IIb), five survived for five years, but seven died; in the conventional treatment group, four patients survived that time interval but eight died.

Discussion

The results of our preliminary trial show that HLI has a certain influence on squamous-cell carcinomas, in terms of decreased β-glucuronidase activity, eliciting of the tumour stromal reaction and lymph node reactivity. Morever, these parameters of reactivity could be used in a prognosis of the disease, since patients with a vague tumour stromal response experienced poor disease outcome. In patients with advanced disease, HLI had no substantial influence, either in terms of reactivity or in terms of prolongation of survival. We conclude that HLI is efficient as an adjuvant chemotherapeutic agent in patients with cervical carcinomas in initial stages.

References

1. BRDAR, B., NAGY, B., JUŠIĆ, D., ŠOOŠ, E., JAKAŠA, V. and KRUŠIĆ, J.: The effect of interferon on the growth of cervical carcinoma in cell culture. In: Proceedings of the Symposium on Clinical Use of Interferon, Yugoslav. Academy of Sciences and Arts, Zagreb, 1—2 October 1975, pp. 245—247
2. KNEŽEVIĆ, M., RODE, B., KNEŽEVIĆ-KRIVAK, Š., IKIĆ, D., MARIĆIĆ, Z., KRUŠIĆ, J., PADOVAN, I., NOLA, P., BRODARED, I., JUŠIĆ, D. and SOOŠ, E. (1979): Histopathologic and histoenzymatic observations in carcinomas treated with human leukocyte interferon. In: Proceedings of the Symposium on Interferon, Yugoslav Academy of Sciences and Arts, Zagreb, 1979, pp. 67—77
3. KRUŠIĆ, J., ŠOOŠ, E., ROGULJIĆ, A., JAKAŠA V. and JUŠIč, D. (1974): Utjecai humanog leuko-citnog interferona na planocelularni karcinom genitalne regije u žena (in Serbo-Croat.). In: Zbornik radova, Savjetovanje o kliničkim ispitivanjima humanog leukocitnog interferona, Zagreb, pp. 112—116
4. STRANDER, H.: Clinical and laboratory investigation on man: Systemic administration of potent interferon to man. J. Nat. Cancer Inst. *51* (1973), 733—742

Dr. Mladen Stojanović University Hospital and Institute of Immunology Zagreb, Yugoslavia

Effect of Interferon on Malignant Head and Neck Tumours

I. Padovan, E. Šooš and I. Brodarec

Introduction

As a result of laboratory and clinical investigations of human leucocyte interferon (HLI) carried at the Institute of Immunology in Zagreb over the past 10 years, topical application of crude HLI was introduced in 1977 for treatment of a group of patients with head and neck tumours.

Interferon exerts a number of biological effects besides its broad antiviral activities; some of these effects are relevant to its antitumour action. Recently, there has been increasing recognition of two major ways in which interferon might exert its antitumour activity:

(I) a direct influence on tumour cells, by inhibiting tumour cell multiplication, enhancing or changing the expression of cell surface antigens, modifying cytoskeletal structure and inhibiting cell motility:

(II) mediation by the host through activation of defence mechanisms, such as enhancement of natural killer cell activity and activation of macrophages.

We have investigated the effect of interferon on skin tumours for the following reasons:

1. Clinical observations of the process and verification of the diagnosis and treatment results are simple and can be measured objectively.
2. Injection of interferon into a skin tumour and the surrounding area is simple and harmless.
3. Removal of tissue for biopsy is easy and non-mutilating.
4. Skin cancers are fairly common.
5. The proven antitumoural properties of interferon justify delaying surgery until the patient has been treated with HLI.

Patients and methods

Between late 1977 and May 1981, 50 patients with cancer were treated with interferon.

The duration of HLI treatment was 1—6 months, depending on the clinical course of the disease. Interferon was administered as infiltration injection into the tumour or the surrounding area, daily for the first 7—9 days and then 2 or 3 times a week. A single daily dose comprised 3×10^5 units of non-purified interferon; in some cases, an ointment containing 3×10^4 units HLI/g was applied.

One patient with cancer of the tongue, who had previously had a laryngeal carcinoma, was given additional therapy with 5×10^5 units twice daily intramuscularly as well as local infiltration into the area of the tongue. Adjuvant therapy was given because a biopsy of the tongue showed absence of immune response in the area surrounding the tumour.

Histologically, there were 21 cases of squamous-cell carcinoma, 23 of basal-cell carcinoma, 1 of neurogenic sarcoma, and 5 of benign skin tumour. Since diagnosis, objective evaluation of tumour and host cell immunity are all based on histological findings, exploratory biopsies were taken from all patients before the start of treatment. The preparations were examined histologically and, in some cases, histochemically. Results of treatment were evaluated by means of clinical observations during the course of HLI applications and from the microscopical appearance of the tumour or tumour residues on completion of treatment.

Results

Histologically, the healing process was similar in all patients: It varied dynamically from complete disappearance of neocytes to blockage of tumour cells by stroma, so that some cells could be identified, while others were ghosts of lysed and necrotic cells. The area of the original lesion showed newly formed connective tissue, which was first filled with immunocytes and gradually became keloid.

Conclusions

Experience in Zagreb and other centres has shown that local infiltration of interferon into tumours and the surrounding area stimulates local immune reaction at the site of the lesion. We suggest that the lymphocytic infiltration observed in all our patients is the morphological equivalent of the cellular immune response of the host to invasion by tumour cells.

According to a number of authors, the immunocompetence of cells in a tumour and in the peritumoural stroma is the most important factor in the long-term survival of cancer patients. B- and T-lymphocytes and macrophages are the classical immunocompetent cells, but there are suggestions that granulocytes are also part of the cellular immune system.

We found that after application of interferon close to the tumour site, the neocytes were blocked, and their dispersal during surgery was thus prevented. Interferon inhibits micrometastatis, thereby reducing the numbers of tumour recurrences and increasing the chance of survival. Without being too optimistic, our experience is that interferon gives favourable results in the treatment of certain malignant tumours. Only after data have been collected on a large number of patients over a long period of time and the results compared with disease recurrence will it be possible to accept this type of therapy on a wider scale in clinical oncology.

West Haven Veterans Administration Medical Center, West Haven, CT 06516,
and
Departments of [1]Internal Medicine and [2] Pharmacology, Yale University School of Medicine, New Haven, CT 06510, USA

Polyamines and Neoplasia:
A Review of Present Knowledge of Their Function
and Therapeutic Potential

P. K. BONDY[1] and Z. NAKOS CANELLAKIS[1,2]

Introduction

The polyamines are small flexible aliphatic linear compounds with a primary amino group at each and which are present in viruses and all living cells. Because they contain at least two amino groups, they are powerful cations at physiological pH. In addition, they are capable of entering into covalent linkages with proteins and possibly other macromolecules, and thus of influencing both the charge and spatial conformation of the product. Their production and intracellular concentration are increased in a circadian manner during cell growth (CANELLAKIS, 1981 B). Although their ubiquity and conservation during evolution imply that they serve an important biological purpose, the exact nature of their activity is still unclear. The availability of enzyme inhibitors wich are capable of modulating the biosynthesis of the polyamines is now making it possible to investigate the practical usefulness of altering the synthesis of these biomolecules in treating a variety of diseases including parasitic infestations and cancer.

Biochemical aspects

The major polyamines present in mammals include 1,4-diaminobutane (putrescine), and its two sequential derivatives, spermidine and spermine (Figure 1). The initial biosynthetic reaction, which also appears to be rate limiting, is the decarboxylation of the amino acid ornithine by the enzyme ornithine decarboxylase (ODC). After this reaction, which yields putrescine, aminopropyl groups made available through the activity of the enzyme S-adenosylmethionine decarboxylase (SAM decarboxylase) are added, mediated by either spermidine or spermine synthese, to yield first spermidine and then spermine. Spermidine and spermine, in turn, can be converted back to putrescine and spermidine respectively by oxidase activity (BOLKENIUS, 1981; Figure 2). The polyamines can also be oxidized to produce carboxylic acids. It is uncertain whether dietary polyamines contribute substantially to the intracellular polyamine pools, but the fact that plant diamines are found in mammalian livers and urine but not in other tissues suggests some absorption and incorporation into hepatic cells from gastrointestinal food and bacterial sources (CANELLAKIS, 1979).

In quiescent, non-dividing cells the activity of ODC is minimal and the concentrations of polyamines are low; but in dividing cells ODC activity increases and the concentration of polyamines rises (TABOR, 1976; WILLIAMS-ASHMAN, 1979). The effect of cell division on ODC activity is seen whether the stimulus is repair of tissue damage,

$$H_3N^+(CH_2)_4N^+H_3$$

Putrescine

$$H_3N^+(CH_2)_3N^+H_2(CH_2)_4N^+H_3$$

Spermidine

$$H_3N^+(CH_2)_3N^+H_2(CH_2)_4N^+H(CH_2)_3N^+H_3$$

Spermine

Fig. 1. The major polyamines of mammals. The compounds are drawn in their protonated form, as they appear at physiological pH.

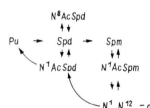

Fig. 2. Pathways for regeneration of putrescine from spermidine and spermine.

neoplasia or cell growth in vivo or in vitro. In specific tissues, influences which stimulate cell activity (but not necessarily cell growth) also increase ODC levels. For example, thyroid stimulating hormone increases thyroid ODC (SCHEINMAN, 1977) and growth hormone increases the ODC activity of liver (JÄNNE, 1969; RUSSELL, 1970).

ODC activity is subject to feed-back inhibition by the polyamines under certain circumstances. Spermidine and spermine suppress the induction of ODC by dibutyryl

Table 1.
Effect of putrescine on half-life of ornithine decarboxylase in induced cells

Concentration of putrescine (M)	Apparent half-life (min) Population density (HTC cells/ml)		p
	5×10^5	5×10^6	
Controll	*	13	0.001
10^{-5}	56	13	0.001
10^{-3}	29	11	0.01
10^{-2}	9	7	N.S.

Cells (5×10^5 cells/ml) were induced for 2 hours with 6×10^{-4} M dibu-cAMP and activity of ODC was measured either in the original culture or after 10-fold concentration of cells (5×10^6 cells/ml). Half-lives were calculated as described in the text. The specific activity of ODC at zero time was 704 pmoles $CO_2/2.5 \times 10^6$ cells/hr at a cell concentration of 5×10^5/ml, and 342 pmoles $CO_2/2.5 \times 10^6$ cells/hr at a cell concentration of 5×10^6 cells per ml. (CANELLA-KIS, 1981 B)
* No significant change in enzyme activity during the 45 minute duration of the experiment.

cyclic AMP in hepatic carcinoma cells in culture, but do not affect ODC activity which has been induced by dexamethasone (THEOHARIDES, 1975). This particular suppressing effect is due to blocking of ODC biosynthesis (CANELLAKIS, 1976). Thus the effect of polyamines in suppressing ODC induction is probably quite specific, and seems to depend on the nature of the inducing agent.

In cells growing in log phase ODC has a relatively long half-life. If the cells are concentrated by gentle centrifugation and resuspension in fresh medium at a cell concentration 10 times higher than their mid-log-phase level (e.g., from 5×10^5 to 5×10^6 per ml) the activity of ODC is abruptly reduced and the apparent half-life of the enzyme is drastically shortened (Table 1, CANELLAKIS, 1981 B). Similar changes are observed when the concentration of cells approaches plateau density (HOGAN, 1971, 1974); but since our studies show that concentrated cells respond similarly whether they are suspended in fresh growth medium or in the medium from which they were removed, this effect cannot be explained by exhaustion of growth components in the medium. We suggest that the cause may be related to factors associated with contact inhibition of growth.

When ODC is induced by feeding cell cultures by dilution with growth medium, suppression of ODC by putrescine occurs over a period of several hours, and is maximal at concentrations of about 10^{-2} M putrescine. In this type of experiment, suppression is associated with the appearance of a low molecular weight protein which appears to be the immediate suppressing agent, and has been called "antizyme" (CANELLAKIS, 1979). Suppression of ODC activity also occurs in the presence of diamines which are not natural products of the reaction, such as diaminopropane and diaminohexane (McCANN, 1980). In the presence of suppressing concentrations of these amines, the apparent half-life of ODC activity is reduced (McCANN, 1979; CANELLAKIS, 1981 B). It has also been suggested that when ODC is subjected to the action of the enzyme transglutaminase (to be discussed later) in the presence of putrescine, putrescine might be covalently incorporated into the enzyme (WILLIAMS-ASHMAN, 1980), and thus be associated with a loss of enzyme activity. Evidence supporting this argument has been reported (RUSSELL, 1981).

Table 2.
Peak stimulatory effect of acetylated di- and polyamines on ornithine decarboxylase activity

Compound	Conc. (M)	Stimulation (% of control)
N-acetylputrescine	5.0×10^{-5}	350
N^1-acetylspermidine	2.5×10^{-6}	1300
N^8-acetylspermidine	2.5×10^{-7}	700
HMBA**	5.0×10^{-5}	550

* Preparation and purity of the acetylated polyamine derivatives is described by BONDY, 1981
** Hexamethylenebisacetamide

In contrast to the suppressing effect of the di- and polyamines on ODC activity, their monoacetyl derivatives stimulate ODC activity when added in concentrations in the micromolar range to rat hepatic carcinoma growing in culture (CANELLAKIS, 1981 A; Table 2). The concentration of the monoacetyl derivatives is too low to measure in resting hepatic cells; however, stimulating growth with partial hepatectomy or the action of thioacetamide causes an increase in the concentration of monoacetylputrescine and N^1-acetylspermidine to levels of 10% and 1% of the parent compounds respectively (SEILER, 1980), which is approximately the level necessary to produce stimulation of ODC. Thus it appears that the polyamines may be involved directly in controlling ODC activity and possibly in modulating the rate of specific protein synthesis and consequently of growth. It therefore seems that the activity of ODC might be under dual control — stimulation by the acetylated derivatives of its products and suppression by the products themselves.

Biological implications

Because of their ubiquitous distribution it is highly likely that these compounds or their derivatives play a central role in cell growth, but their function has not yet been completely elucidated. They increase the rate of transcription of DNA and of translation of RNA to protein in vitro (TABOR, 1976; WILLIAMS-ASHMAN, 1979), effects which are similar to those produced by Mg^{++}. Although the details of the mechanism of these actions are obscure, it has been suggested that the strong cationic nature of the polyamines leads to ionic binding with nucleic acids and nucleoproteins, resulting in stabilization of these entities in an active configuration (TABOR, 1976; WANG, 1981). It is possible that acetylation of ionically associated polyamines, by reducing their net cationic charge, might displace them from their critical position on nucleoproteins and therefore affect their role as regulators of nucleoprotein expression.

The polyamines can also be incorporated into proteins by forming covalent bonds (CANELLAKIS, 1981 C), probably as a result of the activity of the transglutaminase enzymes (FOLK, 1980; WILLIAMS-ASHMAN, 1980). The classic example of the action

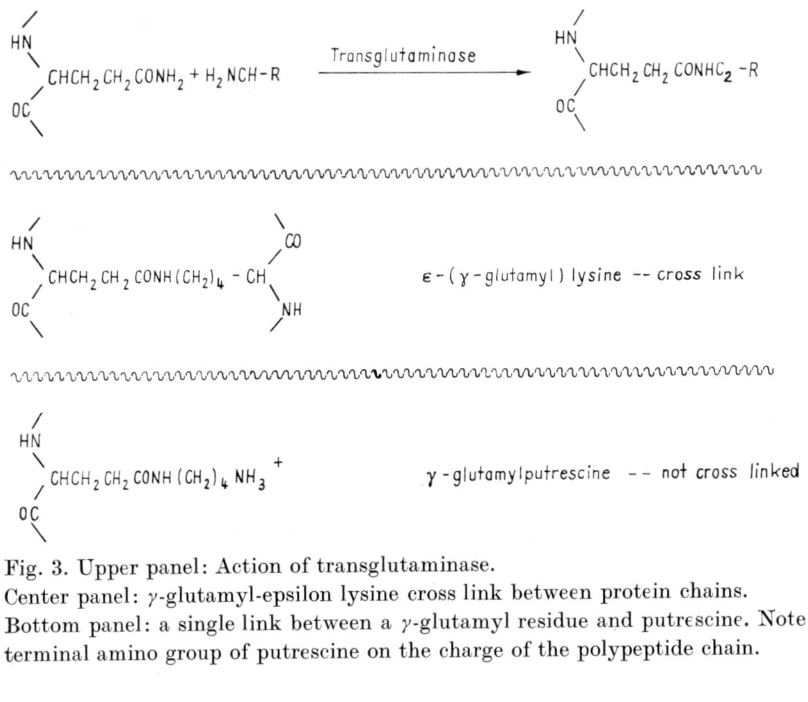

Fig. 3. Upper panel: Action of transglutaminase.
Center panel: γ-glutamyl-epsilon lysine cross link between protein chains.
Bottom panel: a single link between a γ-glutamyl residue and putrescine. Note the effect of the terminal amino group of putrescine on the charge of the polypeptide chain.

of transglutaminase is in providing cross-links between strands of fibrin, by linking the epsilon amino of lysine in one strand with the gamma carboxyl of glutamine in an adjacent one (Figure 3). This is one of the mechanisms by which fibrin cross-linking occurs during blood clotting, through the agency of Factor XIII, a transglutaminase enzyme. The reaction is a general one, by which the amine component of the gamma carboxamide function of peptide-linked glutamine is exchanged for another amine. In addition to the epsilon amino group of lysine, other amines such as the polyamines can also take part in the reaction (Figure 3). This results in effects reflecting changes of both charge and conformation of the protein. Since the polyamines are strong cations at physiological pH, their covalent bonding to a protein alters its electrical charge. After forming the first covalent link, the other terminus of the polyamine remains free to form a second gamma glutamyl derivative, producing a cross-link between two polypeptide strands or between two points in a single strand (Figure 4). Such

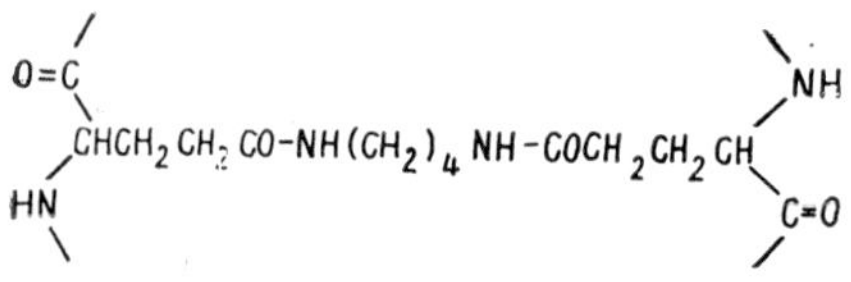

$$O=C$$
$$CHCH_2CH_2CO-NH(CH_2)_4 NH-COCH_2CH_2CH$$
$$HN \qquad NH \qquad C=O$$

Fig. 4. Mechanism of cross link formation between two γ-glutamyl residues and putrescine.

cross-linking would alter the conformation of the molecule and affect its chemical and biological properties. The effect of incorporating putrescine into ODC has already been mentioned. The importance of transglutaminases in producing cross-links has been discussed in recent reviews (WILLIAMS-ASHMAN, 1980). The presence of covalently bound polyamines in cell proteins has been established both by experiments in which labelled polyamines are incorporated into cell proteins (FOLK, 1980 CANELLAKIS, 1981 C) and by demonstration of the presence of polyamines in both cell-associated and extracellular proteins. Digestion experiments have shown that the polyamines are incorporated as cross-links, since both terminal amino groups are combined with gamma glutamyl residues (FOLK, 1980). It seems possible that other acceptors (such as the phosphate of the nucleic acid skeleton) might also form covalent stabilizing links with polyamines.

Relationship of polyamines to cancer

It has recently become apparent that some synthetic congeners of the polyamines can promote differentiation of certain cancer cells in tissue culture (REUBEN, 1980). One of the most potent compounds promoting this effect is N,N'-diacetyl 1,6,-diamino-hexane (Hexamethylene*bis*acetamide; HMBA; (Figure 5)), which can induce the

$$CH_3 CONH(CH_2)_6 HNOCCH_3$$

Hexamethylene<u>bis</u>acetamide

$$CH_3 CONH(CH_2)_4 HNOCCH_3$$

N,N'-diacetylputrescine

Fig. 5. The formulas of hexamethylene*bis*acetamide and N,N'-di-acetylputrescine.

262

Friend murine erythroleukemia line (MELC) to stop dividing and to produce hemo-globin, marks of differentiation into erythrocyte-like cells (REUBEN, 1980). This is a relatively general effect, since HMBA can also induce cell differentiation in other cell types, such as cultured glioblastoma multiforme cells, which differentiate into collagen-producing cells (RABSON, 1977) and promyelocytic human leukemia cells, which assume a mature configuration (COLLINS, 1980).

N,N'-Diacetylputrescine, a compound identical with HMBA except that its skeleton is shorter by two methylene groups, has moderate differentiating ability for MELC in vitro (REUBEN, 1980) but attempts to show an effect of this group of compounds in vivo have been unsuccessful so far (MARKS, 1978). This failure may reflect two types of problems. The diacetyl derivatives may not survive in vivo long enough to have an effect, since they would be subject to the action of esterases; and the differentiating effect, which is not seen in 100% of the cells in vitro, might be undetectable because of the dynamics of cell multiplication in the intact tumour-burdened animal. There are no data defining the concentration of diacetyl derivatives of endogenous poly-amines in vivo. The possibility exists, however, that the acetylated polyamines may be involved in inducing cell differentiation and — by implication — in suppressing or minimizing the development of neoplasms.

Clinical implications of polyamines

Clinical interest in the polyamines was aroused in 1971 by the observation of RUSSELL et al. (1971) that the excretion of putrescine, spermidine and spermine were increased in the urine of patients with cancer. Later studies asserted that plasma concentrations were also elevated (NISHIOKA, 1974). These studies led to the suggestion that the measu-rement of polyamines might provide useful markers for the presence and response of cancer to treatment (RUSSELL, 1971). Extensive further studies of this suggestion have shown that it is without merit. The literature has been reviewed by JÄNNE et al. (1969) and will not be repeated here in detail. It was found that the spread of values in patients with cancer is so wide and overlaps the normal range so frequently that, although the mean value is often higher than normal in populations of cancer patients, this particular determination has little practical usefulness in the individual patient (DESSER, 1980, 1981; NISHIOKA, 1980; TORMEY, 1975; WAALKES, 1975). Attempts to improve the usefulness of the determination by measuring the polyamine content of the affected tissue — e.g., bone marrow — have not been helpful, because elevations appear related more to the rate of cell death than to the mass of tumour cells (NISHIO-KA, 1980). The urinary polyamine levels are not reliably different in patients with lo-calized tumours as compared to those with disseminated disease (LIPTON, 1976), and elevations of serum polyamines are not found in patients during the year before the clinical appearance of cancer (I. M. DUNCAN, pers. commun). Moreover, a host of clinical situations frequently associated with cancer also increases the polyamine excretion or concentration and therefore obscure the specificity of the effect of the neoplasm (Table 3). In highly restricted situations, such as the measurement of polyamines in the cerebrospinal fluid of patients with medulloblastoma (MARTON, 1981) but not other types of brain tumours (FULTON, 1980), the determination may be a useful marker for growth of the tumour. In summary, as compared with better established markers such as CEA (TORMEY, 1975) it appears that "the measurement of polyamines has no reasonable clinical impact" (H. DESSER, pers. commun).

Table 3.

Non-malignant processes associated with elevated polyamine levels

I. Inflammatory processes:	II. Tumour-like:
*polymyositis	polycythemia vera
*pancreatitis	psoriasis
*pneumonia	
*infections	III. Others:
arthritis	*anemia
peptic ulcer	*atherosclerosis
enteritis	*hepatic disease
tuberculosis	cystic fibrosis
systemic lupus	uremia
	acromegaly

* Complications frequently observed in patients with tumours

Since ODC activity and polyamine concentrations increase during active cell growth, attempts have been made to determine whether cells can multiply in their absence. Mutants of *E. coli* which are unable to produce putrescine, spermidine or spermine grow in non-enriched medium at about a third the normal rate, which continues indefinitely as medium is replaced. When putrescine or spermidine is added the growth rate returns to normal. It appears, therefore, that growth of *E. coli* is possible at a reduced rate when polyamine concentrations are reduced to very low levels (HAFNER, 1979).

In contrast to the prokaryote *E. coli*, eukaryotes seem to be much more dependent on the presence of polyamines for growth. Growth is completely eliminated in a mutant of *Saccharomyces cerevisiae* which completely lacks ODC activity unless putrescine is supplied (COHN, 1980).

The opportunity exists of reproducing by blockers the metabolic effects of the mutants just described. It is possible to inhibit ODC with the ornithine analogue, α-difluoro-methylornithine (DFMO), and to inhibit SAM decarboxylase with methylglyoxalbis-(guanylhydrazone) (MGBG; MGGH; Methyl-GAG) (Figure 6). MAMONT (1978) has shown in vitro that the growth of cells in culture is suppressed or eliminated by DFMO. This finding has been confirmed in a line of human pulmonary small cell carcinoma

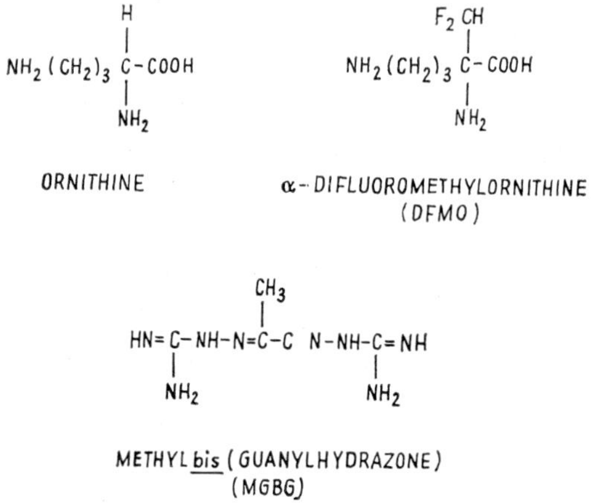

$$NH_2(CH_2)_3\overset{\overset{\displaystyle H}{|}}{\underset{\underset{\displaystyle NH_2}{|}}{C}}-COOH$$

ORNITHINE

$$NH_2(CH_2)_3\overset{\overset{\displaystyle F_2CH}{|}}{\underset{\underset{\displaystyle NH_2}{|}}{C}}-COOH$$

α- DIFLUOROMETHYLORNITHINE
(DFMO)

$$HN=C-NH-N=\overset{\overset{\displaystyle CH_3}{|}}{C}\ N-NH-C=NH$$
$$\underset{NH_2}{|}\qquad\qquad\underset{NH_2}{|}$$

METHYL bis (GUANYLHYDRAZONE)
(MGBG)

Fig. 6. Formulas of some antagonists to the biosynthesis of mammalian polyamines.

264

cells (LUK, 1981). In vivo, DFMO is relatively non-toxic in doses which produce virtually complete depletion of putrescine, and has been used to cure infection with *Trypanosoma brucei* in mice (BACCHI, 1980). The use of DFMO for treatment of tumours is still in its earliest phases of trial, but some experience has been obtained with MGBG. The dose schedules used initially proved too toxic for human use (FREIREICH, 1962), but BURCHENAL (1963) found that it was quite effective, when used in subtoxic doses in combination with stilbamidine in treating mouse leukemias. Recently MGBG has been tried in modest doses in patients with advanced malignant lymphoma, with promising results. WARRELL, 1981). The first report of combining DFMO with MGBG in treating patients (SIIMES, 1981) involves application of a specific schedule: a single dose of MGBG intravenously followed, one or two days later, by DFMO for three to five days. These treatments produced no clinical improvement. If a new infusion of MGBG was added two days later, however, a rapid reduction occurred in the number of blast cells in four pediatric patients with unresponsive lymphoblastic and one with myelogenous leukemia. In each instance, the priming administration of DFMO greatly increased the intracellular concentration of MGBG achieved, suggesting that success of the treatment depends on increasing the tumour uptake of MGBG by prior depletion of intracellular polyamines. This permits use of a non-toxic dose level of both MGBG and DFMO. Although this first report is preliminary, it suggests that further studies are justified.

Abstract

The polyamines are small molecules associated with cell growth which are found in all life forms. Ornithine decarboxylase, the first, rate limiting enzyme in polyamine biosynthesis, has a very short half-life in high density cell populations, but a longer half-life when cells are dispersed. Activity of the enzyme is suppressed by its immediate product, putrescine, and by polyamines and may be induced by many factors, including dilution of cell cultures, increasing the rate of cell proliferation, and cyclic-AMP. It may also be induced by acetyl derivatives of polyamines. The fact that the parent molecules suppress ODC activity, whereas the acetyl derivatives induce it suggests the possibility that antagonistic feed-back loops participate in control of ODC activity.
Since the concentration of polyamines is increased in rapidly growing tissues, they have been suggested as possible clinical markers for the presence of cancer, but the multiplicity of non-neoplastic causes of elevated polyamine levels in plasma and urine makes them of little values for this use.
Polyamines are required in order to sustain normal growth in vitro. The exact reason for this requirement is unclear, but several possibilities have been suggested, including the facts that the polyamines are strong cations at physiological pH and that they can form covalent derivatives with proteins and possibly other macromolecules. Moreover, analogues of the polyamines are capable of inducing differentiation in certain tumour lines in vitro. These properties suggest that they may function by modulating the expression of nucleic acids and the activity of enzymes. These considerations suggest that the growth of tumours might be affected by pharmacological agents influencing polyamine biosynthesis.

References

1. BACCHI, C. J., NATHAN, H. C., HUTNER, S. J., McCANN, P. P. and SJOERDSMA, A.: Polyamine metabolism: a potential target in trypanosomes. Science *210* (1980), 332—334
2. BLANKENSHIP, J. and WALLE, J.: In vitro studies of enzymatic synthesis and metabolism of N-acetylated polyamines. In: Advances in Polyamine Research, vol 2. Ed. R. A. CAMPBELL et al. Raven Press, New York, 1978

3. Bolkenius, F. N. and Seiler, N.: Acetyl derivatives as intermediates in polyamine catabolism. Int. J. Biochem. *13* (1981), 287—292

4. Bondy, P. K. and Canellakis, Z. N.: High-performance liquid chromatography in the separation and measurement of di- and polyamines and their derivatives, and specific preparation of isomers of their monoacetyl derivatives. J. Chrom. *224* (1981), 371—379

5. Burchenal, J. H., Purple, J. R., Bucholz, E. and Straub, P. W.: Potentiation of methyl glyoxal bis(guanylhydrazone) by stilbamidine in transplanted mouse leukemia. Cancer. Chemother. Rep. No. *29* (1963), 85—89

6. Canellakis, E. S., Viceps-Madore, D., Kyriakidis, D. A. and Heller, J. S.: The regulation and function of ornithine decarboxylase and of the polyamines. Current Topics in Cellular Regulation *15* (1979), 155—202

7. Canellakis, Z. N.: Effects of acetylated polyamines on ornithine decarboxylase in rat HTC cells. Biochem. Biophys. Res. Comm. *100* (1981), 929—933

8. Canellakis, Z. N. and Bondy, P. K.: Factors modulating the activity of ornithine decarboxylase in rat HTC cells. Medical. Biol. (1981 B), in press

9. Canellakis, Z. N., Lande, L. A. and Bondy, P. K.: Covalent binding of polyamines to proteins in HTC cells. Biochem. Biophys. Res. Comm. *100* (1981 C), 675—680

10. Canellakis, Z. N. and Theoharides, T. C.: Stimulation of ornithine decarboxylase synthesis and its control by polyamines in regenerating rat liver and cultured rat hepatoma cells. J. Biol. Chem. *251* (1976), 4436—4441

11. Cohn, M. S., Tabor, C. W. and Tabor, H.: Regulatory mutations affecting ornithine decarboxylase activity in *Saccharomyces cerevisiae*. J. Bacteriol. *142* (1980), 791—799

12. Collins, S. J., Bodner, A., Ting, R. and Gallo, R. C.: Induction of morphological and functional differentiation of human promyelocytic leukemia cells (HL-60) by compounds which induce differentiation of murine leukemia cells. Int. J. Cancer *25* (1980), 213—218

13. Desser, H., Frass, M., Kuzmits, R., Aiginger, P., Muller, N. M. and Klaring, W. J.: Assessment of polyamine levels in plasma and urine from patients with carcinoma of the testis. Adv. Polyam. Res. *3* (1981), 431—440

14. Desser, H., Lutz, D., Krieger, O. and Stierer, M.: Rapid detection of polyamines in the sera of patients with colorectal carcinoma by liquid ion-exchange chromatography. Oncolog. *37* (1980), 376—380

15. Folk, J. E., Park, M. H., Chung, S. I., Schrode, J., Lester, E. P. and Cooper, H. L.: Polyamines as physiological substrates for transglutaminases. J. Biol. Chem. *255* (1980), 3695—3700

16. Freireich, E. J., Frei, E. I. I. I. and Karon, M.: Methylglyoxal bis(guanylhydrazone): A new agent active against acute myelocytic leukemia. Cancer Chemother. Rep. *16* (1962), 183—186

17. Fulton, D. S., Levin, V. A., Lubich, W. P., Wilson, C. B. and Marton, L. J.: Cerebrospinal fluid polyamines in patients with glioblastoma multiforme and anaplastic astrocytoma. Cancer. Res. *40* (1980), 3293—3296

18. Hafner, E. W., Tabor, C. W. and Tabor, H.: Mutants of *Escherichia coli* that do not contain 1,4-diaminobutane (putrescine) or spermidine. J. Biol. Chem. *254* (1979), 12419—12426

19. Hogan, B. L. M.: Effect of growth conditions on the ornithine decarboxylase activity of rat hepatoma cells. Biochem. Biophys. Res. Comm. *45* (1971), 301—307

20. Hogan, B. L. M. and Murden, S.: Effect of growth conditions on the activity of ornithine decarboxylase in cultured hepatoma cells. Effect of amino acid supply. J. Cell. Physiol. *83* (1974), 345—352

21. Jänne, J., Pösö, H. and Raina, A.: Polyamines in rapid growth and cancer. Biochim. Biophys. Acta *473* (1978), 241—293

22. Jänne, J. and Raina, A.: On the stimulation of ornithine decarboxylase and RNA polymerase activity in rat liver after treatment with growth hormone. Biochim. Biophys. Acta *174* (1969). 769—772

23. Lipton, A., Sheehan, A., Moertel, R. and Harvey, R. A.: Urinary polyamine levels in patients with localized malignancy. Cancer *38* (1976), 1344—1347

24. LUK, G. D., GOODWIN, G., MARTON, L. J. and BAYLIN, S. B.: Polyamines are necessary for the survival of human small-cell lung carcinoma in culture. Proc. Natl. Acad. Sci. USA *78* (1981), 2355—2358

25. MAMONT, P. S., DUCHENSE, M. C., GROVE, J. and BEY, P.: Anti-proliferative properties of DL-α-difluoromethyl ornithine in cultured cells. A consequence of the irreversible inhibition of ornithine decarboxylase. Biochem. Biophys. Res. Comm. *81* (1978), 58—66

26. MARKS, P. A., REUBEN, R., EPNER, E., BRESLOW, R., COBB, W., BOGDEN, A. E. and RIF-KIND, R. A.: Induction of murine erythroleukemia cells to differentiate: A model for the detection of new anti-tumour drugs. Antibiot. Chemother. *23* (1978), 31—41

27. MARTON, L. J., EDWARDS, M. S., LEVIN, V. A., LUBICH, W. P. and WILSON, C. B.: CSF Polyamines: A new and important means of monitoring patients with medulloblastoma. Cancer *47* (1981), 757—760

28. McCANN, P. P., TARDIF, C., HORNSPERGER, J. M. and BOHLEN, P.: Two distinct mechanisms for ornithine decarboxylase regulation by polyamines in rat hepatoma cells. J. Cell. Physiol. *99* (1979), 183—190

29. McCANN, P. P., TARDIFF, C., PEGG, A. E. and DIEKEMA, K.: The dual action of the non-physiological diamines 1,3 diaminopropane and cadaverine on ornithine decarboxylase of HTC cells. Life Sci. *26* (1980), 2003—2010

30. NISHIOKA, K., EZAKI, K. and HART, J. S.: A preliminary study of polyamines in the bone-marrow plasma of adult patients with leukemia. Clin. Chim. Acta *107* (1980), 59—66

31. NISHIOKA, K. and ROMSDAHL, M. M.: Elevation of putrescine and spermidine in sera of patients with solid tumours. Clin. Chim. Acta *57* (1974), 155—161

32. RABSON, A. S., STERN, R., TRALKA, T. S., COSTA, J. and WILCZEK, J.: Hexamethylene bisacetamide induces morphologic changes and increased synthesis of procollagen in cell line from glioblastoma multiforme. Proc. Nat. Acad. Sci. *74* (1977), 5060—5064

33. REUBEN, R. C., RIFKIND, R. A. and MARKS, P. A.: Chemically induced murine erythroleukemic differentiation. Biochim. Biophys. Acta *605* (1980), 325—346

34. RUSSELL, D. H.: Posttranslation modification of ornithine decarboxylase by its product putrescine. Biochem. Biophys. Res. Comm. *99* (1981), 1167—1172

35. RUSSELL, D. H., LEVY, C. C., SCHIMPF, S. C. and HAWK, I. A.: Urinary polyamines in cancer patients. Cancer Res. *31* (1971), 1555—1558

36. RUSSELL, D. H., SNYDER, S. H. and MEDINA, V J.: Growth hormone induction of ornithine decarboxylase in rat liver. Endocr. *86* (1970), 1414—1419

37. SCHEINMAN, S. J., BURROW, G. N., THEOHARIDES, T. C. and CANELLAKIS, Z. N.: Stimulation of ornithine decarboxylase synthesis in the rat thyroid. Life Sci. *21* (1977), 1143—1148

38. SEILER, N., BOLKENIUS, F. N. and KNODGEN, B.: Acetylation of spermidine in polyamine catabolism. Biochim. Biophys. Acta *633* (1980), 181—190

39. SIIMES, M., SEPPANEN, L., ALHONEN-HONGISTO, L. and JÄNNE, J.: Synergistic action of two polyamine antimetabolites leads to a rapid therapeutic response in childhood leukemia. Int-J. Cancer *28* (1981), in press.

40. TABOR, C. W. and TABOR, H.: 1,4-diaminobutane (putrescine), spermidine, and spermine. Ann. Rev. Biochem. *45* (1976), 285—306

41. THEOHARIDES, T. C. and CANELLAKIS, Z. N.: Spermine inhibits induction of ornithine decarboxylase by cyclic AMP but not by dexamethasone in rat hepatoma cells. Nature *255* (1975), 733—734

42. TORMEY, D. C., WAALKES, T. P., AHMANN, D., GEHRKE, C. W., ZUMWALL, R. W., SNYDER, J. and HANSEN, H.: Biological markers in breast carcinoma. I. Incidence of abnormalities of CEA, HCG, three polyamines and three minor nucleosides. Cancer *35* (1975), 1095—1100

43. WAALKES, T. P., GEHRKE, C. W., TORMEY, D. C., ZUMWALT, R. W., HUESER, J. N., JUO, K. C., LAKINGS, D. B., AHMANN, D. L. and MOERTEL, C. G.: Urinary excretion of polyamines by patients with advanced malignancy. Cancer Chemother. Rep. *59* (1975), 1103—1116

44. WANG, A. H.-J., QUIGLEY, G. J., KOLPAK, F. J., van der MAREL, G., van BOOM, J. H. and RICH, A.: Left-handed double helical DNA: variations in the backbone conformation. Science *211* (1981), 171—176

45. WARRELL, R. P., Jr., LEĖ, B. J., KEMPIN, S. J., LACHER, M. J., STRAUS, D. J. and YOUNG, C. W.: Effectiveness of methyl-GAG (methylglyoxal-bis(guanylhydrazone)) in patients with advanced malignant lymphoma. Blood 57 (1981), 1011—1014

46. WILLIAMS-ASHMANN, H. G. and CANELLAKIS, Z. N.: Polyamines in mammalian biology and medicine. Perspec. Biol. and Med. 22 (1979), 421—453

47. WILLIAMS-ASHMAN, H. G. and CANELLAKIS, Z. N.: Transglutaminase-mediated covalent attachment of polyamines to proteins: mechanisms and potential physiological significance Physiol. Chem. and Phys. 12 (1980), 457—472

Institute for Cancer Research, University of Vienna, Austria

Retinoids

H. WRBA and A. G. RIEDER

As early as 1926 FUJIMAKI et al (3) described the development of stomach cancer in rats after feeding of a Vitamin A deficient diet. More than 70 years since its isolation from egg yolk in 1909, it is now known that Vitamin A has the function of a vital growth regulator in a general sense. Growth control and promotion, differentiation of epithelium and the maintenance of the level of differentiation are phenomena where Vitamin A plays a major role. The most important associations between Vitamin A and cancer appearance are shown in Figure 1.

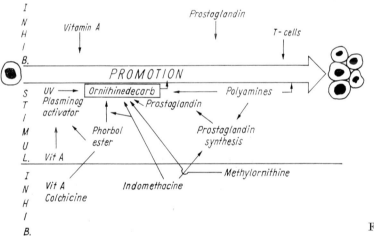

Fig. 1.

A great deal of evidence exists for the correlation of the appearance of premalignant changes in epithelial tissues with the level of Vitamin A. This regulating action is obviously dependent on many circumstances in a complicated equilibrium of influencing factors.

Vitamin A seems to influence the multistep process from the primary transformation to the expression of a malignant growth pattern at various levels.

Maintenance of repression (i. e. inhibition of cancer formation by oncogenes) is the result of many biochemical and biological interactions during the promotion period. Reversion of metaplastic lesions in experimentally-induced hyperplasia of prostata and trachea have been described. Prevention of malignancies by retinoids, mainly by retinolacetate and retinoic acid, is well documented in many animal models for several types of cancer (7).

269

The normal blood level of Vitamin A in humans undergoes variations, which are due to the storage potential of the liver. After saturation, a certain serum level will be reached. Young individuals with a normally filled store have high serum levels. Older persons have a lower serum concentrations and often a bigger tolerance to Vitamin A because of a partly empty liver store.

Analysis of serum levels of retinol shows much lower concentrations for many kinds of malignancies (10). Except for leukemia, tumours of all histological types cause depression of the level of Vitamin A (6).

In addition to the liver store, the supply of Vitamin A in the food is also important. Roughly half of the Vitamin A derives from carotenoids which are constituents of tomatoes, carrots, green vegetables and salads. Several epidemiological studies have shown the connection between Vitamin A content in the food and the appearance of cancer. A clear cut relation between Vitamin A content and appearance of lung cancer is assured by HIRAYAMA (5) who showed in epidemiological approaches that the intake of green and yellow vegetables diminishes the risk of cancer. The main factor in green and yellow vegetables — according to him — is their content of Vitamin A. The same analysis of nutritional habits in relation to cancer formation shows decrease of the lung cancer risk due to smoking with increased intake of Vitamin A. BJELKE (1) established an index of Vitamin A intake, where an increased index caused a relative diminution of the lung cancer risk in smokers.

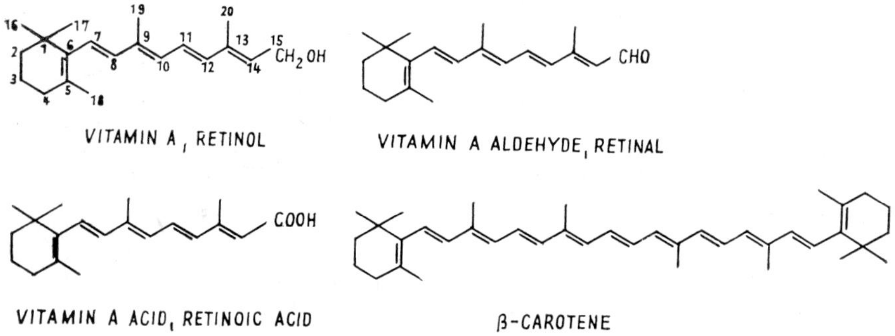

VITAMIN A , RETINOL   VITAMIN A ALDEHYDE, RETINAL

VITAMIN A ACID, RETINOIC ACID   β-CAROTENE

Fig. 2. Chemical structure of Vitamin A and some of its most important naturally occurring derivatives and precursors.

Retinol *per se* is a very unstable, fast-soluble substance. Its esters (mainly palmitate and acetate) are more stable. The molecule is formed of three characteristic elements: a ring roup, a polyene chain and a polar end group (Fig. 2). Substitutions in the three different parts of this molecule are possible and have been systematically performed. Hoffmann — La Roche Co. has more than 3,000 derivatives synthesized in its own laboratories. The aim of this worldwide search is to identify a derivative which would be more water soluble and less toxic, combined with possible increased Vitamin A action in terms of oncolysis and immunopotentiation.

The fat solubility leads to some complications in the use of retinol esters, the most commonly available form. Vitamin A preparations have been used in the past with the addition either of a solubilizer or in the form of oily solutions. Unfortunately, the solubilizer was often more toxic than Vitamin A itself. Injection of preparations made up in oil have resulted in high individual variability of dosage, since a large proportion of the oily material remained unresorbed for a long time. In our laboratory we have used Vitamin A emulsion (A-Mulsin[R]) for clinical purposes and also in ani-

270

mal experiments. The emulsion, which is stable and reliably resorbed through lymphatic channels, contains a very high concentration of Vitamin A.

One ml (= 15 drops) is equivalent to 300,000 units. The resorption of this preparation is complete within 15 min under normal intestinal conditions.

The multiple actions of Vitamin A on the cell metabolism of growth and differentiation explain the observed toxicity at high doses. The main toxic symptoms appear in epithelia and the mucosa. Mice develop conjunctivitis, epithelial disorders, loss of hair and breaking of bones (Fig. 3, Fig. 4), but with different sensitivity according to strain, sex and age.

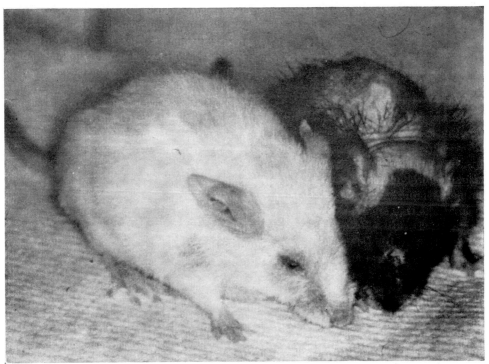

Fig. 3. Toxicity of Vitamin A in different mouse strains (C57 Black, Swiss), 4 months old, after weeks of treatment with a daily dose of 240000 IU A-Mulsin^R/kg mouse.

Fig. 4. Sensitivity of different mouse strains to Vitamin A

Strain	Sex	Age at start of experiment	Units per kg body weight $\times 10^6$	mean survival time (days)
SWA	♂	21	10.2	37
SWA	♂	123	16.6	70
SWA	♀	129	15.1	68
C$_3$H	♂	105	36.1	108
C$_3$H	♀	29	20.0	58
DBA	♀	59	17.8	53
CBA/Ry	♀	59	41.8	140

Vitamin A, given to pregnant animals, produces disorders in differentiation of the embryo. It is logical that a substance that interferes with differentiation, should also be teratogenic. Depending on dose schedule and time of application, malformations of embryos, following treatment of pregnant mice and rats, are very easy to produce (Fig. 5). Pregnancy, therefore, is a contraindication for high doses of Vitamin A.

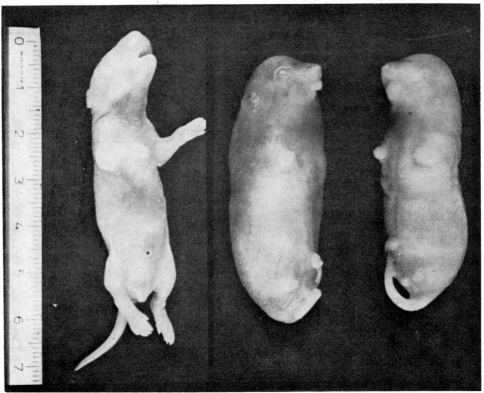

Fig. 5. Teratogenic effect of Vitamin A in rats (Sprague Dawley). Newborn rat after a single dose of 1.5×10^6 IU A-Mulsin[R]/kg body weight on the 13th day of gestation.

In the majority of cancer patients who have been treated with high doses of Vitamin A, the side effects are pronounced, since daily doses of 1.5 million units of Vitamin A for several weeks are necessary for oncolytic action. An effective maintenance daily dose is 300,000 units of Vitamin A. It is striking that the appearance of side effects varies considerably from one patient to the other, and cancer patients obviously tolerate much higher doses than healthy persons. (All the clinical studies presented here were undertaken in cooperation with the Department for Diseases of the Lung and the Boltzmann Institute of Oncology in the City Hospital Lainz — Vienna.)

Desquamation of the dermis is present in 100% of cases above a threshold dose, and is used as an indicator for the initiation of the therapeutic effect, since such a sub-toxic reaction of the epidermis is necessary for oncolytic action. Other clinical symptoms are: nausea in 80% of patients, cheilitis in 70%, headache in 50%, psychical disturbances in 20%, vomiting and loss of hair in 10% (Fig. 6).

Several studies with monotherapy of Vitamin A palmitate and cis-retinoic acid are in progress. In several cases of inoperable cancer, systemic application of Vitamin A in high dosage has produced oncolytic activity, up to a total disappearance of the lesions.

Fig. 6.

High doses of Vitamin A in the treatment of lung cancer
Institute for Cancer Research, University of Vienna Department of Diseases
of the Lung, Municipal Hospital Lainz, Vienna

Toxicity	Clinical Symptoms	Patients (%)
	Desquamation of the dermis	100%
	Nausea	80%
	Cheilitis	70%
Permissible	Headache	50%
	Psychical disturbance	20%
	Vomiting	20%
	Loss of hair	10%
	CNS Symptoms	15%
	Disorientation	
	Somnolence	
	Cephalea	
Severe		
	Coagulopathy	2%
	Generalized petechiasis	
	Mesenteric arterial thromboses	

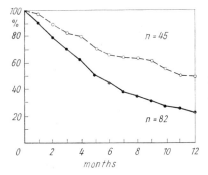

Fig. 7. Survival time of randomized patients with visible
squamous cell lung cancers

●————● Holoxan
○— —○ Holoxan $+ 30 \times 10^6$ IU Vit A (after W. Scheef,
8).

A convincing finding in lung cancer is the improvement of blastic transformation within a period of 6 weeks.
The clinical effects produced in cancer patients may be attributed to several mechanisms. Retinol is certainly a strong stimulator of the humoral immune response. Specific cell-mediated immunity and improvement of cytotoxicity against tumour cells by retinol, and stimulation of natural killer cell activity (as with interferon) by retinoic acid have been described (4). Improvement of cell permeability, lysosome labilization and activation of T-cells, all contribute to the very potent immune stimulating effect of Vitamin A.
A randomized study of patients with squamous cell carcinoma of the lung showed a distinct improvement among patients treated with Vitamin A palmitate in addition to chemotherapy with Holoxan, compared with those receiving Holoxan alone (Fig. 7). The most striking action of retinoids is the protection against carcinogenic factors. In many systems, the induction of cancer by established mechanisms has been inhibited in rate and time. The incidence of carcinomas after DMBA painting is dramatically reduced by a retinoic acid analogue manufactured by Hoffmann — La Roche

RO 10-9395 (2). Treatment with retinylacetate causes a delay in the appearance of NMH-induced mammary tumours in rats.

In our laboratory model system with methylcholanthrene-induced sarcoma in mice, tumour appearance is delayed by adding Vitamin A to the drinking water. From these few examples out of a great number of similar publications, it becomes clear that Vitamin A and its derivatives are possibly suitable preparations for a systematic cancer prevention.

A great deal of activity by several groups is devoted to the analysis and search for the retinol binding proteins (7). In the cell there are different binding proteins and binding sites for retinol and for retinoic acid. There is still no clear correlation between the presence of binding protein and action of retinoids. Further experiments are necessary to determine the specific capacity of the derivatives in this context which would lead to more predictable results. The direction of research should be in the synthesis of less toxic compounds.

Unfortunately, we do not have a simple and reliable test system for the specific antitumour action of Vitamin A. The most reliable method at present available is the evaluation of keratinisation in an organ culture of a hamster trachea. The extension of metaplastic lesions in such an organ culture has been evaluated. SPORN et al. (9) have shown the possibility of using differentiation as a specific action of tested compounds in this system.

The outlook for future progress in this field will depend on an increased knowledge of the specific action of existing compounds, their clinical application, and the elaboration of clear indications and optimal dose schedules.

More effective and less toxic compounds should be sought with retinol specific and, possibly, more oncolytic activity. The known effects of retinoids on growth regulation, control of differentiation, immunostimulation and restoration, labilization of membranes and lysosomes and mitogenic activity, make necessary the investigation of its use in tumour prophylaxis.

Acknowledgements

The authors are indebted to M. MICKSCHE, B. GMEINER, G. ZERLAUTH and A. DUTTER for cooperation and help.

References

1. BJELKE, E.: Dietary Vitamin A and human lung cancer. Int. J. Cancer *15* (1975), 561—565
2. BOLLAG, W.: Prophylaxis of chemically induced epithelial tumours with an aromatic retinoic acid analog (Ro 10-9359). Europ. J. Cancer *11* (1975), 721—724
3. FUJIMAKI, Y.: Formation of carcinoma in albino rats fed on deficient diets. J. Cancer Res. *10* (1926), 469—477
4. GOLDFARB, R. H. & HERBERMAN, R.B.: Natural killer cell reactivity: Regulatory interactions among phorbolester, interferon, cholera toxin and retinoic acid. J. Immunol. *126* (1981), 6
5. HIRAYAMA, T.: Diet and cancer. Nutrition and Cancer *1* (1979), 3
6. KARK, J. D., SMITH, A. H., SWITZER, B. R. and HAMES, C. G.: Serum Vitamin A (retinol) and cancer incidence in Evans County, Georgia. J. Natl. Cancer Inst. *66* (1981), 41
7. LOTAN, R.: Effects of Vitamin A and its analogs (retinoids) on normal and neoplastic cells. Biochim. Biophys. Acta *605* (1980), 33—91
8. SCHEEF, W.: Fachklinik für Tumorerkrankungen, Bonn; personal communication (1973)
9. SPORN, M. B. et al: Retinoids and cancer prevention. In "Carcinogens: Identification and Mechanism of Action" ed. A. C. GRIFFIN & C. R. SHAW, Raven Press N.Y., p. 441 (1979)
10. WALD, N., IDLE, M., BOREHAM, J. and BAILEY, A.: Low serum Vitamin A and subsequent risk of cancer. The Lancet 1810 (1980), 813

274

Roswell Park Memorial Institute, 666 Elm Street, Buffalo, New York 14263, USA

The Role of Drug-Induced Differentiation
in the Control of Tumour Growth

K. Takeda, J. Minowada and A. Bloch

The clinical therapy of cancer has, in the past, been predicated on the proposition that the direct killing of tumour cells is the major objective of drug therapy. This view needs to be amended by taking into consideration other drug effects that can also lead to the control of tumour-cell growth, including the ability of various chemical agents to induce the differentiation of tumour cells into mature, non-proliferating elements. It is the objective of this presentation to demonstrate the potentiality of this approach, on the basis of information we have accumulated with ML-1, a human myeloblastic leukaemia cell line recently isolated from a patient with acute myelogenous leukaemia.

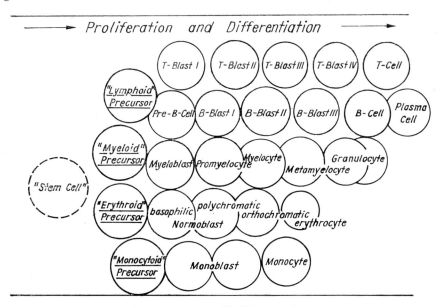

Fig. 1. Scheme of human haematopoietic cell differentiation

It is by now well established that mature human lymphoid, myeloid and erythroid cells proceed from a common stem cell (Fig. 1) (1) and that their development is controlled by a variety of factors, which include erythropoietin, various lymphokines and diverse macrophage and granulocyte inducers (2).

The stage of differentiation are identifiable not only from their morphological characteristics, but also by various markers that pertain to cellular antigens or to cell function (Fig. 2) (1). The antigenic markers include a variety of surface and cytoplasmic

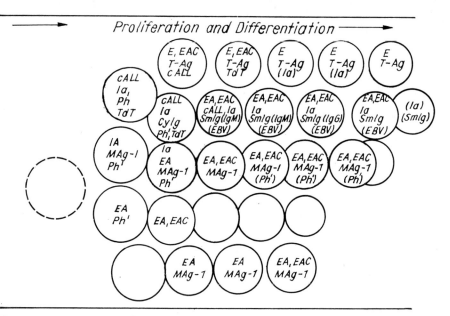

Fig. 2. Marker expression during haematopoietic cell differentiation. Abbreviations used: cALL common ALL associated antigen; Ia, p28,30 glycoprotein antigen; Ph', Philadelphia chromosome; TdT, terminal deoxynucleotidyl transferase; E, sheep erythrocyte rosette; EA, rosette formed by bovine erythrocyte-IgG antibody complex; EAC, rosette formed by bovine erythrocyte-IgM antibody complement complex; T-Ag, T-cell antigen; CyIg, cytoplasmic immunoglobulin; SmIg, surface membrane immunoglobulin (G or M); EBV, Epstein-Barr virus.

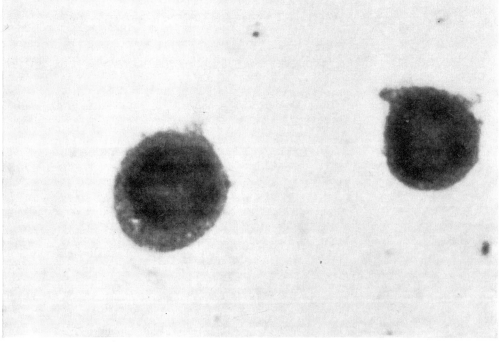

Fig. 3. Untreated ML-1 cells grown in culture for 6 days showing large nuclei and scant cytoplasm (Wright-Giemsa; × 1,000).

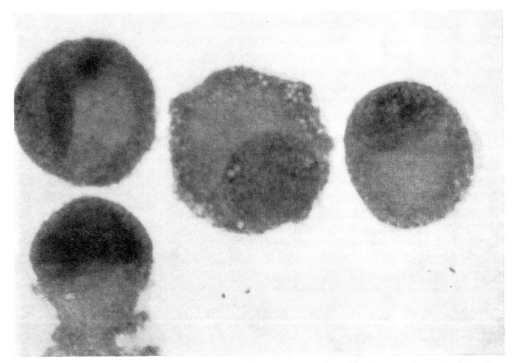

Fig. 4. ML-1 cells after culture for 6 days in the presence of arabinofuranosylcytosine (Ara C), exhibiting the morphological appearance of macrophages (Wright-Giemsa; × 1,000).

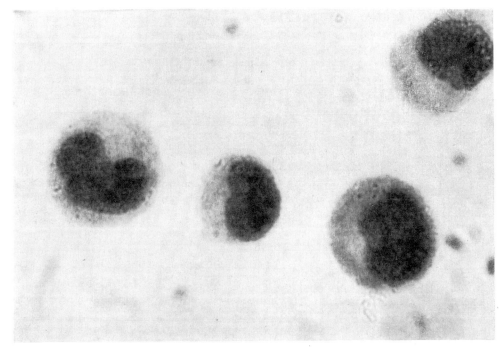

Fig. 5. ML-1 cells after culture for 6 days in the presence of dimethylsulfoxide (1.6%), exhibiting the morphological appearance of maturing myeloid cells (Wright-Giemsa; × 1,000).

277

immunoglobulins and glycoproteins (1, 3); and the functional indicators comprise diverse changes in the metabolism of the differentiating cells, including an increase in oxidative reactions as expressed by their enhanced capacity to reduce nitroblue tetrazolium dye (4) and an increase in their phagocytic activity as demonstrated by their enhanced capability to engulf latex particles (5).

On the basis of such characteristics, the human leukaemias can be classified as to the stage at which they are arrested in their development, the ML-1 cells being blocked at the myeloblast stage (1).

Under normal conditions, haematopoietic cell differentiation is tightly linked to cell proliferation; this linkage is absent in the leukaemic state, leading to proliferation without differentiation. The question therefore arises whether leukaemic cells, such as ML-1, have lost their ability to differentiate, or whether they retain this capacity and which could then possibly be exploited for the control of tumour cell growth.

During prolonged culture in vitro, only about 3—5% of ML-1 cells, which are characterized by a large nucleus and scant cytoplasm (Fig. 3), convert spontaneously to more mature forms. However, when treated with various compounds, including clinically effective antitumour agents, a high percentage of the cells is converted to macrophages (Fig. 4) or to myeloid cells of intermediate maturity (Fig. 5) (6, 7). Macrophage-like cells are induced by drugs such as 6-mercaptopurine or arabinofuranosylcytosine (Ara C); myeloid elements emerge upon treatment with dimethylsulfoxide.

The kinetics by which differentiation of the ML-1 cells is induced is shown in Figures 5—8 for the case of Ara C. Surface receptors for the F_c portion of IgG begin to appear within 24 hours after exposure to the drug (Fig. 6), and increase steadily during the ensuing incubation period. The increased ability of the treated cells to reduce nitroblue tetrazolium dye (Fig. 7) and to engulf latex particles (Fig. 8) manifests itself after some delay. These functional alteration are accompanied by morphological changes towards more mature forms. On day 7, approximately 45% of the viable cells are ma-

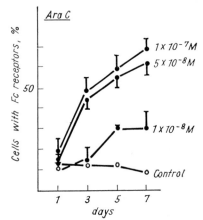

Fig. 6. Increase in the number of cells containing F_c-IgG surface receptors after treatment of a culture of ML-1 cells with arabinofuranosylcytosine (Ara C).

ture macrophages (Fig. 9), whereas 35—45% of the cells are present at intermediate stages of maturation. It is important to note (Fig. 10) that with an optimal concentration of Ara C (5 × 10⁻⁸ M) the inhibition of population growth is due predominantly to cell differentiation: thus, apprximately 40% of the cells are dead, and close to 50% are differentiated. The fate of the residual viable cell fraction has not yet been assessed. Such analysis are important for assessing the mechanism by which clinically effective agents may cause long-term remission, cell kill being only one of the mediating factors (6).

278

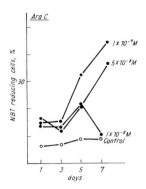

Fig. 7. Increase in the number of cells with nitroblue tetrazolium (NBT)-reducing ability after treatment of a culture of ML-1 cells with arabinofuranosylcytosine (Ara C).

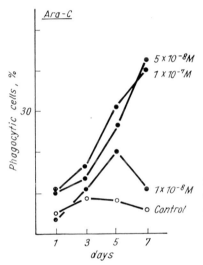

Fig. 8. Increase in the number of phagocytic cells after treatment of a culture of ML-1 cells with arabinofuranosylcytosine (Ara C). Phagocytic activity was measured by ingestion of latex particles.

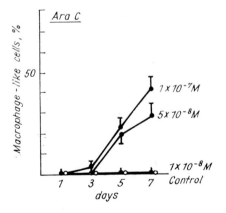

Fig. 9. Increase in the number of macrophage-like cells after treatment of a culture of ML-1 cells with arabinofuranosylcytosine (Ara C). The data shown do not include cells at intermediate stages of maturation; at day 7, these comprise 35—45% of the viable cell population.

Of therapeutic importance is the finding (Table 1) that the compounds capable of inducing differentiation are inhibitors of DNA synthesis or function. Agents that interfere with RNA synthesis, such as cordycepin, or those that interfere with protein synthesis, such as puromycin and cycloheximide, cannot induce differentiation.

This inability undoutedly relates to the need for RNA and protein synthesis required for bringing about the structural and functional changes that accompany cell differentiation.

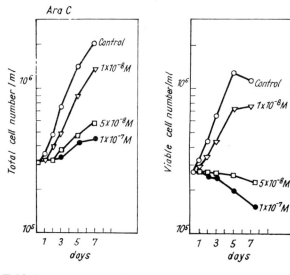

Fig. 10. Concentration-dependent effect of arabinosylcytosine (Ara C) on the proliferation and viability as measured by dye exclusion of ML-1 cells in culture.

Table 1.
Ability of various agents to induce differentiation of human myeloblastic leukaemia cells (ML-1) in vitro

Compound	Concentration (M)	Macrophages (%) Intermediate	Mature
Control		4	0
6-Mercaptopurine	5×10^{-7}	42	38
Arabinosylcytosine	5×10^{-8}	51	28
Actinomycin D	1×10^{-11}	53	7
Cordycepin	1×10^{-3}	2	0
Pyromycin	1×10^{-7}	5	0
Cycloheximide	1×10^{-6}	5	1

Although the mechanism by which inhibition of DNA synthesis translates into the expression of genetic information associated with differentiation is not yet understood, the observations made by the use of these drugs demonstrate that the differentiating potential of leukaemic cells has not been lost.

In conclusion, these results demonstrate that drug-induced differentiation may constitute a significant factor in the control of tumour growth. Further exploration is required to establish its clinical utility.

References

1. MINOWADA, J. (1981): Immunology of leukemia. Gunz, F. and Henderson, E., eds., New York, Bourne and Stratton
2. CLARKSON, B., MARKS, P. A. and TILL, J. E. (1978): Differentiation of Normal and Neoplastic Hematopoietic Cells. Cold Spring Harbor Laboratory

3. FERRARINI, M., MORETTA, L., ABRILE, R. and DURANTE, M. L.: Receptors for IgG molecules on human lymphocytes forming spontaneous rosettes with sheep red cells. Eur. J. Immunol. 5 (1975), 70—72

4. BAEHNER, R. L., BOXER, L. A. and DAVIS, J.: The biochemical basis of nitroblue tetrazolium reduction in normal human and chronic granulomatous disease polymorphonuclear leukocytes. Blood 48 (1976), 309—313

5. MICHL, J., OHLBAUM, D. J. and SILVERSTEIN, S. C.: 2-Deoxyglucose selectively inhibits F_c and complement receptor-mediated phagocytosis in mouse peritoneal macrophages. J. Exp. Med. 144 (1976), 1465—1483

6. TAKEDA, K., LEASURE, J., LOK, M. S., MINOWADA, J. and BLOCH, A.: Appearance of differentiation associated characteristics in human myeloblastic leukemia cells (ML-1) treated with dimethylsulfoxide, 12-0-tetradecanoyl phorbol 13-acetate and arabinofuranosyl cytosine. Proc. Am. Assoc. Cancer Res. 22 (1981), 224

7. TAKEDA, K., MINOWADA, J. and BLOCH, A.: Kinetics of appearance of differentiation associated characteristics in a line of human myeloblastic leukemia cells (ML-1) treated with tetradecanoylphorbol acetate, dimethylsulfoxide or with arabinofuranosyl cytosine. Cancer Research, (in press)

281

Departments of Radiology and Pathology, The Pritzker School of Medicine, University of Chicago, Chicago, Illinois (60637), USA

Modifying Effect of the Sex Hormonal Environment on the Growth of Basophilic Foci and Hepatocellular Carcinoma[1]

S. D. Vesselinovitch and N. Mihailovich

High sensitivity of the new-born and infant mouse to hepatocarcinogenesis has been demonstrated repeatedly in our laboratory (7, 11). Thus even single low dose treatments of $B6C3F_1$ mice with diethylnitrosamine (DEN) induced hepatocellular carcinomas in all animals. The latent periods were, however, related indirectly to the carcinogenic dose (8). Dealkylation of DEN represents the essential step in its biochemical activation to ultimate carcinogenic entity. Our earlier studies have shown that livers of infant mice dealkylate effectively DEN with similar rates in both sexes (5), and hepatocellular carcinomas develop with the same incidence although after a longer latency in females than in males. Thus, although the rapid replication of the macromolecules during the growth period (2, 3) facilitated equally in both sexes the fixation of the original biochemical lesion (7, 8), the rate of neoplastic expression was dependent upon the sex hormonal environment of the host (9).

The objective of the present study was to define the effects of gonadectomy on the onset, kinetics, and growth of both microscopic and gross focal hepatocellular lesions in relation to the development of carcinomas. These lesions were induced by a single hepatocarcinogenic dose of diethylnitrosamine.

Materials and methods

Fifteen-day-old $B6C3F_1$ mice of both sexes were injected once intraperitoneally with DEN (2.5 µg/g body weight). Groups of mice were gonadectomized after 4, 14 and 24 weeks. Six-week-old sham-gonadectomized mice served as carcinogen-treated controls. Groups of 8 to 25 mice were killed at 10-week intervals and the focal liver lesions were identified on H.-E. stained 5 µm thick sections. The images of histological sections were projected onto the Hewlett-Packard 9874 digitizer and the foci were outlined by a cursor. The digitizer has been interphased with a basic mini computer and a Neo-Palmer Leitz projecting microscope. The images of the focal lesions were quantitated as to their number per unit transection area (cm^2), the number per unit volume of the liver (cm^3), and the percentage of transection area occupied by foci. The number of foci per unit volume were computed using the formula developed by Fullman (1) and used recently by Moore et al (4).

Results and discussion

The original studies (10) showed that the early focal lesions induced by DEN were characterized by cells showing increased cytoplasmic basophilia owing to elevated

[1] These studies were supported in part by grants 5 R01 CA-25549 and 5 R01 CA-25522 from the National Cancer Institute.

282

RNA, increased ^{3}H-TdR labeling index, and deficiency of glucose-6-phosphatase. The superceding hyperplastic nodules, hepatocellular adenomas, and carcinomas were characterized as described earlier (6). In random liver transections, 9% of such basophilic foci showed protrusions into central and intercalated veins which extended up to 200 μm beyond the point of entry. The vascular obstructions were absent and no hepatic cell emboli were observed in the serial sections of the lungs of mice showing the above phenomenon. Intravascular protrusions and variations in diameters of the early lesions suggested the heterogeneity in their biologic behaviour. However, cellular and histoid morphology and the lack of dissemination to new sites with the establish-

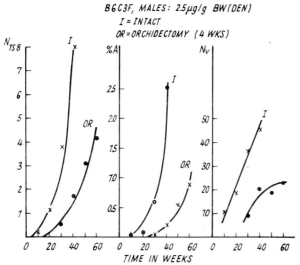

Fig. 1. Delay in the development of focal and nodular lesions due to orchidectomy. Lesions were induced by DEN in 15-day-old mice. Carcinomas were seen at 60 weeks in 100% of intact and in 18.7% of orchidectomized males.

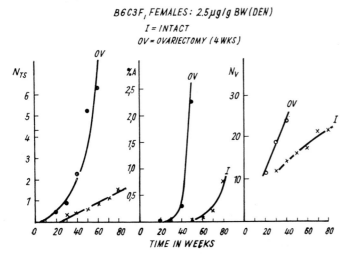

Fig. 2. Acceleration of the emergence of focal and nodular lesions following ovariectomy. Lesions were induced by DEN in 15-day-old females. Carcinomas were seen at 60 weeks in none of the intact and 40.0% of ovariectomized females.

283

ment of cell proliferation suggests the non-neoplastic nature of the basophilic foci including those which showed intravascular protrusion. In the course of growth only few foxi may acquire the essential characteristics of neoplasia (6) which appear to occur in a random fashion. Thus it is not possible to predict which one, if any, of the early focal lesions may represent potential carcinoma.

Figures 1 and 2 illustrate the kinetics of the basophilic foci (first 28 and 48 weeks in males and females respectively), hyperplastic nodules, and hepatocellular adenomas and carcinomas. The latter lesions emerged after 40 weeks in males and after 60 weeks in females. The orchidectomy (OR) delayed the onset and slowed the rate of the development and growth of the basophilic foci (Fig. 1). This is shown in the number of foci per unit of transection (N_{TS}), in the percent of the focal area per transection (%A), and in the estimated number of foci per unit volume (N_V). In contrast, the ovariectomy (OV) advanced the onset and accelerated the development of the basophilic foci in all three above-mentioned endpoints (Fig. 2). This implies that the physiologic levels of androgen enhanced the development of the early emerging basophilic cell populations in the intact males and that the normal levels of estrogen suppressed the development of the basophilic foci in the intact females.

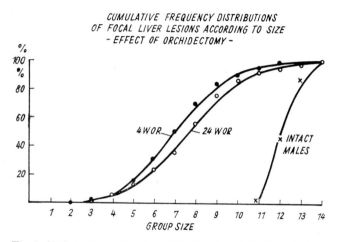

Fig. 3. Shift in the radial size of focal and nodular liver lesions towards smaller class groups due to orchidectomy.

Table 1.
Incidence of hepatocellular carcinomas 60 weeks after DEN treatment[a]

	Males		Females	
	Ratio	Percent	Ratio	Percent
Sham-gonadectomized	25/25	100	0/23	0
Gonadectomized at weeks:[b]				
4	3/25	12	11/25	44
14	5/25	20	11/25	44
24	6/25	24	8/25	32

[a] DEN: 2.5 µg/g BW at 15 days of age.
[b] After DEN administration.

284

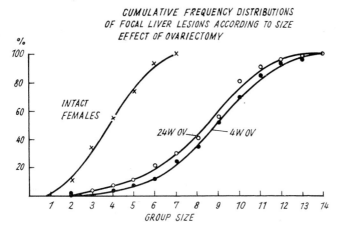

Fig. 4. Shift in the radial size of focal and nodular liver lesions towards greater class groups due to ovariectomy.

In order to assess the effect of the sex hormone environment on the growth of focal and nodular liver lesions, we calculated cumulative frequency distributions according to their radial sizes [from 40 μm (group 1) to greater than 2500 μm (group 14)] at the time of terminal sacrifice. Orchidectomy led to a shift in the radial size towards smaller class groups (Fig. 3) and to a decrease in the incidence of hepatocellular carcinomas from 100% to 18.7% (Table 1). Ovariectomy resulted in a shift in the radial size towards greater class groups (Fig. 4) and to an increase in the incidence of the hepatocellular carcinomas from 0% to 40% (Table 1). The size of hepatocellular carcinomas was decreased by orchidectomy and increased by ovariectomy. On the average, only 3.6% of all observed lesions in intact and gonadectomized animals were hepatocellular carcinomas. The change in the incidence of hepatocellular carcinomas was thus dependent upon the number of overall lesions which emerged.

Conclusions

The foregoing observations demonstrated that: (a) orchidectomy delayed the onset and slowed the rate of development and growth of the basophilic foci and of the hepatocellular carcinomas, and (b) ovariectomy advanced the onset and accelerated the development and growth of the basophilic foci and the hepatocellular carcinomas. Carcinogenesis can be divided into at least two stages: initiation and promotion. Since gonadectomy was performed following initiation, it may be conceived that the change in the hormonal environment modified the promoting phase of hepatocarcinogenesis by influencing the time of onset and the rate of development of basophilic foci, which in turn was related directly to the rate of neoplastic expression of hepatocellular carcinomas (10). This explanation assumes that the neoplastic expression was dependent upon the growth rate of the foci which, because of their different neoplastic potential, were limiting the probability at which time the carcinomas would occur. An equally likely possibility is that the expression of the neoplastic potential governed both the growth rate of the basophilic foci and the neoplastic nature of the superceding lesions. Regardless of this dilemma, the present study demonstrated that the sex-hormone environment already operates at the level of the basophilic foci, even when instituted late in their development (24-week gonadectomy). Further studies are required to establish whether or not the hormonal environment would effectively modulate hepatocarcinogenesis when restricted to the period during which carcinomas emerge.

References

1. FULLMAN, R. L.: Measurement of particle size in opaque bodies. Trans. AIME *197* (1953), 447—452
2. ITZE, L., VESSELINOVITCH, S. D. and RAO, K. V. N.: Estimation of the rate of DNA synthesis in newborn, regenerating and intact mouse livers. Physiol. Bohemoslov. *22* (1973), 457—460
3. ITZE, L., VESSELINOVITCH, S. D. and RAO, K. V. N.: Inter and intra diurnal variations of DNA, RNA and protein synthetic activity in newborn, infant and young adult mouse livers. Physiol. Bohemoslov. *25* (1976), 289—293
4. MOORE, M. P., DRINKWATER, N. R., MILLER, E. C., MILLER, J. A., and PITOT, H. C.: Quantitative analysis of the time-dependent development of glucose-6-phosphate deficient foci in the livers of mice treated neonatally with diethylnitrosamine. Cancer Res. *41* (1981), 1585—1598
5. RAO, K. V. N., and VESSELINOVITCH, S. D.: Age- and sex-associated diethylnitrosamine dealkylation activity of the mouse liver and hepatocarcinogenesis. Cancer Res. *33* (1973), 1625 to 1627
6. VESSELINOVITCH, S. D.: Morphology and metastatic nature of induced hepatic nodular lesions in C57BL × C3H F₁ mice. Cancer Res. *38* (1978), 2003—2010
7. VESSELINOVITCH, S. D.: Factors modulating response to carcinogenic mutagens. In: Progress in Environmental Mutagenesis, pp. 281—296. Edited by M. ALACEVIC. Elsevier/North Holland Biomedical Press, 1980.
8. VESSELINOVITCH, S. D.: Infant mouse as a sensitive bioassay system for carcinogenicity of N-nitroso compounds. In: N-Nitroso Compounds: Analysis, Formation and Occurrence, pp. 645—655. Edited by E. A. WALKER, M. CASTEGNARO, L. GRICIUTE, and M. BÖRZSÖNTI. IARC Scientific Publication No. 31, Lyon, 1980.
9. VESSELINOVITCH, S.D., and MIHAILOVICH, N.: The effect of gonadectomy on the development of hepatomas induced by urethan. Cancer Res. *27* (1967), 1788—1791
10. VESSELINOVITCH, S. D., MIHAILOVICH, N., RAO, K. V. N., and GOLDFARB, S.: Relevance of basophilic foci to promoting effect of sex hormones on hepatocarcinogenesis. In: Carcinogenesis, vol. 7, pp. 127—131. Edited by E. HECKER et al. Raven Press, New York, 1982.
11. VESSELINOVITCH, S. D., RAO, K. V. N., and MIHAILOVICH, N.: Neoplastic response of mouse tissues during perinatal age periods and its significance in chemical carcinogenesis. J. Natl. Cancer Inst. Monograph *51* (1979), 239—250

Department of Chemotherapy and Neurosurgery, Central Institute for Tumours and Allied Diseases, Ilica 197, 41000 Zagreb, Yugoslavia

Phase II Clinical Trial of cis-Dichlorodiammine Platinum (cis-DDP) in Metastatic Brain Tumours — a Preliminary Report

K. Kolarić, A. Roth, I. Jeličić and A. Matković

Summary

Although pharmacokinetic studies have shown that only traces of cis-DDP reach brain tissue, a cytotoxic action of this drug in primary brain tumours was reported recently. The purpose of this study was to examine whether cis-DDP also has antitumoural properties in metastatic brain tumours. Twenty-two consecutive untreated patients with brain metastases, recorded by computerized axial tomographic scans or radionuclide scans plus neurological examinations, underwent treatment. Pathohistology of the primary tumours showed six bronchial, seven breast, one gastric and one colorectal carcinoma, and four melanomas, one soft-tissue sarcoma, one hypernephroma and one carcinoma of the suprarenal gland. Cis-DDP was administered in doses of 30 mg/m² body surface daily for four days. All the patients received at least three cycles and were evaluated. An objective response (five complete and six partial remissions) was observed in 11 of the 22 patients (response rate, 50%). Five cases of stable disease were also noted; however, in the remaining six patients the brain tumour progressed. Complete remissions (5+, 6+ and 7+ months) were seen in three breast cancer patients, in one (6 months) lung cancer patient and in one (7+ months) melanoma patient. Six partial remissions (in lung, breast and melanoma cases) lasted 2—5 months. An antitumoural activity of cis-DDP was also seen in extracerebral tumours (breast, lung and melanoma patients). Toxicity was moderate but tolerable for the patients. The preliminary results of this study show for the first time that cis-DDP also has antitumourigenic properties in patients with metastatic brain tumours.

Introduction

Few chemotherapeutic agents penetrate the brain tissue and cerebrospinal fluid sufficiently to attain therapeutic concentrations. Nitrosoureas (bischloroethylnitrosourea (BCNU), 1-(2-chloroethyl)-3-cyclohexyl-1-nitrosourea (CCNU), 1-(2-chloroethyl)-3-(4-methyl-cyclohexyl)-1-nitrosourea (MeCCNU) and methylnitrosourea (MNU)), which are liposoluble, are, of course, the most important group of cytostatic agents that cross the blood-brain barrier and act on primary and metastatic brain tumours (2, 3, 4, 8, 9, 14). An ability to cross the blood-brain barrier, however, may not be essential for a drug to be effective in the treatment of intracerebral tumours, in view of their leaky vasculature and the fact that the blood-brain barrier does not exist in tumorous tissue of the brain (5, 11, 13, 15). The potential antitumorigenic action of cis-DDP on tumorigenic processes in the brain is a case in point. Thus, cis-DDP does not cross the blood-brain barrier, or does so very slightly, and only trace concentrations are found in the cerebrospinal fluid and in normal brain tissue (1, 10, 12). Nevertheless, the latest clinical observations have shown that cis-DDP has antitumorigenic activity even in primary cerebral tumours (6, 7). Because there are still

287

scant and inadequate clinical data regarding the action of cis-DDP on tumourigenic processes in the brain, and particularly on metastatic tumours (for which no clinical data are available), a clinical study was undertaken to investigate the action of cis-DDP on metastatic brain tumours. The preliminary results are reported below.

Patients and methods

Twenty-two patients, 13 women and 9 men, average age, 41 years (24—63), entered the study. In all patients, metastatic processes in the brain were confirmed by neurological examination, computerized axial tomography (CAT), brain scintiscan, eye fundus examination, and electroencephalography. The examinations were made prior to therapy, and after the second and fifth cycles of chemotherapy. The primary tumour of all patients was examined pathohistologically, and six carcinomas of the bronchi (all microcellular), seven carcinomas of the breast, four melanomas, one carcinoma of the stomach, one carcinoma of the colon, one soft-tissue sarcoma, one hypernephroma and one carcinoma of the suprarenal gland were established. Twelve patients had solitary brain metastases, and the other 10 had multiple metastases. All the patients also had metastases in other tissues and organs. The patients had not been treated before entering the study, either by cytostatic drugs or by radiotherapy.

Only patients under 70 years of age, with normal function of the cardiorespiratory system, kidney and liver and a normal blood cell count were entered into the study. Patients in the terminal stage of the disease or in cerebral coma (life expectancy 4 week were also excluded. The performance status of the patients, according to the Karnofsky scale, was 3 to 10: three patients were grade 8—10, 10 patients grade 5—7 and nine patients grade 3—4.

Cis-DDP was given in a daily intravenous dose of 30 mg/m^2 of body area on four days (total dose per cycle, 120 mg/m^2). Before administration of the drug, patients were given an infusion of 500 ml of 5% glucose; in order to enhance diuresis, cis-DDP was then given in a 500 ml 5% glucose infusion over eight hours. Patients were then administered 500 ml of mannitol. The interval between cycles was three weeks; in the case of a fall in leucocyte or thrombocyte counts, renewal of the cycle was postponed.

All toxic side effects, and in particular nephrotoxicity, were monitored regularly. Creatinine was determined before therapy, every day during the cycle, and upon completion of chemotherapy. Diuresis was monitored round the clock throughout the cycle. An audiogram was also made before therapy and after the fourth cycle of cis-DDP. During chemotherapy, no corticoids were given.

The patients were evaluated by criteria recommended by the WHO, and classed into the unmeasurable but evaluable disease group (16); treatment results were judged by objective (CAT scan or radionuclide scan) brain examinations. The following classifications were made: complete remission, complete disappearance of all neurological signs and complete disappearance of pathological changes, as established by CAT or radionuclide scan, for at least one month; partial regression, estimated $> 50\%$ reduction of CAT or brain scan changes and a respective improvement in neurological findings, for at least one month; stable disease, no sign of progression or $< 50\%$ reduction of tumorous lesions; and, finally, progression, increase of metastatic changes. The effect of cis-DDP with regard to other metastatic sites in the body was also evaluated.

288

The results of treatment were evaluated after two chemotherapy cycles, i. e., when the patient was about to receive the third cycle. Treatment was continued only in those who responded to treatment. If the disease showed signs of progressing, patients were administered a nitrosourea derivative, mainly BCNU plus corticosteroids.

Results

All patients were administered at least two (up to six) chemotherapy cycles, so that the results could be evaluated in all 22 cases (Table 1). Eleven of the 22 treated patients responded to cis-DDP, giving a response rate of 50%. In five patients, a complete remission of brain metastases was observed, whereas in six patients the remission was partial. In five cases the disease remained stable; and in six it progressed in spite of therapy. Both complete and partial remissions were achieved in cases of carcinoma of the lung, and breast and of melanoma. Interestingly, an objective regression of brain metastases was achieved in three out of six patients with microcellular lung carcinoma; and six out of seven female patients with carcinoma of the breast and two of the four melanoma patients had regression of brain metastases. The durations of the complete remissions were 5+, 6+ and 7+ months in breast cancer patients, 6 months in the lung cancer patient and 7+ months in the case of melanoma. The six partial remissions were of shorter duration (mean 4 months). During the average follow-up period of 10 months, six patients died: four did not respond to therapy, and the remaining two were in the group evaluated as stable disease.

Table 1.
Antitumorigenic activity of cis-DDP in metastatic brain tumours

Primary tumour	No. of patients	Complete response	Partial response	Stable disease	Progression	Response rate
Lung	6	1	2	1	2	3/6
Breast	7	3	3	1	—	6/7
Melanoma	4	1	1	—	2	2/4
Colon	1	—	—	1	—	0/1
Hypernephroma	1	—	—	—	1	0/1
Stomach	1	—	—	1	—	0/1
Suprarenal gland carcinoma	1	—	—	1	—	0/1
Soft-tissue sarcoma	1	—	—	—	1	0/1
Total	22	5	6	5	6	11/22 (50%)

The therapeutic response at metastatic sites other than the brain, was also evaluated (Table 2): five complete responses were noted in lymph node, subcutaneous and lung metastases in patients with primary lung and breast cancer, and partial responses were seen in liver, lung, lymph node and subcutaneous metastases. Breast cancer patients had the highest response (5/7).

The toxic side effects were also evaluated. Nausea and vomiting were seen in all 22 patients, particularly on the first day of the cycle; vomiting occurred four to

Table 2.

Responses[a] of extracerebral-tumour lesions in patients treated with cis-DDP

Primary tumour	No. of patients	Secondary tumour					Response rate
		Liver	Lung	Lymph nodes	Cutis-subcutis	Bone	
Lung	6	—	1 CR 1 PR 1 SD	—	—	—	2/6
Breast	7	1 PR	2 CR 1 SD	1 CR	1 CR	1 SD	5/7
Melanoma	4	—	—	1 PR 1 SD	1 PR	—	2/4
Colon	1	—	—	—	—	—	—
Stomach	1	—	—	—	—	—	—
Soft-tissue sarcoma	1	—	—	—	—	—	—
Suprarenal-gland carcinoma	1	—	—	—	—	—	—
Hypernephroma	1	—	—	—	—	—	—

[a] CR, complete response; PR, partial response; SD, stable disease

five hours after administration of cis-DDP and was very persistent, lasting six to eight hours despite the administration of antiemetics (Largactil, Torecan). In two patients, after the third and fourth chemotherapy cycles, respectively, temporary increases in serum creatinine levels (to 120 and 150 mmol/l) occurred; therapy was not discontinued, but the amounts of glucose mannitol were increased. Two patients displayed marked thrombocytopenia (2.1 and 45) with a severe hemorrhagic syndrome after the second and fourth cycles, respectively; thrombocyte transfusions were made, and chemotherapy was discontinued until the blood counts recovered, at two and three weeks, respectively. Leucopenia (2.6, 3.2, 1.5, 1.2) was observed in four cases. No signs of ototoxicity or peripheral neuropathy were noted. In one patient, a palmar fibrosis appeared after the second cis-DDP cycle, and lasted throughout the drug therapy; this side effect had not previously been reported.

Discussion

Following administration of cis-DDP to 22 previously untreated patients with brain metastases, regression was observed in 11 (five complete and six partial remissions), pointing to a marked antitumorigenic effect of this cytostatic agent on metastatic brain tumours. Regressions were observed in metastases from carcinomas of the bronchi and breast and from melanoma but not in those from gastrointestinal tumours. Extracerebral metastatic sites in patients with cancer of the breast and lung and melanoma also showed complete and partial remissions.

These preliminary results show that cytostatic agents that do not cross the blood-brain barrier can also have an antitumorigenic effect on brain metastases. Similar results were obtained by KAHN et al (7), who reported regression of primary recurrent glioblastoma in six of eight (75%) patients treated with cis-DDP (although the doses were different from those used here). An analysis of available references produced no other examples of application of cis-DDP to brain tumours in humans. In our view brain tumours represent an area in which cis-DDP could be used and studied — both as a single agent and in polychemotherapy, particularly in combination with nitrosoureas. The present study is still under way, and we hope soon to be able to publish definitive results on a larger group of patients.

References

1. BELT, R. J., HIMMELSTEIN, K. J., PATTON, T. F., BANISTER, S. J., STERNSON, L. A. and REPTA, A. J.: Pharmacokinetics of non-protein bound platinum species following administration or cis-dichlorodiamine platinum (II). Cancer Treat. Rep. *63* (1979), 1515—1523
2. CARTER, S. and WASSERMAN, T. H.: The nitrosoureas — thoughts for the future, Cancer Treat. Rep. *60* (1976), 389—408
3. GUTIN, P. and WILSON, C. B.: Modern concepts in brain tumour therapy. Surg. Neurol. *8* (1977), 392—396
4. HILDEBRAND, J., BRIHAYE, J., WAGENKNECHT, L., MICHEL, J. and KENIS, Y.: Combination chemotherapy with CCNU, vincristin and methotrexate in primary and metastatic brain tumours. Eur. J. Cancer *11* (1979), 585—588
5. HIRANO, S. and MATSUI, T.: Vascular structures in brain tumours. Human Pathol. *6* (1975), 611—621
6. KHAN, A., McCULLOUGH, D., BORTS, F. and SINKS, L. F.: Update on use of cis platinum in CNS malignancies. ASCO Abstracts (1979), 326
7. KHAN, A., McCULLOUGH, D., BORTS, F. and SINKS, L. F.: Update on use of cis platinum in CNS-malignancies. ASCO Abstracts (1980), 390
8. KOLARIĆ, K. and ROTH, A.: Treatment of metastatic brain tumours with the combination of 1-methyl-1-nitrosourea (MNU) and cyclophosphamide. J. Cancer Res. Clin. Oncol. *97* (1980), 193—198
9. LEVIN, V. A., HOFFMAN, V. F., PISCHER, T. K., SEAGER, M. L., BOLDREY, E. B. and WILSON, C.: BCNU-5-fluorouracil combination chemotherapy for recurrent malignant brain tumours. Cancer Treat. Rep. *62* (1978), 2071—2076
10. LITTERST, C. L., LEROY, A. F. and GUARINO, A. M.: Disposition and distribution of platinum following parenteral administration of cis dichlorodiamine platinum (II) to animals. Cancer Treat. Rep. *63* (1979), 1485—1493
11. PINEDO, H. M. (1979): Cancer Chemotherapy, Amsterdam, Excerpta Medica, pp. 107—124
12. SEIFERT, W., CAPRIOLI, R., BENJAMIN, R. and HESTER, J. P.: Energy dispersive X-ray fluorescence determination of platinum in plasma, urine and cerebrospinal fluid of patients administered cis dichlorodiamine platinum (DDP). AACR Abstracts (1979), 168
13. SHAPIRO, W. R., POSNER, J. B., USHIO, Y., CHERNIK, N. and YOUNG, D. F.: Treatment of meningeal neoplasmas. Cancer Treat. Rep. *61* (1977), 733—743
14. STAQUET, M. J. (1978): Randomized Trial in Cancer: A Critical Review by Site, New York, Raven Press, pp. 377—390
15. STEWART, D. J., BENVENUTO, J. A., LEAVENS, M., HALL, S. W., BENJAMIN, R. S., PLUNKETT, W., McCREDIE, K. B., BURGESS, M. A. and Ti Li Loo: Penetration of 3-deazauridine into human brain, intracerebral tumour and cerebrospinal fluid. Cancer Res. *39* (1979), 4119—4122
16. WHO: WHO Handbook for Reporting Results of Cancer Treatment. Antitumour Drug Ther. Rep. *6* (1980), 31—61

Institute of Oncology, Bologna, Italy

Adriamycin: Experimental Evidence of Carcinogenicity

P. Chieco and C. Maltoni

Adriamycin (ADM), an antibiotic originally derived from a culture of *Streptomyces peucetius* (Arcamone et al, 1969), has been one of the most widely used drugs for the prevention of recurrences in patients with resectable neoplasms (adjuvant therapy). In particular, children with Wilms' tumours, osteosarcomas and rhabdomyosarcomas, and adults with bronchogenic carcinomas, breast cancer and gastric and testicular tumours, have been treated with ADM, alone or in combination with other antiblastic compounds, mainly to prevent the development of metastases (Bonadonna et al, 1978). Since, after surgery either with or without adjuvant therapy, such patients often have a long survival, consideration must be taken of the adverse effects, particularly chronic effects such as toxicity and carcinogenicity, of antiblastic drugs.

ADM is known to cause severe cardiomyopathy; moreoever, it has been reported to induce malignant transformation and mutagenesis in cell cultures, and to produce genetic toxicity in humans (Price et al, 1975; Marquard et al, 1976; Picciano, 1979). Drugs in adjuvant therapy — several alkylating agents, antimetabolites and antibiotics — have been proven to be carcinogenic in experimental rodents (Schmähl and Habs, 1978).

The carcinogenic effects of ADM have been studied in long-term carcinogenic bioassays on rats in our laboratory (Maltoni and Chieco, 1975; Chieco, 1979) and in those of others (Bertolazzi et al, 1971; Marquard et al, 1976; Solcia et al 1979; Bucciarelli, 1981). In the studies performed in other laboratories, ADM was administered intravenously to rats, and the surviving animals were sacrificed one year after treatment. In those studies, mammary carcinomas were the only tumours correlated to ADM treatment (Table 1). Only the report of Solcia et al (1979) showed significant positive results. The importance of Bucciarelli's data (1981) is reduced by

Table 1.

Long-term bioassays performed in other laboratories of intravenously administered adriamycin in virgin female Sprague-Dawley rats

Reference	Dose (mg/kg)	Animals with mammary carcinomas	
		Treated	Controls
Bertazzoli et al (1971)	8	1/25	0/25
Marquard et al (1976)	5	3/17	2/20
Solcia et al (1979)	8	10/63	0/31
Bucciarelli (1981)	10	10/35	5/38
	5	16/24	5/38

292

the high incidence of mammary carcinomas in the controls, and by the fact that the incidence of the malignancies is evaluated on the basis of the total number of mammary carcinomas, and not of the number of mammary carcinoma-bearing animals. (It is known that one rat can bear multiple mammary malignant tumours.)

The carcinogenic potential of ADM was tested in our laboratory by a single subcutaneous injection. This method of testing is valid for chemicals that are eliminated from the injection site slowly enough to allow carcinogenic properties to express themselves (PEACOCK et al, 1949). The incidence, prevalence, histologic type and grading of the tumours arising at the site of injection are indications of the carcinogenic properties of the compound being tested. Preliminary results of these experiments were reported previously (MALTONI and CHIECO, 1975; CHIECO, 1979).

Material and methods

Male and female, 13-week-old Sprague-Dawley rats were used. The animals were separated by sex and distributed at random in two groups, one treated and one control. They were housed in solid-bottom Makrolon cages, with stainless-steel wire tops and had hardwood shavings for bedding. Each cage contained five animals. Temperature was maintained at $22-24$ °C, with a relative humidity of $60-70\%$. Drinking-water and diet (of the standard type used in our laboratory) were given ad libitum.

The injections were made into the subcutaneous tissue of the anterior right flank, after local shaving. Test animals were injected with 1 ml of a freshly made $2^0/_{00}$ w/v suspension of ADM chlorohydrate from Farmitalia (Milan, Italy) in olive oil (Olearia Toscana, Florence, Italy), corresponding to a dose of 8 mg/kg bw ADM. In preliminary experiments, this dose caused no general toxic effects; only a mild inflammatory reaction was seen at the site of injection, which decreased gradually, within three weeks, to a small subcutaneous nodule ($2-5$ mm in diameter), barely detectable by clinical examination. Control animals were injected similarly with 1 ml of olive oil.

Animals were observed two to three times daily, and examined clinically every two weeks for pathological lesions. They were weighed every four weeks during the first 40 weeks, and then every eight weeks. All detectable pathological lesions, and especially those at the site of injection, were recorded. The latent period of tumours was considered to be the time between injection and early observation of a neoplasia. In general, all animals were kept under observation up to spontaneous death. Only in a few instances were rats with massive tumours killed when moribund.

A complete autopsy was performed on each animal. Specimens for histological examination were taken from reactive nodules around injected material (two specimens), tumour masses (at least three specimens), thymus, lungs, liver, spleen, left kidney, testes and any other pathological organ. The specimens were fixed in alcohol, and sections were stained with haematoxylin-eosin and, when necessary, with Mallory, Van Gieson or PAS stains.

The chi-Square, Fisher exact test and actuarial method (PIKE and ROE, 1963) were adopted for analysis of tumour incidence and survival. Weight gain was analysed by linear regression. Mammary tumour latencies were compared by the two-sample Wilcoxon test (ARMITAGE, 1971). Values expressed as mean $\pm$ SE ($\bar{x}$); '50% survival time' is the number of weeks at which 50% of rats were still alive. The doubling time of tumours was calculated using measurements of tumour diameters taken at two weeks (starting point) and at four weeks (end point) from their appearance, since during that interval tumour size was not too small to be measured and masses were not ulcerated. For calculation, BLUM's correction (1944) was applied to the exponential function.

Results

The results are shown in Table 2. The higher mortality that can be observed in the treated group was due to the onset of tumours at the site of injection.

Table 2.
Incidences of tumours in Sprague-Dawley rats 107 weeks after receiving a single subcutaneous injection of 2 mg of adriamycin (ADM) in 1 ml of olive oil at 13 weeks of age

Treat-ment	Animals			Animals with tumours											
				Local sarcomas			Mammary tumours				Other tumours				
							Total		Average latency (weeks)	Malig-nant %^{a}	Total	Benign	Malignant		Types
	Sex	No.	50% survival (weeks)	No.	%	Average latency (weeks)	No.	%			No.	No.	No.	%	
ADM 2 mg in 1 ml of olive oil	M	40	60	31	78	40 ± 1	3	7.5	56 ± 9^b	0	1	1	0	—	1 pheochromocy-toma
	F	42	60	24	57	41 ± 3	22	52	52 ± 5^b	9	6	3	3	7	1 dermal angio-sarcoma 1 lung carcino-sarcoma 1 adrenal adenoma 1 kidney carcinoma 2 uterine angiomas
	M and F	82	60	55	67	40 ± 2	25	30	53 ± 4^b	8	7	4	3	4	

Olive oil alone (controls)	M	40	100	0	—	—	8	20	89 ± 9	12.5	5	4	1	2.5	3 meningiomas 1 oligodendroglioma 1 leukaemia
	F	40	104	0	—	—	24	60	73 ± 5	27	5	1	4	10	1 Zymbal gland carcinoma 1 rhabdomyosarcoma of the arm 1 uterine leoimyo-sarcoma 1 meningioma 1 leukaemia
	M and F	80	102	0	—	—	32	40	77 ± 5	22	10	5	5	6	

[a] to total mammary-tumour-bearing animals with respect

[b] p < 0.01 when compared with the corresponding control group

Linear regression analysis showed a significant (p < 0.01) decrease in weight gain up to 60 weeks of age in male treated rats, when compared with matched controls. No such difference was observed in females.

The reactive subcutaneous nodules around the injection site were studied microscopically in animals without tumours which died between 21—105 weeks after treatment. The deposits of ADM are easily recognizable within the reactive tissue by the bright orange-red colour of the compound. At 21 weeks, the nodule appeared to be composed of a capsule of reactive tissue surrounding a core made of crypts, separated by hyalinotic collagen trabecula, containing the oil solution of ADM and homogeneous protein material with calcium deposits. The reactive tissue is made up of more or less mature fibrogenic cells, reticular and collagen fibres, macrophages (often containing granules of ADM), and many regenerative rhabdomyoblasts (originating from the panniculus carnosus) (Fig. 1, 2).

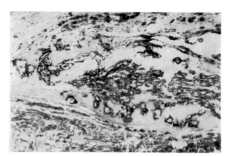

Fig. 1. Fibrous and rhabdomyoblastic cell reaction at the site of subcutaneous injection of adriamycin in oil. H.-E. × 80.

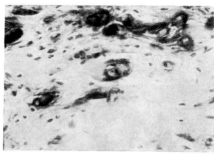

Fig. 2. A detail of Figure 1 showing regenerating rhabdomyoblastic cells. H.-E. × 520.

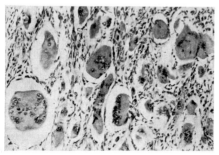

Fig. 3. Regenerating rhabdomyoblstic cells within a subcutaneous tumour arising at the site of the injection of adriamycin. H.-E. × 200.

After 40 weeks, no ADM deposits were found. From 21 weeks the reactive tissue gradually became more and more fibrotic: the collagen fibres grew more thickly and were more closely packed, and the number of fibroblasts and macrophages decreased. Regenerative rhabdomyoblasts were then also found within the sarcomas arising at the site of the injection (Fig. 3).

The incidence and frequency distribution of sarcomas at the site of injection, and of mammary tumours and other types of neoplasia are shown in Table 2 and Figure 4.

In the experimental group, 78% of males and 57% of females developed tumours at the injection site, starting at 19 weeks after treatment. Nearly 90% of the local tumours were diagnosed as rhabdomyosarcomas, with various degrees of differentiation (SAXÉN, 1953; MALTONI, unpublished data) (Fig. 5—8). Some of these tumours metastasized to the lungs (Fig. 9) and to local nodes. Three of the local tumours were fibrosarcomas, one was a neurinosarcoma (arising after 103 weeks), and the others

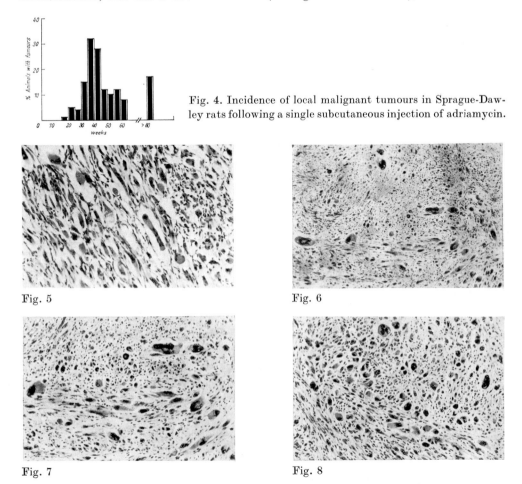

Fig. 4. Incidence of local malignant tumours in Sprague-Dawley rats following a single subcutaneous injection of adriamycin.

Fig. 5

Fig. 6

Fig. 7

Fig. 8

Fig. 5. Well-differentiated rhabdomyosarcoma at the site of injection of adriamycin. H.-E. ×200

Fig. 6. Rhabdomyosarcoma at the site of the injection of adriamycin. H.-E. × 130.

Fig. 7. A detail of Figure 6. H.-E. × 200.

Fig. 8. Rhabdomyosarcoma at the site of the injection of adriamycin. H.-E. × 200.

presented the pattern of mixed mesodermal sarcomas with histiocytic, fibroblastic and myoblastic elements.

Latency for all local sarcomas ranged from 19 to 65 weeks, with a mean of 42 ± 2; the mean latency for rhabdomyosarcomas was 37 ± 1 weeks. The frequency distribution curve for local tumours shows a high concentration around the mean, with a kurtosis at 12.25. With the exception of the late-arising neurinosarcoma, the tumours originating at the site of the injection were rapidly growing sarcomas with a mean doubling time of 8.8 ± 0.7 days. No significant differences were found when the latency and the growing rate of different types of sarcomas were compared.

In nearly 90% of the animals bearing sarcomas at the site of injection, death occurred from cachexia due to the presence of tumour masses (which in several instances reached a volume greater than 80 cm³). In only seven animals that died with local sarcomas was the tumour mass too small to account for death.

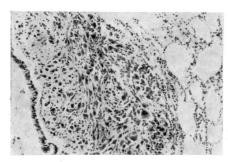

Fig. 9. Pulmonary metastasis of a rhabdomyosarcoma following injection of adriamycin. H.-E. × 200.

The higher incidence and higher final malignant:benign ratio of mammary tumours in the control group are due to the earlier high mortality of treated rats, caused by local sarcomas. However, the latency of mammary tumours in experimental animals was significantly ($p < 0.01$) less than that in matched controls (Table 2) and in a group of historical controls in our laboratory. At the 53rd week, which represents the mean latency of mammary tumours in the experimental group, only five matched controls had developed mammary lumps.

Tumours other than sarcomas at the site of injection and mammary neoplasias were observed in all groups. They were of the types usually observed in untreated animals of the strain used. The slightly higher incidence of these tumours in the control group may again be explained by their longer survival.

Discussion

The potency of ADM in causing subcutaneous sarcomas in rats may be compared with that one of the most potent carcinogenic polycyclic aromatic hydrocarbons. The simple formula of IBALL (1939) — $K = N_t/L_t$ — can be used to compare the relative power of carcinogens, particularly in those long-term animal bioassays in which the same tumour type is produced (as in the case of local sarcomas in the subcutaneous test). In the above equation, N_t represents the incidence of local sarcomas, L_t the latency expressed in days, and K an arbitrary carcinogenic index. In the experiment reported here, the K value was 0.2. K values for comparable doses of dibenzanthracene, benzopyrene and methylcholanthrene, using the same subcutaneous test (DUNNING et al, 1940; ROUSSY et al, 1942; MALTONI, unpublished data) ranged from 0.12 to 0.33.

Other parameters which demonstrate the strong carcinogenic activity of ADM, are the homogeneity of tumour types (nearly 90% of the local sarcomas were rhabdomyosarcomas), the concentration of the latency of these tumours around the mean (56% of local sarcomas arose between 35 and 45 weeks) (Fig. 4), and, finally, the decreased latency of the mammary tumours (Table 2).

Under our experimental conditions, ADM appears to be carcinogenic mainly towards rhabdomyoblasts. This observation is of particular interest in view of the selective cardiac toxicity shown by ADM in humans, as well as in rats (LEFRAK et al, 1973; OLSON and CAPEN, 1978).

References

1. ARCAMONE, F., CASSINELLI, G., FANTINI, G., GREIN, A., OREZZI, P., POL, C. and SPALLA, C.: Adriamycin, 14 hydroxydaunomycin, a new antitumour antibiotic from *Streptomcyes peucetius* var. caesius. Biotechnol. Bioeng. *11* (1969), 1101—1110
2. ARMITAGE, P. (1971): Statistical Methods in Medical Research, Oxford, Blackwell Scientific Publications
3. BERTAZZOLI, C., CHIELI, T. and SOLCIA, E.: Different incidence of breast carcinomas or fibroadenomas in daunomycin or adriamycin treated rats. Experientia *27* (1971), 1209—1210
4. BLUM, H. F.: Estimation of growth rates of tumours. J. Natl. Cancer Inst. *4* (1944), 21—24
5. BONADONNA, G., TANCINI, G., ROSSI, A. and GASPARINI, M.: Chemotherapy in prevention of the recurrence of resectable cancer. Ann. Rev. Med. *29* (1978), 149—175
6. BUCIARELLI, E.: Mammary tumour induction in male and female Sprague-Dawley rats by adriamycin and daunomycin. J. Natl. Cancer Inst. *66* (1981), 81—84
7. CHIECO, P. (1979): Adriamycin: subcutaneous carcinogenicity in rodents. In: Annual Meeting, Southwestern Section, American Association for Cancer Research, Albuquerque, November 16—17
8. DUNNING, W. F., CURTIS, M. R. and EISEN, J. J.: The carcinogenic activity of methylcholanthrene in rats. Am. J. Cancer *40* (1940), 85—127
9. IBALL, J. (1939): The relative potency of carcinogenic compounds. Am. J. Cancer *35* (1939), 188—190
10. LEFRAK, E. A., PITHA, J., ROSENHEIM, S. and GOTTLIEB, J. A.: A clinicopathologic analysis of adriamycin cardiotoxicity. Cancer *32* (1973), 302—314
11. MALTONI, C. and CHIECO, P.: Adriamicina: un nuovo potente cancerogeno. Osp. Vita *2/6* (1975), 107—109
12. MARQUARD, H., PHILIPS, F. S. and STENBERG, S. S.: Tumorigenicity in vivo and induction of malignant transformation and mutagenesis in cell cultures by adriamycin and daunomycin. Cancer Res. *36* (1976), 2065—2069
13. OLSON, H. M. and CAPEN, C. C.: Chronic cardiotoxicity of doxorubicin (adrimycin) in the rat: morphologic and biochemical investigations. Toxicol. Appl. Pharmacol. *44* (1978), 605—616
14. PEACOCK, P. R., BECK, S. and ANDERSON, W.: The influence of solvents on tissue response to carcinogenic hydrocarbons. Br. J. Cancer *3* (1949), 296—305
15. PICCIANO, D. (1979): Communication at the 4th Annual Course in the Principle and Practice of Genetic Toxicology, Galveston, October 22—26
16. PIKE, M. C. and ROE, F. J.: An actuarial method of analysis of an experiment in two-stage carcinogenesis. Br. J. Cancer *17* (1963), 605—610
17. PRICE, P. J., SUK, W. A. and SKEEN, P. C.: Transforming potential of the anticancer drug adriamycin. Science *187* (1975), 1200—1201
18. ROUSSY, G., GUERIN, M. and GUÉRIN, P.: Comparison de quelques hydrocarbures cancérigènes au point du vue de leur activité. C. R. Sci. Soc. Biol. *136* (1942), 374—375
19. SAXÉN, E. A.: On the factor of age in the production of subcutaneous sarcomas in mice by 20 methylcholanthrene. J. Natl. Cancer Inst. *14* (1953), 547—569
20. SCHMÄHL, D. and HABS, M.: Experimental carcinogenesis of antitumour drugs. Cancer Treat. Rev. *5* (1978), 175—184
21. SOLCIA, E., BALLERINI, L., BELLINI, O., SALA, L. and BERTAZZOLI, C.: Mammary tumours induced in rats by adriamycin and daunomycin. Cancer Res. *38* (1979), 1444—1446

Istituto di Farmacologia della Università degli Studi di Bologna, Italy

Electroreduction, Mutagenicity and Antimicrobial Activity of 5-Nitroimidazole Derivatives

G. Aicardi, G. Cantelli Forti, M. C. Guerra, A. M. Barbaro and G. L. Biagi

The nitroimidazoles, which have been used frequently as chemotherapeutic agents in human and veterinary medicine (1, 2), were introduced more recently in the therapy of noeplastic disease. It has been shown that they sensitize hypoxic cells to the lethal effects of ionizing radiation (3); however, for that particular use, large amounts of drug are required, increasing the risk of toxic effects. Several of these compounds have mutagenic activity and some of them are weak carcinogens. Although the mechanism of the cytotoxic and mutagenic action of the nitroimidazoles is still under investigation, it is generally assumed that their activities are dependent on a mechanism of action which proceeds first through a reduction of the nitrogroup and then through an interaction of highly reactive derivatives, possibly by binding to DNA and other biopolymers (4).

Edwards et al (5) have demonstrated that reduction of the nitrogroup is a necessary step in the action of the 5-nitroimidazoles against anaerobic bacteria such as *Clostridium* and *protozoa* such as *Trichomonas vaginalis*. A relationship between antibacterial activity and electroreduction has been discussed by Chien et al (6). Adams et al (7) pointed out a relationship between one-electron reduction potential and efficiency as a radiosensitizer. Chien et al (8) studied the influence of one-electron attachment potential on the mutagenic activity of nitrocompounds.

The purpose of the present work was to investigate whether the redox process plays a role in the mutagenicity of 25 nitroimidazoles and of two nitrothiazole derivatives, in view of the finding that the mutagenic and antibacterial activities of nitroimidazoles are intimately related at the molecular level (1).

The details of the mutagenic and antibacterial assay will be published elsewhere (9).

Material and methods

The structural formulae of the compounds tested are given in Table 1. While nimorazole, metronidazole, tinidazole and azanidazole are commercial drugs used to treat infections due to anaerobic protozoa and bacteria, the D A and M Y series include derivatives synthesized as radiosensitizers. Mutagenic activitiy was determined by means of the Ames test in *Salmonella typhimurium* TA100 strain (10, 11). Antimicrobial activity was assayed against the same microorganism by means of the cylinder-plate method (12). The electroreduction potential of all 27 compounds was determined at pH 7.4 by means of cyclic voltametry, using a mercury-dropping electrode *versus* a saturated calomel electrode (13). Only peaks between -200 and -900 mV were considered.

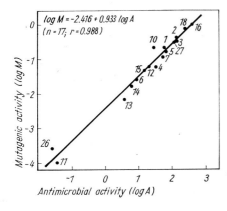

Fig. 1. Relationship between mutagenic and antibacterial activity of 15 nitroimidazoles and two nitrothiazole derivatives (25, 26).

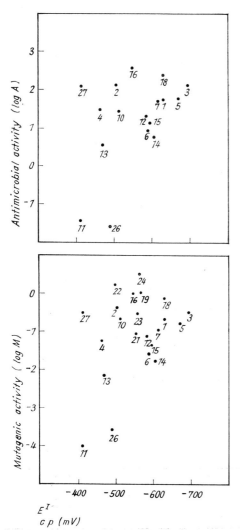

Fig. 2. Relationship between antimicrobial activity and electroreduction potential (E_{cp}^{I}) and between mutagenic activity and E_{cp}^{I}.

301

Table 1.
Biological activies and electroreduction potential for 25 nitroimidazoles and two nitrothiazole derivatives

Compound

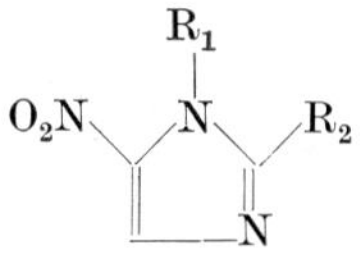

$$O_2N \quad \overset{R_1}{\underset{N}{\overset{N}{\diamond}}} R_2$$

No.	Name	R_1	R_2
1	1-[α-(chloromethyl)- -hydroxyethyl]-2-me- thyl-5-nitroimidazole (Ornidazole)	CH_2Cl $\mid$ $CH—CH_2OH$	$—CH_3$
2	1-(2-N-morpholinyl- ethyl)-5-nitroimidazole (Nimorazole)	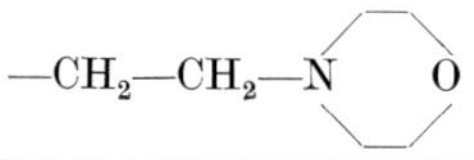 $—CH_2—CH_2—N\bigcirc O$	$—H$
3	1-(2-hydroxyethyl)-2- -methyl-5-nitroimidazole (Metronidazole)	$—CH_2—CH_2OH$	$—CH_3$
4	1-methyl-2-formyl-5- -nitroimidazole	$—CH_3$	$—CHO$
5	1-[2-(ethylsulfonyl)- -ethyl]-2-methyl-5- -nitroimidazole (Tinidazole)	$—CH_2—CH_2—SO_2—CH_2—CH_3$	$—CH_3$
6	1-methyl-2-[(carbamoyl- oxy)-methyl]-5-nitro- imidazole (Ronidazole)	$—CH_3$	$—CH_2OOCNH_2$
7	1-methyl-2-hydroxy- methyl-5-nitroimidazole	$—CH_3$	$—CH_2OH$
8	2-methyl-5-nitro- imidazole	$—H$	$—CH_3$
9	5-nitroimidazole	$—H$	$—H$
10	1-(2-ethylcarbamothioic acid O-methyl ester)-2- -methyl-5-nitroimida- zole (Carnidazole)	$—CH_2—CH_2—NH—\overset{\underset{\|}{S}}{C}—OCH_3$	$—CH_3$
11	1-methyl-2-(2-amino-4- -ethinyl-pyrimidine)- -5-nitroimidazole (Azanidazole)	$—CH_3$	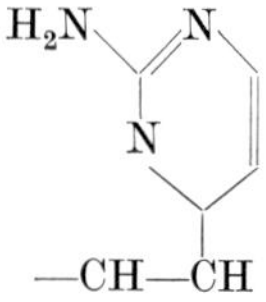 $H_2N\diagdown{\underset{N}{\overset{N}{\diamond}}}$ $—CH—CH$
12	1-methyl-2-(1-methyl- ethyl)-5-nitro- imidazole (Ipronidazole)	$—CH_3$	$—CH{<}{\overset{CH_3}{\underset{CH_3}{}}}$

302

Mutagenic assay				Antimicrobial assay				E_{cp}^{I} (mV)[c]
log dose/effect equation			log M[a]	log dose/effect equation			log A[b]	
a	b	r		a	b	r		
−85.23	38.80	1.000	−0.680	8.28	12.40	0.998	1.752	−630
−38.19	16.46	0.976	−0.380	3.35	12.49	0.999	2.120	−505
−67.25	28.90	1.000	−0.500	3.74	12.35	0.998	2.126	−695
−43.19	27.33	0.998	−1.237	11.30	12.64	0.985	1.498	−465
−69.26	33.58	1.000	−0.790	9.46	11.47	0.989	1.791	−670
−53.32	41.19	1.000	−1.580	18.61	12.30	0.997	0.928	−590
−20.67	12.52	0.993	−0.951	7.73	13.02	0.998	1.710	−615
—	—	—	—	—	—	—	—	−790
—	—	—	—	—	—	—	—	−760
−97.85	44.09	1.000	−0.670	7.42	15.68	0.997	1.440	−515
34.31	29.60	0.980	−3.991	48.55	12.87	0.997	−1.439	−410
−53.62	31.31	0.992	−1.131	12.78	13.24	0.998	1.300	−585

Compound

$$\begin{array}{c} R^1 \\ O_2N \diagdown \ N \diagup R_2 \\ N \end{array}$$

No.	Name	R₁	R₂
13	DA 3832	$-CH_2-CH_2OH$	$-CH=CH-$ (benzene ring with methylenedioxy, $O\diagdown CH_2\diagup O$)
14	MY 40/20	$-CH_2-CH_2-SO_2CH_3$	$-CH_3$
15	DA 3851	$-CH_3$	$-CH\diagup$ (cyclopropyl, CH_2–CH_2)
16	DA 3804	$-CH_3$	$-CH_2-N\diagup\diagdown N-CH_3$ (piperazine)
17	DA 3829	$-CH_2-\overset{OH}{\underset{\vert}{CH}}-CH_2-N\big\langle{}^{CH_2CH_3}_{CH_2CH_3}$	$-CH_3$
18	DA 3838	$-CH_2-\overset{OH}{\underset{\vert}{CH}}-CH_2OH$	$-CH_3$
19	DA 3831	$-CH_3$	$-CH=C\big\langle{}^{COOH}_{O-}$ (O–phenyl)
20	DA 3837	$-CH_2-CH_2-OSO_3Na$	$-CH_3$
21	DA 3839	$-CH_2-CO-NH-$ (pyrimidine ring, N, N)	$-CH_3$
22	DA 3840	$-CH_2-CO-N\diagup\diagdown N-CO-CH_2$ (piperazine); O_2N, CH_3, imidazole/pyrrole N	$-CH_3$
23	DA 38 53	$-CH_2-\overset{OH}{\underset{\vert}{CH}}-CH_2-N\diagup\diagdown N$ with CH_3 and O_2N (nitroimidazole)	$-CH_3$
24	DA 3854	$-CH_2-CH_2-O-CH_2-CH_2-N\big\langle{}^{CH_2CH_3}_{CH_2CH_3}$	$-CH_3$

| Mutagenic assay | | | | Antimicrobial assay | | | | E_{cp}^{I} (mV)[c] |
| log dose/effect equation | | | log M[a] | log dose/effect equation | | | log A[b] | |
a	b	r		a	b	r		
−23.89	34.34	0.977	−2.161	23.01	12.59	0.990	0.555	−470
−38,18	34.83	0.973	−1.759	20.40	12.57	0.996	0.763	−605
−57.88	37.50	0.964	−1.320	14.48	13.54	0.982	1.146	−597
−8.69	4.55	1.000	0.000	1.87	11.63	0.996	2.570	−550
—	—	—	—	—	—	—	—	−545
−12.52	6.07	0.997	−0.120	−4.29	14.43	0.996	2.376	−630
−4.25	3.06	0.999	0.030	—	—	—	—	−568
—	—	—	—	—	—	—	—	−712
−51.44	28.69	0.996	−1.030	—	—	—	—	−555
−44.22	15.30	1.000	0.220	—	—	—	—	−500
−37.63	17.37	1.000	−0.550	—	—	—	—	−560
−21.95	7.67	1.000	0.510	—	—	—	—	−565

Compound		

O$_2$N, N—R$_1$, R$_2$, N (fused ring structure)

No.	Name	R$_1$	R$_2$
25	DA 3915	—CH$_2$—CH$_2$—N⟨ ⟩N—CH$_3$	—H
26	1-(5-nitro-2-thiazolyl)--2-imidazolidinone (Niridazole)	O$_2$N—S—N structure with O, N, H imidazolidinone	
27	2-amino-5-(*p*-nitro-phenyl sulfonyl)--thiazole	O$_2$N—⟨ ⟩—S(=O)(=O)—S, NH$_2$ thiazole	

[a] M, concentration (mM/l) that increases the number of revertants by five fold
[b] A, concentration (mM/l) giving an inhibition diameter of 30 mm
[c] E_{cp}^I, electroreduction potential determined at pH 7.4 by means of cyclic voltametry using a mercury dropping electrode *vs* a saturated calomel electrode

Results and discussion

Dose-effect relationships were shown for most of the compounds under study, in both the mutagenic and antibacterial assays. From the equations describing the linear relationship between the log dose and the mutagenic or antibacterial effect (given in Table 1), it was possible to calculate for each compound the concentration that caused a five-fold increase in the number of revertants in the Ames test and which gave an inhibition diameter of 30 mm in the antibacterial assay. The relative potencies in the mutagenic and antibacterial assays showed a close correlation (Fig. 1), supporting the hypothesis that the two activities occur via the same mechanism.

The eletroreduction potentials (E_{cp}^I) at pH 7.4 were between -790 and -410 mV. The E_{cp}^I for metronidazole was -695 mV, a value fairly close to that of about -623 mV calculated at the same pH by CHIEN et al (6).

In Figure 2, E_{cp}^I values are plotted against antibacterial and against mutagenic activity. The compounds most active in the mutagenic assay, i. e., azanidazole, niridazole and DA 3832, are those with the least negative electroreduction values; and compounds no. 8 and no. 9, for which no mutagenic effect could be determined, have the most negative electroreduction values. This finding indicates that all active compounds must be reducible and that reductive biotransformation is an essential step in their mechanism of action; and in *S. typhimurium*, reduction of the nitro group is carried out by a reductase. However, compounds no. 4 and no. 27, which had electroreduction values similar to those of compounds no. 11, 26 and 13, were much less active; and

Mutagenic assay				Antimicrobial assay				E_{cp}^I (mV)[c]
log dose/effect equation			log M[a]	log dose/effect equation			log A[b]	
a	b	r		a	b	r		
—	—	—	—	—	—	—	—	−543
11.15	10.66	0.970	−3.577	49.63	12.15	0.995	−1.587	−490
−15.83	8.38	0.973	−0.514	7.15	10.80	0.992	2.084	−415

the remaining compounds showed a large scattering of E_{cp}^I values. Thus, significant relationship was seen between E_{cp}^I values and mutagenic activity.

The same was true with regard to the antibacterial activity. These results are in substantial agreement with those of CHIEN et al (8).

Thus the reduction step is necessary but is not sufficient to explain the mechanism of action of nitroimidazoles, and it must be concluded that other properties of these molecules play a major role in determining the interaction of the reduced products with cell components.

In particular, an important role might be played by the lipophilic character of the molecules; this is evident in the chromatographic R_m values, which have been determined in our laboratory (14). Structure-activity relationships indicated the influence of lipophilic character and of the electronegativity of the R_1 groups for antischistosomal and antiprotozoal activity (15, 16); and frontier electron density is important in the protein binding of metronidazole derivatives (17).

We are now undertaking a multiple regression analysis of the R_m values and other physico-chemical parameters in order to obtain a better correlation with mutagenic or antibacterial activity.

Acknowledgement

We are grateful to Professor A. BRECCIA and his coworkers for help in the determination of the E_{cp}^I values.

References

1. BAMBURY, E. R. (1979): Synthetic antibacterial agents. In: WOLFF, M. E., ed., Burger's Medical Chemistry, part II, New York, John Wiley & Sons, p. 63
2. ROSS, W. J. (1979): Antiamebic agents. In: WOLFF, M. E., ed., Burger's Medical Chemistry, parts II, New York, John Wiley & Sons, p. 428
3. BRECCIA, A., RIMONDI, C. and ADAMS, G. E. (1979): Radiosensitizers of Hypoxid Cells, Amsterdam, Elsevier/North-Holland
4. LINDMARK, D. G. and MULLER, M.: Antitrichomonas action, mutagenicity and reduction of metronidazole and other nitroimidazoles. Antimicrob. Agents Chemother. *10* (1976), 476
5. EDWARDS, D. I., DYE, M. and CARNE, H.: The selective toxicity of antimicrobial nitroheterocyclic drugs. J. Gen. Microbiol. *76* (1973), 135
6. CHIEN, Y. W. and MIZUBA, S. S.: Activity-electroreduction relationship of antimicrobial metronidazole analogues. J. Med. Chem. *21* (1978), 374
7. ADAMS, G. E., FLOCKHART, I. R., SMITHEN, C. E., STRATFORD, I. J., WARDMAN, P. and WATTS, M. E.: Electron-affinic sensitization. VII. A correlation between structures, one-electron reduction potentials, and efficiencies of nitroimidazoles as hypoxic cell radiosensitizers. Radiat. Res. *67* (1976), 9
8. CHIEN, J. B., SHEININ, D. H. K. and RANTH, A. M.: Screening for the mutagenicity of nitrogroup containing hypoxic cell radiosensitizers using *Salmonella typhimurium* strain TA-100 and TA-98. Mutat. Res. *58* (1978), 1
9. CANTELLI FORTI, G., AICARDI, G., GUERRA, M. C., BARBARO, A. M. and BIAGI, G. L.: Mutagenicity of 25 nitroimidazoles and 2 nitrothiazoles in *Salmonella typhimurium*. Terat. Carc. Mutag. (Submitted for publication)
10. AMES, B. N., LEE, F. D. and DURSTON, W. E.: An improved bacterial test system for the detection and classification of mutagens and carcinogens. Proc. Natl. Acad. Sci. USA *70* (1973), 782
11. AMES, B. N., MCCANN, J. C. and YAMASAKI, E.: Method for detecting carcinogens and mutagens with the *Salmonella*/mammalian microsome mutagenicity test. Mutat. Res. *31* (1975), 347
12. GRAVE, D. C. and RANDALL, W. A. (1955): Assay Methods of Antibiotics: A Laboratory Manual, New York, Medical Encyclopedia Inc.
13. BOND, A. M. (1980): Modern Polarographic Methods in Analytical Chemistry, New York, M. Dekker, p. 201
14. GUERRA, M. C., BARBARO, A. M., CANTELLI FORTI, G., FOFFANI, M. T., BIAGI, G. L., BOREA, P. A., and FINI, A.: R_m and log P values of 5-nitroimidazoles. J. Chromatogr. *216* (1981), 93
15. LIN, Y., HULBERT, P. B., BUEDING, E. and ROBINSON, C. N.: Structure and antischistosomal activity in the nitrofurylinyl and the niridazoles series. Noninterchangeability of the nitroheterocyclic rings. J. Med. Chem. *17* (1974), 835
16. MILLER, M. W., HOWES, H. L., KASUBICK, R. V. and ENGLISH, A. R.: Alkylation of 2-methyl-5-nitroimidazole. Some potent antiprotozoal agents. J. Med. Chem. *13* (1970), 849
17. SANVORDEKER, D. R., CHIEN, Y. W., LIN, T. K. and LAMBERT, H. J.: Binding of metronidazole and its derivatives to plasma proteins: an assessment of drug binding phenomenon. J. Pharm. Sci. *64* (1975), 1797

Istituto di Farmacologia and Istituto di Chimica Farmaceutica (*), Università di Trieste, I-34100 Trieste, Italy

Mechanism of the Antileukemic Action of DTIC and its Benzenoid Analog DM-COOK in mice

G. Sava, T. Giraldi, L. Lassiani* and C. Nisi*

Introduction

The imidazole dimethyltriazene DTIC possessess antitumour activity against several rodent transplantable tumours (1), and is also clinically employed against human malignancies (2, 3). The structurally related aryldimethyltriazenes also possess antitumour activity in experimental models, equal or greater than that of DTIC in some instances (4—6). It has been suggested that dimethyltriazenes exert their antitumour effects after conversion to cytotoxic metabolites generated either by proton catalysed hydrolysis, or after oxidative N-demethylation by liver microsomes. The former pathway, which generates diazonium cations, appears of marginal importance since compounds practically resistant to hydrolysis possess antitumour activity when tested in vivo. Connors et al (4) and Abel et al (7), on the other hand, provided evidence suggesting that the conversion to monomethylderivatives may lead to the activation of aryldimethyltriazenes to cytotoxic products.

The aim of this investigation was therefore that of examining the mechanism of the antileukemic action of the dimethyltriazenes, DTIC and p-(3,3-dimethyl-1-triazeno)-benzoic acid potassium salt (DM-COOK), in comparison with cyclophosphamide in mice bearing P 388 leukemia.

Experimental

DM-COOK was synthesized following already reported procedures (8), whereas DTIC and cyclophosphamide were kindly provided by the Drug Synthesis and Chemistry Branch, Division of Cancer Treatment, National Cancer Institute, Bethesda, Md. A first series of experiments was performed in order to determine the increase of survival time and the number of peritoneal tumour cells at the end of treatment. The highest dosage employed is the maximum tolerated one for each drug, and cause a similar body weight reduction of $10-15\%$. All the three substances cause a significant increase of the survival time of the treated animals at the highest dosage used; for DM-COOK and cyclophosphamide a significant prolongation of the life-span is caused also at the lower dosage. DTIC and DM-COOK reduce the number of peritoneal tumour cells only to about $50-75\%$ of that of controls, at 100 and 50 mg/kg respectively, while cyclophosphamide cause the absence of detectable tumour cells in the peritonael cavity of the treated mice at both dose levels emploeyd. In these conditions, the viability of peritoneal tumour cells is unmodified by DTIC and DM-COOK, whereas a significant reduction of clonogenic tumour cells in the brains of the treated animals is

Table 1.
Effects of the treatment of P388 leukemia with DTIC, DM-COOK and cyclophosphamide on the survival time, on the number of peritoneal tumour cells, on their viability and on the presence of clonogenic tumour cells in the brains of the treated mice.

Compound	Dose	Effects on the treated mice		Effects on the bioassay of		
				peritoneal tumour cells	whole brain	
	mg/kg/day	A	B	A	A	C
—	—	12.3 ± 0.3	978 ± 97	12.9 ± 0.5	15.1 ± 0.9	0/11
DTIC	50	14.3 ± 1.1	661 ± 59	12.6 ± 1.1	16.0 ± 1.3	0/5
	100	19.1 ± 2.0*	493 ± 41*	13.7 ± 0.3	18.5	3/5
DM-COOK	50	19.3 ± 0.9*	738 ± 72	12.1 ± 0.5	21.4 ± 2.1*	3/8
	100	21.5 ± 0.8*	517 ± 87*	13.0 ± 0.4	> 120	10/10
Cyclo-phosphamide	12.5	17.5 ± 1.3*	0	ND	> 120	5/5
	25	22.0 ± 0.6*	0	ND	> 120	5/5

A: survival time (days); B: total number of peritoneal tumour cells ($\times 10^6$); C: animals surviving at four months; ND: not determined.
Each value is the mean ± SE obtained in groups of 5—11 BDF1 mice transplanted i. p. with 10^6 P388 tumour cells treated daily on days 1—7 after tumour transplantation. The determination of the total number of peritoneal tumour cells was performed measuring the tumour cell concentration in the ascitic fluid by means of a Coulter Counter, and relating it to the total volume of the ascitic fluid. The experiments on the bioassays have been performed by transplanting 10^6 P388 tumour cells obtained from the peritoneal cavity, or whole brains of the treated animals, i. p. into normal mice whose survival time has been recorded. The statistical analysis performed is the Student-Newman-Keuls Test (15), * means significantly different from the controls ($p = 0.05$).

observed. In particular, DM-COOK at 100 mg/kg causes the absence of clonogenic tumour cells in the brain of all treated animals. For cyclophosphamide, the bioassay of peritoneal tumour cells was not performed because of the absence of tumour cells in the peritoneal cavity at the end of treatment, whereas the transplantation of the brains indicates the absence of clonogenic tumour cells in that organ at both dose levels used.

Discussion

The data reported so far indicate that the antitumour activity of cyclophosphamide is related with a drastic reduction of the number of peritoneal tumour cells, consistent with the growth kinetics of the tumour employed. The prolongation of the survival time and the absence of viable tumour cells in the brains of the animals treated with DTIC and DM-COOK therefore seems to be caused with a mechanism different from a purely cytotoxic effect, since the number and viability of the peritoneal tumour cells is unaffected by the treatment.
Similar experiments have been performed with DTIC and DM-COOK using the TLX5 lymphoma growing in CBA/LAC mice. The results are identical to those obtained with P388 leukemia and confirm that the antileukemic activity of dimethyltriazenes is not due to cytotoxic effects for tumour cells (9).

The presently reported data thus indicate that the treatment of mice bearing P388 leukemia with dimethyltriazenes cause a significant prolongation of the survival time unrelated to cytotoxic effects for tumour cells. The lack of cytotoxic effects on peritoneal tumour cells suggests that the mechanism of the antileukemic action of DTIC and DM-COOK might consist in the prevention of the arrival of tumour cells in crucial organs such as the brain, as observed in the present investigation. It thus seems that dimethyltriazenes such as DTIC and DM-COOK prevent tumour cells dissemination also in leukemic animals, as already observed in mice bearing the solid metastasizing tumour Lewis lung carcinoma (10—12). In this experimental model, dimethyltriazenes proved to prevent lung metastasis formation without any significant cytotoxic effect for tumour cells located either in the subcutaneous tumour or in lung metastases (10, 12).

These findings suggest that the treatment with dimethyltriazenes might be usefully employed in order to prevent tumour infiltration of the central nervous system in leukemic patients, thus overcoming the establishment of tumour reservoirs poorly responsive to chemotherapy with cytotoxic agents (13, 14).

Summary

The antitumour effects of DTIC (Dacarbazine) and p-(3,3-dimethyl-1-triazeno)benzoic acid potassium salt (DM-COOK) have been tested in BDF1 mice bearing P338 leukemia. The treatment performed on days 1—7 after tumour transplantation, significantly increased the life-span of the animals. At the same time, at the end of treatment no significant reduction in the number and viability of peritoneal tumour cells was detected. In these conditions, cyclophosphamide caused the absence of detectable peritoneal tumour cells.

This finding indicates that the antileukemic effects of the triazenes are not due to cytotoxicity for tumour cells, as conversely evidenced for cyclophosphamide. The increased survival time caused by DTIC and DM-COOK might thus be due to the prevention of leukemic cell dissemination, as already observed for a larger series of aryldimethyltriazenes in mice bearing Lewis lung carcinoma. The migration of leukemic cells has been studied by transplanting the brains of tumour bearing animals into normal recipients. The treatment with triazenes caused a significant prolongation in the life-span of these recipients, whereas the survival time of normal mice receiving peritoneal tumour cells from the treated animals was not affected.

These data indicate that the triazenes tested act in leukemic mice inhibiting the invasion of a crucial organ, the brain, rather than exerting cytotoxic effects on tumour cells.

Acknowledgement

This work was supported by a Grant from the University of Trieste, and by Italian National Research Council Special Project 'Control of Neoplastic Growth', contract n° 80.01562.96.

References

1. VENDITTI, J. M.: Antitumour activity of DTIC (NSC-45388) in animals. Cancer Treat. Rep. *60* (1976), 135—140
2. SLAVIK, M.: Clinical studies with DTIC (NSC-45388) in various malignancies. Cancer Treat. Rep. *60* (1976), 213—214
3. RÜMKE, P. (1979): Malignant melanoma. In: "Cancer Chemotherapy", 412—423. Editor: PINEDO, H. M., Excerpta Medica, Amsterdam.

4. CONNORS, T. A., GODDARD, P. M., MERAI, K., ROSS, W. C. J. and WILMAN, D. E. V.: Tumour inhibitory triazenes: structural requirements for an active metabolite. Biochem. Pharmacol. *25* (1976), 241—246

5. GIRALDI, T., NISI, C., CONNORS, T. A. and GODDARD, P. M.: Preparation and antitumour activity of 1-aryl-3,3-dimethyltriazene derivatives. J. Med. Chem. *20* (1977), 850—853

6. GIRALDI, T., GODDARD, P. M., NISI, C. and SIGON, F.: Antitumour activity on hydrazones and adducts between aromatic aldehydes and p-(3,3-dimethyl-1-triazeno)benzoic acid hydrazide. J. Pharm. Sci. *69* (1980), 97—98

7. ABEL, G., CONNORS, T. A. and GIRALDI, T.: In vitro metabolic activation of 1-p-carboxamido-phenyl-3,3-dimethyl triazene to cytotoxic products. Cancer Letters *3* (1977), 259—264

8. KOLAR, G. F.: Synthesis of biologically active triazenes from isolable diazonium salts. Z. Naturforsch. (B) *27* (1972), 1183—1185

9. SAVA, G., GIRALDI, T., CUMAN, R., LASSIANI, L. and NISI, C. (1981): Mechanism of the anti-leukemic actixity of dimethyltriazenes in mice. Proceedings of the 12th International Congress of Chemotherapy, Florence, in press.

10. GIRALDI, T., GUARINO, A. M., NISI, C. and SAVA, G.: Antitumour and antimetastatic effects of benzenoid triazenes in mice bearing Lewis lung carcinoma. Pharmacol. Res. Commun. *12* (1980), 1—11

11. GIRALDI, T., HOUGHTON, P. J., TAYLOR, D. M. and NISI, C.: Antimetastatic action of some triazene derivatives against the Lewis lung carcinoma in mice. Cancer Treat. Rep. *62* (1978), 721—725

12. SAVA, G., GIRALDI, T., LASSIANI, L. and NISI, C.: Mechanism of the antimetastatic action of dimethyltriazenes. Cancer Treat. Rep. *63* (1979), 93—98

13. PERK, K. and PEARSON, J. W.: Me-CCNU in the treatment of an animal analog of meningeal leukemia. Israel J. Med. Sci. *13* (1977), 460—465

14. POUILLART, P., SCHWARZENBERG, L., BELPOMME, D., DE VASSAL, F., HAYAT, M., AMIEL, J. L. and MATHÉ, G.: La prévention des meningites leucemiques. Bull. du Cancer *61* (1974), 403—410

15. SOKAL, R. R. and ROHLF, F. J. (1969): Single classification analysis of variance. In: "Biometry", 204—252. Editor FREEMAN, W. H., San Francisco

312

Laboratory Assessment of Therapeutic Activity

Central Institute of Cancer Research, Academy of Sciences, German Democratic Republic

The Role of In Vitro Techniques in Assessing Antineoplastic Therapeutic Activities

St. Tanneberger and E. Nissen

At present, in vitro techniques are widely used for screening new antineoplastic drugs (40) and for radiobiological studies. In such studies cell lines are acceptable models.

In vitro techniques seem also to be the most promising approach for predicting drug sensitivity of human tumours and for individualizing cancer chemotherapy. For more than 15 years we have stressed the biological individuality of human tumours (52, 55, 56), which demands individualized, biologically-adapted cancer treatment. This has been proved both on a clinical and a cell biological level (59).

Efforts to predict the drug sensitivity of human tumours by the use of in vitro investigation of biopsy material date back to 1955 when Cobb studied the effect of TEM against human tumours in plasma clot cultures. Later, using new methodological approaches the groups of Limburg (28), Ambrose (2) and others, continued the pioneer work in this field. Our own studies on human tumour drug sensitivity prediction began in 1964.

The history of predictive tests

The long history of predictive tests has been repeatedly reviewed (6, 40, 53, 60) and is summarized in Table 1, where the most important predictive tests are classified.

The history of predictive tests is characterized by a very optimistic beginning of some groups in the early sixties with relatively insufficient methodology (monolayer or plasma clot cultures with morphological evaluation of drug effects).

Later on, every advance in tissue culture techniques and biochemistry (organ culture, metabolic monitoring of cultures) has been used to elaborate effective in vitro predictive tests, but in spite of that, no final solution ot the problem has been achieved. As can be seen in Table 1, but majority of authors evaluated their assays very positive, but the fact that, up to now, no assay achieved general clinical application is evidence enough that, often, the evaluation was overoptimistic. This tendency seems also to be true for the in vitro soft-agar human tumour stem cell assay which has been strongly recommended during the last few years (15), and which received a very precise and realistic evaluation by Rupniak and Hill (46).

Our own experiences of the use of in vitro methods to predict tumour response to antineoplastic chemotherapy are quite similar to the described international situation. In 1964 we started very optimistically with a cell culture technique, evaluating drug effects by morphological criteria. Cultivating some hundred tumour specimens, we recognized that the preparation of single cells, their characterization in vitro and

Table 1.

Prediction of human tumour drug sensitivity conclusion: + = valuable; — = non-valuable

Approach	Method	Clinical value patients	correl. %	concl.	Authors, year
Long-term tissue cultures + drug	Cell cultures/ morphology	102		(+)	LICKISS et al, 1974
		188		(+)	COBB, et al 1964
		85	65	+	LIMBURG, 1973
		88	63	(+)	TANNEBERGER et al, 1967
		41	46	+	KRAFFT et al, 1973
		96	83	+	KRAFFT et al, 1981
		33	81	+	TERENTIEVA et al, 1976
		39		+	IZSAK et al, 1971
		201		+	MARZOTKO et al, 1976
	Cell cultures/ transmembrane potential	25		+	WALLISER et al, 1981
	Cell cultures/ cell counting	36	92	+	HOLMES et al, 1974
	Cell cultures/ autoradiography	48	100	+	MURPHY et al, 1975
		53	77	+	ZITTOUN et al, 1975
		40	79	+	LIVINGSTONE et al, 1980
	Cell cultures/ DNA or RNA synthesis	450		(+)	MITCHEL et al, 1972
		55		+	WHEELER et al. 1974
		5		+	SHRISTAV et al, 1980
				(+)	TSCHAO et al, 1962
	Organ cultures/ DNA synthesis	108		(+)	TANNEBERGER et al, 1977
		74		(+)	NISSEN et al, 1978
		152		(+)	PEEK et al, 1981
	Organ cultures/ histochemistry	10	45	+	HECKER et al, 1976
	Tumour slices/ DNA, RNA, protein-synthesis, respiration, glycolysis	211		+	DICKSON, 1976
	In-vitro-soft agar human tumour stem cell assay	18		(+)	SALMON et al, 1978
		66	100	+	v. HOFF, 1979
		5	100	+	TVEIT et al, 1980
		40	62/99	+	ALBERTS et al, 1980
Short-term tissue incubation + drug	Cell suspension/ morphology	48	73	+	DENDY et al, 1973
		148	55	+	WRIGHT et al, 1973
	Biopsy/ autoradiography	25	27	—	WOLBERG, 1971
	Cell suspension/	15			
	autoradiography	15	93	+	THIRLWELL et al, 1976
	Cell suspension/	50	92	+	ANDRYSEK, 1973
	DNA or RNA synthesis	23	50	(+)	HIRSCHMANN, 1973
		24	100	+	POSSINGER et al, 1976
		24	40	+	MATTERN et al, 1976
		125		+	BASTERT et al, 1975
		23	90	+	VOLM, 1975
		114	85	+	VOLM, 1980
		69		(+)	SCHLAG, 1979

Table 1 continued

Approach	Method	Clinical value patients	correl. %	concl.	Authors, year
	Biopsy/				
	DNA synthesis	21		(+)	Kaufmann et al, 1971
	Cell suspension/	22	83	+	Kondo, 1971
	enzyme assay	89	27	(+)	Di Paolo, 1971
		60	70	+	Knock et al, 1974
	Bone marrow + cell suspension/ DNA synthesis	11		(+)	Tisman, 1973
Determination of drug-inacti-vating or target enzymes	SH groups			+	Kulik, 1977
	DNA dependent RNA polymerase (Bleomycin inacti-vating enzymes)	23	45	+	Müller, 1977
	TMP-Synthetase FdUMP d-UMP			+	Moran et al, 1979
Cell kinetic data	Clumps/biopsy/ labeling index	34			Kirmiss et al, 1976
	Cell suspensions/ cytophotometry	23	82	+	Smets et al, 1976
In vivo test	Diffusion chamber/ cell suspension	47		+	Heckmann, 1967
	Xenografts/	3/3(5)	100	+	Batemann, 1980
	colony assay	5	100	+	Tveit, 1980
		2	100	+	Siegel, 1980

finally their cultivation as monolayer was possible only in a limited number of cases (Fig. 1). Furthermore, the effects of antimetabolites could not be detected definitely by morphological methods (55). Taking into account the experiences of the first period of our studies in 1969—70 we developed a second type of assay using the organ culture

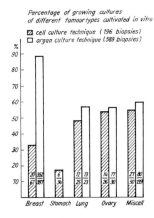

Fig. 1

technique and evaluating the drug effects by DNA-synthesis measurement (56). Without any doubt, this organ culture assay was a real advance compared with the former technique of in vitro drug prediction. As can be seen in Fig. 1 for example the rate of in vitro maintenance for breast cancer specimens was 88.7% in organ culture and 32.8% in monolayer cell culture. Furthermore, the detection of cell viability by the aid of DNA-synthesis measurement is much more precise than the use of a morphological method. Another unsolved problem in this assay arises because the material investigated cannot be adequately characterized as typically neoplastic. Due to the inhomogeneity of human tumours this is a major limitation of the assay.

The results of some clinical trials were performed using the organ culture predictive assay were in good agreement with our theoretical expectations. In 1972, two randomized clinical trials (UICC registered trials No. 72-020, 72-053) evaluating individualized drug treatment using the organ culture assay were initiated in our institute. In the first of these trials, 50 patients with ovarian cancer (40 palliatively operated, 10 non-operated) were treated with Trenimon (one of the most recommended drugs when we started this trial) and 37 (31 palliatively operated, 6 non-operated) were treated with the predicted drug. The survival rate of the patients treated individually had a tendency to be higher but the difference was not significant statistically (60). No difference was found either between non-individualized (31 patients) and individualized (33 patients) surgical adjuvant chemotherapy in lung cancer in the second trial we performed.

A very promising result was obtained with individualized surgical adjuvant chemotherapy in breast cancer stage III (UICC registered trial No. 77-051) (43). From January 1974 to February 1981 200 patients entered this study. For the first 110 patients the control-to-treatment ratio was 1:1, thereafter for ethical reasons, 1:2. 193 patients can be evaluated now. According to the protocol, all patients (control and treatment groups) were investigated in vitro for drug sensitivity and estrogen receptor content

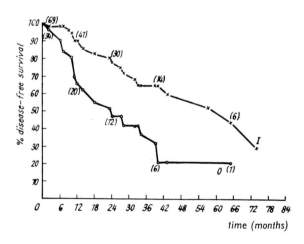

Fig. 2. ZIK 2/81 P. High Risk Breast Cancer CCT CICR Berlin Buch 1974—1980. In vitro sensitive tumours, irrespective of age, menopausal and estrogen receptor state. Results of surgical adjuvant therapy, disease-free survifal (dfs). Total 107; treatment 72 (I); control 35 (0); patients at risk ( ) $X^2 = 8,99$; p $= < 0.005$, significant.

of the tumour. The control group was treated by radical mastectomy only, the treatment group received the predicted hormone-chemotherapy in case of sensitivity and
ER$^+$, and no hormone-chemotherapy in case of drug resistance and ER$^-$. Where there
were insufficient in vitro data for technical reasons, patients of the treatment arm received surgical adjuvant treatment with cyclophosphamide. As shown in Fig. 2, a
statistically significantly longer relapse-free survival was achieved when drug sensitive, ER$^\pm$ patients were treated with the predicted hormone-chemotherapy (72 patients), compared with the relapse-free survival of drug sensitive, ER$^\pm$ patients, who
received no surgical adjuvant treatment, as control (35 patients). This difference could
not be confirmed (Fig. 3), when the total of controls (85 patients) were compared
with the total treatment group (105 patients).

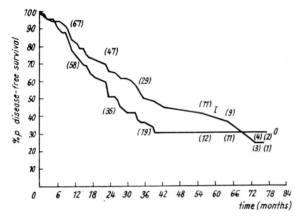

Fig. 3. ZIK 2/81 P. High Risk Breast Cancer CCT CICR Berlin Buch 1974—1980. All cases irrespective of age, menopausal state and results of ER-assay and oncobiogram. Disease-free survival
(dfs) of patients with surgical adjuvant therapy according to predictive tests, resistant tumours
included (12/80). Total 193; treatment 105 (1); control 85 (0); ( ) patients at risk ( ); $X^2 = 2.25$;
p = > 0.1. not significant.

Of course, the value of this trial, relevant to the problem of correlation between in
vitro drug prediction and clinical response, was limited because of the combination
of hormone- and chemotherapy. Furthermore, in our view, premenopausal controls
should always receive standard CMF surgical adjuvant chemotherapy, rather than
non-individualized. Nevertheless this trial, which was designed to approach the general
problem of individualized cancer treatment, was useful in confirming our present
position regarding the antineoplastic drug prediction problem.

Some conclusions from 20 years of international history
of in vitro drug predictive tests and our own results

There are some biologically and pharmacologically acceptable approaches of proved
predictive value for antineoplastic drug efficacy in experimental systems and also in
man. But these approaches are complicated, time-consuming and need special laboratory facilities. In contrast to some over- optimistic evaluations in the past, there is
no assay for prediction of antineoplastic drug efficacy available at present, which
could be recommended for use in clinical practice. Accordingly, human tumour drug

sensitivity prediction and individualized cancer chemotherapy remain one of the more important problems for applied cancer research. Because we are entering a period in which there is growing interest in surgical adjuvant chemotherapy, the importance of this problem is still increasing.

Some obstacles to the elaboration of an effective predictive test

The obstacles to the elaboration of effective predictive tests result mainly from the non-homogeneity of human tumours in space and time (17).
This non-homogeneity affects both the sampling and maintenance of human tumours in vitro.

1. *Isolated cells* for short-term studies, monolayer cultures or soft-agar cloning are often not obtainable in sufficient amount, particularly in such clinically important tumour types as breast and stomach cancer (10). Furthermore, as underlined by DENDY (7), the identification of isolated cells as neoplastic, which is essential for a successful assay, is still an unsolved problem. Moreover, the risk of selection in mixed cell populations should never be forgotten. A final and critical point is the fact that, of necessity, the cell kinetic status of isolated single cells is very different from that of tissue cells, and this can influence the drug sensitivity (10).

2. *Tumour biopsies* as used particularly in the proposed short-term incubation techniques, avoid tissue disaggregation or digestion of the tumour, but have the disadvantage that "dying tissue" is no longer representative of a proliferating tumour. Another crucial point is the characterization and identification of the biopsies. Due to the heterogeneity of human tumours, there is a high risk of working with connective tissue instead of neoplastic tissue. To know that is in the test tube is essential for a successful in vitro assay, but this may prove difficult when working with biopsies.

3. *Organ cultures* provide stronger evidence that vital tumour tissue is under investigation.
   The tumour cells metabolize in the normal biological environment, and the original biological architecture is maintained. There are only minimal deviations of the cell behaviour from the in vivo situation. In these respects, organ cultures offer considerable advantages in comparison with other in vitro approaches. There is no difference between conventional organ culture techniques and tumour biopsy techniques as far as the characterization and identification of the test object.

4. *Instability*
   A problem of all in vitro techniques is the instability of human tumour properties in biological systems. As we demonstrated with an in vitro nude mouse model (39), fundamental properties of tumours such as growth rate, karyotype and also drug sensitivity, change promptly in response to the biological environment of the cells.

Some critical problems in detecting antineoplastic drug effects in vitro

1. *Morphological methods* are the simplest techniques for detecting cell damaging and cell death. To measure the multiplication rate of a cell population, without any doubt, provides definitive information on the viability of that cell population.

Unfortunately, the measurement of the multiplication rate of a given cell population is difficult to standardize and time-consuming. Furthermore, as discussed above, cell populations are difficult to obtain from most solid tumours. Morphological criteria of cell damage and death, such as shrinking, granulation etc. can be used to detect the effects of some antineoplastic drugs, but, unfortunately, some compounds (e. g. antimetabolites) only cause late but not early changes of cells and cell properties.

2. *Biochemical techniques* are widely used for the measurement of cell damage and death. Without any doubt, the maesurement of changes in DNA-, RNA- or protein synthesis satisfactorily reflects cellular defects. However, not all antineoplastic compounds act directly on the DNA-, RNA- or protein synthesis. It seems justifiable to expect alterations in the nucleic acid or protein synthesis after 1—2 days of drug influence on metabolizing cells, but such alterations could not be expected for all drugs within a few hours. Therefore, the so-called short-time incubation tests need a critical evaluation. Short-term incubation assays can work only if target reactions or metabolites of the drug tested are measured.

3. *Cloning ability*
   The measurement of the cloning ability of tumour cells in soft-agar, theoretically, is a promising approach. On the one hand, cloning gives a greater chance that from a mixed cell population, neoplastic cells will be selectively cloned because of their higher potential for cloning in soft-agar (11, 21, 45). On the other hand, cloning is a very precise test for cell viability. The crucial points concerning cloning techniques for the detection of antineoplastic drug effects are: the limitations for the preparation of single cell suspensions from solid tumours; the limitations of the cloning ability also of tumour cells (10, 31); and, last but not least, the long duration of a cloning assay (10 days on the average).

4. *Physical conditions of an in vitro system*
   A more general problem playing a role in all approaches to in vitro drug sensitivity detection is the dependency of drug effects on a number of conditions of in vitro systems. These include the influence of medium composition, medium pH, serum quality etc. (42).

5. *The problem of pre-activation*
   Finally, it should be underlined that drugs that need to be activated in vivo before interaction with neoplastic cells, like cyclophosphamide, have to be activated in vitro, too, if a realistic assay is to be performed. There are a number of approaches in this direction, including the application of post-injection serum of patients (30) but no complete solution has yet been achieved (10).

The requirements for an effective in-vitro assay

Summarizing this critical consideration of the main obstacles for developing an effective in vitro sensitivity prediction assay, the following requirement for the elaboration of such an assay could be formulated:

1. The method of sampling and maintaining a human tumour for drug prediction should guarantee that well-characterized, representative neoplastic cells are investigated which behave biologically and biochemically, in a similar way to the cells in vivo. Particularly, the cells should metabolize and proliferate as in vivo, having comparable cell kinetic parameters.

2. The in-vitro system should guarantee an acceptable stability of the main properties of the tumour cells.
3. The method of detecting the antineoplastic drug effects in vitro should objectively reflect the viability of the neoplastic cells.
4. The antineoplastic drugs should be tested in concentration comparable to the in vivo situation, and in the in vivo active form.
5. The whole assay should take no more than 1 week before results are given to the clinician.
6. Drug resistance should be predicted with at least 90% probability, and drug sensitivity, with 75% probability.
7. The assay should be cheap enough to be used for the majority of patients in all hospitals.

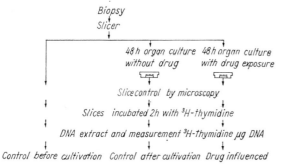

Fig. 4.

Table 2.
DNA synthesis of human breast cancer (dpm ³H-Thymidine/µg DNA) measured before and after (48 hours) organ culture of biopsies and slices

Patient	Histology	Tumour biopsies		Tumour slices	
		before culture	after culture	before culture	after culture
F. I.	Simple,	64,6	75,6	2335,8	3142,3
	undifferentiated	100,9	82,8	2006,4	3941,6
St. E.		126,1	63,6	1949,5	4197,6
		94.7	89.3	2271.8	3838.5
F. R.		291.3	191.6	3377.8	2175.5
		304.1	206.7	3885.0	3731.9
Sch. D.		220.1	402.1	2697.6	2266.2
		169.5	206.6	3689.5	2548.7
P. A.		166.4	119.5	2308.3	3990.2
		134.1	115.0	4383.3	4909.8
L. I.		291.4	472.9	2338.2	1162.8
		244.3	308.5	1459.0	1439.9
Sch. E.		350.8	541.6	2191.2	3039.7
		468.5	813.4	4524.4	4413.5
E. S.		119.3	151.8	10624.2	2420.8
		205.3	182.8	7860.2	3882.5
Sp. S.	Medullary	331.3	895.5	1889.4	15743.7
		234.5	836.2	1758.0	17701.7
U. I.		1091.7	292.6	29773.3	6445.6
		1624.4	193.1	28087.5	3245.1

Based on these demands, in our institute a new predictive test has been developed in 1979—80 (Fig. 4).

Our main concern in elaborating this new test was focused on the problem of using our positive experiences with organ cultures, and overcoming the very critical point of an insufficient characterization of the tumour samples, when using the conventional organ culture technique. Based on earlier experience (54) in the use of tissue slices, instead of human tumour biopsies for organ culture, a new technique has been developed (41), in which vital slices of human tumours are prepared which can be characterized morphologically and cultivated in organ culture. The technique guarantees, in contrast to the conventional organ culture technique, a strict morphological control of all cultures. Furthermore, as shown in Table 2 the metabolic activity of the tissue slices, maintained in vitro, is much higher than in maintained biopsies, due to an improved cell-medium interaction and an improved oxygenation. Because we had already developed an optimal detection technique for cell viability with the DNA-synthesis measurement after 48 hour drug exposure, this technique has also been used successfully in our new assay. As shown in Table 3, antineoplastic drug effects and the individual tumour sensitivity are very well demonstrated by the DNA-synthesis measurement of drug-exposed tumour slices cultivated in organ culture. The effects are even more precise than in the conventional organ culture assay.

Summarizing our first experiences with the new assay, we believe that this new approach is a realistic advance towards a strictly predicted individualized cancer chemo-

Table 3.
Tumour drug response in vitro measured by conventional organ culture assay (COCA) or slice organ culture assay (SOCA)
Patient: H. A.
Histology: non-diff., medull., simple breast cancer

Drug	Concentration µg/l	DNA-synthesis dpm/µg DNA (% control) COCA		SOCA	
VLB	2.0	74.7	(78.3%)	321.0	(32.8%)
	0.2	112.4	(119.4%)	544.0	(55.6%)
FU	220.0	56.2	(59.7)	438.3	(44.8%)
	20.0	555.6	(590.1%)	1166.1	(119.2%)
DBL	10.0	175.9	(186.8%)	161.4	(26.5%)
	1.0	208.6	(221.6%)	389.3	(39.8%)
MTX	6.0	52.0	(55.2%)	646.1	(66.0%)
	0.6	391.8	(416.1%)	1824.7	(186.5%)
L-PAM	60.0	69.6	(73.9%)	170.0	(17.4%)
		218.3	(231.9%)	318.9	(32.6%)
Control after culture		94.2	(91.7%)	978.3	(164.2%)
Control before culture		102.7	(100.0%)	595.9	(100%)

therapy. It should never be forgotten, however, that drug prediction is only a part of individualized antineoplastic drug treatment. As shown in Fig. 5, individualized cancer chemotherapy means much more and includes also consideration of drug pharmacokinetics, and tumour-host relationships.

Tumour Drug Host Interaction in Cancer Chemotherapy

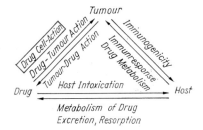

Fig. 5.

References

1. ALBERTS, D. S., CHEN, H. S. G., SOEHNLEN, B., SALMON, S. E., SURWIT, E. A. and YOUNG, L.: Lancet (1980), 340—342
2. AMBROSE, E. J.: In: Europ. J. Cancer 4 (1968), 39—44
3. ANDRYSEK, O. (1973): In: Aktuelle Probleme der Therapie maligner Tumoren. G. WÜST, Ed., Georg Thieme, Stuttgart, 80—85
4. BASTERT, G., SCHMIDT-MATTHIESEN, H., GERNER, R., MICHEL, R. T., NORD, D. and LEPPIEN, G.: Dtsch. med. Wschr. 100 (1975), 2035—2043
5. COBB, J. P. and WALER, D. G.: Unio internationalis contra cancerum. Acta 20 (1964),206—211
6. DENDY, P. P., DAWSON, M. P. A. and HONESS, D. J.: In: Aktuelle Probleme der Therapie maligner Tumoren, G. WÜST, Ed., Georg Thieme, Stuttgart, 34—45
7. DENDY, P. P.: Br. J. Cancer 41 Suppl. IV (1980), 195—198
8. DI PAOLO, J. A.: Nat. Cancer Inst. Monogr. 34 (1971), 240—247
9. DICKSON, J. A. and SUZANGAR, M. (1976): In: Human tumours in short term culture. P. P. DENDY, Academic Press, 107—137
10. FREI III, E. and LAZARUS, H.: New Engl. J. Med., 298, 24 (1978), 1358—1359
11. HAMBURGER, A. W. and SALMON, S. E.: Sciences 197 (1977), 461—463
12. HECKER, D., SAUL, G. and WOLF, G.: Arch. Geschwulstforsch. 46 (1976), 34—43
13. HECKMANN, U.: Dtsch. med. Wschr. 92 (1967), 932—943
14. HIRSCHMANN, W. D. (1973): In: Aktuelle Probleme der Therapie maligner Tumoren, G. WÜST Ed., Georg Thieme, Stuttgart, 108—115
15. HOFF, D. D. von: J. Amer. Med. Assoc. 242 (1979), 501—508
16. HOLMES, H. L. and LITTLE, J. M.: Lancet II (1974), 985—986
17. IVERSON, O. H. (1975): Excerpta Medica International Congress, Series n. 375. Proceedings of the Sixth Int. Symposium on the Biological Characterization of Human Tumours, Copenhagen
18. IZSAK, F. Ch., EYLAN, E., GAZITH, A., SHAPIRO, J., NATTARIN, S. and RAANANI, Ch.: Europ. J. Cancer 7 (1971), 33—39
19. KAUFMANN, M., VOLM, M. and GOERTLER, K.: Klin. Wochenschr. 49 (1971), 219—224
20. KIRMISS, K., GÜRTLER, R., LANGEN, P., DE HEUREUSE, R., and ARNDT, K.: Dt. Gesundh.— Wesen, 31 (1976), 2056—2060
21. KLEIN, J. C.: Arch. Geschwulstforsch. 51 (1981), 58—62
22. KNOCK, F. E., GALT, R. M., OESTER, Y. T. and SYLVESTER, R.: Oncology 30 (1974), 1—22
23. KONDO, K.: Nat. Cancer Inst. Monogr. 34 (1971), 251—256
24. KRAFFT, W., PREIBSCH, W. and MARZOTKO, F.: Arch. Geschwulstforsch. 41 (1973), 241—247
25. KRAFFT, W., BRÜCKMANN, D., PREIBSCH, W., BEHLING, H., and KADEMANN, J.: Arch. Geschwulstforsch. 51 (1981), 133—139
26. KULIK, G. I., KOROL, W. S. and KADETZKI, R. I.: Mitteilungen der Akademie der Wissenschaften der UdSSR — Ministerium für Gesundheitswesen.
27. LICKISS, J. N., CANE, K. A. and BAIKIE, A. G.: Europ. J. Cancer 10 (1974), 809—815
28. LIMBURG, H. and KRAHE, M.: Dt. med. Wochenschr., 89 (1964), 1938—1943

29. LIMBURG, H. (1973): In: Aktuelle Probleme der Therapie maligner Tumoren. G. WÜST, Ed., Georg Thieme, Stuttgart, 7—17

30. LIVINGSTON, R. B., TITUS, G. A. and HEILBRUN, L. K.: Cancer Res. *40* (1980), 2209—2217

31. MARSHALL, C. J., FRANKS, L. M. and CARBONELL, A. W.: J. Nat. Cancer Inst., *58* (1977) 1743—1747

32. MARZOTKO, F., KRAFFT, W., PREIBSCH, W. and SCHRÖDER, M.: Arch. Geschwulstforsch. *46* (1976), 140—149

33. MATTERN, J., KAUFMANN, M., WAYSS, K., VOLM, M., KLECKOW, M., MOSTHAGI, M. and VOGT-MOYKOPF, I.: Klin. Wochenschr. *54* (1976), 665—673

34. MITCHEL, J. S., DENDY, P. P., DAWSON, M. P. A. and WHEELER, T. K.: Lancet I (1972), 955—958

35. MORAN, R. G. and HEIDELBERGER, C.: Bull. Cancer (Paris) *66*, 1 (1979), 79—83

36. MÜLLER, W. E. G.: Cancer *40* (1977), 2787—2792

37. MURPHY, W. K., LIVINGSTON, R. B., RUIZ, V. G., GERCOVICH, F. G., GEORGE, S. L., HART J. S. and FREIREICH, E. J.: Cancer Res. *35* (1975), 1438—1446

38. NISSEN, E., TANNEBERGER, St., PROJAN, A., MORACK, G. and PEEK, U.: Arch. Geschwlstforsch. *48* (1978), 667—672

39. NISSEN, E., ARNOLD, W., WEISS, H. and TANNEBERGER, St. (1980): In: Cell movement and neoplasia, Ed. M. DE BRABANDER, Pergamon Press Oxford and New York, 171—177

40. NISSEN, E. and PROJAN, A. (1980): In: Experimentelle und klinische Tumorchemotherapie, Ed. St. TANNEBERGER, Akademie-Verlag, Berlin, 103—116

41. NISSEN, E., SCHÄLIKE, W. and TANNEBERGER, St. (in preparation): Exp. Cell Res.

42. NISSEN, E. and TANNEBERGER, St.: Arch. Geschwulstforsch. *51* (1981), 152—156

43. PEEK, U., TANNEBERGER, St., HEISE, E., GÖRLICH, M., NISSEN, E., MARX, G., PROJAN, A., WINKLER, R., KUNDE, D. and BODEK, B.: Arch. Geschwulstforsch. *51* (1981), 139—152

44. POSSINGER, K., HARTENSTEIN, R. and EHRHART, H.: Klin. Wochenschr., *54* (1976), 349—361

45. PUCK, T. T. and MARCUS, P. L.: Proc. Natl. Acad. Sci. USA *41* (1955), 432—437

46. RUPNIAK, T. and HILL, B. T.: Cell Biology International Rep. *4*, 5 (1980), 479—486

47. SALMON, S. E., HAMBURGER, A. W., SOEHNLEIN, B., DURIE, B. G. M., ALBERTS, D. S. and MOON, Th. E.: New Engl. J. Med. *298* (1978), 1321—1327

48. SCHLAG, P., VESER, J., BREITIG, D. and MERKLE, P.: J. Cancer Res. Clin. Oncol. *95* (1979), 273—280

49. SHRISTAV, S., BONAR, R. A., STONE, K. R. and PAULSON, D. F.: Cancer Res. *40* (1980), 4438 — 4442

50. SMETS, L. A., MULDER, E., DE WAAL, F. C., CLETON, F. J. and BLOK, J.: Br. J. Cancer *35* (1976), 153—161

51. SIEGEL, M. M., CHUNG, H. S., RUNCKER, N., SIEGEL, St. E., SEEGER, R. C., ISAACS, H. and BENEDICT, W. F.: Cancer Chemotherap. Rep. *64* (1980), 975—983

52. TANNEBERGER, St. and BACIGALUPO, G.: Dt. Gesundh.-Wesen *22* (1967), 11—19

53. TANNEBERGER, St.: Arch. Geschwulstforsch. *31* (1968), 387—400

54. TANNEBERGER, St.: Experientia *25* (1969), 334

55. TANNEBERGER, St. and BACIGALUPO, G.: Arch. Geschwulstforsch. *35* (1970), 44—53

56. TANNEBERGER, St. and MOHR, A. (1973): Arch. Geschwulstforsch. *42* (1973), 307—315

57. TANNEBERGER, St., RIECHE, K., BUTSCHAK, G., GÖRLICH, M. and MAGDON, E.: Arch. Geschwulstforsch. *41* (1973), 177—196

58. TANNEBERGER, St.: Arch. Geschwulstforsch. *47* (1977), 755—756

59. TANNEBERGER, St. (1979): In: Chemotherapy of solid tumours. Ed. F. PANNUTI, Patron Editore, Bologna, Italia, 27—44

60. TANNEBERGER, St., NISSEN, E., SCHÄLIKE, W. (1979): In: Advances in medical oncology, research and education, Vol. 5, Basis for cancer therapy 1, Ed. B. W. Fox, Pergamon Press Oxford/New York, 197—211

61. TERENTIEVA, T. G., BUKHNY, T. G., DURNOV, A. F. and IVANITZKAJA, M. A.: Antibiotiki *21* (1976), 1011—1015

62. THIRLWELL, M. P., LIVINGSTON, R. B., MURPHY, W. K. and HART, J. S.: Cancer Res. *36* (1976), 3279—3283
63. TISMAN, G., HERBERT, V. and EDLIS, H.: Cancer Chemotherapy Reports *57* (1973), 11—19
64. TSCHAO, E., EASTY, G. C., AMBROSE, E. J., RAVEN, R. W. and BLOOM, H. J.: Europ. J. Cancer *4* (1962), 39—44
65. TVEIT, K. M., FODSTAD, O., OLSNES, S. and PHIL, A.: Int. J. Cancer *26* (1980), 717—722
66. VOLM, M.: Langenbecks Arch. Chirurgie *339* (1975), 4—12
67. VOLM, M., WAYSS, K., KAUFMANN, M. and MATTERN, J.: Europ. J. Cancer *15* (1979), 983—993
68. VOLM, M.: Dt. med. Wochenschr. *43* (1980), 1493—1496
69. WALLISER, S. and REDMANN, K.: Arch. Geschwulstforsch. *51* (1981), 125—133
70. WHEELER, T. K., DENDY, P. P. and DAWSON, A.: Oncology *30* (1974), 362—376
71. WOLBERG, W. H.: Cancer Res. *31* (1971), 448—453
72. WRIGHT, J. C. and WALKER, D. (1973): In: Aktuelle Probleme der Therapie maligner Tumoren. Ed. G. WÜST, Georg Thieme, Stuttgart, 17—28
73. ZITTOUN, R., BONCHARD, M., PACQUET-DANIS, J., PERCIA-DU-SERT, M. and BOUSSER, J.: Cancer *35* (1975), 507—514

I. Institute of Pathology and Experimental Cancer Research of the Semmelweis Medical School, Budapest, Hungary

In Vivo Tests — Xenografts

K. Lapis and L. Kopper

The use of human tumour xenografts as in vivo test system have become quite popular in experimental oncology, although, clear evidence is still needed that xenografted tumours offer more advantages for learning about the behaviour and therapeutic sensitivity of human neoplasias' than syngeneic animal tumours.

To evaluate critically the value of human tumour xenografts, the following points will be reviewed briefly:

1. hosts available for xenografting and the take rate,
2. maintenance of characteristics of the parental tumour,
3. therapeutic approaches.

1a. Hosts for human tumour xenografts

Human tumours have been transplanted either into those anatomical sites, where the immune activity was expected to be low, or into such recipients where immune response was — congenitally or artificially — deficient. Recently most research groups favoured congenitally thymusless nude mice or prepared immune-suppressed animals as recipients. In the latter case, the preparation usually means adult thymectomy, whole-body irradiation and bone marrow reconstitution. Some authors tried to modify this process and obtained a higher take rate of primary or serial transplants (e. g. ara-C protection technique (1); carrageenan pretreatment (2)). Athymic-asplenic (Lasat) mice (3) or nude rats (4) are also available. At the present time there are no data sufficient to make a choice between nude and immune-suppressed mice.

1b. Take rate of xenografts

Transplants from in vitro cultured tumour cell lines showed a higher take rate than the tumours transplanted from the surgical specimen directly to the recipient (Table 1) (2, 5, 6, 7). Some tumour types show a relatively high proportion of growing implants (e. g. colorectal tumours, melanomas), while others have a much lower capacity to take (e. g. breast carcinomas). Benign tumours were also successfully transplanted into nude mice (e. g. breast (8), prostate (9), pituitary adenoma (10)). The main reasons responsible for graft rejection could be an insufficiency of the tumour fragment or suspension (i. e. the number of viable cells was too low, the angiogenesis stimulating effect was insufficient) or the residual host defence (presumably non-specific cytotoxi-

Table 1.
Take rate of human tumour xenografts

	Primary implants		Serially transplanted tumours	
	attempted	successful	attempted	successful
GIOVANELLA et al. (1978) nude mice	277	154 (56%)	78	57 (73%)
SHIMOSATO et al. (1976) nude mice	91	22 (24%)	18	14 (78%)
POVLSEN et al. (1978) nude mice	102	42 (41%)	42	26 (62%)
FOGH et al. (1979) nude mice — colonic	24	13 (54%)	13	9 (69%)
DAVIES et al. (1981) nude rat — colonic	12	7 (58%)		
STEEL (1978) mice — colonic	65	40		
IPCR immune-suppressed mice				
— colorectal	12	7 (58%)	7	6 (86%)
— breast	5	1	1	0
— melanoma	2	1	1	1
— kidney	5	1	1	1
— misc.	7	0		
total	31	10 (32%)	10	8 (80%)

Table 2.
Take rate of serially transplanted human colorectal tumour xenografts

	Number of mice received bilateral implants	Number of takes per mice		
		0	1	2
Six colorectal tumour lines	652	212	77	363
	Overall take probability: 61.58			
	Expected t. p.	0.14	0.47	0.38
	Observed t. p.	0.32	0.12	0.56

On the basis of a binominal distribution, if p is the take probability for single implant, the expected proportions of 0, 1 or 2 takes out of 2 implants per mouse are $(1 - p)^2$, $2 p(1 - p)$ and p^2 respectively

city of macrophages and natural killer cells). The heterogeneity of artificially immune-suppressed recipients was indicated by a significantly lower proportion of single takes after bilateral grafting (Table 2, Fig. 1) than expected on a binominal distribution (11, 12). The most favoured sites for transplantation are the subcutaneous area and the subrenal capsule. Concerning preferential sites of growth of human tumours in nude mice, KYRIAZIS and KYRIAZIS (13) observed that tumours transplanted in the anterior lateral thoracic wall grew faster than did tumours transplanted in the posterior aspect of the trunk.

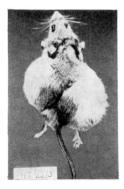

2. Maintenance of characteristics of the parental tumour

If the main reason for using human tumour xenografts is their resemblance to cancer in man, the extent to which a xenograft maintains the properties of the parental tumour is crucial.

In this context, most of the studies revealed the morphological identity of xenografts. Obviously this is valid only on the parenchymal elements, since the tumour stroma is provided by the recipient. Dedifferentiation is rather infrequent. Surprisingly, SHARKEY et al (14) claimed that in about 25% of xenografts the light microscopic appearance became more differentiated and so the origin of tumours with uncertain histogenesis could be recognised after xenotransplantation.

TAKÁCS et al (15) studied the ultrastructure of 5 serially transplanted colorectal xenografts compared to the primary tumour, and supported the view on the maintenance of morphological characteristics even after 10 passages (Figs. 2, 3). The adenomatous and mucinous tumours showed some distinct features. In the adenomatous tumours (Fig. 4) the cells surrounding acinus-like lumina were covered by microvilli and were connected to each other by well-developed intercellular junctions. Basal membrane separated the tumour cells from the stromal elements. On the contrary, in the mucinous tumours the cells were situated as single cells or were attached loosely to each other with an almost complete lack of the basal membrane and cell junction

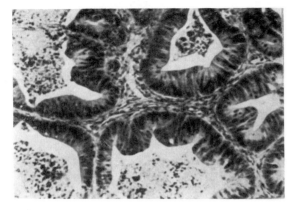

Fig. 2.

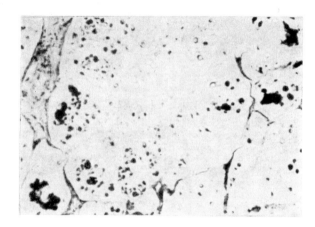

Fig. 3

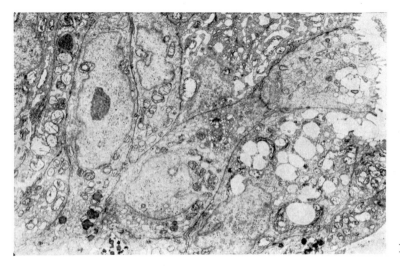

Fig. 4.

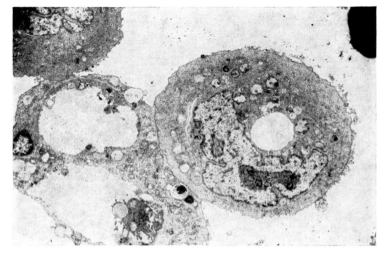

Fig. 5.

structures (Fig. 5). In these tumours, the cells were practically free of microvilli on the surface. Ultrastructural studies provide a tool, not only to obtain more exact knowledge on the morphological features of certain tumours, but also to follow the treatment-induced alterations at subcellular level.

The human origin of xenografted tumours and their similarity to their parental tumours, as shown by the light- and electronmicroscopic features, can also be confirmed by karyotype studies (16, 17, 18) and by their characteristic lactic dehydrogenase or glucose-6-phosphate dehydrogenase isoenzyme activities (19, 20, 21). Naturally, mouse-originated karyotypes and isoenzymes could also be present, since the stroma derives from the recipient.

Table 3.
Tumour products in human tumour xenografts-bearing mice

Human choriogonadotropin	—choriocarcinoma	—KAMEYA et al. (1976)
(ectopic)	—lung tumour	—LIEBLICH et al. (1977)
CEA	—colon tumours	—MACH et al. (1974)
		MITCHLEY et al. (1977)
		HOUGHTON and TAYLOR (1978)
Ectopic plasmaproteins	—kidney, colon,	
	maxilla tumours	—YOSHIMURA et al. (1978)
Alpha-foetoprotein	—hepatoblastoma	—HIROHASHI et al. (1979)
Immunoglobulins	—myeloma	—MITCHELL et al. (1974)
Dopamine-hydroxylase	—neuroblastoma	—HELSON et al. (1975)
β_2-microglobulin	—panreactic,	
	colon; bladder	—Di PERTIO et al. (1980)
CEA (CIS kit) —control		12 ng/ml
—colon tumours		
HT 6 adenom.		320 ng/ml
HT 17 adenom.		38 ng/ml/patient: 20—61 ng/ml
HT 22 adenom.		
mucinous		300 ng/ml
HT 8 mucinous		320 ng/ml

Several reports identified tumour products (Table 3) in xenograft tumour-bearing animals (e. g. human choriogonadotropin (21, 22, 23); carcinoembryogenic antigen (24, 25); ectopic plasmaproteins, alpha-foetoprotein (26, 27); immunoglobulins (28)). POULSEN et al (29) reported the preserved antigenic properties of Burkitt's lymphoma growing in nude mice. The capacity of xenografts to express their "functional" activity (i. e. to carry on the synthesis of various tumour products) makes it possible to use this model to search for new tumour markers.

The implanted tumours start to grow and remain localised in most instances. Metastasis formation from xenografts is rather difficult to assess. It occurs infrequently, mainly in the regional lymph nodes or in the lung (30, 31, 32, 33, 34, 35, 36). The tumours xenografted from in vitro lines tend to metastasise better than direct implants of primary tumour. SKOV et al (37) injected tumour cells intravenously into nude mice and observed no metastasis in the lung. The loss or decrease of metastatic capacity could be due to the residual host defense or the disadvantage of the implantation site (usually subcutaneous).

Since the therapeutic response of tumours may be influenced by their growth rate, it is interesting to consider how far the xenografts maintain the cell kinetic charac-

Table 4.
Cell kinetic parameters of human and xenografted human colorectal tumours

	T_d (days)	T_c (hr)	T_{g1} (hr)	T_s (hr)	T_{g2} (hr)	LI (%)	GF (%)	∅ (%)	MI (%)	References
Human — primer	138—1155									WELIN et al. (1963)
		66.4		17.0		7.1	30			LESHER et al. (1977)
		26.0	5.0	14.0	5.7	23.1	49			TERZ et al. (1971)
— metastases (lung)	34—120									COLLINS (1962)
Xenografted human		24.8 —				9.0 —	29 —		0.4 —	PICKARD et al. (1975)
		34.4				27.0	50		3.2	
	6.0	26.1	7.6	11.9	2.5	19.0	46	66	1.0	KOPPER and STEEL (1975)
	11.8	35.0	13.1	17.0	4.6	22.0	47	80	1.1	
	6.5	23.6	8.7	9.0	3.8	20.0	65	86	2.3	HOUGHTON and TAYLOR (1978)
	17.0					25.3			1.5	
	27.0					13.7			0.7	KOPPER et al. (1978)
	13.7	38.2	8.9	14.2		12.9	24	63	2.8	STRAGAND et al. (1980)

teristics upon transplantation. Tumours start to grow — more or less exponentially — after a latency period which is needed to induce stroma for blood supply. This interval ranged from 3 to 33 weeks (mean value 12.8) in 76 different xenografts (14) and from 4 to 16 weeks in our 6 colorectal tumours (Fig. 6) (38). Comparing the tumour volume doubling times and cell cycle times of colorectal xenografts (Table 4) to those observed in man (11, 21, 39, 40, 41, 42, 43, 44), only a tentative conclusion can be made because

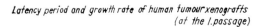

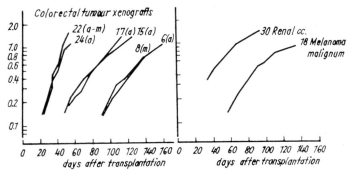

Fig. 6.

lines represent median growth curves
(a) adenomatous
(m) mucinous
colorectal tumours derived from primary carcinomas
renal oc. and melanoma derived from metastatic lesions

there are no detailed comparisons between the tumour growing in the patient and its xenografts. It seems that in the xenografts the growth rate is faster, which is indicated rather by the shorter tumour volume doubling times, while the cell cycle parameters are not much different from those of human tumours. The longer doubling time in a patient's tumour, compared to xenografts (passage 1) was confirmed by MATTERN et al (45) in 4 lung epidermoid carcinomas. It could be that a lower cell loss rate in xenografts is responsible for the faster growth rate. Another explanation is that the sizes of tumours studied in patients were perhaps larger than those measured in mice, and since the doubling time of tumours often increases with increasing size, this could contribute to the discrepancy in growth rate.

3. Therapeutic approaches

Seeing that xenografts maintain much of the characteristics of their parental tumour, they could also be expected to display the same therapeutic sensitivity, which after all, is the salient question of the usefulness of the xenograft system. In most experiments, the therapeutic response seen in xenograft systems was compared only to the general clinical experience concerning the therapeutic response of the given tumour type. Only very few reports are available in which therapeutic response of xenograft and its parental tumour were compared. For the assessment of therapeutic response, two approaches are being used: tumour volume measurements in vivo (we are at present using this method) and clonogenic cell survival assays in vitro. Somewhat surprising, nude mice tolerated high doses of different agents as well as conventional mice of the same strain (46).

Table 5.
Chemotherapeutic experiments on human colorectal xenografts

Drugs studied	Drugs found to be active	References
5-FU, BCNU, MTX, UC 51	5-FU	Cobb and Mitchley (1974)
5-FU, CCNU, MeCCNU, CY, ADR, DTIC	5-FU, CY	Kopper and Steel (1975)
5-FU, BCNU, CY, ADR, HMM, cis-dichlorodiammineplatinum	5-FU, BCNU	Mitchley et al. (1977)
5-FU, BCNU, CY, MTX, FUdR, Mitomycin-C	BCNU	Ovejera et al. (1977)
MeCCNU, chlorozotoxin, PALA, AMSA, Baker's antifol, maytansine	MeCCNU	Osieka et al. (1977)
5-FU, MeCCNU, CY, Act. D., doxorubicin, pentamethyl-melamine cis-dichlorodiammine-platinum	5-FU, MeCCNU, CY	Houghton and Houghton (1978)
5-FU, MeCCNU, CY, MTX, HMM, Act., D., Melph., Cis-DDP	5-FU, HMM, Melph.	Nowak et al. (1978)
5-FU, MeCCNU, BCNU, ADR, Dianhydrogalactitol, Dibromo-dulcitol	5-FU, BCNU, MeCCNU	Kopper et al. (1980)
5-FU, BCNU, 4'-deoxydoxorubicin (DDR) 4'-0-methyldoxorubicin (MDR)	DDR, MDR	Giuliani et al. (1981)

Several groups have reported on the effect of chemotherapy on colorectal tumour xenografts (Table 5). Generally, only a temporary inhibition of tumour growth was achieved by the various agents with rare exceptions of total tumour regression. Such effect was achieved, moreover, only by those drugs which were already known to be effective against colonic tumours in patients (e. g. nitrosoureas and 5-fluorouracil) (11, 38, 47, 48, 49). We have studied the effect of several agents on colorectal xenograft. The changes in volume doubling time following treatment with one single dose of the agents used are shown in Figure 7. 5-FU and MeCCNU, as well as larger doses of BCNU all proved to be effective. Studying the response of a tumour panel (10 colorectal tumour xenografts) to 8 different chemotherapeutic agents, Nowak et al (50) con-

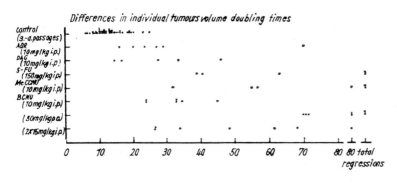

Table 6.
Response of colorectal tumour xenografts on 5-fluorouracil treatment

	Dose	Tumour volume doubling time		Growth delay
	mg/kg	control	treated	
HX 18/10 anaplastic	175 i.p.	4.0	20.0	4.0
	100 i. p.		14.0	2.5
HT 6/3 adenomatous	150 i. p.	10.5	40.5	2.9
HT 13/4 adenomatous	200 i. p.	7.5	28.8	2.8
HT 17/3 adenomatous	150 i. p.	15.0	29.3	1.0
HT 22/13 adenomatous				
mucinous	100 i. p.	15.5	22.8	0.5
HT 8/3 mucinous	150 i. p.	22.5	34.0	0.5
/16	100 i. p.	23.5	28.5	0.6

$$\text{Growth delay} = \frac{TD_{treated} - TD_{control}}{TD_{control}}$$

cluded that there was no tumour sensitive to all drugs and no drug effective against all tumours. Comparing the response of adenomatous and mucinous colorectal tumours, it has been found that the former group was more sensitive to BCNU, MeCCNU and 5-FU than the latter (38). The growth delay was calculated from the median tumour doubling time and was considered as a parameter for drug evaluation (11). Growth delay expresses the number of doublings which can be prevented by the treatment (Table 6).

Studying panel of tumours having the same anatomical origin may give some insight into the reasons for therapeutic responsiveness or unresponsiveness. For example, OSIEKA and THOMAS (51) found a direct relationship in 3 colorectal xenografts between the sensitivity to MeCCNU and the rate of its cross-binding capacity to DNA. HOUGHTON and HOUGHTON (52) and KOPPER et al (38) failed, however, to show differences in the uptake of ³H-5-fluorouracil between 5-fluorouracil-resistant and -sensitive colorectal xenografts. In further studies, there were no marked differences in the metabolism of 5-fluoruracil or of the analogues of 5-fluorouridine and 5-fluoro-2'-deoxyuridine between tumour lines responsive or non-responsive to these agents (in: HOUGHTON et al — 53). A detailed analysis of the activity of different enzymes in slowly and rapidly growing colorectal xenografts demonstrated a profound biochemical imbalance in these tumours (54). The authors concluded that the increased activities of both de novo and salvage pathway enzymes, and the remarkably enlarged pools of purine and pyrimidine ribonucleotides, should confer selective advantages for replication of human colon carcinoma cells. Such a study clearly predicts the hopelessness of single agent therapy with drugs available at present, and calls for an enzyme pattern-targeted approach in the design of chemotherapeutic agents.

The similarity of the therapeutic response of xenografts to the general clinical experience has also been reported for tumour xenografts derived from tumours other than colorectal.

Limited information is available on individual comparisons of patient's and xenograft's responses (50, 55, 56, 57). Although all the available information supports the chemotherapeutic validity of xenografts, the question remains: what is the best way to evaluate accurately the clinical response in those patients whose tumour is growing as xenograft?

One of the major problems in experimental chemotherapy is the choice of a proper screening system for selecting newly-developed drugs, that might be promising for clinical use. In this respect, the xenografted human tumours provided a new approach for drug selection. The Screening Program at the Division of Cancer Treatment (National Cancer Institute, U.S.A.) incorporates three human xenografted tumours (breast, lung, and colon) growing subcutaneously or in the subrenal capsule in nude mice. GOLDIN et al (58) surveyed the results they experienced in the last few years, and concluded that animal tumour systems rated a higher percentage of drugs as active, than did the human xenografts. Since some of the xenograft models, particularly the colon tumours, are rather resistant to therapy, they might prove to be useful in selecting drugs which will produce less disappointment in clinical practice. Although it remains to be answered, whether xenograft positives are more active in the clinic than those drugs selected by animal models, the results so far, indicate the importance of clinical testing of drugs that have definitive activity in the xenograft system. Interestingly enough, xenografts transplanted underneath the renal capsule have been shown to be more sensitive than the subcutaneously growing xenografts, and may be more useful as an initial xenograft test system.

Radiation therapy of xenografts has received less attention than chemotherapy. It is too early to draw conclusions from the scattered data but some efforts indicate the usefulness of the xenograft system in this area (e. g. study on the hypoxic cell radiosensitizer, misonidazole (59. 60, 61), radiation sensitivity of ovarian carcinoma xenografts seeming to be in good agreement with clinical response (62), and exploration of drug-radiation interaction (63, 64)).

4. Conclusions

This brief review presents those experiences which indicate that human tumour xenografts are an essential tool in the armoury of experimental oncology and especially chemotherapy. The maintenance of some characteristics of the parental tumour and the resemblance of the therapeutic response of tumours in man and xenografts with the same anatomical origin are encouraging evidence indeed. The problems of the interaction between recipient host and xenografts, as well as their therapeutic response to treatment with various drugs need to be studied further. The comparison of the pharmacokinetics of drugs in man and xenograft-bearing animals is not less important, and should be studied intensively, particularly in the light of treatment schedules, ranking different drugs against a particular tumour.

References

1. STEEL, G. G., COURTENAY, L. D. and ROSTOM, A. Y.: Brit. J. Cancer 37 (1978), 224
2. KOPPER, L., TRAN VAN HANH, LAPIS, K. and TIMÁR, J.: Europ. J. Cancer 16 (1980a), 671
3. LOZZIO, B. B.: Biomedicine 24 (1976), 144
4. COLSTON, M. J., FIELDSTEEL, A. H. and DAWSON, P. J.: J. Natl. Cancer Inst. 66 (1981), 843
5. SHIMOSATO, Y., KAMAYA, T., NAGAI, K., HOVHASHI, S., KOIDE, T., HAYASHI, H. and NOMURA, T.: J. Natl. Cancer Inst. 56 (1976), 1251
6. FOGH, J., FOGH, J. M. and ORFEO, T.: J. Natl. Cancer Inst. 59 (1977), 221

7. GIOVANELLA, B. C., STEHLIN, J. S., WILLIAM, L. J., LEE, S. S. and SHEPARD, R. C.: Cancer *42* (1978), 2269
8. McMANUS, M. J., DEMBROSKÉ, S. E., PIENKOWSKI, M. M., ANDÉRSON, T. J., MANN, L. C., SCHUSTER, J. S., VOLLWILER, L. L. and WELSCH, C. W.: Cancer Res. *38* (1978), 2343
9. OKADA, K., SCHROEDER, F. H., JELLINGHAUS, W., WILLSTEIN, H. K. and HEINEMEYER, H. M.: Invest. Urol. *13* (1976), 395
10. O'SULLIVAN, J. P., ALEXANDER, K. M. and JENKINS, J. S.: J. Endocrinol. *79* (1978), 139
11. KOPPER, L. and STEEL, G. G.: Cancer Res. *35* (1975), 2704
12. HOUGHTON, J. A. and TAYLOR, D. M.: Brit. J. Cancer *37* (1978), 213
13. KYRIAZIS, A. A. and KYRIAZIS, A. P.: Cancer Res. *40* (1980), 4509
14. SHARKEY, F. E., FOGH, J. M., HAJDU, S. I., FITZGERALD, P. J. and FOGH, J.: In: The Nude Mice in Experimental and Clinical Research, p. 187. Editors: J. FOGH and B. C. GIOVANELLA. Gustav Fischer Verlag, Stuttgart.
15. TAKÁCS, J., KOPPER, L., LAPIS, K. and HEGEDÜS, Cs.: Acta Morphol. Acad. Sci. Hung., in press
16. VISFELDT, J., POULSEN, C. O. and RYGAARD, J.: Acta pathol. microbiol. Scand. *80* (1972), 169
17. UEYAMA, Y., MORITA, K., KONDO, Y., SATO, N., ASANO, S., OHSAWA, N., SAKURAI, M., NAGUMO, F., IIJIMA, K. and TAMAOKI, N.: Brit. J. Cancer *36* (1977), 523
18. REEVES, B. R. and HOUGHTON, J. A.: Brit. J. Cancer *37* (1978), 612
19. KLEIN, G., GIOVANELLA, B. C., LINDAHL, T., FIALKOW, P. J., SINGH, S. and STEHLIN, J. S.: Proc. Natl. Acad. Sci. U.S. *71* (1974), 4737
20. PESCE, A. J., BUBEL, H. C., DIPERSIO, L. and MICHAEL, J. G.: Cancer Res. *37* (1977), 1998
21. HOUGHTON, J. A. and TAYLOR, D. M.: Brit. J. Cancer *37* (1978), 199
22. KAMEYA, T., SHIMOSATO, Y., TUMURAYA, N., OSHAWA, N. and NOMURA, T.: J. Natl. Cancer Inst. *56* (1976), 325
23. LIEBLICH, J. M., ROSEN, S. W., WEINTRAU, B. B. D., SINDELAR, U. F., TRALKA, T. S. and ROBSON, A. S.: J. Natl. Cancer Inst. *59* (1977), 1285
24. MACH, J. P., CARREL, S., MERENDA, C., SORDAT, B. and CEROTTINI, J. C.: Nature *248* (1974), 705
25. MITCHLEY, B. C. U., CLARKE, S. A., CONNORS, T. A., CARTER, S. M. and NEVILLE, A. M.: Cancer Treat. Rep. *61* (1977), 451
26. YOSHIMURA, S., TAMAOKI, N., UEYAMA, Y. and MATA, J.: Cancer Res. *38* (1978), 3474
27. HIROHASKI, S., SKIMOSATO, Y., KAMEYA, T., KOIDE, T., MUKOJIMA, T., TAGUCHI, Y. and KAGEYAMA, K.: Cancer Res. *39* (1979), 1819
28. MITCHELL, D. N., REES, J. W. and SALSBURY, A. J.: Brit. J. Cancer *30* (1974), 33
29. POULSON, C. O., FIALKOW, P. J., KLEIN, G., RYGAARD, J. and WIENER, F.: Int. J. Cancer *11* (1973), 30
30. COBB, L. M.: Brit. J. Cancer *26* (1972), 183
31. GIOVANELLA, B. C., YIM, S. O., MORGAN, A. C., STEHLIN, S. S. and WILLIAMS, L. J.: J. Natl. Cancer Inst. *50* (1973), 1051
32. FRANKS, C. R., BOULGER, L. G., GARRETT, A. J., BISHOP, D., REESON, D. and PERKINS, F. T.: Europ. J. Cancer *11* (1975), 619
33. SINGH, I., HATHEWAY, J. M., TSANG, K. Y., BLAKEMORE, W. S. and McALLISTER, R. M.: Surgery *81* (1977), 168
34. TIBBETS, L. M., CHU, M. Y., HAGER, J. C., DEXTER, D. L. and CALABRESI, P.: Cancer *40* (1977), 2651
35. HATA, J. I., UEYAMA, Y., TAMAOKI, N., FURUKAWA, T. and MORITA, K.: Cancer *42* (1978), 468
36. ROSTOM, A. Y., THOMAS, J. M., PECKHAM, M. J. and STEEL, G. G.: Lancet II (1978), 428
37. SKOV, C. B., HOLLAND, J. M. and PERKINS, E. H.: J. Natl. Cancer Inst. *56* (1976), 193
38. KOPPER, L., LAPIS, K. and HEGEDÜS, Cs.: Oncology *37* (1980b), 42
39. COLLINS, V. P.: Cancer *15* (1962), 387
40. WELIN, S., YOVKER, J. and SPRATT, J. S.: Amer. J. Roentgenol. *90* (1963), 672

41. Terz, J. J., Curutchet, P. and Lawrence, W. Jr.: Cancer 28 (1971), 1100

42. Pickard, R. G., Cobb, L. M. and Steel, G. G.: Brit. J. Cancer 31 (1975), 36

43. Steel, G. G.: Bull. Cancer 65 (1978), 465

44. Lesher, S., Schiffer, L. M. and Phause, M.: Cancer 40 (1977), 2706

45. Mattern, J., Haag, D., Wayss, K. and Volm, M.: Exp. Cell Biol. 49 (1981), 34

46. Houchens, D. P., Johnson, R. K., Gaston, M. R. and Goldin, A.: Cancer Treat. Rep. 61 (1977), 103

47. Osieka, R., Houchens, D. P., Goldin, A. and Johnson, R. K.: Cancer 40 (1977), 2640

48. Ovejera, A. A., Houchens, D. P., and Barker, A. D. (1977): In: Proc. Int. Workshop on Nude Mice, p. 451. Univ. Tokyo Press, Gustav Fischer Verlag, Stuttgart

49. Giuliani, F. C., Zirvi, K. A., Kaplan, N. O. and Goldin, A.: Int. J. Cancer 27 (1981), 5

50. Nowak, K., Peckham, M. J. and Steel, G. G.: Brit. J. Cancer 37 (1981), 576

51. Osieka, R. and Thomas, C. B.: (1978) In: Proc. Symp. on Use of Athymic (Nude) Mice in Cancer Research, p. 225. Gustav Fischer, New York, Stuttgart

52. Houghton, P. J. and Houghton, J. A.: Brit. J. Cancer 37 (1978), 833

53. Houghton, J. A., Makoda, S. J., Phillips, J. O. and Houghton, P. J.: Cancer Res. 41 (1981), 144

54. Weber, G., Hager, J. C., Lui, M. S., Prajda, N., Tzeng, D. Y., Jackson, R. C., Takeda, E. and Eble, J. N.: Cancer Res. 41 (1981), 854

55. Giovanella, B. C., Stehlin, J. S. and Shepard, R. C. (1977): In: Proc. Int. Workshop on Nude Mice. Univ. Tokyo Press, Gustav Fischer Verlag, Stuttgart

56. Hayashi, H., Kameya, T., Shimosato, Y. and Mukojima, T.: Amer. J. Obstet. Gynecol. 131 (1978), 548

57. Shorthouse, A. J., Peckham, M. J., Smyth, J. F. and Steel, G. G.: Brit. J. Cancer 41 (1980) SIV. 142

58. Goldin, A., Venditti, J. M., MacDonald, J. S., Muggia, F. M., Henney, J. E. and Deutta, V. T.: Europ. J. Cancer 17 (1981), 129

59. Courtenay, L. D., Smith, I. E. and Steel, G. G.: Brit. J. Cancer 37 (1978), SIII. 225

60. Rofstad, E. K. and Brustad, T·: Brit. J. Radiol. 52 (1979), 393

61. Guichard, M., De Langen-Omri, F. and Malaise, E.-P.: Int. J. Rad. Oncol. Biol. Phys. 5 (1979), 487

62. Davy, M., Brustad, T. and Mossage, J. (1977): In: Proc. Int. Workshop on Nude Mice, p. 491. Univ. Tokyo Press, Gustav Fischer Verlag, Stuttgart

63. Rofstad, E. K., Brustad, T., Johannessen, J. V. and Mossige, J.: Brit. J. Radiol. 50 (1977), 314

64. Bateman, A. E., Fu, K. K. and Towse, G. D. W.: Int. J. Rad. Oncol. (in press)

Institute of Oncology, Bologna, Italy

Suitable Models for Long-Term Bioassays on the Therapeutic and Toxic effects of Antiblastic Drugs: Liver Angiosarcomas Produced in Sprague-Dawley Rats by Vinyl Chloride

C. Maltoni, G. Cotti, L. Valgimigli and A. Mandrioli

There is currently a need for suitable animal tumour models on which to test the therapeutic and toxic activities of antiblastic drugs, in order better to evaluate their efficacy against different types of tumours. Such models must fulfill the following prerequisites:

1. the tumours must be of the same histotype and have the same localization as the human equivalent;
2. they must have a similar natural history as their human counterparts;
3. they must be easily reproducible, in a sufficient number, at a chosen time.

Many human-equivalent animal tumours have already been made available by experimental oncology; however, there are rate and peculiar tumours for which it may be difficult to provide such models.

In this report, we present a suitable experimental model of liver angiosarcoma, a rare neoplasia in humans and in experimental animals. This model seems to us to be particularly important, because liver angiosarcoma has in recent years presented an increasing clinical problem due to its steadily rising frequency among people exposed to a series of agents, namely vinyl chloride, inorganic arsenicals, thorotrast and androgenic/anabolic steroids (Popper et al, 1981). Moreover, with regard to this neoplasia very little is known about its therapy in general and chemotherapy in particular.

It is known that vinyl chloride causes liver angiosarcomas in rats similar to those in

Table 1.
Incidence of liver angiosarcomas in Sprague-Dawley rats exposed from 12-day embryo life for 57 weeks to vinyl chloride in air at 2500 ppm, 4—7 hours daily, 5 days weekly

Animals used			Animals with liver angiosarcoma		Average latency (weeks)[c]	Animals with lung metastases	
Sex	No. at start	Corrected no.[a]	No.	%[b]		No.	%[d]
M	63	56	32	57.1	50.5	13	40.6
F	65	55	38	69.1	49.4	16	42.1
M and F	128	111	70	63.1	49.9	29	41.4

[a] animals alive at 35 weeks, when the first tumour was observed
[b] with respect to the corrected number
[c] from start of treatment
[d] with respect to the total number of liver angiosarcoma bearing animals

22*

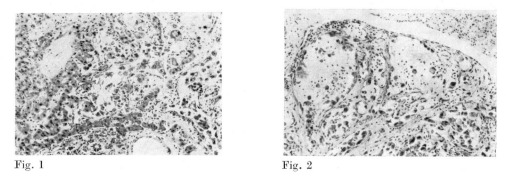

Fig. 1   Fig. 2

Fig. 1. Liver angiosarcoma in Sprague-Dawley rat, following exposure to vinyl chloride by inhalation. H.-E. × 200.

Fig. 2. Pulmonary metastasis of the liver angiosarcoma shown in Figure 1. H.-E. × 200.

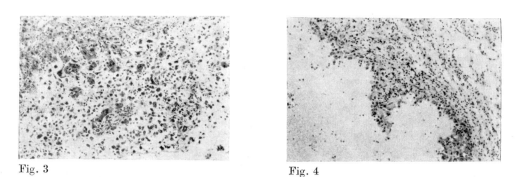

Fig. 3   Fig. 4

Fig. 3. Liver angiosarcoma in Sprague-Dawley rat, following exposure to vinyl chloride by inhalation .H.-E. × 200.

Fig. 4. Pulmonary metastasis of the liver angiosarcoma shown in Figure 3. H.-E. × 200.

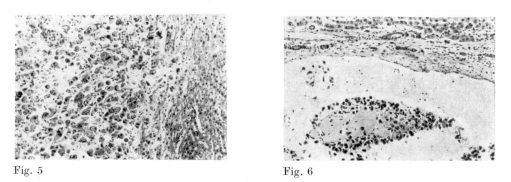

Fig. 5   Fig. 6

Fig. 5. Liver angiosarcoma in Sprague-Dawley rat, following exposure to vinyl chloride by inhalation. H.-E. × 200.

Fig. 6. Liver angiosarcoma in Sprague-Dawley rat, following exposure to vinyl chloride by inhalation. H.-E. × 200.

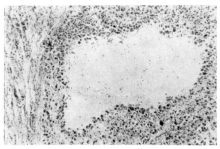 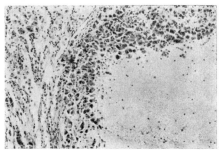

Fig. 7   Fig. 8

Fig. 7. Pulmonary metastasis of the liver angiosarcoma shown in Figure 6. H.-E. × 130.

Fig. 8. A detail of Figure 7. × 200.

humans (MALTONI and LEFEMINE, 1975; MALTONI, 1977; MALTONI et al, 1980). Under the experimental conditions described in this report, we were able to obtain a high incidence of these tumours, in a shorter period, with little variation in their histopathological picture or biological behaviour.

Sprague-Dawley rats were exposed by inhalation to 2500 ppm of the monomer, from the 12th day of embryonal development to one year of age: Breeders were exposed 4 hours daily, from the 13th day of pregnancy to delivery; offspring were exposed 4 hours daily, 5 days weekly, for 5 weeks, and then 7 hours daily, 6 days weekly, for 50 weeks.

The incidence and latency of the liver angiosarcomas obtained are shown in Table 1. The tumours are readily detected by laparoscopy.

They were generally multicentric and often metastasized, mainly to the lungs: pulmonary metastases were found in 29 out of 70 tumour-bearing animals. Microscope pictures of these experimental angiosarcomas are shown in Figures 1—8.

Comparisons of the angiosarcomas obtained in rats and those observed in humans (occupational cases studied at our Institute) showed surprising analogies with respect to gross pathology, histological picture and spread.

References

1. MALTONI, C. (1977): Vinyl chloride carcinogenicity: an experimental model for carcinogenesis studies. In: HIAT, H. H., Watson, J. D. & WILSON, I. C., eds., Origins of Human Cancer, Cold Spring Harbor, NY, Cold Spring Harbor Laboratory, pp. 119—146
2. MALTONI, C. and LEFEMINE, G. (1975): Carcinogenicity bioassays of vinyl chloride: current results. In: SELIKOFF, I. J. & HAMMOND, E. C., eds., Toxicity of Vinyl Chloride-Polyvinyl Chloride, New York, New York Academy of Sciences, pp. 195—218
3. MALTONI, C., LEFEMINE, G., CILIBERTI, A., COTTI, G. and CARRETTI, D. (1980): Vinyl chloride carcinogenicity bioassays (BT project) as an experimental model for risk identification and assessment in environmental and occupational carcinogenesis. In: Epidémiologie animale et épidémiologie humaine: le Cas du Chlorure de Vinyle monomere, Paris, Publications Essentielles, pp. 15—112
4. POPPER, H., MALTONI, C. and SELIKOFF, I. J.: Vinyl chloride induced hepatic lesions in man and rodents. A comparison. Liver 1 (1981), 7—20

Research Institute of Oncopathology, National Institute of Oncology, Budapest, Hungary

Role of some Biological Parameters in Drug Sensitivity and Resistance of Tumour Cells

J. Sugár, O. Csuka, I. Pályi and E. Oláh

There are two main limiting factors to successful chemotherapy of neoplasia, the toxicity of antitumour agents, and natural or acquired resistance of the tumour to chemotherapy. Sensitivity of a tumour cell population to an anticancer agent and the selective effect of a chemotherapeutic on a target are of multifactorial nature.

Some biological parameters of acquired resistance

Various pharmacological factors are known to influence the development of resistance. The most important factor is the active drug concentration achieved in the tumour, and this depends on the route and schedule of drug administration, as well as the inactivation and excretion of the drug. Location and vascularization of the tumour may also modify the attainable drug concentration.

Kinetic considerations, including such factors as cell cycle, phase specificity, recovery rates, and the size of the non-proliferating pool also play a part (6).

An important factor of the biochemical activity is the intracellular concentration of drug, which may be affected by reduced transport, decrease of activating enzymes, induction or activation of drug-catabolizing enzymes. Another factor is the decreased effect of antitumour agents on target enzymes.

Tumour cells may survive, following exposure to drug, by improved repair resulting from induction or activation of repair mechanism.

Resistance to Cholchicine and Actinomycin D, Adriamycin, and Daunorubicin may be attributed to the alterations of the cellmembrane resulting in decreased drug uptake (8, 10). Resistance to antimetabolites may result from the deletion of drug activating enzymes, such as uridine phosphorylase and uridine kinase which convert 5-fluorouracil to its nucleoside (16). In case of ara C, there may be a decrease in deoxycytidine kinase activity or an increase in the activity of catabolic enzymes, such as pyrimidine nucleoside deaminase (1, 9). In the methotrexate resistant cell the concentration of the target enzyme dihydrofolate reductase is elevated (11).

Resistance to alkylating agents may result from an increase in thiol content in the target cells, and thiols, having a high affinity for alkylating agents, would prevent active drug from reaching the target DNA (2).

Natural resistance

Some important questions related to the mechanisms of drug resistance were raised at the Workshop on Drug Resistance organized by UICC in 1975 (17). These included: the role of heterogeneity of a tumour cell population in the determination of drug sensitivity or resistance; the relative importance of transport mechanisms through the plasma membrane; and a requirement to elucidate the mechanism of cell death caused by the drugs. Our recently performed studies relate to these topics of drug resistance.

Heterogeneity may be related to the difference in ploidy or to cell kinetic properties. In our studies, the sensitivity of clonal lines isolated from heteroploid, heterogeneous cell population was compared with the target line. The sensitivity of growing and resting cell populations was also examined.

For a better understanding of the mode of action of vinca alkaloids, the uptake and intracellular distribution of these drugs have been determined.

There is an increasing body of evidence that tumour cell populations are heterogeneous, from a number of points of view including drug sensitivity (7). To test for the presence of cell with "natural" resistance, clonal lines were isolated from a heteroploid, hetero-geneous cell population of the NK/Ly mouse ascites lymphoma, and the sensitivity to vincristine (VCR) and to other drugs of the separate clones and the parent line were compared (14). Drug sensitivity was studied by the plating efficiency method using soft agar. Of the clones, one was diploid (P_1), and two others, hypotetraploid (P_3, P_4). In dose response studied, the cells were treated with different doses of VCR for 3 h. The parent line showed the lowest sensitivity to VCR, while clone P_3 was the most sensitive to the drug. (Fig. 1) Sensitivity of the proliferating and resting popu-lations was also studied.

A major stumbling block in the treatment of human neoplasia is the large fraction of the tumour cell population which is in the resting phase (i. e. G_0 or very long G_1) but nevertheless able to reenter the active cycle. In the resting state the cells may be quite insensitive to anticancer agents, and so attempts have been made to influence

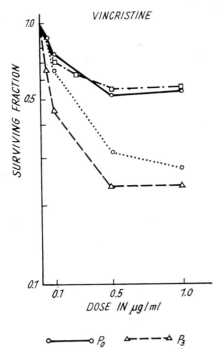

Fig. 1. Dose response curves of P clones treated with VCR for 3 h.

343

these cells. Such in vitro studies were inspired largely by the observations of Hahn and Little (5), who suggested that, from a kinetic viewpoint, the resting or plateau phase cultures may represent a better model of in vivo populations of tumour cells than do cultures in the exponential phase of growth. In this paper we present the chemotherapeutic response of Morris hepatoma cells 3924A to vinca alkaloids, vincristine and Vinblastine. Dose-response curves were evaluated after 3 h treatment. Resting state was induced by unfed culturing (13), and defined as the time period during which the cell number was constant, the mitotic activity and cell loss were practically zero, and about 4% the nuclei were labeled. Our earlier studies (12) demonstrated that VCR was able to kill preferentially non-proliferating Chinese hamster cells. The rapidly prowing Morris hepatoma cell line proved to be more sensitive to VCR in the actively groliferating phase (Fig. 2). Vinblastine (VLB) was equally toxic to proliferating and resting cells (Fig. 3).

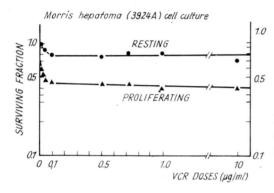

Fig. 2. Dose response curves of proliferating and resting hepatoma cells treated with VCR for 3 h.

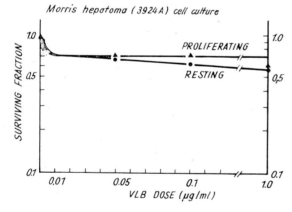

Fig. 3. Dose response curves of proliferating and resting hepatoma cells treated with VLB for 3h.

The apparent efficiency of vinca alkaloids in killing non-proliferating cells in vitro does not necessarily mean that G_0 tumour cells in vivo will exhibit a similar response, although similar examples have been published on the cytotoxicity of vinca alkaloids (3, 4).

Drug resistance can easily be induced by first giving small doses of the drug, and then with gradual increase of the dose, a resistant tumour develops. Such a VCR-resistant subline of the P388 mouse lymphoma has been induced. It is, however, important to know, whether the host organism plays any role in the lowered sensitivity of the tumour to VCR. Therefore the distribution with time of ^{14}C-VCR in the tumours and host tissues was determined. The tissue distribution of ^{14}C-VCR was almost the same in mice transplanted either with sensitive or resistant P388 leukaemias, but the uptake of the labeled drug, however, was more pronounced in the sensitive than in the resistant tumour cells. These data suggest that altered properties of the tumour cells and not those of the host are responsible for the resistance.

Further studies were carried out on the in vitro established sensitive (P388/S) and resistant (P388/R) tumour cells, and drug sensitivity was determined by colony-forming ability in soft agar. The cells were treated for 3 h with VCR. It was shown that P388/R cells retained their resistance to the drug in vitro.

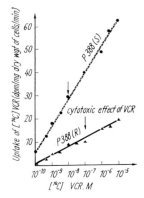

Fig. 4. The rate of VCR uptake by P388 tumour cells growing in tissue culture.

It was, also noted that the sensitive cells took up three times, as much labelled VCR as the resistant cells (Fig. 4). Decreased drug uptake in the resistant line was probably caused by changes in the composition and/or structure of the cell membrane. In order to get direct evidence for the interaction of vinca alkaloids and membrane constituents, the radioactive VCR binding capacity of membrane fraction prepared from P388 leukaemia has been determined. The ratio of VCR in the plasma membrane obtained from the sensitive tumour cells, to that obtained from the resistant cells was 1.6. The ratio of binding of VCR by tubulin isolated from the sensitive cells to that derived from the resistant tumours was 3.1 (Table 1). We think that the different VCR binding capacity of the cell membrane in the sensitive and resistant tumours, as well as their different drug uptake, may be the bases of drug resistance.

In the following experiments, the nature of this resistant phenotype was studied. The hybridization method was used to detect the dominant or recessive character of drug resistance (15).

Table 1.
Distribution of ^{14}C-VCR in isolated cell fractions of P388 leukemias

Cell fractions	Bound ^{14}C-VCR dpm/mg protein		Ratio
	P388/S	P388/R	
Crude homogenate	7,478	2,624	2,85
Golgi fraction	2,600	1,745	1,49
Plasma membrane I.	3,750	2,260	1,66
Plasma membrane II.	3,408	2,130	1,6
Purified tubulin	8,900	2,870	3,1

Intraspecific hybrids were constructed from both the sensitive and resistant lines. A thymidine kinase (TK)-deficient, bromodeoxyuridine (BUdR)-resistant clone was isolated from the VCR-sensitive line, and a hypoxanthineguanine phosphoribosyl transferase-deficient (HPRT), 6-thioguanine-resistant (6-TG) clone, from the VCR-resistant line. The two clones were hybridized with polyethylene glycol, and the true hybrid cells were selected in HAT medium.

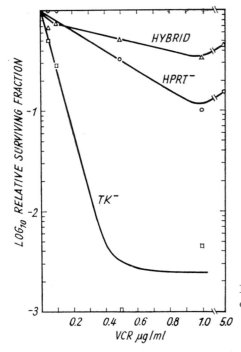

Fig. 5. Dose response curves of mutants and hybrid cells treated with VCR for 3 h.

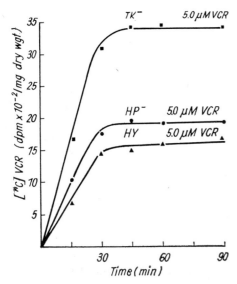

Fig. 6. ^{14}C-VCR uptake by the VCR-sensitive (TK⁻) and VCR-resistant (HPRT⁻) parent P388 cells and by their hybrids (HY).

346

Direct enzyme measurements showed deficiency of the enzymes in the deficient clones. The hybrid cells showed a lower chromosome number than the sum of those of the two component cells.

Dose response studies were carried out similarly to those outlined previously. The hybrid cells were as resistant to VCR, as was the parent VCR-resistant line (Fig. 5).

Drug uptake studies have also supported the supposition that it is the membrane which is responsible for the decreased drug sensitivity, because the hybrid cells were found to take up half as much ^{14}C-VCR as the TK$^-$VCR-sensitive line (Fig. 6). The resistant phenotype proved to be of dominant character in the intraspecific hybrid cells.

Chromosomal alterations undoubtedly play an important role in resistance at cellular level. Resistance to antimetabolites is due to mutation. There is no proof, however, that all types of resistance are related to changes in the genome. The appearance or disappearance of chromosome markers can be both the cause, and the consequence of changes in drug sensitivity of cells.

Conclusions

Among the various pharmacological factors influencing drug resistance, the most important is the active drug concentration in the tumour. In addition, cell kinetics and the ratio of resting to proliferating pools of the tumour may also have some influence. The biochemical factors influencing drug resistance include reduced transport and decrease of the activating enzymes, as well as the reduced effect of the antitumour agents on target enzymes themselves.

In our own studies resistance to vinca alkaloids was investigated. Clones isolated from NK/Ly mouse ascites lymphoma exhibited varying sensitivity to Vincristine. The Morris hepatoma (3924 A) cell culture proved to be more sensitive to VCR in the actively proliferating phase, while VLB was equally toxic against both the proliferating and resting cells. The sensitive subline of P388 mouse lymphoma took up more ^{14}C-VCR both in vivo and in vitro. The decreased VCR binding capacity of the cell membrane in the resistant tumour may be related to reduced drug uptake. Intraspecific hybrids were constructed from the sensitive and resistant P388 tumour culture. The VCR resistant phenotype proved to be of dominant character.

References

 1. Chu, M. Y. and Fischer, G. A.: Biochem. Pharmacol. *13* (1965), 333
 2 Connors, T. A.: Eur. J. Cancer 2 (1966), 293
 3. Drewinko, B. and Barlogie, B.: AACR Abstr. (1980), 284
 4. Gage, A., Orengo, A. and Drewinko, B.: AACR Abstr. (1980), 286
 5. Hahn, G. M. and Little, J. B.: Current Topics Radiat. Res. *8* (1972), 39
 6. Hill, B. T.: Biochem. Biophys. Acta. *516* (1978), 389
 7. Holczinger, L., Turi, G., Oláh, E. and Gál, F.: Acta morph. hung. *24* (1976), 351
 8. Inaba, M. and Johnson, R. K.: Biochem. Pharmacol. *27* (1978), 2123
 9. Kessel, D., Hall, T. C. and Rosenthal, D.: Cancer Res. *29* (1969), 459
10. Ling, V.: Canad. J. Genet. Cytol. *17* (1975), 503
11. Misra, D. K., Humphreys, S. R., Friedhin, M., Goldin, A. and Crawford, E. J.: Nature *189* (1961), 39
12. Oláh, E., Lui, M. S., Tzeng, D. Y. and Weber, G.: Cancer Res. *40* (1980), 2869

347

13. Oláh, E., Pályi, I. and Sugár, J.: Europ. J. Cancer *14* (1978), 895
14. Pályi, I., Oláh, E. and Sugár, J.: Int. J. Cancer *19* (1977), 859
15. Pályi, I., Turi, G., Szikla, K. and Dallmann, L.: Arch. Geschwulstforsch. *61* (1981), 119
16. Sköld, O., Magnusson, P. H. and Révész, L.: Cancer Res. *22* (1962), 1226
17. UICC Workshop on Drug Resistance and Selectivity in Cancer Chemotherapy (1976) UICC Technical Report Series, 21

Department of Clinical Oncology, University of Glasgow and Beatson Institute for Cancer Research, Glasgow, U. K.

Analysis of Cytotoxic and Cytostatic Effects

R. I. Freshney, F. Celik and D. Morgan

One of the major problems which faces the individualised chemosensitivity testing of human tumours is that the results must be known within a few weeks if they are to be of any value in directing subsequent chemotherapy. The determination of plating efficiency was clearly established some years ago as the generally accepted method for measuring cytotoxicity and the inhibition of cell proliferation (cytostasis). Unfortunately, due to the low plating efficiencies which prevail in studies on cells freshly isolated from human tumours and, for that matter, with cells derived from early passage cell lines from human tumours, there is some doubt as to whether the results would be representative of the tumour cell population. This has given rise to the speculation that cells which will form colonies in suspension may be regarded as the stem cells or repopulating cells of the tumour from which the culture was derived (Hamburger and Salmon, 1977). Although there is considerable evidence in the literature to confirm that transformed or malignant cells clone in suspension with a very much higher efficiency than normal cells (Macpherson and Montagnier, 1964), the evidence of a distinction in cloning efficiency between normal cells and malignant cells freshly explanted is not so clear. In recent studies with human glioma and melanoma we have found that the plating efficiencies of normal glia and normal human fibroblasts, cloned in suspension, are similar to that of glioma and melanoma derived cell lines. Both are extremely low (in the order of 0.5%) and do not approach the magnitude observed with transformed rodent cell lines. While it may yet be possible that cells cloning in suspension represent a specific stem cell compartment, currently the evidence is lacking that these are necessarily tumour cells. We have therefore concentrated on the comparison of microtitration and cloning efficiency of cells growing in monolayer to determine whether these give similar measurements of drug sensitivity. It is hoped that at some stage in the future we may make a similar comparison between cloning efficiency in monolayer and in suspension.

Although many different tests have been used to predict chemosensitivity, those in common use can be divided into three major categories. (1) The short term assay (4—24 hours) of chopped fragments or slices from the tumour, the effect of drugs being assessed by isotope incorporation (e. g. Volm et al, 1978). (2) Monolayers of either primary or subcultures from the tumour where drug sensitivity is measured using cell proliferation (Berry et al, 1975), cloning efficiency (Berry et al, 1975; Wallen et al, 1981) or isotope incorporation (Dendy and Bozman, 1970; Wolberg and Ansfield, 1971). Because of the time taken to set up the culture, for the culture to initiate proliferation. and for the necessary characterisation to be performed, this type of test usually takes between 2 and 6 weeks. (3) "Stem cell" assay, performed on cell suspensions prepared directly from the tumour, and cloned in suspension, with

349

the assumption that this will select neoplastic cells (HAMBURGER and SALMON, 1977 OZOLS et al, 1980). This type of test may take between 2 and 4 weeks. The experiments that I would like to describe today have been performed on monolayer cultures derived from human anaplastic astrocytoma and maintained in culture as cell lines. Drug sensitivity assays have been performed between the third and the tenth passage. The microtitration assay was developed based on the measurement of protein synthesis after exposure to drugs (FRESHNEY, PAUL and KANE, 1975) and was shown to be capable of discriminating between different cell lines and their sensitivity to a variety of cytostatic and cytotoxic drugs (THOMAS et al, 1979). This type of assay, however, was always open to the question of whether isotope incorporation was measuring survival in terms of the number of surviving cells or the residual capability of protein synthesis in all the cells in the population. The morphological appearance of the culture after drug treatment confirm that in most cases a drop in protein synthesis was accompanied by cell loss in the culture but it was felt that this relationship required to be established more clearly by comparison with a clonogenic assay. Consequently a series of experiments were performed on six drugs, 5-fluorouracil, vincristine, bleomycin, methyl CCNU, mithramycin and VM26, and five cell lines, IJK, EME, GMS, JPT and 496/5. Each cell line was assayed for drug sensitivity by microtitration and by cloning and the results compared.

The microtitration assay (FRESHNEY and MORGAN, 1978) was performed by trypsinising the secondary, or later, stage culture and seeding cells into microtitration plates at 2×10^4 cells/ml (2×10^3/well), allowing the cells a minimum of 48 hours to recover from the trauma of trypsinisation and then adding drugs in a range of concentrations across the plate. Drugs were replaced after 24 and 48 hours, removed at 72 hours, and the plate cultured for a further 5 days with regular medium changes before assaying for survival with [^{35}S]methionine. The [^{35}S]methionine was added for 4 hours, removed, the plate washed, and the cells fixed in methanol and dried. After acid soluble extraction of unincorporated [^{35}S]methionine, the plate was again dried and scintillation fluid added directly to the wells. This was dried by spinning the plate in a centrifuge for 1 hour at approximately $800 \times g$. The dried plate was bound up with X-ray film (Kodak Royal RP14) and exposed in the dark for between 24 hours and 3 days at -70 °C. Development of the plate showed spots of varying intensity proportional to the amount of [^{35}S] incorporated per well and this was quantified by running the autofluorogram through a densitometer. The densitometer scan enabled calculation of the ID_{50}, i. e. that concentration of drug reducing [^{35}S]methionine incorporation (optical density of the spots) by 50%. The distribution of ID_{50}'s are illustrated in Fig. 1. We have previously obtained data with procarbazine, methyl CCNU and vincristine for a series of twenty anaplastic astrocytomas (MORGAN et al, in preparation) suggesting that, on the whole, very little sensitivity could be demonstrated to methyl CCNU or CCNU, that a small proportion (3 out of 20 cell lines) could be demonstrated as sensitive to vincristine, and while procarbazine was effective in inhibiting [^{35}S]methionine incorporation, cells recovered from this within a few days. The current series of observations confirmed that differences in drug sensitivity could be demonstrated between individual cell lines and that in some cases these differences amounted to more than two orders of magnitude. Vincristine and bleomycin were found to be particularly effective both in terms of their absolute ID50's and the ratios of the ID50's to the predicted plasma levels.

The same series of 5 cell lines were then exposed to drugs in regular monolayer culture following the same routine as used for microtitration, i. e. cells were seeded at 2×10^4

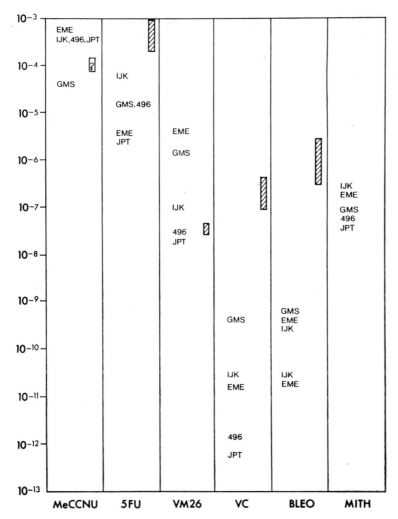

Fig. 1. Distribution of ID_{50}'s by microtitration assay. Each point, indicated by the three letter designation of the culture, is the mean of duplicate drug titrations, measured by autofluorography 5 days after removal of the drugs. The shaded bars are the estimated ranges of the peak plasma concentration for each drug taken from the following reports: Bleomycin — ALBERTS et al, 1978, ALBERTS et al, 1979; VM-26, epipodophyllotoxin — ALLEN and CREAVEN, 1975; Vincristine — DYKE and NELSON, 1977, OWELLEN et al, 1977; 5-fluorouracil — FINN and SADEE, 1975, MAC-MILLAN et al, 1978.

Figures for the peak plasma concentration of methyl CCNU were difficult to obtain (SPONZO et al, 1973) and BCNU is given in its place (LEVIN et al, 1978).

per ml, 48—72 hours later drugs were added at a range of concentrations and replaced daily for 3 days. On the third day drugs were removed, the culture was trypsinised and plated out at 200 cells/ml in 9 cm petri dishes. Half of the cultures were placed on homologous feeder layers of mitomycin-C treated cells which had been seeded at 2500 cells/ml. After 3 weeks stained colonies were counted by eye, the surviving fraction counted and results plotted as in Figs. 2—7.

In Fig. 2. it can be seen that following treatment with 5-fluorouracil cell line 496/5 had an ID50 of approximately 10^{-4} M and showed evidence of a surviving fraction of approximately 4% up to 10^{-2} M. When results were compared with clones forming in the absence of a feeder layer the ID50 was similar although the surviving fraction was reduced. The effect of the feeder layer was more noticeable, however, with the antibiotics bleomycin and mithramycin on the cell GMS. A 2—3% surviving fraction after exposure to mithramycin was only detectable in the presence of a feeder layer

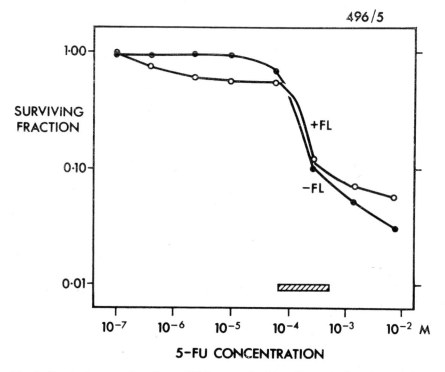

Fig. 2. Survival curves for glioma 496/5 treated with 5-fluorouracil as in test. Open circles and solid line, treated cells cloned in the presence of 790 homologous feeder cells per cm^2, filled circles and solid line, treated cells cloned in the absence of feeder cells. The shaded bar represents the approximate range for the peak plasma concentration as in Fig. 1. The 496/5 cell line was derived from a human anaplastic astrocytoma passaged in immune-deprived mice by Dr. Nick BRADLEY of the Chester Beatty Research Institute, Fulham, Road, London.

but not in its absence (Fig. 3). When the results with IJK and GMS are compared after exposure to bleomycin, GMS is apparently more sensitive to the antibiotic than IJK; however, in the presence of a feeder layer a significant resistant fraction becomes apparent in GMS which persists up to around 3×10^{-8} M (Fig. 4). Although GMS still appears to be more sensitive than IJK at low drug concentrations, the position is reversed at higher drug concentrations due to the persistence of a resistant fraction in GMS. Clearly this could make a great difference to the interpretation of clonogenic assays and emphasizes the need to maintain an adequate cell concentration in plates during cloning.

Figs. 5, 6 and 7 illustrate the differences in sensitivity to 5-FU, vincristine and methyl CCNU demonstrated by the clonogenic assay. Examination of the results from 5-FU shows that cell line EME was marginally more sensitive than the others studied but, at a drug concentration which could be expected in vivo, the cell survival remained high. The position was similar with vincristine where, although differences could be demonstrated in ID50, a substantial resistant fraction was present with 3 out of 4 of the cell lines illustrated and only in one case did this fall below 10%.

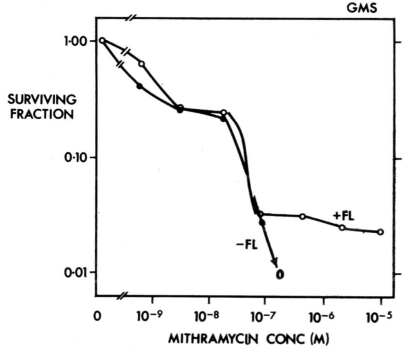

Fig. 3. Survival curve for GMS cells following exposure to different concentrations of mithramycin. Treated cells were cloned in the presence and absence of a feeder layer as in Fig. 2.

The results shown in Fig. 7 demonstrate that the sensitivity of the lines to methyl CCNU was very low, as had been indicated by the results obtained by microtitration. All the three lines illustrated in Fig. 7 show virtually no sensitivity to methyl CCNU whatsoever, unless cloned in the absence of feeder layer, where some sensitivity was demonstrable with line 496/5, but apparently only about 50% of the population were sensitive.

It is apparent from the results of the clonogenic assays that, while some distinctions may be made between the cell lines on the basis of the ID50, as demonstrated previously with microtitration, much more information can be derived from the clonogenic assays in terms of the size of the resistant fraction present in each cell population. Comparing the clonogenic assay with the microtitration assay, on the basis of the ID50, showed a very good correlation as demonstrated in Fig. 8. All the available data with the six drugs and five cell lines are presented here and give a correlation coefficient of 0.96. It was interesting to note that most of the outlying points belonged to one cell line GMS which has been shown subsequently to have been contaminated by endothelial cells. When the ID90's were compared the correlation coefficient dropped to 0.82 implying less agreement between the two assays. This may imply a higher resolving power of the clonogenic assay at higher inhibitory doses where small resistant fractions may be identified more accurately than with microtitration.

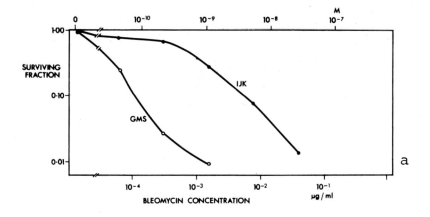

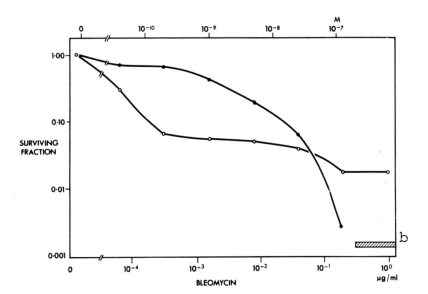

Fig. 4. Comparison of survival curves for GMS and IJK cells after treatment with Bleomycin. (a) Treated cells cloned in the absence of a feeder layer. (b) Treated cells cloned on feeder layer as described in text and in legend to Fig. 2.

It is important to realise that the identification of small resistant fractions by the clonogenic assay was only possible in some cases where a feeder layer had been incorporated. Conventional practice attempts to adjust the number of colonies forming per dish in a clonogenic assay such that the cell concentrations at different drug levels will be approximately the same at the end of the assay. It is perhaps necessary to take this procedure a step further and ensure that the cell concentration remains high and independent of drug action, i. e. by employing a feeder layer, the cell concentration of which is greatly in excess of that of the clonogenic cell population. Further evidence for the effect of cell density on the measurement of drug sensitivity has been obtained in observations on sensitivity to steroids. Glucocorticoids are used

354

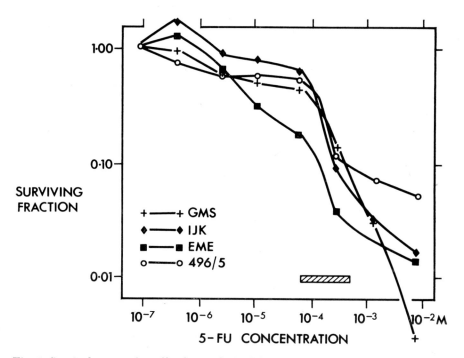

Fig. 5. Survival curves for cell cultures derived from four different anaplastic astrocytomas, cloned on feeder layers after treatment with a range of concentrations of 5-FU. The shaded bar represents the approximate peak plasma concentration as in Fig. 1.

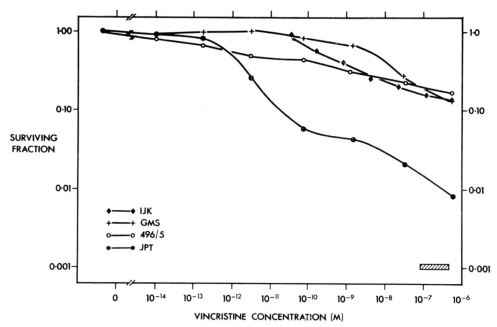

Fig. 6. Survival curves for cultures from four anaplastic astrocytomas, cloned on feeder layers after treatment with vincristine. The shaded bar repesents the approximate peak plasma concentration as in Fig. 1.

in the treatment of glioma to reduce cerebral oedema and enhance post-operative recovery. It has been suggested that steroids may also be cytostatic. When cultures of glioma, grown to saturation density in the presence or absence of steroids, were compared, it was seen that methyl prednisolone, betamethasone and dexamethasone were all equally effective in reducing the saturation density of the culture (FRESHNEY et al, 1980). When cells were taken from saturation density, after labelling overnight with [³H]thymidine, and autoradiographs prepared, a difference in the labelling index

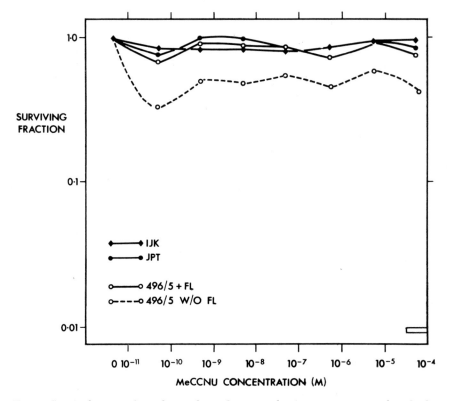

Fig. 7. Survival curves for cultures from three anaplastic astrocytomas, cloned after treatment with Methyl-CCNU. All three cultures were cloned on feeder layers. The lowest curve (0 —·— 0) was obtained by cloning 496/5 cells in the absence of a feeder layer. The bar represents the approximate peak plasma concentration range for BCNU (See Fig. 1).

was also observed, implying a reduction in cell proliferation in the presence of steroids. However, when these cultures were exposed to dexamethasone in a clonogenic assay both cell survival and cell proliferation were enhanced (FRESHNEY et al, 1980; GUNER et al, 1977). The presence of a feeder layer did not alter the stimulation of clonal growth by steroids, and cytostasis was only observed when cells were densely packed. While the advantages of a clonogenic assay can be appreciated in terms of analysis of both survival and cell proliferation, it must be recognized that the necessity to plate cells at low densities may alter their response quite dramatically. Elevation of cell concentration by adding a homologous feeder layer to the culture may in part correct for this error, but observations with glucocorticoids imply that it is the density of the culture, i. e. intimate cell-cell contact, which is important rather than the absolute numbers of cells present.

Although there is as yet insufficient data to correlate these observations with clinical outcome, it may be possible that assays of cytotoxicity, such as the microtitration assay described above, may be good indicators of the response in vivo, but that survival rate may require analysis of clonal growth. This demands further investigations of the effects of cell density.

	Correlation Coefficient	y/x
ID_{50} ●--●	0.96 p ≲ 0.001	0.90
ID_{90} ○—○	0.82 p ≲ 0.001	0.98

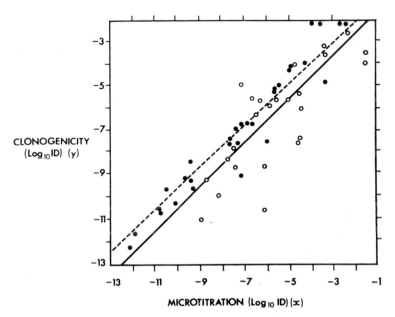

Fig. 8. Correlation curves for the ID_{50}'s and ID_{90}'s of all of the cell lines with the six drugs, obtained by microtitration and by cloning. The filled circles are ID_{90}'s and the open circles ID_{50}'s. The broken line is the regression line drawn through the ID_{90}'s, the solid line through the ID_{50}'s.

Acknowledgements

This work was supported by the Nuffield Foundation, the Medical Research Council, the Cancer Research Campaign and the Humane Research Trust. The authors are indebted to Dr. D. I. Graham and members of the staff of the Neuropathology Department of the Southern General Hospital, Glasgow for helpful collaboration.

References

1. Alberts, S. D., Chen, H.-S. G., Liu, R., Himmelstein, K. J., Mayersohn, M., Perrier, D., Gross, J., Moon, T., Broughton, A. and Salmon, S. E.: Cancer Chemother. Pharmacol. 1 (1978), 177—181
2. Alberts, D. S., Chen, H.-S., G. Mayersohn, M., Perrier, D., Moon, T. E. and Gross, F. J.: Cancer Chemother. Pharmacol. 2 (1979), 127—132

357

3. ALLEN, I. M. and CREAVEN, P. J.: Europ. J. Cancer *11* (1975), 697—707
4. BERRY, R. J., LAING, A. H. and WELLS, J.: Br. J. Cancer *31* (1975), 218—227
5. DENDY, P. P. and BOZMAN, G.: (1970) The Lancet 68—72
6. DYKE, R. W. and NELSON, R. L.: Cancer Treat. Rev. *4* (1977), 135—142
7. FINN, C. and SADEE, W.: Cancer Chemother. Rep. Part 1 *59* (1975), 279—286
8. FRESHNEY, R. I., PAUL, J. and KANE, I. M.: Br. J. Cancer *31* (1975), 89—99
9. FRESHNEY, R. I. and MORGAN, D.: Cell Biology International Reports. Vol. 2 No. *4* (1978), 375—380
10. FRESHNEY, R. I., SHERRY, A., HASSANZADAM, M., FRESHNEY, M., CRILLY, P. and MORGAN, D.: Brit. J. Cancer *41* (1980), 857—866
11. GUNER, M., FRESHNEY, R. I., MORGAN, D., FRESHNEY, M. G., THOMAS, D. G. T. and GRAHAM, D. I.: Br. J. Cancer *35* (1977), 439—447
12. HAMBURGER, A. W. and SALMON, S. E.: Science. Vol. 197 (1977), 461—463
13. LEVIN, V. A., HOFFMAN, W. and WEINKAM, R. J.: Cancer Treat. Rep. *62* (1978), 1305—1312
14. MacMILLAN, W. I., WOLBERG, W. H. and WELLING, P. E.: Cancer Res. *38* (1978), 3479—3482
15. MACPHERSON, I. and MONTAGNIER, L.: Virology *23* (1964), 291—294
16. OZOLS, R. F., WILLISON, J. K. V., WALTZ, M. D., GROTZINGER, K. R., MYERS, C. E. and YOUNG, R. C.: Cancer Research *40* (1980), 4109—4112
17. OWELLEN, R. J., ROOT, M. A. and HAINS, F. O.: Cancer Research *37* (1977), 2603—2607
18. ROSENBLUM, M. L., VASQUEZ, D. A., HOSHINO, T., WILSON, C. B.: Cancer *41* (1978), 2305
19. SPONZO, R. W., DEVITA, V. T. and OLIVERIO, V. T.: Cancer *31* (1973), 1154—1159
20. THOMAS, D. G. T., DARLING, J. L., FRESHNEY, R. I. and MORGAN, D. (1979): In: Multidisciplinary Aspects of Brain Tumour Therapy. Eds. P. PAOLETTI, M. D. WALKER, G. BUTTI and R. KNERICH. Elsevier/North Holland Biomedical Press
21. VOLM, M., WAYSS, K., KAUFMANN, M. and MATTERN, J.: Europ. J. Cancer *15* (1978), 983—993
22. WOLBERG, W. H. and ANSFIELD, F. J.: Cancer Research *31* (1971), 448—450

Department of Biochemical Pharmacology, Institute of Cancer Research, Belmont, Sutton, Surrey, England

An Appraisal of Current In Vivo and In Vitro Screening Methods

A. H. Calvert and K. R. Harrap

Introduction

In the last few years a number of methods have become available which may be used to test for antitumour activity in unknown compounds. In particular the use of human tumours rather than the transplantable tumours of rodents is becoming more widespread. Two of the most popular techniques are human tumour xenografts in which a human tumour may be transplanted serially in immune-suppressed or nude mice and the in vitro clonogenic assay, which has recently been the subject of much attention due to the work of Salmon and his collaborators (1). This article examines these two methods in the context of more traditional rodent screens and discusses their potential contribution towards the selection of new drugs which may provide a better treatment for human cancer.

Achievements of screening with rodent tumours

There are a number of forms of human cancer in which chemotherapy has met with some success. Between one third and one half of children with acute lymphoblastic leukaemia now survive for long periods (2) and are probably cured. A higher proportion of patients with Hodgkin's disease, certain non-Hodgkin's lymphomas and testicular tumours seem to be cured (3, 4), and it is even possible for a few patients with ovarian adenocarcinoma or small cell bronchial tumours to survive in the long term (5, 6). The derisory attitude which maintains that these results make only a trivial impact upon the toll of human cancer is perhaps not entirely justified if the age of cancer sufferers with diseases treatable by chemotherapy is considered. These are mostly children or young adults, so that the number of "man years" saved per individual is greater than the number which would be saved were we able to treat, for example, carcinoma of the colon. The facts that there has been a considerable degree of success in the development of cancer chemotherapy and that the drugs by which this success has been achieved have been selected exclusively by the use of rodent screens, suggest that these screens should be very carefully considered in any future selection process.

Limitations of rodent tumour screens

There is, however, evidence to suggest that the uncritical use of rodent screens has frequently failed to select the more active and less toxic drugs which are so clearly needed to improve the treatment of human cancer. Table 1 summarises the results

Table 1.
Clinical activity of selected drugs which performed well in rodent screens

Drug	Activity in rodent screens	Activity against human tumours
Nitrosoureas	Broad spectrum activity in most systems	Minor activity in some tumours. No established role in any curative therapy
PALA	Lewis lung B16 melanoma Glioma 26 Colon 26 FANFT bladder	No clinical activity in over 200 patients
Pyrazofurin	Walker 256 755 mammary Gardner X 5563 plasma cell tumour DMBA mammary	Clinical responses very rare
DON	P388 and L1210 C26 and C38 colon CD8F1 mammary	Clinical responses very rate
Maytansine	B16 melanoma	0/23 metastatic melanoma

obtained both experimentally and clinically with several drugs which have emerged during the past ten years. It is particularly disappointing that examples can be shown of drugs which are highly active in a broad spectrum of animal tumours, but which have a clinical role which is extremely limited or non-existent. This is not to say that the clinical evaluation of new drugs has been insufficient to determine their role. Several other drugs, notably Adriamycin, VP16 and Cisplatinum have established themselves are a part of curative treatment in the same period. Thus the use of rodent screening systems has on occasions led to the selection of drugs with no clinical value. A more important defect of a screen would be if it had rejected a drug which would in fact be of great value. An example of this is difficult to find since activity in the rodent models has usually been a prerequisite for clinical trial. However, 6-mercapto-purine may be such an example. It is a drug with a clinical role in the maintenance of acute lymphatic leukaemia (2), has very limited activity in most rodent tumours and would probably not now be selected for clinical trial. In the next few years we may expect to see the clinical results obtained with a number of new drugs selected for their activity in either the human tumour xenograft system or in a clonogenic assay. It will be of great interest to compare these results with those obtained on drugs selected in a conventional manner. However, there are already a number of examples in the experience of the authors and others where these two screening methods seem not to be predictive for human activity. The reasons for this are known to a degree and serve as a useful illustration of how to interpret these models.

The use of the in-vitro human tumour stem cell assay

In this technique, by which single cell suspensions of human tumour biopsy specimens are cloned in agar may be used to assay drug activity by the inhibition of colony format-ion. SALMON et al published a paper in which in vitro activity of certain drugs against ovarian cancer or myeloma cells was shown to correlate with clinical activity of the same drugs(s) in the patient from whom the original cells were derived (1). Since that time there has been wide interest in the technique which has been applied by numerous workers, not only to the problem of predicting a response for an individual patient, but also for evaluation unknown drugs for their supposed activity against human tumours (7). Surprisingly, in spite of all this activity, good evidence for the in vitro—in vivo correlation has been lacking. The original data was based on small numbers of patients, not all of whom were treated with the same drugs as those tested in vitro. For example cyclophosphamide cannot be tested in vitro without activation by hepatic microsomes. For this reason in vitro sensitivity was measured using melphalan, while in some cases the patients were treated with cyclophosphamide. In many cases patients were treated with a combination therapy demanded by a clinical protocol, where in vitro testing was of course done with a single agent. Subsequent reports have presented data to the effect that the clinical response rate to protocol designed in the basis of in vitro sensitivity is greater than that achieved using an empirical scheme (8). Nevertheless, extensive prospective studies of the correlation between in vitro and in vivo response, necessary if the in vitro assay is to be adopted as a means of drug selection, have still not been performed.

A number of authors have studied the in vitro—in vivo correlation using the human tumour xenograft systems (9, 10). The advantages of this technique are that experiments can be repeated and confirmed using the same system and further, that the in vivo treatment is not hampered by clinical ethical constraints. Although some authors have reported a good correlation (9), others have shown that there is not correlation with all drugs. In particular, BATEMAN et al have shown that in vitro response to adriamycin does not correlate with the in vivo result in melanoma xenografts (10). A dramatic example of the lack of in vitro—in vivo correlation was encountered recently in the development of a new antifolate, CB 3717. Fig. 1 shows the in vitro dose response of two rodent cell lines, the L1210 tumour and the TLX/5 lymphoma in vitro. It is apparent that the TLX/5 lymphoma is somewhat more sensitive than

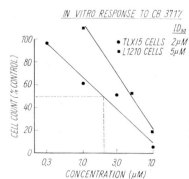

Fig. 1. Dose response curve for TLX/5 lymphoma cells and L1210 cells to CB 3717 in vitro. Data — personal communication, A. L. JACKMAN.

the L1210. However, the converse applied in vivo (Fig. 2), where the drug was curative to the L1210 tumour but had no effect on the TLX/5 lymphoma. The reason for this disparity is not known, but could be due to differences in the ability of the two cell lines to salvage circulatory thymidine in vivo. Thymidine reverses the antitumour effect of CB 3717 in vitro but was not present in the in vitro assay system used.

From the examples cited above it can be seen that, even if an in vitro—in vivo correlation could be demonstrated for certain drugs, it could not be applied generally

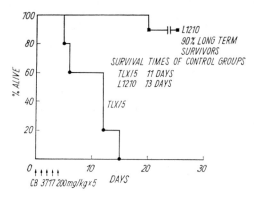

Fig. 2. Survival of mice bearing the L1210 or the TLX/5 tumour treated with equal doses of CB 3717.

to drugs requiring metabolic activation or to antimetabolites whose action may be modulated by circulating nucleosides. In view of the fact that major disparities between in vitro and in vivo response are not predictable with current knowledge even for well known drugs, it seems that in vitro techniques will at most make only a very limited contribution to the characterization of new and unknown compounds.

The use of human tumour xenografts

This technique is applicable to a wider range of drugs than an in vitro technique since metabolic activation is not a problem. It also has the advantage that experiments may be repeated on the same tumour. Its obvious disadvantages are that it is slow and expensive, but a more serious shortcoming is that it may still either predict activity in drugs which are inactive clinically or vice versa. These problems seem to relate to differences in the normal metabolism and in drug metabolism existing between mouse and man.

Differences in drug metabolism

This problem is well exemplified by the history of pentamethylmelamine. Pentamethylmelamine is active in several human tumour xenografts, and has recently been the subject of several Phase I studies (11) treating a total of about 150 patients. Although the objective of a Phase I study is not to demonstrate antitumour activity, it is surprising that out of all these patients no complete or partial responses were seen. Pentamethylmelamine undergoes oxidative demethylation, with N-hydroxymethyl derivatives being formed as intermediates. Subsequent to the clinical studies, animal studies have shown that the formation of hydroxymethyl compounds appear to be a prerequisite for antitumour activity. Studies of patients included in Phase I studies have demonstrated that there is virtually none of this intermediate formed in man (11).

362

Differences in normal metabolism and pharmacokinetics

SHORTHOUSE et al, in an excellent correlative study, were unable to establish 18 xeno-graft lines from patients with lung cancer (12). The response of the patients to a com-bination therapy correlated exactly with the response of the xenograft to the same combination. In the majority of patients the combination comprised methotrexate, CCNU and cyclophosphamide. However, none of the xenograft lines were sensitive to methotrexate given as a single agent (SHORTHOUSE, personal communication). Although none of the patients received methotrexate as a single agent, it seems un-likely that treatment of consecutive patients with methotrexate would result in no therapeutic results. The fact that methotrexate may be less active against a human tumour growing in a mouse than against a human tumour in man might be anticipated. Normal rodent tissues are rather more sensitive to methotrexate than those of man (13, 14), so that high levels of the drug cannot be maintained for so long in the mouse. The half-life of methotrexate in the mouse is about four times shorter than that in man (15, 16), further compromising the exposure of the human tumour. Finally, plasma thymidine levels in mice are considerably higher than those found in man (see Table 2).

Table 2.
Plasma thymidine levels (μM)

MICE:	CBA	0.53	
	BDF1	1.54	
	BalbC	1.85	
	Nude	1.00	
	DBA2	1.80	
MAN:	Normal Volunteers		0.43 ± 0.063
	12 Cancer patients		$5, < 0.1$
	Remaining		$7, 0.10-2.0$
	Median		0.17

Data — personal communication, G. A. TAYLOR

Summary and conclusions

Two interesting new methods of screening potential anticancer drugs against human tumours have been discussed. Although both can clearly add to the information gained by the use of conventional rodent antitumour screens, examples have been cited in which either system can lead to a spurious prediction of activity or inactivity. These tests should therefore be used not to replace, but to supplement those already existing. The final arbiter of activity in human cancer will be clinical trial itself. In view of the fact that the predictive accuracy of all the test systems is poor it seems reasonable to adopt a scheme which expedites both the preclinical and clinical evaluation of interesting new agents. One possible scheme currently under study is as follows. A drug is selected for study clinically if it satisfied the following three conditions:

a. There is a satisfactory rationale for its use. A novel chemical structure, or bioche-mical mode of action would be considered suitable, or an analogue of an existing drug which showed less cross-resistance or reduced toxicity.

b. There is evidence for antitumour activity in some test systems. A novel compound would not be required to have extensive testing, but a close analogue of an existing compound would need to be at least as good as the parent experimentally. Broad spectrum animal activity in say a nitrosourea would not be considered an adequate reason for clinical study, since many all nitrosoureas show excellent activity in animal screens, but are extremely disappointing in man.

c. Appropriate toxicity testing in one or two species, as an indicator of the starting dose for use in a clinical study.

The clinical studies may be speeded up on two ways:

a. Escalation of doses in successive courses within patients. This allows the majority of the patients entering the study to receive a dose high enough to have the possibility of being therapeutic, and may assist in achieving objective (b) below.

b. Selection of patients carefully who may be ethically treated with a new agent, but who have the possibility of achieving a clinical response and thus vindicating or refuting the rationale for the use of the drug. For example, in a study of an analogue which was not cross-resistant with the parent drug experimentally, patients would be selected who had relapsed from prior treatment. If a drug was specifically designed for say melanoma, patients with metastatic melanoma could be given the new drug as a first line of therapy since no satisfactory chemotherapy for this condition is known.

It is to be hoped, that by such a scheme it will be possible to test drugs which otherwise would not have been tested and by this means to discover additional useful therapies for human cancer.

Acknowledgements

We are extremely grateful to A. L. Jackman and G. A. Taylor for permission to show their data in this review. We would also like to thank Dr. A. Jones and Mr. A. Shorthouse for their helpful advice and discussion in preparing this manuscript.

References

1. Salmon, S. E., Hamburger, A. W., Soehnlen, B., Durie, B. G. M., Alberts, S. D. and Moon, T. E.: New Eng. J. Med. *298* (1978), 1321
2. Simone, J. V., Aur, R. J. A., Hustu, H. O. and Pinkel, D.: Cancer *30* (1972), 1488
3. DeVita, V. T. Jr., Serpick, A. A. and Carbone, P. P.: Ann. Int. Med. *71* (1970), 881
4. Peckham, M. (ed.): Management of Testicular Tumours. Edward Arnold, London (1981),
5. Young, R. C., Chabner, B. A., Hubbard, S. P., Fisher, R. I., Bender, R. A., Anderson, T. Simon, R. M., Canellos, G. P. and DeVita, V. T.: New Eng. J. Med. *299* (1978), 1261
6. Smith, I. E., Sappeno, A. P., Bondy, P. K. and Gilby, E. D.: Europ. J. Cancer *17* (1981), 1249
7. Salmon, S. E., Meyskens, F. L., Alberts, D. S., Soehnlen, B. and Young, L.: Cancer Treat. Rep. *65* (1981), 1
8. Alberts, D. S., Salmon, S. E., Chen, H. S. G., Surwit, E. A., Soehnlen, B., Young, L. and Moon, T. E.: Lancet ii (1980), 340
9. Tveit, K. M., Fodstad, O., Olsnes, S. and Pihl, A.: Int. J. Cancer *26* (1980), 717—722
10. Bateman, A. E., Selby, P. J., Steel, P. J. and Towse, G. D. W.: Br. J. Cancer *41* (1980), 189

11. RUTTY, C. J., NEWELL, D. R., MUINDI, J. F. R. and HARRAP, K. R.: This volume

12. SHORTHOUSE, A. J., SMYTH, J. F., STEEL, G. G., ELLISON, M., MILLS, J. and PECKHAM, M. J.: Br. J. Surg. *67* (1980), 715

13. SKEEL, R. T., SAWICKI, W. L., CASHMORE, A. R. and BERTINO, J. R.: Cancer Res. *36* (1976), 3659

14. CHABNER, B. A., STOLLER, R. G. and HANDE, K.: Drug Metab. Rev. *8* (1978), 107

15. BISCHOFF, K. B., DEDRICK, R. L., ZAHARKO, D. S. and LONGSTRETH, J. A.: J. Pharm. Sci. *60* (1971), 1128

16. CALVERT, A. H., BONDY, P. K. and HARRAP, K. R.: Cancer Treat. Rep. *61* (1977), 1647

Department of Gynaecology and Obstetrics
Erfurt Medical Academy, German Democratic Republic

Clinical Relevance of some Useful Methods for In-Vitro Testing of Cytostatic Sensitivity in Cases of Ovarian Cancers

W. KRAFFT, D. BRÜCKMANN, J. BRÜCKMANN, H. BEHLING, W. PREIBSCH and J. KADEMANN

Introduction

Ever the method of cell cultivation as a means of pretherapeutic testing of cytostatic effectiveness was introduced into clinical practice by COBB, DULBECCO, VOIGT, WALKER and WRIGHT more than 25 years ago, discussions about its value have continued. So far, no definite decision has been reached.

Advocates consider pretherapeutic cytostatic testing as a way to individualize tumour chemotherapy. Critics of the testing methods doubt if the results obtained apply to clinical reality, since probleme of duration of cytostatic influence and activation, the dedifferentiation of tumour cells, and interpretation of test results have never been convincingly solved. No doubt, the in vitro testing system cannot imitate perfectly the biological processes of cytostatic action. Apart from the possibility of methodological error, the spatially and temporally heterogeneous structure of the tumour itself (IVERSEN) is a factor that cannot be overcome. Therefore, all test results obtained reflect only part of the whole, and show the limits of the present testing systems.

Even the application of additional methods such as short-term incubation, implantation of diffusion chambers in the rat peritoneum (HECKMANN) or the use of nude mice, did not markedly alter the situation.

Materials and methods

Seven hundred and forty patients with gynecologic tumours have been treated with individualized chemotherapy over a 13-year period. This paper based on clinical observations and the results obtained in by vitro tests over the past 5 years (1976—1981). During this period 125 patients suffering from ovarian cancer were treated. One hundred and sixty-one tumours were cultivated according to the cell culture method of TANNEBERGER, after being trypsinized. Cytostatics were applied for 48 h. The cytostatic effects in cell culture were observed microscopically or by determination of ^{3}H-thymidine or ^{3}H-cytidine incorporation, and compared with non-treated controls. The effects were classified into 3 groups, according to clinical experience (see Fig. 2). This evaluation was important for rating the so-called correlation between the in vitro test results and the effects obtained in clinical therapy. The evaluation is seldom uniform, and has led to differences between correlation rates reported by different authors. The most active cytostatics in vitro are CPM, ADM, RBM, VBL, and they have proved their effectiveness in clinical therapy, too. The cytostatic DDP however, which is effective clinically, seems to be quite inactive in vitro.

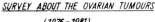

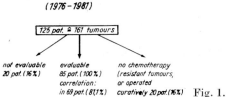

SURVEY ABOUT THE OVARIAN TUMOURS
(1976 – 1981)

125 pat. ≙ 161 tumours

not evaluable 20 pat. (16%)

evaluable 85 pat. (100%)
correlation:
in 69 pat. (81,1%)

no chemotherapy (resistant tumours, or operated curatively 20 pat. (16%)

Fig. 1.

EVALUATION OF IN VITRO TEST RESULTS

decrease of the 3H-thymidine (3H-cytidine) uptake in comparison to the control

"S" = sensitive tumours — > 75 %

"s" = less sensitive tumours — > 25 – 75 %

"r" = resistant tumours — no change or < 25 %

Fig. 2.

CONDITIONS FOR THE EVALUATION OF THE
SO CALLED CORRELATION RATE:

in vitro test result	expected therapeutic effect
"sensitivity" (S)	survival time: at least 16 months (CR, PR)
"less sensitivity" (s)	survival time: 9–12 months (PR, NR, SD) mostly
"resistant" (r)	survival time: 6 months (SD, P) like untreated tumours

Fig. 3.

The conditions for evaluating the correlations observed in this study are given in Figure 3.

Greater importance was attached to survival time, rather than to remission or "response", which is unreliable in cases of ovarian carcinomata. The correlation between results obtained in cell culture in vitro tests and clinical therapy was 81.2% for 85 patients evaluated.

Correlation of some cytostatic drugs in vitro and the response of ovarian cancers under chemotherapy (85 pat. 1976 – 1981)

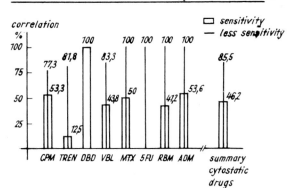

Fig. 4.

Correlation of some in vitro methods [18 pat]

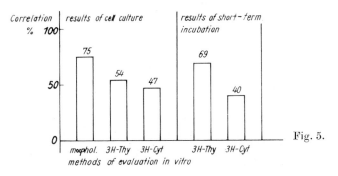

Fig. 5.

CPM and ADM correlated most frequently (about 80%), TREN and 5-FU had the lowest correlation rates (11%) (Figure 4). In order to evaluate the relevance of the in vitro test methods used, the tumours of 18 patients were tested simultaneously in cell culture and in short-term incubation. Cytostatic effects were determined in cell culture by comparative microscopic observations and ^{3}H-thymidine and ^{3}H-cytidine incorporation. The cytostatic effects of the short-term incubation were ascertained only by determination of ^{3}H-cytidine and ^{3}H-thymidine uptake. All test results were compared with clinical response. Results are given in Figure 5.

Microscopic, morphological observation of cell cultures gave the best correlation, and ^{3}H-cytidine uptake in short-term incubation was the worst. The results obtained in the short-term incubation with ^{3}H-thymidine were, however quite useful. It seems to be important that cytostatics can influence 4 h and the ^{3}H-thymidine 1—2 h. We prefer to use the cell culture method, but have found the short-term incubation test useful in cases where the tumours could not be cultured, provided ^{3}H-thymidine uptake was measured.

Experience has shown that in vitro tests may help in: individualizing post-operative tumour chemotherapy by the selection of suitable cytostatics; determining therapy duration by repeated in vitro testing of tumour cells; recognizing secondary resistance development with consequent change or abandoning the chemotherapy; and in making cautious predictions.

Hippocration General Hospital, Athens, Greece

Immunoglobulin Producing Cell Infiltration in Colorectal Cancer Tissues Correlated with Patients Survival

G. P. Stathopoulos, Ch. Pathouli, A. Manouras, A. Delladetsika, K. Pratsika-Uguroglou and M. Phillipakis

Introduction

Colorectal carcinoma is effectively treated by surgery. Five-year and ten-year survival of 51.4% and 51% respectively have been reported, with ten-year survival of 58.9% for cancer of the colon and 32.8% for cancer of the rectum (1). When the tumour is confined within the bowel wall, cure rates of 80% or more can be anticipated (2), but when the tumour penetrates to the serosa and then metastasized to regional lymph nodes, cure rates drop to a range of 27—58% (3, 4, 5).

Various factors may have a bearing on the prognosis of cancer of the large bowel, such as: duration of symptoms (6), tumour fixation, sex (6, 7), age (8, 9), degree of differentiation (10) and vein invasion by the tumour (11). But the local extent of the tumour according to Dukes' classification is still the major prognostic factor.

It has been shown that some carcinomas may present a "pushing" border with infiltration of plasma cells and lymphocytes at the interface between the tumour and the surrounding structures, while others may present diffusely infiltrating borders (12). The former are expected to metastasize less frequently than the latter.

Patients however in the same stage, according to Dukes' classification, and with cancers of the same histological differentiation may have different prognosis, and this justifies the need for new prognostic factors.

It has been shown that immunoglobulin-producing cells in colorectal cancer tissue differ quantitatively between patients (13). The estimation of cytoplasmic immunoglobulin in colorectal cancer tissues has, therefore, been developed as a possible prognostic factor. Immunocytochemical methods are now available for the demonstration of many substances including immunoglobulins, hormones and oncofetal antigens in fixed tissue sections (14). The presence of the reaction product, together with the facility for simultaneous pathological diagnosis, make the immunoperoxidase method the technique of choice in histopathology at the present time (15). This technique has been used in recent years for the detection of epithelial membrane antigens such as carcinoembryonic antigen, especially in colon cancer tissues, but also in other tumour tissues (16). In the present study the immunoperoxidase method is used to demonstrate plasma-cell cytoplasmic immunoglobulins in colorectal cancer tissues. Quantitative differences of plasma-cell immunoglobulins were then correlated to the disease evolution and the patients' survival.

Material and Methods

52 patients with colorectal cancer were included in the study. They had been operated with tumour resection in Hippocration Hospital, Athens, during the years 1973—1977. 31 were males and 21, females. Their age range is given in Table 1.

Surgical specimens of all tumour tissue were routinely taken for formalin fixation, paraffin embedding and haematoxylin-eosin staining. All the specimens included in the study were, histologically, adenocarcinomas. Undifferentiated cancers were not included. The staging according to Dukes' classification is given in Table 2.

Table 1.
Number of patients studied

	No. of patients	Age	Median age
Male	31	34—77	63
Female	21	37—80	59
Total	52	34—80	63

Table 2.
Colorectal cancer patients studied

Dukes classification	No. of patients
A	7
B	24
C	21
Total	52

Histopathological sections were submitted to the immunoperoxidase technique to identify the intracellular plasma-cell immunoglobulin. Plasma cells identified as characteristic mononuclear cells containing immunoglobulins were found surrounding or infiltrating the tumour mass.

Immunoperoxidase technique: The sensitive immunoperoxidase bridging technique (Pap-technique) that was originally described by TAYLOR (17) was used in combination with the immunoperoxidase or histological methods described by MASON, PAPADIMITRIOU, THUNG, BURCK and others (18, 19, 20, 21). This combination was used to overcome certain limitations of the histological material due to the long storing such as the folding of the paraffin sections on the glass slides, unsticking and loss of the sections, and dehydration and dryness.

The paraffin slides were dried slowly overnight in a 56 °C oven. Sections were deparaffinized by warming in a 37 °C xylene bath twice for ten minutes each time. Sections were then transferred to first 95% ethanol for 3 min, then to 70% ethanol for 3 min, and finally to 50% ethanol for 3 min in order to rehydrate them. Post fixation of the sections was done with acetone-formol phosphate for 90 sec (20 mg Na_2HPO_4, 100 mg KH_2PO_4, 45 ml acetone, 25 ml concentrated formalin, 30 ml distilled water). Sections were rinsed in distilled water for a few minutes, then washed twice in baths of tris buffered saline 0.15 M, pH 7.6 for 3 min each time. This was followed by blocking of endogeneous peroxidase in tris saline buffer, 0.15 M, pH 7.6 containing 3% hydrogen peroxidase, for 30 min; washing twice in tris saline buffer bath for 5 min each time; incubating in −20 °C overnight; transferring to room temperature for a few minutes and rinsing in tris saline buffer for 5 min; incubating of the sections with normal swine serum (Dakopatts, Denmark) diluted 1/10 in tris saline buffer for 10 min. Without further washing, the sections were incubated with specific rabbit anti-human immunoglobulins antisera (Dakopatts) diluted 1/200 to 1/400 in tris HCl buffer 0.15 M, pH 7.6 for 24 h at room temperature, and washed 3 × 10 min with tris saline buffer. The sections were then incubated with swine anti-rabbit immunoglobulin (Dakopatts) diluted 1/20 in tris HCl buffer for 1 h, washed 3 × 10 min with tris saline buffer, and incubated with horseradish rabbit anti-horseradisch complex (PAP) (Dakopatts) diluted 1/60 in tris HCl buffer for 45 min, followed by washing 3 × 10 min with saline buffer. Development of the enzyme activity with DAB solution was continued for 10 min. Diaminobenzidine tetrahydrochloride salt (Serva, FRG) was dissolved in tris HCl 0.15 M, pH 7.6 buffer immediately before use. After filtration of this solution, hydrogen peroxide was added to make a concentration of 0.01% and then sodium azide in a concentration of 0.01 M to remove resting endogeneous peroxidase activity. After washing in tap water for a few minutes, counterstaining followed with Harris haematoxylin (Merck, FRG) for 30 sec and differentiation with acid alcohol for a few seconds, then again washing in tap water for a few seconds and dehydration in 50% ethanol for 3 min, 70% ethanol for 3 min, 95% ethanol for 3 min, absolute ethanol for 5 min, and xylene for 5 min, before mounting in Enkitt (FRG).

The microscopical estimation of the cancer tissue infiltration by plasma cells was done under 10 × 40 and 10 × 100 magnification. The plasma-cell immunoglobulins (Ig) were shown by a

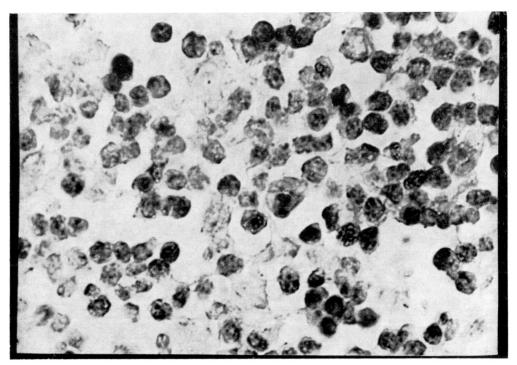

Fig. 1

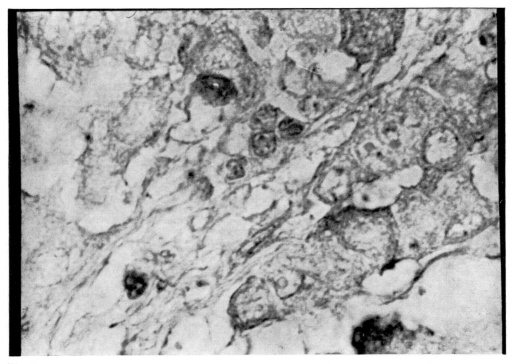

Fig. 2

brown stained cytoplasm. The slides were divided into three groups: those that had 30 or more plasma cells per field with intensive staining were considered as high Ig (Fig. 1); those that had 10 or less and pale staining were considered as low Ig (Fig. 2); and those containing between 10 and 30 plasma cells as moderate Ig.

Results

The distribution of the patients according to high and low Ig and Dukes' staging is shown in Table 3.

Table 4 shows the number and percentage of patients, grouped according to Dukes' classification, that survived after four-eight years of follow-up. In Dukes' A stage three out of seven patients were in the high Ig group, and they were all alive after four or more years while of the two patients in the low Ig group one had died (Table 5).

Table 3.
Colorectal cancer patients distribution to cytoplastic Ig and DUKES classification

	High Ig	Low Ig	Moderate Ig	Total
Dukes A	3	2	2	7
Dukes B	13	6	5	24
Dukes C	8	9	4	21
Total	24	17	11	52

Table 4.
Colorectal cancer patients survival on the basis of Dukes classification

Dukes	Alive disease-free	Alive with disease	Died from disease	Total
A	6 (85.7%)	—	1 (14.2%)	7
B	18 (75.0%)	—	6	24
C	10 (47.6%)	1 (4.7%) G	10 (47.6%)	21
Total	34	1	17	52

Table 5.
Colorectal cancer patients with high and low cytoplasmic Ig

	Dukes A patients survival			
	High Ig	Low Ig	Mod Ig	Total
Alive and disease-free	3	1	2	6
Died from the disease	—	1	—	1
Total	3	2	2	7

Table 6.
Colorectal cancer patients with high and low cytoplasmic Ig

| | Dukes B patients survival | | | |
	High Ig	Low Ig	Mod Ig	Total
Alive and disease-free	12	3	3	18
Died from the disease	1	3	2	6
Total	13	6	5	24

Table 7.
Colorectal cancer patients with high and low cytoplasmic Ig

| | Dukes C patients survival | | | |
	High Ig	Low Ig	Mod Ig	Total
Alive disease-free	5	4	1	10
Alive with disaese	—	—	1	1
Died from disease	3	5	2	10
Total	8	9	4	21

Table 8.
Colorectal cancer patients survival on the basis of high and low cytoplasmic Ig

	Alive disease-free	Alive with disease	Died from disease	Total
High Ig	20 (83.0%)	—	4 (16.6%)	24
Low Ig	8 (47.0%)	—	9 (52.9%)	17
Moderate Ig	6 (54.5%)	1 (9%)	4 (36.3%)	11
Total	34	1	17	52

Out of the twenty-four patients in Dukes' B stage, 13 were in the high Ig and six in the low Ig group. In the high Ig group all patients but one were still alive and disease-free, while only half of the patients in the low Ig group were alive by the end of this study (Table 6).

In Dukes' C stage, there were 21 patients, eight in the high Ig and nine in the low Ig group. In the high Ig group the majority, and in the low Ig group, the minority of the patients were alive and disease-free by the end of this study (Table 7). One patient out of two in the group of moderate Ig was still alive with disease after four years. Comparing the percentage of surviving patients of all Dukes' stages in the groups of high Ig and low Ig we found that 83% of the high Ig group patients were alive and disease-free while in the low Ig group 47% of the patients were surviving (Table 8).

Discussion

The plasma-cell and lymphocyte presence in cancer involved tissues has in the past been considered of some significance in the protection from metastases, particularly when these cells form a border between the tumour and the normal tissue (12). In a small number of colorectal cancer patients the abundant presence of Ig-producing cells has been shown, furthermore, to be correlated with the absence of regional lymph node metastases (13). In the present study we found that the Ig-producing cells, and the intensity of cytoplasmic Ig in colorectal cancer tissues vary from patient to patient. The variability of Ig-producing cells is found in all the Dukes' stages. The correlation of the amount of Ig-producing cells with the patients survival shows that there is a significantly higher survival in the group of patients with higher infiltration of Ig-producing cells. The difference of survival is more significant in Dukes' B stage. The Ig production has been interpreted as a reaction to metabolic products of the neoplastic cells (22).

The present study does not claim to interpret the difference in the amount of Ig-producing cells in the cancer tissue of different patients. The possibility of having cancers of different antigenicity however might imply different Ig production as one of the mechanisms of the host immune response.

The number of patients is not big enough to draw statistically significant conclusions, but it is indicative though, that the amount of plasma-cells and the intensity of cytoplasmic Ig may be of some prognostic value in colorectal cancer patients.

References

1. BERGE, T. H., EKELUND, G., MELLNER, C., PIHL, B. and WENCKERT, A.: Carcinoma of the colon and rectum in a defined population. Acta Chir. Scand. (Supp.) *438* (1973), 1—86
2. MOERTEL, C. G.: Chemotherapy of cancer of the colon and rectum. Human Cancer: Its Characterization and Treatment. Vol. 5. Amsterdam, Excerpta Medica, 1980
3. DIXON, W. J., LONGMIRE, W. P. Jr. and HOLDEN, W. D.: Use of triethylthiophosphoramide as an adjuvant to the surgical resection of gastric and colorectal carcinoma. Ann. Surg. *173* (1971), 26—39
4. SILVERBERG, E.: Cancer of the colon and rectum. New York, American Cancer Society Inc., 1970
5. SILVERBERG, E.: Cancer Statistics, 1978. Cancer *28* (1978), 17—32
6. SCUDAMORE, H.: Cancer of the colon and rectum — general aspects, diagnosis, treatment and prognosis. Dis. Colon Rectum *12* (1969), 105—114
7. CUTLER, S. J., et al.: End results in cancer, Report no. 3, National Cancer Institute, End Results Section of Biometry Branch, Washington, D. C., 1968, U.S. Government Printing Office
8. ADAM, Y. G., CALABRESE, C. and VOLK, H.: Colorectal cancer in patients over 80 years of age. Surg. Clin. North. Am. *52* (1972), 883—889
9. JENSEN, H. E., NIELSEN, T. and SALSLEV, I.: Carcinoma of the colon in old age. Ann. Surg. *171* (1970), 107—115
10. ACKERMANN, L. V., and REGATO: Cancer digestive tract — large bowel. St. Louis, The C.V. Mosby Company, 1977, pp. 510—547
11. BROWN, C. E., WARREN, and SHIELDS: Visceral metastasis from rectal carcinoma. Surg. Gynecol. Obstet. *66* (1938), 611—621
12. ACKERMANN, L. V.: Pathological evidence of host immunity in cancer: lymphocyte plasma-cell infiltrate in malignant neoplasms. In: CLAR, R. L. et al.; eds.: Oncology 1970; Proceedings of the Tenth International Cancer Congress, Chicago, Year Book Medical Publishers Inc., 1971

13. MANOUSOS, N. O.: Some immunological disturbances in carcinoma of colon and rectum. A thesis. Athens, 1972

14. HEYDERMAN, E.: Immunoperoxidase technique in histopathology: applications, methods and controls, J. Clin. Path. *32* (1979), 971—978

15. DeLELLIS, R. A., STEMBERGER, L. A., MANN, R. B., BANKS, P. M. and NAKANE, P. K.: Immunoperoxidase techniques in diagnostic pathology. Amer. J. Clin. Path. *71* (1979), 483—488

16. HEYDERMAN, E., STEELE, K. and ORMEROD, M. G.: A new antigen on the epithelial membrane: its immunoperoxidase localisation in normal and neoplastic tissue. J. Clin. Path. *32* (1979), 35—39

17. TAYLOR, C. R.: The nature of Reed-Sternberg cells, and other malignant "reticulum" cells. Lancet *II* (1974), 802

18. MASON, D. Y., FARRELL, C. and TAYLOR, C. R.: The detection of intracellular antigens in human leucocytes by immunoperoxidase staining. Brit. J. Haemat. *31* (1975), 361

19. PAPADIMITRIOU, C. S.: Ig-production by reactive follicular centers and malignant lymphomas of a follicular center origin. A thesis. Athens, 1978

20. THUNG, S. N., GERBER, M. A., SARYO, E. and POPPER, H.: Distribution of 5 antigens in hepatocellular carcinoma. Lab. Invest. (1979)

21. BURCK, H. C.: Histologische Technik. Leitfaden für die Herstellung mikroskopischer Präparate in Unterricht und Praxis. Stuttgart, Georg Thieme Verlag, 1969

22. BURTIN, P., LOISILLIER, F., BUFFE, D., GUILLERM, M. and GLUCKMAN, E.: Immunoglobulin producing cells in human cancerous lymph nodes. Cancer *23* (1969), 80

Institute of Oncology, Bologna, Italy

Suitable Models for Long-Term Bioassays of Therapeutic and Toxic Effects of Antiblastic Drugs: Brain Tumours of Neuronal Cells and Primitive Bipotential Precursors Produced in Sprague-Dawley Rats by Vinyl Chloride

G. Cotti, L. Valgimigli, A. Mandrioli and C. Maltoni

At present, very little is known about the chemotherapy of brain tumours of neuronal cells and of their primitive bipotential precursors, i. e., of medulloepitheliomas, medulloblastomas and neuroblastomas. A suitable experimental model, providing an animal equivalent to the human situation, would be a useful tool to improve our knowledge in this field.

It has been shown in our Institute that exposure by inhalation to vinyl chloride, at doses varying from 2,500 to 10,000 ppm, can induce tumours of neuronal cells and of their precursors in Sprague-Dawley and Wistar rats (Maltoni and Lefemine, 1975; Maltoni, 1977; Maltoni et al, 1980). In this report we describe experimental means of inducing a high incidence of these tumours over a relatively short period, and therefore of making available a sufficient number of these tumours for testing antiblastic drugs.

Sprague-Dawley rats were exposed by inhalation to 2,500 ppm of the monomer from the 12th day of embryonal development to one year of age: Breeders were exposed 4 hours daily, from the 13th day of pregnancy to delivery; offspring were exposed 4 hours daily, 5 days weekly, for 5 weeks, and then 7 hours daily, 5 days weekly, for 50 weeks.

The incidence and the latency of the tumours obtained are shown in Table 1. Microscopically, the tumours displayed different potentialities, which varied from tumour to tumour and in different areas of the same tumour, and which represent the equi-

Table 1.

Incidence of brain tumours of neuronal cells and primitive bipotential precursors in Sprague-Dawley rats exposed from 12-day embryonal life for 57 weeks to vinyl chloride in air at 2,500 ppm, 4—7 hours daily, 5 days weekly

Animals used			Animals with brain tumours		
Sex	No. at start	Corrected no.[a]	No.	%[b]	Average latency (weeks)[c]
M	63	57	27	47.4	45.5
F	65	57	28	49.1	48.4
M and F	128	114	55	48.2	47.0

[a] Animals alive at 35 weeks, when the first tumour was observed
[b] with respect to the corrected number
[c] From start of treatment

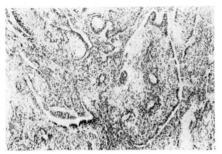 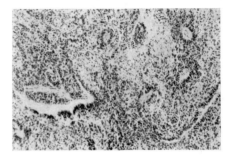

Fig. 1   Fig. 2

Fig. 1. Medulloepithelioma in Sprague-Dawley rat, following exposure to vinyl chloride by inhalation. H.-E. × 80.

Fig. 2. A detail of Figure 1. × 130.

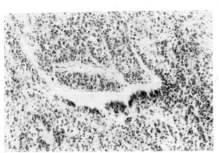 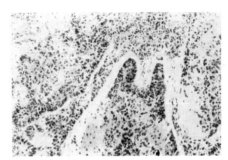

Fig. 3   Fig. 4

Fig. 3. A detail of Figures 1 and 2. × 200.

Fig. 4. A detail of Figure 1. × 200.

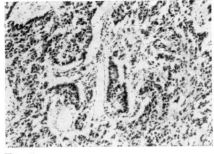 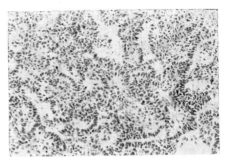

Fig. 5   Fig. 6

Fig. 5. Medulloepithelioma in Sprague-Dawley rat, following exposure to vinyl chloride by inhalation. H.-E. × 200.

Fig. 6. Medulloblastoma in Sprague-Dawley rat, following exposure to vinyl chloride by inhalation. H.-E. × 200.

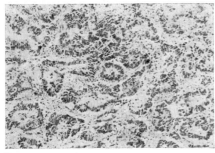 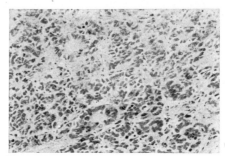

Fig. 7 Fig. 8

Fig. 7. Medulloblastoma in Sprague-Dawley rat, following exposure to vinyl chloride by inhalation. H.-E. × 200.

Fig. 8. Medulloblastoma in Sprague-Dawley rat, following exposure to vinyl chloride by inhalation. H.-E. × 320.

valent of the human medulloepithelioma, medulloblastoma and neuroblastoma. Typical pictures are shown in Figures 1—8.

It is of particular interest for the testing of drugs that these tumours manifest themselves with characteristic symptoms several days before the death of the animal. The major symptoms are a reduction in muscle tone, hypomotility, ruffling of hair, reduction in food intake, loss of body weight and exophthalmia.

References

1. MALTONI, C. (1977): Vinyl chloride carcinogenicity: an experimental model for carcinogenesis studies. In: HIATT, H. H., WATSON, I. D. & WILSON, J. C., eds., Origins of Human Cancer, Cold Spring Harbor, NY, Cold Spring Harbor Laboratory, pp. 119—146
2. MALTONI, C. and LEFEMINE, G. (1975): Carcinogenicity bioassays of vinyl chloride: current results. In: SELIKOFF, I. J. & HAMMOND, E. C., eds., Toxicity of Vinyl Chloride - Polyvinyl Chloride, New York, New York Academy of Sciences, pp. 195—218
3. MALTONI, C., LEFEMINE, G., CILIBERTI, A., COTTI, G. and CARRETTI, D. (1980): Vinyl chloride carcinogenesis bioassays (BT project) as an experimental model for risk identification and assessment in environmental and occupational carcinogenesis. In: Epidémiologie animale et épidémiologie humaine: le Cas du Chlorure de Vinyle monomère, Paris, Publications Essentielles, pp 15—112

Institute of Oncology, Bologna, Italy

Laboratory Assessment of Therapeutic Activity (with Particular Regard to Chemotherapy): Relevant Animal Models

C. Maltoni

Introduction

The current protocol for selecting and evaluating potentially active drugs in cancer chemotherapy is based on a sequence of steps, which may be summarized as shown in Table 1.

The experimental approach, as routinely performed nowadays, is insufficient (to be euphemistic). As far as toxicological studies are concerned, the observation period is generally limited to 28 days for mice and 60 days for dogs: Under such conditions it is not possible to determine subchronic or chronic effects, including carcinogenicity. Furthermore, mutagenicity and teratogenicity studies are not done systematically. In experimental determinations of therapeutic activity, compounds are usually tested on transplanted tumours (including xenografts) in mice. The tumours most commonly used, listed in Table 2, are mainly tumours which grow fast and produce artificial host-tumour interrelationships. This type of experimental model in no way reproduces human situations, and its predictive value for human neoplastic pathology is very low indeed. Under these circumstances, the knowledge that can be obtained about the biological effects of drugs before clinical evaluation is approximately nil.

Table 1.
Protocol for selecting and evaluating potentially active drugs in cancer chemotherapy

---

I. Evaluation in experimental animals:
   1) Toxicity
   2) Therapeutic activity
II. Clinical evaluation:
   1) Phase 1: toxicity, with particular regard to determination of the maximum tolerated dose
   2) Phase 2: efficacy on different tumours, aiming at eliminating drugs with a low probability of therapeutic utility
   3) Phase 3: comparative randomized studies, often multi-centred, in order to compare the effects of the regimen under study and pre-existing treatments already in use in therapeutic practice

---

The clinical procedures for evaluating potentially active drugs present major difficulties and have substantial limitations, which must be taken into proper account before reaching conclusions about the clinical effectiveness of a drug in terms of risk-benefit assessment (Table 3). Further, the well-known ethical aspects must not be underestimated.

Table 2.
The tumours most commonly used for the experimental
evaluation of therapeutic activity of drugs, and parameters on which the selection of new drugs for human
use is based

Tumour	Parameter
Leukaemia P388	Survival
Leukaemia L1210	Survival
Melanoma B16	Survival
Lewis lung carcinoma	Survival
Colon carcinoma 38	Survival
Mammary carcinoma CD8F1	Tumour weight
Mammary Mx1 (xenografts)	Tumour weight
Lung Lx1 (xenografts)	Tumour weight
Colon Cx1 (xenografts)	Tumour weight

Table 3.
The difficulties and limits of clinical procedures for evaluating potentially active drugs in cancer
chemotherapy

  I. It is difficult, or even impossible, to obtain homogeneous and comparable groups of patients
     in whom to test the efficacy of drugs in absolute and relative terms.
 II. The clinical evaluation of the effects of drugs is more inaccurate and subjective than stati-
     sticians or pharmacologists or other non-clinical students of chemotherapy may think. This
     factor must be taken into proper consideration, particularly with regard to results of multi-
     centred trials.
III. The natural history and characterization of tumours, which heavily condition their prog-
     nosis, are rarely, if ever, available in a homogeneous way, even for patients of the same group
     (since, given to long evolution of the disease and the multidisciplinary approach to its the-
     rapy, patients are evaluated, characterized and treated at various times, in different hospitals,
     by different specialists, using different parameters and different terminologies).
 IV. Clinical procedures, as they are presently carried out, do not provide data on the long-term
     adverse effects of drugs.

One may conclude that the entire strategy for evaluating new drugs is, at present,
rather precarious, and may lead to inconclusive or unrealistic results. Furthermore,
as limited as it may be, this procedure is usually foreseen and carried out only for
single drugs and not in the case of an association of drugs, for which clinical Phase
III, is, at present, the only trial procedure.

The role of proper animal models in risk-benefit assessment
of cancer chemotherapy

In every field of medicine, the availability of proper experimental models speeds research and makes it possible to produce objective results, while avoiding inadequate
and often unethical trials in humans. In recent years, the demonstration that adequate
long-term carcinogenicity bioassays are highly predictive for identifying and quanti-
fying oncogenic risks for mankind has brought about tremendous progress in the

prevention of environmental tumours. This is not yet the case for cancer therapy, and particularly for cancer chemotherapy.

Nowadays, there is a wide range of experimental systems to test cancer chemotherapeutic drugs (singly or in association) (Table 4). The systems usually studied, i. e., transplantable tumours and, in a few instances, autochthonous tumours induced by agents producing strong toxic effects, are far from meeting the prerequisites for extrapolation of results to humans.

Table 4.
Experimental systems for testing cancer chemotherapeutic drugs

Type	Constraints and potentialities
I. In-vitro systems	Artificial
II. Transplantable tumours	Artificial
III. Autochthonous tumours induced by viruses	Artificial; often strongly antigenic
IV. Autochthonous tumours induced by strong carcinogenic, physical or chemical agents, producing strong toxic effects	Interference of toxic effects in the evaluation of results
V. Autochthonous tumours induced by physical and chemical agents, producing mild, if any, otherwise pathological effects	Potential human equivalent
VI. Spontaneous autochthonous tumours, frequently occurring in selected strains of small rodents	Potential human equivalent

In our opinion, there is an urgent need to introduce, in the protocol for selecting and evaluating cancer drugs, animal models that better represent human equivalents. Such models that are presently available are mainly spontaneous tumours in selected strains of experimental animals and the autochthonous tumours produced by physical and chemical treatment, with little, if any, otherwise associated pathological effects.

Experimental tumours and animals bearing tumours that better reproduce human equivalents must be studied using the same clinical, histopathological and laboratory investigations adopted for cancer patients. With this type of approach, highly predictive experimental results can be expected. It is surprising that many people now

Table 5.
The biological and experimental prerequisites of human-equivalent animal models for selecting and evaluating potentially active drugs in cancer chemotherapy

   I. The histotype of the tumour must be the same as that in humans.

  II. The localization of the primary site must also be the same as that in humans.

 III. The natural history of the animal neoplasia must be similar to that of the equivalent tumour in humans.

 IV. The animal tumours and hosts must be characterized by the same parameters and methodologies as the equivalent human tumours and patients (tumours: grading and staging; hosts: performance status, laboratory — hematological and urinary — parameters, objective symptomatology, food intake, loss of body weight, etc.).

  V. The experimental model must be readily reproducible and provide a high incidence of tumour cases distributed over a reasonable period of time.

 VI. There must be adequate data on the behaviour of the tumour in historical controls, providing information on the range of natural fluctuations.

 VII. There must be adequate data on the changes produced by the tumour per se in the host.

VIII. For each type of tumour a characterization card must be made available.

working in chemotherapy are, on principle, negativistic regarding the use of experimental tools, without considering that the experimental tools studied so far are so inadequate.

The prerequisites and the availability
of human-equivalent animal models: some examples

Suitable animal models must fulfil the prerequisites listed in Table 5. Many tumours, both spontaneous and induced, are available in small rodents, such as mice, rats and

Table 6.
Examples of animal tumour suitable for selecting and evaluating active drugs in cancer chemotherapy, available at the Institute of Oncology of Bologna

---

    I. Skin tumour in mice produced by repeated low doses of aromatic hydrocarbons

   II. Soft (subcutaneous)-tissue sarcomas (rhabdomyosarcomas and fibrosarcomas) in rats produced by a single local injection of inorganic pigments (e. g., molybdenum orange)

 III. Spotaneous mammary tumours (fibromas, fibroadenomas, cystosarcoma phyllodes, different types of carcinomas, sarcomas) in rats

 IV. Forestomach epithelial tumours (equivalent to human oesophageal tumours) produced in rats by styrene oxide

   V. Hepatocarcinomas produced in rats by vinyl chloride

  VI. Liver angiosarcomas produced in rats by vinyl chloride

 VII. Kidney adenocarcinomas produced in mice by vinylidene chloride

VIII. Nephroblastomas produced in rats by vinyl chloride

 IX. Spontaneous pheochromocytomas and pheocromoblastomas in rats

   X. Tumour of neuronal cells and primitive bipotential precursors produced in rats by vinyl chloride

 XI. Gliomas produced in rats by acrylonitrile

 XII. Spontaneous neoplastic diseases of haematopoietic and lymphoid tissue in rats, including non-Hodgkin's and Hodgkin's lymphomas and malignant histiocytosis.

XIII. Mesotheliomas of pleura and peritoneum, produced by asbestos and erionite

---

Table 7.
Spotaneous mammary tumours: identification card

    I. *Species and strain*: Sprague-Dawley rats

   II. *Sex*: female

 III. *Treatment and other experimental factors*: —

 IV. *Incidence of tumours[a]*: 53.3% (total tumours)

   V. *Distribution of different types of tumours[b]*:
       — fibromas and fibroadenomas: 87%
       — carcinomas: 21.8%
       — sarcomas   2.3%
       — carcinosarcomas: 1%

 VI. *Age distribution[c]*:
       — fibromas and fibroadenomas: Table 7 A
       — carcinomas: Table 7 B

 VII. *Most frequent sites of metastases*: regional nodes, lung

VIII. *Morphological picture*: Figures 1—12

 IX. *Detection*: clinical examination (inspection and palpation)

---

[a] Percentage of tumour-bearing animals

[b] Percentage of animals bearing a particular type of mammary tumour, in relation to the total number of mammary tumour-bearing animals. One animal may bear more than one type of tumour.

[c] At detection of first tumour

382

Table 7 A.
Age distribution of 935 female Sprague-Dawley rats bearing fibromas and fibroadenomas

Rats' age (weeks)	8	16	24	32	40	48	56	64	72	80	88	96	104	112	120	128	136	144
No.	0	0	5	11	18	29	74	115	140	159	154	113	57	42	13	1	3	1
%	—	—	0.5	1.2	1.9	3.1	7.9	12.3	15.0	17.0	16.5	12.1	6.1	4.5	1.4	0.1	0.3	0.1
Equivalent women's age (years)	5	10	15	20	25	30	35	40	45	50	55	60	65	70	75	80	85	90

Table 7 B.
Age distribution of 232 female Sprague-Dawley rats bearing mammary carcinomas

Rats' age (weeks)	8	16	24	32	40	48	56	64	72	80	88	96	104	112	120	128	136	144
No.	0	1	4	3	5	14	19	29	28	38	25	22	19	13	6	6	0	0
%	—	0.4	1.7	1.3	2.1	6.0	8.2	12.5	12.1	16.4	10.8	9.5	8.2	5.6	2.6	2.6	—	—
Equivalent women's age (years)	5	10	15	20	25	30	35	40	45	50	55	60	65	70	75	80	85	90

Table 8.

Induced forestomach epithelial tumours: identification card

I. *Species and strain*: Sprague-Dawley rats

II. *Sex*: male and female

III. *Treatment and other experimental factors*:
   - exposure by ingestion (stomach tube) to styrene oxide, in olive oil at 250 mg/kg b. w., once daily, 4—5 days weekly, for 52 weeks
   - age of animals at start: 13 weeks
   - length of biophase: 116 weeks

IV. *Incidence of tumours*:
   - total tumours: 51.9% [a]
   - papillomas and acanthomas: 15.6% [b]
   - squamous-cell carcinomas: 46.7% [b]

V. *Latency*[c]:
   - total: 107 weeks
   - papillomas and acanthomas: 108 weeks
   - squamous-cell carcinomas: 107 weeks

VI. *Site of metastases*: liver

VII. *Morphological picture*: Figures 12—20

VIII. *Detection*: weight loss, reduction in food intake, gastroscopy (?), laparoscopy

[a] Percentage of tumour-bearing animals

[b] Percentage of animals bearing a particular type of forestomach tumour, in relation to the total number of forestomach tumour-bearing animals. One animal may bear more than one type of tumour.

[c] Period from start of treatment to death

Table 9.

Induced liver angiosarcomas: identification card

I. *Species and strain*: Sprague-Dawley rats

II. *Sex*: male and female

III. *Treatment and other experimental factors*:
   - exposure by inhalation to vinyl chloride in air at 2,500 ppm, 4—7 hours daily, 5 days weekly, for 54 weeks
   - age of animals at start: 12-day embryos
   - length of biophase: 57 weeks

IV. *Incidence of tumours*[a]: 63.1%

V. *Latency*[b]: 50 weeks

VI. *Site of metastases*: abdominal cavity and lung

VII. *Morphological picture*: Figures 21—24

VIII. *Detection*: laparoscopy

[a] Percentage of tumour-bearing animals

[b] Period from start of treatment to death

hamsters. Any general or experimental oncologist can easily list a few dozen of them. These tumours include those that occur frequently in humans and animals pathology and very rare ones.

A list of the animal tumours available at present in our Institute is given in Table 6. The following data are provided on these tumours:

1) optimal carcinogenic treatment and other experimental factors for those that are induced;

384

Table 10.
Brain tumours of neuronal cells and primitive bipotential precursors: identification card

   I. *Species and strain*: Sprague-Dawley rats
  II. *Sex*: male and female
 III. *Treatment and other experimental factors*:
  - exposure by inhalation to vinyl chloride in air at 2,500 ppm, 4—7 hours daily, 5 days weekly, for 54 weeks
  - age of animals at start:12-day embryos
  - length of biophase: 57 weeks
 IV. *Incidence of tumours*[a]: 48.2%
  V. *Latency*[b]: 47 weeks
 VI. *Site of metastases*: in nodes and lungs (very rare)
VII. *Morphological picture*: Figures 25—28
VIII. *Detection*: consistent, specific symptoms

[a] Percentage of tumour-bearing animals
[b] Period from start of treatment to death

Table 11.
Nephroblastomas: identification card

   I. *Species and strain*: Sprague-Dawley rats
  II. *Sex*: male and female
 III. *Treatment and other experimental factors*:
  - exposure by inhalation to vinyl chloride in air at 100 ppm, 4 hours daily, 5 days weekly, for 52 weeks
  - age of animals at start: 13 weeks
  - length of biophase: 143 weeks
 IV. *Incidence of the tumours*[a]: 9.2%
  V. *Latency*[b]: 83.3 weeks
 VI. *Site of metastases*: adrenals, regional nodes, liver, spleen, lung
VII. *Morphological picture*: Figures 29—32.
VIII. *Detection*: laparoscopy

[a] Percentage of tumour-bearing animals
[b] Period from start of treatment to death

2) time of latency and/or age distribution
3) histiotype
4) clinical progression of the primary tumour;
5) metastatic spread;
6) associated pathological changes;
7) and, for many, time from first clinical observation to death.

Examples of such characterization cards, for spontaneous mammary tumours, induced forestomach epithelial tumours (equivalent to human oesophageal tumours), induced liver angiosarcomas, induced neuroblastomas and induced nephroblastomas, all in rats, are given in Table 7—11.

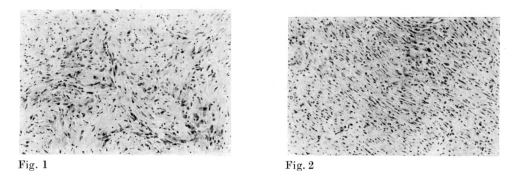

Fig. 1   Fig. 2

Fig. 1 and 2. Spontaneous mammary fibroma in female Sprague-Dawley rat. H.-E. × 200.

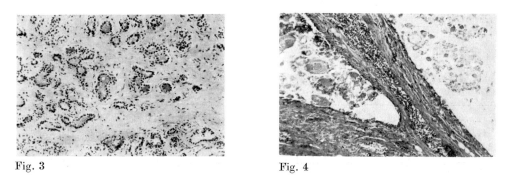

Fig. 3   Fig. 4

Fig. 3. Spontaneous mammary fibroadenoma in female Sprague-Dawley rat. H.-E. × 200.

Fig. 4. Spontaneous secreting mammary fibroadenoma in female Sprague-Dawley rat. H.-E. × 130.

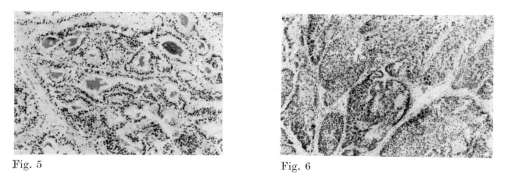

Fig. 5   Fig. 6

Fig. 5. Spontaneous, well-differentiated secreting mammary adenocarcinoma in female Sprague-Dawley rat. H.-E. × 200.

Fig. 6. Spontaneous, poorly-differentiated mammary adenocarcinoma in female Sprague-Dawley rat. H.-E. × 130.

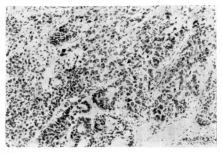
Fig. 7

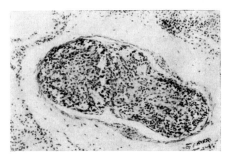
Fig. 8

Fig. 7. A detail of Figure 6. × 200.

Fig. 8. Pulmonary metastasis of the adenocarcinoma shown in Figures 6 and 7. H.-E. × 200.

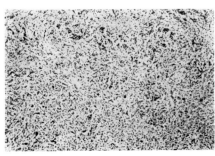
Fig. 9

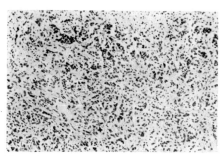
Fig. 10

Fig. 9. Spontaneous undifferentiated mammary adenocarcinoma in female Sprague-Dawley rat. H.-E. × 130.

Fig. 10. A detail of Figure 9. × 200.

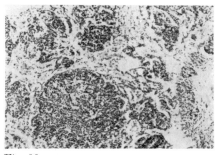
Fig. 11

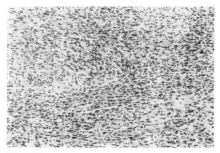
Fig. 12

Fig. 11. Pulmonary metastases of the adenocarcinoma shown in Figures 9 and 10. H.-E. × 130.

Fig. 12. Spontaneous mammary fibrosarcoma in female Sprague-Dawley rat. H.-E. × 130.

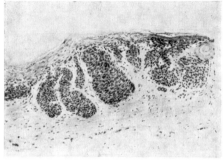
Fig. 13

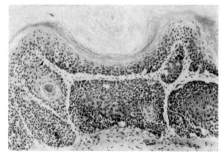
Fig. 14

Fig. 13. Forestomach squamous carcinoma *in situ* in Sprague-Dawley rat, following administration of styrene oxide by ingestion. H.-E. × 200.

Fig. 14. Forestomach microinvasive squamous carcinoma in Sprague-Dawley rat, following administration of styrene oxide by ingestion. H.-E. × 200.

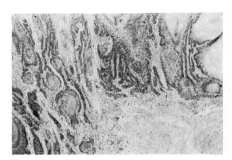
Fig. 15

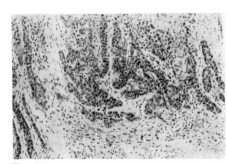
Fig. 16

Fig. 15. Forestomach invasive squamous carcinoma in Sprague-Dawley rat, following administration of styrene oxide by ingestion. H.-E. × 80.

Fig. 16. A detail of Figure 15. × 200.

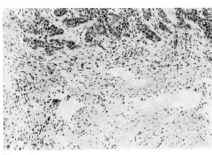
Fig. 17

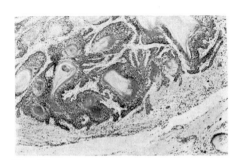
Fig. 18

Fig. 17. A detail of Figure 15, showing early invasion of the muscular wall. × 200.

Fig. 18. Same tumour as in Figures 15—17, showing invasion of serosa. × 80

388

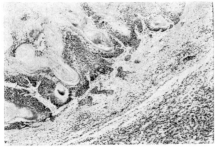

Fig. 19   Fig. 20

Fig. 19. Liver metastasis of the carcinoma shown in Figures 15—18. H.-E. × 80.

Fig. 20. A detail of Figure 19. × 200.

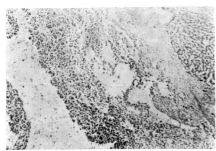
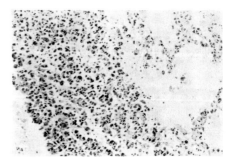

Fig. 21   Fig. 22

Fig. 21. Liver angiosarcoma in Sprague-Dawley rat, following exposure to vinyl chloride by inhalation. H.-E. × 80.

Fig. 22. A detail of Figure 21. × 200.

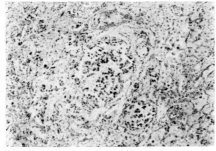
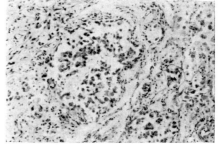

Fig. 23   Fig. 24

Fig. 23. Pulmonary metastases of the liver angiosarcoma shown in Figures 21 and 22. H.-E. × 130.

Fig. 24. A detail of Figure 23. × 200.

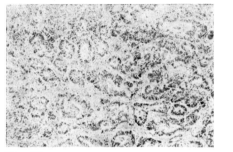

Fig. 25   Fig. 26

Fig. 25. Medulloblastoma in Sprague-Dawley rat, following exposure to vinyl chloride by inhalation. H.-E. × 130.

Fig. 26. A detail of Figure 25. × 200.

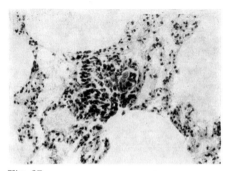

Fig. 27   Fig. 28

Fig. 27. Pulmonary metastases of the medulloblastoma shown in Figure 25. H.-E. × 200.

Fig. 28. A detail of Figure 27. × 520.

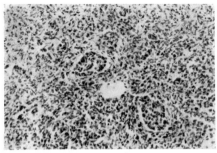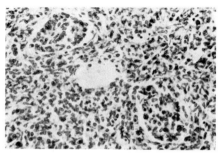

Fig. 29   Fig. 30

Fig. 29. Nephroblastoma in Sprague-Dawley rat, following exposure to vinyl chloride by inhalation. H.-E. × 320.

Fig. 30. A detail of Figure 29. × 520.

390

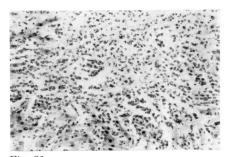
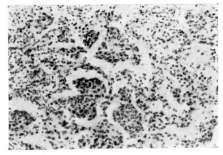

Fig. 31   Fig. 32

Fig. 31. Liver metastasis of the nephroblastoma shown in Figure 29. H.-E. × 320.

Fig. 32. Pulmonary metastases of the nephroblastoma shown in Figure 29. H.-E. × 320.

Table 12.

Protocol for the experimental evaluation of chronic toxicity, carcinogenicity and therapeutic efficacy of antiblastic drugs (singly or in association with others)

I. *Chronic toxicity* (in Sprague-Dawley rats):
  1) *Treatment*:
    — maximum tolerated doses during long-term treatment
    — clinical regimen
  2) *Duration of biophase*: 2 years
  3) *Parameters observed*:
    — survival
    — behaviour
    — clinical history
    — body weight
    — histopathology
    — laboratory parameters

II. *Carcinogenicity* (in Sprague-Dawley rats):
  Treatment:
    — subcutaneous injection
    — miaxmum tolerated doses during long-term treatment by the route(s) chosen for clinical chemotherapy
    — clinical regimen

III. *Therapeutic activity, and further information on acute and chronic toxicity and carcinogenicity (in animals bearing test tumours)*:
  1) *Treatment*:
    — maximum tolerated doses during long-term treatment by the routes chosen for clinical chemotherapy
    — clinical regimen
  2) *Parameters observed*:
    — survival
    — reduction of tumour mass
    — inhibition of tumour growth
    — regressive and necrotic changes in neoplastic tissues
    — behaviour, body weight, and clinical and histopathological parameters for evaluating therapeutic effects and toxicity
    — carcinogenic effects: induction of unexpected tumours, enhancement of the incidence or malignancy of expected tumours (other than that under test), or accelerated progression of the tumour under study

Of course, many further details, particularly relating to clinical progression, associated pathological changes, and time between detection to death, must be evaluated a posteriori in individual animals and added to each card.

The project, and the protocols of experimental bioassays for the evaluation of antiblastic drugs at the Institute of Oncology of Bologna

A systematic, integrated project to develop experimental bioassays for evaluating antiblastic drugs in animal models, in order to provide predictive information for cancer chemotherapy is now part of the programmes of our Institute. The project includes bioassays for monitoring long-term toxicity and carcinogenicity and the therapeutic activity of single drugs or associations of drugs. The protocol of the standard bioassays is shown in Table 12. The first drugs to be tested were some of those already widely used in mono- and polychemotherapy, both for prophylactic and therapeutic purposes.

Immunopathology Department, INO and Andrology Clinic, University Hospital, Madrid, Spain

Biological Significance and Dose-Dependent Effect of 'Resistocell' on Peripheral Blood Leucocytes In Vitro

S. Perez-Cuadrado, M. C. Moreno-Koch and A. Uson-Calvo

Introduction

Tumour immunology is now in a phase of reappraisal. The immune competence of cancer patients is usually depressed both by the disease itself and by treatment with surgery, radiation, chemotherapy, etc. (Cochran, 1978). It is closely related to prognosis; and the early return of host immune function is of great importance for the successful control of cancer and for preventing secondary infectious diseases resulting from immunosuppression (Eilber and Morton, 1970; Israel, 1973; Hersh et al, 1975, 1978).

Much of the enthusiasm for tumour immunotherapy with which the last decade began has recently diminished, as clinical trials have shown that it offers no dramatic answer to the management of cancer patients, although the use of bacille Calmette-Guérin appears to be promising. Positive results have been reported for adjuvant immunotherapy of malignant tumours, with modest but clinically and scientifically important improvements in long-term, disease-free survival (Mathé et al, 1969; Beretta et al, 1978; Hersh et al, 1978; Holland and Bekesi, 1978; Mckneally et al, 1978; Morton et al, 1978); while some of the reports described as negative had insufficient numbers of patients to allow a definitive negative conclusion (Cunningham et al, 1978; Pinsky et al, 1978).

The growth of modern tumour immunology has paralleled, to some extent, the expantion of basic immunological knowledge; and recent progress in cellular immunology suggests various basic strategies that ought to be tested for application to cancer. Augmentation of host immunity by various agents used either alone or in combination with other modalities of cancer treatment has been described. However, the two agents that have been most widely studied so far — levamisol and thymosine — do not stimulate immune responses above the normal phytohaemagglutinin (PHA) base-line or above physiological levels (Symoens, 1978; Hersh et al, 1978); and their use must be approached with caution, since it might have harmful as well as beneficial effects (Hersh et al, 1978). In this report we evaluate data on the biological significance and dose-dependent effect of resistocell (RSTL), a biological agent used by some cancer therapists as an immunomodulator, on the PHA base-line of cultured leucocytes from symptomless adults.

Material and methods

Population studied:

One hundred and twenty consecutive symptomless adults (sterile couples), 64 men (53.33%) and 56 women (46.66%), 29.20 ± 4.54 years old (range, 21—40 years), seen at the Andrology Department of the University Hospital of Saint Carlos, Madrid, were entered into the study.

393

Peripheral blood leucocytes (PBL) were separated from heparinized blood by centrifugation and incubation with PHA (0.08%) at 4 °C for 45 min. Then, 0.8 ± 0.2 ml (mean) of autologous plasma containing 5×10^6 PBL (2×10^6 lymphocytes, average), from the same aliquot in each control, were transferred to each of experimental models B, C, D and E, which contained 10 ml of TC-199 medium; 0.10, 0.15 and 0.20 ml of RSTL (7 mg/ml) were added to models C, D and E, respectively.

Number and distribution of controls and tests:
Two hundred and forty-nine sequential controls, 129 (51.81%) from men and 120 (48.19%) from women, were carried out at three-month intervals, to total of 896 tests. Their distribution as to experimental models and controls is shown in Table 1. (Six tests were excluded as outliners $\overline{X} \pm 2$ Sx.)

Table 1.
Distribution of tests

Exp. model	Sequential controls				
	First	Second	Third	Fourth	Total
B	117	65	40	21	243
C	117	65	40	21	243
D	95	54	21	7	177
E	114	64	35	20	233
Total tests	443	248	136	69	896

[a] Excluding outliners $> \overline{X} \pm 3$ Sx

Lymphocyte response in vitro:
The proliferative response of lymphocytes in vitro was evaluated by the number of lymphoblastoid cells (immunoblasts) found in each experimental model after three-days' incubation at 37 °C, and is given as number of immunoblasts $\times 10^4$.

The PHA response in model B represents the so-called PHA base-line or index, sometimes used here as the PHA immune competence index (IIC-PHA). The joint PHA-RSTL response in models C, D and E is referred as the response of the respective model; the highest PHA + RSTL response obtained in each test, regardless of the model, has been designated the RSTL combined response (RSTL CR). The true effect of RSTL in each model was estimated by subtracting the PHA response from the respective joint PHA + RSTL response. The relative increment of the PHA + RSTL effect above the IIC-PHA was calculated by the formula: (PHA + RSTL response/PHA response) $- 1 \times 100$.

Results

The blastogenic response of PBL in vitro assessed in this study, varied widely among individuals, and for the same individual, among experimental models and controls. The joint PHA + RSTL response in model C was higher than that in models D and E in 49.8% of tests; and the PHA response of model B was higher in 61.81%. The RSTL CR was greater than the model B PHA response in 74.70% of tests and in 74% of persons during the first test. However, the effect of RSTL became positive for at least one of the controls in 95 to 100% of cases where two, three and four sequential tests were available.

The difference between the mean values for PHA and PHA + RSTL response of the four assay levels (mean inter-assay difference of models) was not significant, except for tests 1 vs. 4 and 2 vs. 4 in the case of model B and tests 1 vs. 2 and 1 vs. 3 of model D (Table 2). Thus, the statistical evaluation included all of the tests in sequential assays.

The sampling distribution of frequencies for models B and C and for RSTL CR fits that of the expected normal curve fairly well, with three or more degrees of freedom (model B: $X_3^2 = 6.90 < 7.81$; model C: $X_5^2 = 5.66 < 11.07$; RSTL CR: $X_6^2 = 11.09 < 12.59$). There was a good concentration of individual values around the mean, and a relatively low standard error of the mean in every model (Table 3). The RSTL CR showed the highest mean PHA + RSTL value, followed by the responses of models C, B, D, and E; and it represented a significant 30% increase over the IIC − PHA.

Table 2.
Mean inter-assay difference of models — statistical significance

Assay	Experimental model				
Group	B	C	D	E	RSTL CR[a]
T − 1	0.617	0.841	0.067	0.549	0.549
T − 2	0.368	0.368	0.162	0.941	0.549
T − 3	0.549	0.764	0.194	0.424	0.920
T − 4	0.028	0.317	0.889	0.920	0.617
1 − 2	0.549	0.368	0.016	0.548	0.368
1 − 3	0.368	0.841	0.021	0.271	0.617
1 − 4	0.016	0.368	0.271	0.689	0.484
2 − 3	0.230	0.368	0.921	0.617	0.617
2 − 4	0.012	0.194	0.617	0.020	0.920
3 − 4	0.110	0.424	0.617	0.617	0.689

[a] The highest phytohaemagglutinin + resistocell response in each assay, regardless of the model — RSTL combined Response

Table 3.
PHA and PHA + RSTL response

Exp. model	Statistical evaluation				
	N	$\overline{X}$[a]	Sx[a]	$S\overline{x}$[a]	CV
B	243	130	63	4	48
C	243	144	69	4	48
D	177	126	69	5	55
E	233	122	72	5	59
RSTL CR[b]	243	169	74	5	44

[a] Number of immunoblasts $\times 10^4$
[b] Combined maximal individual PHA + RSTL responses from models C, D and E

The mean responses of model C differed significantly from those of models B, D and E, which were higher by 11, 14 and 18%, respectively. The highly significant relative increase of the mean RSTL CR value over those of models C, B, D and E was 17, 30, 34 (39%). The differences between the mean responses of models B, D and E were not significant (Table 4).

When the data were grouped according to PHA response a two-fold effect of RSTL was reen. The highest positive effect was observed in the lowest interval (PHA index sange: $31-60 \times 10^4$ immunoblasts), and represented significant increases of 155, 114, 76 and 63% over the mean IIC $-$ PHA value of that interval ($\bar{X}$: 49×10^4 immunoblasts), for the RSTL CR and models C, D and E, respectively. In all cases, the PHA $+$ RSTL response decreased progressively as the IIC $-$ PHA increased. It became progressively more negative from the fifth interval on, for models C, D and E; it became negative for the RSTL CR only in the last (or highest) IIC $-$ PHA interval (PHA responses $> 220 \times 10^4$ immunoblasts). The most negative effect of RSTL observed represented significant decreases, of 37, 25, 22 and 15% of the IIC $-$ PHA in the last interval ($\bar{X}$: 259×10^4 immunoblasts), for models E, C and D and RSTL CR, respectively (Tables 5 and 6 and Fig. 1).

Table 4.
Difference between the means of experimental models
— statistical significance —

All tests

	B	C	D	E	RSTL CR
B	—	0.016	0.484	0.194	0.001
C	0.016	—	0.005	0.001	0.001
D	0.484	0.005	—	0.617	0.001
E	0.194	0.001	0.617	—	0.001

Table 5.
Relative effect of RSTL on IIC-PHA in vitro[a] (data grouped into intervals according to PHA response)

Model	IIC-PHA interval							All data
	31−60	61−90	91−120	121−150	151−180	181−220	> 220	
C	114	45	36	17	−1	−10	−25	11
D	76	21	21	11	−11	−32	−22	−3
E	63	21	14	2	−12	−24	−37	−6
RSTL CR	155	74	53	41	16	2	−15	30
Class IIC-PHA								
$\bar{X}$	49	77	104	133	163	201	259	130

[a] [(PHA + RSTL/PHA) − 1] × 100; figures represent the number of immunoblasts $\times 10^4$

Table 6.
Relative effect of RSTL on IIC-PHA in vitro
— statistical significance —

Mean difference between models	IIC-PHA interval						
	31−60	61−90	91−120	121−150	151−180	181−220	> 220
C vs. B	0.001	0.001	0.001	0.046	0.841	0.134	0.001
D vs. B	0.001	0.028	0.110	0.317	0.016	0.001	0.003
E vs. B	0.036	0.057	0.089	0.764	0.110	0.003	0.001
RSTL CR, vs B	0.001	0.001	0.001	0.001	0.016	0.764	0.007

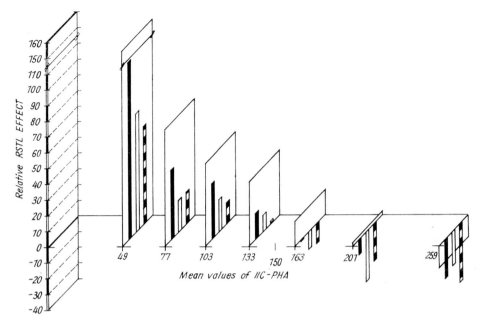

Fig. 1. Relative effects of resistocell (RSTL) as a function of the phytohaemagglutinin immune competence index (IIC-PHA). □, highest combined effect of PHA + RSTL; ▮, effect on model C (0.7 mg RSTL/5 × 10^6 peripheral blood leucocytes); ▯, effect on model D (1.05 mg); ▣, effect on model E (1.4 mg).

There is a certain correlation between the IIC — PHA and the true effect of RSTL, but only for the grouped data. The correlation changes from positive to negative with the IIC — PHA intervals established; and in all instances the coefficient was low (< 0.50). When all the data are taken together (range of PHA response: 31—400 × 10^4 immunoblasts), the coefficient was —0.42 for the RSTL CR and —0.47 for models E and C, which are significant at the 1% level (Fig. 2).

When the correlation coefficient is calculated for the IIC — PHA intervals and arranged in ascending order of magnitude, the true picture emerges. As is seen in Figure 2, points for the intervals representing mean IIC — PHA values of 133 and above fit fairly well the corresponding straight lines M, C and E, which represent the RSTL CR and responses of models C and E, respectively. However, the points representing lower mean IIC — PHA intervals diverge more and more from the line with decreasing values. Within the intervals 61—90, a positive correlation between the two variables, significant at the 5% level, was found for model E and RSTL CR.

Discussion

The data presented here show that RSTL (unlike levamisol and thymosine, the two agents used most widely) may induce a significant increase in the PHA index of PBL in vitro over the "normal" physiological level in 100% of symptomless adults. This effect depends on the dose of RSTL and on the kinetics of lymphocyte subpopulations that are sensitive to it. Thus, variations are to be expected among individuals and in the same individual among assays, as was observed in this study.

There is a dual effect of RSTL on the PHA index of PBL, which becomes clear when the data are separated into groups. In general, the lower the RSTL dose and the PHA index, the higher the effect of RSTL and vice versa. The mean value of the negative effect of RSTL showed a direct correlation with PHA index and with dose of RSTL. However, model C, which contained the lowest dose of RSTL (0.7 mg), gave its hi-

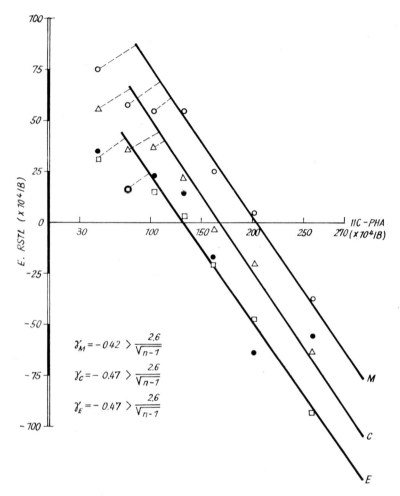

Fig. 2. Correlations between the effect of resistocell (E. RSTL) and the phytohaemagglutinin immune competence index (IIC-PHA). IB, immunoblasts; M, highest combined effect of PHA + + RSTL; C, effect on model C (0.7 mg RSTL/5 × 10⁶ peripheral blood leucocytes); E, effect on model E (1.4 mg).

ghest PHA + RSTL response in only half of the assays (49.8%), and models D and E in about 25%. Therefore, the positive effect of RSTL is represented better by the RSTL CR than by the PHA + RSTL response for all of the models.
The overall data indicate a significant positive effect of RSTL in model C and in the RSTL CR, with 11 and 30% increases over the PHA index, respectively. When the data are separated into intervals it can be seen that the effect of RSTL was as much as 155 and 114% over the mean PHA interval for the RSTL CR and model C, respectively; that is, about five times greater than the relative RSTL effect calculated

398

for the data as a whole. In models D and E, there was a significant effect of RSTL on the PHA index in two and one of the intervals, respectively, although the mean PHA + RSTL in the data as a whole were lower than the PHA index.

The RSTL-induced increase in the non-specific PHA immune competence index shown in this study is a real and important biological phenomenon. Its mechanism of action and target cells are unknown; none the less, those cells appear to be insensitive to either PHA or RSTL alone. It would appear that such cells and the PHA-sensitive T-lymphocyte subpopulations counterbalance each other, so that when one increases, the other diminishes. It is therefore postulated that they are T-lymphocyte precursors, which can be induced to active proliferation in vitro by PHA, like normal immuno-competent T-lymphocytes, under the direct action of RSTL or indirectly, via lymphokines from PHA-sensitive T-lymphocytes. The negative effect of RSTL is probably due to a direct killing action of RSTL on PHA-sensitive T-lymphocytes.

If this hypothesis is established, the situation would be unique since the therapeutic use of RSTL, unlike the usual agents used, could really increase the host repertoire above the normal physiological level and hopefully provide the cancer therapist with a useful immunomodulator for developing different combined treatment regimens.

Summary

The biological effects and dose dependence of RSTL on the PHA index of PBL from symptomless adults have been studied. A total of 249 assays were performed in vitro. Each usually included four experimental models, all containing the same amount of autologous plasma, PBL and PHA, with 0.7, 1.0 and 1.4 mg of RSTL added to three of them.

Evaluation of the data has shown that addition of RSTL to PBL in culture may induce significant increases in the PHA index, over and above the physiological level. The effect of RSTL may be positive or negative and depends critically on the dose of RSTL, on the PHA index and on the kinetics of the lymphocyte subpopulations sensitive to it, as best shown by analysis of the grouped data. The lower the RSTL dose and the PHA index, the higher the effect of RSTL; and the higher the RSTL dose and PHA index, the lower the effect of RSTL.

The highest RSTL CR was highly significant representing a 30% increase over the mean PHA index for the group as a whole ($\overline{X} = 130 \times 10^4$ immunoblasts) and 155% over the lowest PHA index ($\overline{X} = 49 \times 10^4$ immunoblasts). The lowest RSTL effect was seen with the highest PHA index ($\overline{X} = 259 \times 10^4$ immunoblasts), representing a 37% decrease in the mean PHA index.

A positive effect of RSTL was observed in 74% of cases in the first assay and was positive for at least one of four sequential assays.

Although the mechanism(s) of action is (are) unknown, it has been postulated that the target cells for the positive and negative effects of RSTL are the T-cell precursors and PHA-sensitive T-lymphocytes, respectively.

Acknowledgement

We gratefully acknowledge the collaboration of Misses M. Gómez, M. F. Castaño, P. Lapuente, A. Cortes and M. A. Alonso and Mr F. Cortizo, for their skillful technical assistance and typing of the manuscript. We thank also to Mrs A. C. Gianoli and J. Stein for their scientific advice and for kindly supplying the RSTL preparations from Cybila Laboratories.

This work was partially supported by the Fondacion Cientifica of the AECC.

References

1. BERETTA, G. et al (1978): Controlled study for prolonged chemotherapy. Immunotherapy and chemotherapy plus immunotherapy as an adjuvant to surgery in stage I—II malignant melanoma. Preliminary report. International Group for the Study of Melanoma. In: TERRY, W. D. & WINDHORST, D. eds., Immunotherapy of Cancer: Present Status of Trials in Man, New York, Raven Press, p. 65

2. COCHRAN, A. J. (1978): Man, Cancer and Immunity. The effects of treatment on the immune system. New York, Academic Press, pp. 145—159

3. CUNNINGHAM, D. J. et al (1978): A controlled study of adjuvant therapy in patients with stage I and II malignant melanoma. In: TERRY, W. D. & WINDHORST, D., eds., Immunotherapy of Cancer: Present Status of Trials in Man, New York, Raven Press, p. 191

4. EILBER, F. R. and MORTON, D. L.: Impaired immunologic reactivity and recurrence following cancer surgery. Cancer 25 (1970), 362—367

5. HERSH, E. M., CUTTERMAN, J. U. and MAVLIGIT, G. M. (1975): Cancer and host defense mechanisms. In: IOACHIM, H. L., ed., Pathobiology Annual, New York, Appleton Century Crofts, pp. 133—167

6. HERSH, E. M., GUTTERMAN, J. U. et al (1978): Clinical rationale for immunotherapy and its role in cancer treatment. In: TERRY, W. D. & WINDHORST, D., eds., Immunotherapy of Human Cancer: Present Status and Trials in Man, New York, Raven Press, pp. 83—97

7. HOLLAND, J. F. and BEKESI, G. (1978): Comparation of chemotherapy plus VCN-treated cells in acute myeloblastic leukemia. In: TERRY, W. D. & WINDHORST, D., eds., Immunotherapy of Human Cancer: Present Status and Trials in Man, New York, Raven Press

8. ISRAEL, L.: Cell-mediated immunity in lung cancer: Data, problems and propositions. Cancer Chemother. Rep. 4 (1973), 279—281

9. MATHÉ, G. et al: Active immunotherapy for acute lymphoblastic leukemia. Lancet L (1969), 697—699

10. MCKNEALLY, M. F. et al (1978): Regional immunotherapy of lung cancer using postoperative intrapleural BCG. In: TERRY, W. D. & WINDHORST, D., eds., Immunotherapy of Human Cancer: Present Status of Trials in Man, New York, Raven Press, p. 161

11. MORTON, D. L. et al (1978): Adjuvant immunotherapy of malignant melanoma: Preliminary results of a randomized trial in patients with lymph node metastases. In: TERRY, W. D. & WINDHORST, D., eds., Immunotherapy of Human Cancer: Present Status of Trials in Man, New York, Raven Press, pp. 58, 81

12. PINSKY, C. M. et al (1978): Surgical adjuvant immunotherapy with BCG in patients with malignant melanoma: Results of a prospective randomized trial. In: TERRY, W. D. & WINDHORST, D., eds., Immunotherapy of Human Cancer: Present Status of Trials in Man, New York, Raven Press, p. 27

13. SYMOENS, J. (1978): Treatment of the compromised host with levamisol—a synthetic immunotherapeutic agent. In: CHIRIGOS, M. A., ed., Immune Modulation and Control of Neoplasia by Adjuvant Therapy, New York, Raven Press, pp. 1—9

[1] Institute of Cell and Tumour Biology, German Cancer Research Center, Heidelberg, and

[2] Department of Obstetrics and Gynecology, Mannheim, University of Heidelberg, FRG

Human Serum Ribonuclease Activity as a Marker for Therapeutic Success in Ovarian Carcinoma

H. G. Schleich[1], W. W. Wiest[2] and R. Pohl[2]

Ovarian carcinoma is usually not diagnosed until the disease reaches an advanced stage, and only 25% of patients have localized disease at the time of diagnosis. In cases of ovarian carcinoma that are detected and treated early, however, three out of four patients survive more than five years, whereas the mean survival time for all patients drops to only 18 months.

Unfortunately precise methods for diagnosis and surveillance of ovarian cancer, indispensable for better success in therapy, do not yet exist.

It has been shown, however, that serum ribonucleolytic activity increases significantly in patients with florid carcinoma of the ovary.

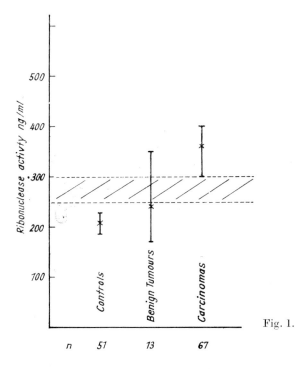

Fig. 1.

Figure 1 shows the medians with the confidence intervals of the serum ribonuclease activity of 51 controls, 13 patients with benign tumours of the ovary and 67 patients with histologically confirmed ovarian carcinoma. The ordinate gives the ribonuclease activity, equivalent to the amount of RNase A from bovine pancreas in ng/ml serum. The shaded area depicts the transition range from normal to increased serum ribonuclease activity, an indication of a malignant process. The difference between the control group and the ovarian carcinoma group is significant at the 1% level. Benign tumours of the ovary demonstrate a median in the normal range, however, the confidence interval reaches the area indicating a malignant process. Figure 2 refers to a 66 year old patient with an endometrioid ovarian carcinoma, stage $T_4N_XM_{1b}$. The behaviour of the serum ribonuclease activity is characteristic of an advanced ovarian carcinoma. The ordinate gives the ribonuclease activity, the abscissa the duration of surveillance. Arrows indicate a four day cyclophosphamide cure. Transition area is again shaded, and the serum ribonuclease activity is in the malignant area.

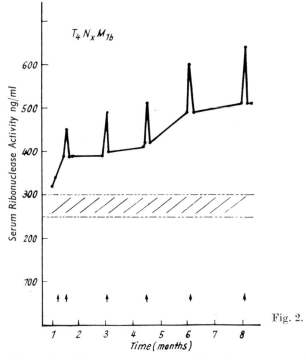

Fig. 2.

Clinically, the tumour progressed despite of cytostatic therapy, and this was clearly indicated by the increase of serum ribonuclease activity.

The cyclophosphamide therapy itself consistently produced a spike of increased activity immediately following treatment, a maximum being reached on the third or fourth day of treatment. This was superimposed on the already increased level of serum ribonuclease activity, and was definitely less pronounced in patients without a detectable tumour burden. The results suggest that this additional sudden increase of serum ribonuclease activity is mainly due to the therapy-induced tumour cell destruction. A direct inhibition of the serum ribonucleases by cyclophosphamide can be excluded.

Figure 3 shows the behaviour of the serum ribonuclease activity in a 58 year old patient with an endometrioid ovarian carcinoma, stage $T_4N_0M_{1b}$. The activity was in the transition area at first, but increased continuously after twelve months of relative stability. The effect of the cyclophosphamide treatment was significantly less pronounced. Despite the further cytostatic treatment the disease progressed after 14 months. This was also indicated by the increase of serum ribonuclease activity.

Figure 4 refers to a 36 year old patient with a papillary cystadenocarcinoma of the ovary, stage $T_4N_XM_{1b}$, and shows the course of the serum ribonuclease activity following a successful therapy. The activity never exceeded the normal range, and the effect of the cyclophosphamide treatment was not comparable with that observed in florid carcinoma. The arrow indicates the time of surgical intervention. A laparotomy confirmed the absence of any tumour residues.

With more than 3,000 serum analyses completed, the determination of serum ribonuclease activity appears to be a very reliable diagnostic tool for surveillance of non-invasive ovarian carcinoma.

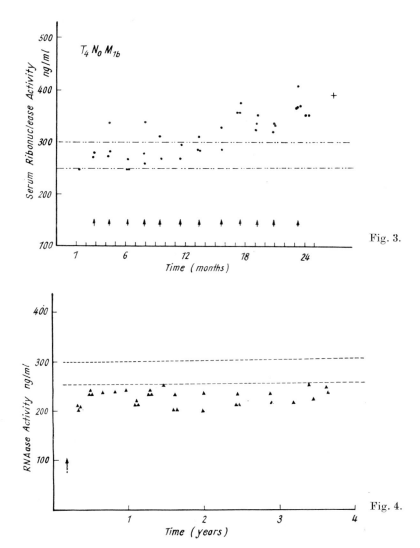

Fig. 3.

Fig. 4.

Department of Biochemical Pharmacology, Institute of Cancer Research, Belmont, Sutton, Surrey, England

Biological Properties of the New Quinazoline Inhibitor of Thymidylate Synthetase CB 3717

A. L. Jackman, A. H. Calvert, G. A. Taylor and K. R. Harrap

Introduction

CB 3717 (N-(4 (N-((2-amino-4-hydroxy-6-quinazolinyl)methyl) prop-2-ynylamino)-benzoyl)-L-glutamic acid) is a new quinazoline antifolate that is an inhibitor of the enzyme thymidylate synthetase (TS) [EC 2.1.1.45]. Exceptional results obtained against the L1210 tumour in vivo and its activity against cells resistant to methotrexate in vitro led to a more detailed investigation into its biochemical and antitumour properties (1). This, together with its toxicological evaluation has resulted in a clinical study at the Royal Marsden Hospital.

The inhibition of the de novo synthesis of thymidylate is an attractive target for the design of an antiproliferative drug and this objective may be achieved with an inhibitor of TS. This enzyme catalyses a bi-substrate reaction, one substrate being the reduced folate, 5,10-methylene tetrahydrofolate and the other being the pyrimidine mononucleotide, deoxyuridylate (dUMP). Inhibition of this step may be achieved indirectly by antifolates such as methotrexate (2, 3) or directly by active metabolites of pyrimidine analogues such as 5-fluorouracil (2). 5-Fluorodeoxyuridylate (FdUMP), an active metabolite of 5-fluorouracil is a potent inhibitor of isolated TS enzyme although it is controversial whether this is its prime site of action in cells (2). 5-Fluorouracil is incorporated into RNA which may account for much of the drug's toxicity (4,5)

All antifolates currently available are inhibitors of dihydrofolate reductase (DHFR). Inhibition of this enzyme results in the accumulation of intracellular folates as the inactive dihydrofolate. The depletion in the one-carbon carrying tetrahydrofolate pool leads to the reduction of 5,10-methylene tetrahydrofolate dependent thymidylate synthesis. In addition, the synthesis of purines may be inhibited and evidence exists to suggest that this is detrimental to achieving a good cytotoxic effect in some cell lines (6) and may also contribute to toxicity in vivo (7).

A folate-based inhibitor of TS such as CB 3717 should possess certain advantages due to being a vitamin analogue. Unlike pyrimidines folates cannot be synthesised de novo so that the natural substrate for the enzyme should not build up significantly and compete with the inhibitor for binding. A folate analogue usually does not need metabolic activation, is not easily catabolised and cannot be incorporated into nucleic acids.

Thus, a folate-based TS inhibitor would be expected to lead to a specific inhibition of TS without affecting other processes.

We aim here to review our current knowledge of the biochemistry of CB 3717 and to present some additional data that supports the hypothesis that CB 3717 acts solely as a TS inhibitor in vitro. Results of further antitumour testing and evidence for the drug's in vivo locus is also presented here.

Methods

Antitumour testing

CB 3717 was screened against two solid tumours, the TLX/5 lymphoma (8) and the PC6 plasmacytoma (9).

In addition to our previously reported L1210 i. p. tumour model (1) we screened CB 3717 against the same tumour injected intravenously. 10^4 cells were injected into the tail vein on Day 0 and the course of 5 daily injections (i. p.) started on Day 3.

In all these screens, methotrexate given at an optimal dose was included for comparison.

CB 3717 was injected as a solution of the disodium salt in isotonic saline. The pH of this preparation was approximately 8.5.

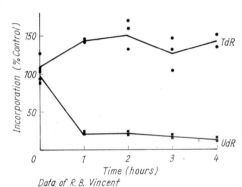

Fig. 1. TdR and UdR incorporation by L1210 cells exposed to CB 3717 (25 μM).

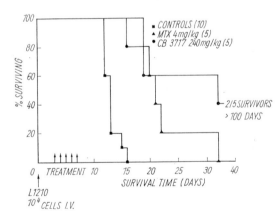

Fig. 2. I. v. L1210 tumour test.

Plasma deoxyuridine measurements

$DBA_2 \times C57 F_1$ hybrius were injected with 5×10^4 L1210 cells on Day 0. A course of 5 daily injections (i. p.) of CB 3717 started on Day 3. Groups of 5 mice were bled by cardiac puncture at the times indicated in Figure 3. Control mice (tumour-bearing) received 0.15 M sodium bicarbonate pH 9.0.

Deoxyuridine was determined by a modification of the high performance liquid chromatographic method of TAYLOR et al (10). Neutralised perchlorate extracts were applied to a μ Bondapak 10 μ C18 reversed phase column (Waters Associates) running isocratically in 0.025 M ammonium acetate pH 5.0. Fractions corresponding to deoxyuridine were collected and applied to an Apex 5 μ C18 reversed phase column (Jones Chromatography) running isocratically in 90% 0.025 M ammonium succinate pH 5.8:10% methanol.

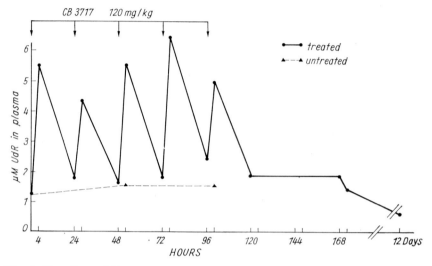

Fig. 3. The effect of CB 3717 on plasma deoxyuridine in L1210 tumour-bearing mice.

Incorporation of radiolabelled precursors

Incorporation of radiolabelled precursors into acid-precipitable material was measured as described by BROWMAN et al (11).

Cell culture

L1210 cell culture with thymidine protection experiments were performed as described previously (1).

Results and discussion

CB3717 is a tight-binding inhibitor of TS competitive with the folate co-substrate, 5,10-methylene tetrahydrofolate. The Ki for the enzyme purified from W1L2 human lymphoblastoid cells is 5 nM (12).
Having shown that CB 3717 is a tight-binding inhibitor of TS is was necessary to determine whether this is its intracellular locus of cytotoxicity.

Identification of the cytotoxic locus of CB 3717

Quinazoline antifolates which inhibit TS are also fairly potent DHFR inhibitors (1 and references therein). CB 3717 has a Ki for W1L2 DHFR of 23 nM (12). However consideration of the kinetic parameters, concentrations of the two enzymes and their natural substrates strongly suggests that in the presence of CB 3717 TS is rate-limiting

406

Table 1.

Ki's of CB 3717 and methotrexate for L1210 thymidylate synthetase and dihydrofolate reductase.

	TS Ki (nM)	DHFR Ki (nM)	Ki TS/DHFR
MTX	15,000*	0.005+	3×10^6
CB 3717	1++	14++	0.07

DHFR rate-limiting only if Ki TS/DHFR > 3,000

* Harrap et al (17)

\+ Jackson et al (18)

++ Jones et al (1)

and inhibition of DHFR is inconsequential. The mathematical model demonstrates that a dual inhibitor of TS and DHFR will be rate-limiting on TS even if the affinity of the inhibitor for TS is 3,000 weaker than for DHFR (12). Table 1 illustrates how the two dual inhibitors, MTXrand CB 3717 may each be expected to have a different locus as demonstrated by this model.

Experiments with cells in culture exposed to MTX or CB 3717 support the prediction that these drugs each have a different intracellular locus. A mutant L1210 cell line, the L1210:R71 has a 230-fold increase in DHFR and this raised enzyme confers a high degree of resistance to methotrexate upon these cells (600-fold resistant) (13). However, these cells are only 3-fold resistant to CB 3717, evidence consistent with DHFR not being the cytotoxic locus (1).

Cells that have their DHFR inhibited and active TS should accumulate intracellular folates as dihydrofolate while those where TS only is inhibited should not. This is demonstrated clearly by methotrexate and CB 3717 in W1L2 cells where only the former results in raised dihydrofolate (12).

As the biochemical lesions in cells treated with methotrexate is the decrease in fully reduced folates necessary for de novo purine and thymidylate synthesis, full protection from cytotoxicity is possible by repleting the folate pool with the addition of folinic acid or by-passing the de novo thymidine and purine pathways by supplying salvageable precursors (14).

CB 3717 cytotoxicity is prevented by thymidine alone (1, 12) but only by folinic acid at very high concentrations (10 μM) (1). In the latter case the raised intracellular pool of 5,10-methylene tetrahydrofolate may then compete with the inhibitor.

These results are consistent with the mathematical prediction that DHFR is not the cytotoxic locus for CB 3717, at least in the cell lines studied.

There are a number of other folate-dependent enzymes which are potential targets for CB 3717. However if L1210 cells are treated with a high dose of CB 3717 (500 μM) which is 100-times the ID_{50}, cytotoxicity is largely prevented by thymidine alone (74%) suggesting that there is probably not an additional weaker locus of action in these cells (Table 2).

Incorporation of radiolabelled precursors into acid precipitable material also gives qualitative evidence that the synthesis of thymidylate alone is affected by CB 3717. Figure 1 clearly demonstrates that deoxyuridine incorporation into cells treated with the drug falls while that of thymidine increases slightly, consistent with inhibition of

Table 2.

The effect of TdR on high dose CB 3717 in L1210 cells grown in culture.

	Cell count as % controls at 48 hr
CB 3717 alone (500 μM)	0
CB 3717 + 10^{-5} M thymidine	74

TS. The incorporation of leucine and uridine were unchanged suggesting that protein and RNA synthesis were unaffected (data not shown). Similarly, measurement of nucleotide and deoxynucleotide pools in WIL2 cells treated with CB 3717 exhibited changes attributable only to the antithymidylate properties of the drug (12). Thymine nucleotides decreased while dUMP (the co-substrate for TS) increased, indicating inhibition of TS. Although methotrexate caused similar changes, due to the indirect inhibition of the same step, it also caused a decrease in ATP and GTP consistent with the drug's additional antipurine effect (12).

Evidence that inhibition of thymidylate synthetase is achieved better with a folate analogue rather than a pyrimidine

The expansion of the dUMP pool after treatment with CB 3717 emphasises the advantage that a folate-based inhibitor of TS has over a pyrimidine-based inhibitor such as FdUMP. The dUMP levels reported after treatment with an ID_{50} dose of CB 3717 or methotrexate showed an increase from 11 nmoles/10^9 cells to 490 and to 323 nmoles/10^9 cells respectively (12). Levels as high as 1.22 μmoles/10^9 cells have been reported for human lymphoblastoid (8866) treated with a substantial concentration of methotrexate (10 μM) (15). Thus dUMP levels can rise very significantly when the synthesis of thymidylate is inhibited.

The intracellular concentrations of the natural substrates for TS and their kinetic constants are critical when considering the effectiveness of a competitive inhibitor. L1210 TS has a Km value of 0.7 μM for dUMP and 17 μM for 5,10-methylene tetrahydrofolate (data not shown). As the Km for dUMP is low and the potential intracellular concentration of this substrate is very high a pyrimidine-based inhibitor of TS e. g. FdUMP is unlikely to achieve significant inhibition. Even though the ternary complex, when formed in cell-free systems is covalently bound, high intracellular levels of dUMP would inhibit the initial competitive binding (2). Intracellular folates are unlikely to accumulate as 5,10-methylene tetrahydrofolate as this cofactor is also an intermediate in other pathways. However it has been calculated that if they did accumulate, the concentration could not exceed 20 μM (16) since de novo synthesis of folates is not possible. As this concentration is only approximately the Km value it is clear that inhibition by CB 3717 is unlikely to be reversed by substrate competition.

Inhibition of TS in vivo

Having established that specific inhibitors of TS and consequently DNA synthesis has been achieved in vitro it is necessary to establish whether the cytotoxic locus is the same in vivo. We know that CB 3717 is an active antitumour agent against the i. p. L1210 tumour where 90% "cures" are consistently obtained with non-toxic

Table 3.
ADJ/PC6 tumour test.

CB 3717 dose (mg/kg/day × 5 days)	Animals surviving treatment	% inhibition of tumour growth
300	0/3	—
150	3/3	84
75	3/3	57
37.5	3/3	51
18.75	3/3	16
9.375	3/3	32

Methotrexate dose (mg/kg/day × 5 days)	Animals surviving treatment	% inhibition of tumour growth
24	0/3	—
12	1/3	80
6	2/3	50
3	3/3	43
1.5	3/3	36
0.75	3/3	−5

Table 4.
TLX/5 lymphoma test.

CB 3717 dose (mg/kg/day × 5 days)	% increase in lifespan
300	18
150	22
75	9
37.5	11
18.75	9
9.375	−1

Methotrexate dose (mg/kg/day × 5 days)	% increase in lifespan
24	−19
12	−13
6	73
3	71
1.5	71
0.75	50

Data of P. M. GODDARD

doses of the drug (125 mg/kg) (1). We have demonstrated recently that the same percentage cures can be obtained with 50 mg/kg (LD_{50} = 300 mg/kg) (data not shown). The results of further antitumour testing against the L1210 leukaemia injected i. v., the PC6 plasmacytoma and the TLX/5 lymphoma are shown in Figure 2 and Tables 3 and 4. In only the TLX/5 lymphoma did CB 3717 show activity inferior to that of methotrexate.

So far we have two pieces of evidence to suggest that the antitumour activity is attributable to inhibition of TS. First is the lack of metabolic activation. HPLC analysis fails to show any metabolite of CB 3717 in the plasma. The drug is excreted predominantly in the faeces ($> 50\%$) while less than 20% is excreted in the urine (D. R. NEWELL, personal communication). So it seems unlikely that CB 3717 is metabolised to a compound which might have a different locus.

The large intracellular concentration of dUMP found in vitro may lead to a similar increase in the corresponding nucleoside, deoxyuridine. We monitored plasma deoxyuridine in L1210 tumour-bearing mice treated with 120 mg/kg of CB 3717 daily $\times$ 5 for evidence that TS is inhibited in vivo. Deoxyuridine was found to peak at approximately 4 hours following injection, falling to basal levels by 24 hours. Figure 3 demonstrates this throughout the 5 day injection period.

In conclusion, CB 3717 was designed as a folate-based inhibitor of TS that would have this enzyme as its sole cytotoxic locus and would not require metabolic activation. The objectives so clearly shown to have been achieved in vitro also appear to have been achieved in vivo probably accounting for its excellent antitumour properties in some animal models.

Biochemical investigations on the patients receiving CB 3717 are underway to establish whether the "thymineless" state is being achieved. Correlation of these results with clinical activity should be of great interest as a test of the applicability of this particular biochemical rationale.

References

1. JONES, T. R., CALVERT, A. H., JACKMAN, A. L., BROWN, S. J., JONES, M. and HARRAP, K. R.: Europ. J. Cancer *17* (1981), 11
2. CHABNER, B. A.: In: Cancer Chemotherapy. The EORTC Cancer Chemotherapy Annual 2 (Edited by H. M. PINEDO) p. 1. Excerpta Medica, Amsterdam, Oxford (1980).
3. ENSMINGER, W. D., GRINDEY, G. B. and HOGLIND, J. A.: Adv. Cancer Chemother. *1* (1979), 61
4. MARTIN, D. S.: Cancer Bull. (Tex.) *30* (1978), 219
5. HOUGHTON, J. A., HOUGHTON, P. J. and WOOTEN, R. S.: Cancer Res. *39* (1979), 2406
6. BORSA, J. and WHITMORE, G. F.: Cancer Res. *29* (1969), 737
7. HARRAP, K. R., TAYLOR, G. A. and BROWMAN, G. P.: Chem.-Biol. Interactions *18* (1977), 119
8. CONNORS, T. A. and JONES, M.: Rec. Res. Cancer Res. *33* (1970), 181
9. ROSENOER, V. M., MITCHLEY, B. C. V., ROE, F. J. C. and CONNORS, T. A.: Cancer Res. *26* Suppl.) (1966), 957
10. TAYLOR, G. A., DADY, P. J. and HARRAP, K. R.: J. Chromatog. *183* (1980), 421
11. BROWMAN, G. P., CALVERT, A. H., TAYLOR, G. A., HART, L. I. and HARRAP, K. R.: Europ. J. Cancer *16* (1980), 1547
12. JACKSON, R. C., CALVERT, A. H., JACKMAN, A. L. and HARRAP, K. R.: In preparation.
13. JACKSON, R. C., NIETHAMMER, D. and HUENNEKENS, F. M.: Cancer Biochem. Biophys. *1* (1975), 151
14. TATTERSALL, M. H. N., JACKSON, R. C., JACKSON, S. T. M. and HARRAP, K. R.: Europ. J. Cancer *10* (1974), 819
15. GOULIAN, M., BLEILE, B. and TSENG, B. Y.: J. Biol. Chem. *255* (1980), 10 630
16. JACKSON, R. C., NIETHAMMER, D. and HART, L. I.: Arch. Biochem. Biophys. *182* (1977), 646
17. HARRAP, K. R., HILL, B. T., FURNESS, M. E. and HART, L. I.: In: Ann. N.Y. Acad. Sci. (Ed. J. R., BERTINO) 186, p. 312. New York Academy of Sciences (1971)
18. JACKSON, R. C., HART, L. I. and HARRAP, K. R.: Cancer Res. *36* (1976), 1991

Miscellaneous

Central Institute for Tumours and Allied Diseases, Zagreb, Yugoslavia

Reactivation of Alkylation-Damaged Adenovirus 3 by Cell Cultures Derived from Human Tumours

B. Brdar and J. Sorić

Introduction

It has been reported that low-passage human astrocytoma cell cultures prepared from a series of tumours show wide variation in susceptibility to killing by a derivative of nitrosourea (4). Consequently, it has been postulated that tumours that respond well to alkylation chemotherapy are composed of cells which are defective in repairing DNA damage due to alkylating agents. This hypothesis was recently tested by Day and collaborators (3), who found that some human cell strains derived from a series of tumours are deficient in repairing alkylation-damaged DNA of adenovirus 5. These include astrocytomas, lung, colon and epidermoid carcinomas and melanoma, suggesting that alkylation repair-deficient tumours arise in different organs. To test this assumption further, we examined host cell reactivation of N-methyl-N-nitrosourea(MNU)-damaged adenovirus 3 by primary and early-passage cell cultures derived from the following human tumours: ovarian and cervical carcinomas, glioblastomas and melanomas. In some experiments, another alkylating agent, nitrogen mustard (HN_2), was used.

In the course of this work, the question arose whether alkylation reactivation of adenovirus 3 is inducible in mammalian cells. We therefore investigated whether pretreatment of HeLa or KB cells in culture with either alkylating agent enhanced alkylation-damaged survival of adenovirus, similar to that observed when ultraviolet-irradiated DNA viruses were plated on ultra-violet irradiated hosts (1, 2, 7).

Material and methods

Adenovirus 3 and poliovirus 2 were grown on KB or HeLa cells and were purified in the following way: Cell monolayers were infected with the two viruses at a high multiplicity of infection (10 plaque-forming units (PFU/cell)); and after a period of virus adsorption (1 hour at 37 °C) cultures were thoroughly washed with culture medium. Minimal essential medium containing 2% foetal bovine serum was then added, and incubation proceeded until a cytopathogenic effect appeared in infected cultures. After three cycles of freezing and thawing, cell debris was removed by centrifugation at 2,000 g for 10 min, and an equal volume of a saturated solution of $(NH_4)_2$-SO_4 was added to the supernatant in the cold. The precipitate was obtained by centrifugation at 16,000 g for 10 min, dissolved in a small volume of 0.01 M Tris, pH 8.0 and layered on a discontinuous gradient of sucrose (20%) and CsCl ($\varrho' = 1.43$). After centrifugation at 25,000 rpm for 60 min (MSE-super speed centrifuge, SW), the interphase was collected and dialysed against three changes of 0.01 M Tris, pH 8.0. The virus was titered by a plaque assay as described previously (2).

Inactivation of adenovirus 3 or poliovirus 2 with MNU (1, 2, 3, 4 mg/ml) or HN_2 was carried out as described by DAY et al (3).

Primary cultures of human neoplastic and normal cells were derived from histologically determined surgical specimens of ovarian and cervical carcinomas, glioblastoma, melanoma and a normal ovary and skin. The procedure used in isolating the cell cultures was described previously (6). Cultures were propagated in Dullbecco's medium supplemented with 10% foetal bovine serum.

To test for alkylation-induced Weighle's reactivation, KB or HeLa cells were pretreated with either MNU (200 µg/ml) or HN_2 (0.1 µg/ml) for 3 hours and were infected 24 hours later with inactivated adenovirus 3 (see above).

The media for cell culturing, foetal bovine serum and plastic Petri dishes were purchased from Flow Laboratories, Irvine, Scotland. MNU was obtained through the generosity of Dr. D. Ivankovic of the Institut für Toxikologie und Chemotherapie, Deutsches Krebsforschungszentrum, Heidelberg, FRG. MNU was dissolved in absolute ethanol (10—40 mg/ml) and kept in liquid nitrogen. The human glioblastoma cell strain, U-105-MG, was generously provided by Dr J. FOGH, Sloan-Kettering, New York, USA.

Results

Figure 1 shows the results of an experiment in which the reactivation of MNU-damaged adenovirus 3 was examined in low-passage human cell cultures derived from a meningioma (P.S.), a melanoma (K.I.) and an astrocytoma (V.M.). None of these cultures showed deficient repair of damaged virus as compared to that of a cell strain of human glioblastoma (U-105 MG), which had previously been shown to be deficient in repairing alkylation-damaged adenovirus 5 (3). Comparable results were obtained with human cell cultures of skin and of two cervical carcinomas (S.R. and K.D.) (Fig. 2). Figure 3 shows the high level of reactivation of MNU-damaged adenovirus by one normal and

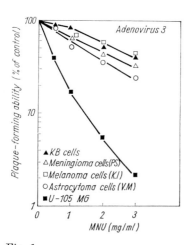

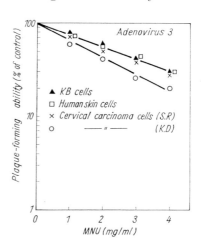

Fig. 1   Fig. 2

Fig. 1. Reactivation of MNU-treated adenovirus 3 by human tumour cells in culture. Purified adenovirus 3 was diluted 1:100 in 0.3 M Tris, pH 8.0 and treated with the indicated concentrations of MNU by incubation at 37 °C for 30 min. The virus plaque-forming ability was then determined on confluent monolayers of the cell cultures indicated.

Fig. 2. Reactivation of MNU-treated adenovirus 3 by human tumour cells in culture. Experimental conditions as in the legend to Fig. 1.

two ovarian tumour cell cultures (P.V. and B.R.) and the poor reactivity of one ovarian carcinoma (P.M.) cell culture.

We reported previously (2) that MNU inhibits the growth of DNA (herpes simplex virus)- and RNA(poliovirus)-containing viruses to an equal extent. It was therefore of some interest to compare the host-cell reactivation of MNU-damaged adenovirus 3 and poliovirus by KB cells. The results (Fig. 4) show that survival of MNU-treated poliovirus in KB cells is very low as compared with that of adenovirus 3. They also show that MNU lesions in the RNA of damaged poliovirus cannot be reactivated by the host.

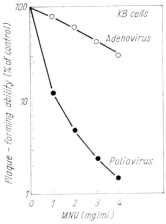
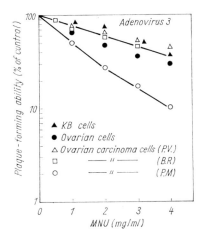

Fig. 3   Fig. 4

Fig. 3. Reactivation of MNU-treated adenovirus 3 by human tumour cells in culture. Experimental conditions as in the legend to Fig. 1.

Fig. 4. Reactivation of MNU-treated adenovirus 3 and poliovirus by KB cells in culture. Experimental conditions as in the legend to Fig. 1.

Table 1.
Survival of adenovirus 3 in alkylating agent-treated and untreated host cells[a]

Host cells and pretreatment	Treated virus (PFU/ml) $\times 10^5$	Untreated virus (PFU/ml) $\times 10^5$	Survival (%)
KB cells untreated	MNU 7.5	19.3	39
KB cells pretreated with 200 µg/ml MNU	9.0	13.5	67
HeLa cells untreated	HN$_2$ 10.5	20.5	53
HeLa cells pretreated with 0.1 µg/ml HN$_2$	15.8	16.2	98

[a] Cells were plated at a concentration of 8×10^5/60-mm Petri dish and were treated 12 hours later by addition of alkylating agent, or were left untreated. Cells were washed after 3-h treatment and further incubated for 24 h in fresh medium. Purified adenovirus 3 was diluted 1:100 in 0.3 m Tris, pH 8.0 and treated with 3000 µg/ml MNU or 1000 µg/ml HN$_2$ by incubation at 37° C for 30 min. The virus plaque-forming ability was determined on confluent monolayers of each cell culture.

Some evidence suggests that mammalian cells respond to DNA-damage by inducing a high survival of ultraviolet-damaged virus. For instance, ultraviolet-irradiated cells of monkey, rat and man show induced virus reactivation when infected with DNA-damaged viruses (1, 5, 7). We thus attempted to determine whether a similar induced reactivation could be obtained with adenovirus 3 damaged by either MNU or HN_2. Cultures of KB or HeLa cells were pretreated for 24 hours with MNU (200 µg/ml) or HN_2 (0.1 µg/ml), respectively, under conditions in which cell survival was about 50%. The results (Table 1) show that the survival of MNU-damaged (3,000 µg/ml) adenovirus 3 increased by a factor of 1.7 in MNU-treated KB cells as compared with untreated control cells. In a parallel experiment, greater host-cell reactivation (a factor of 1.9) was also found when HN_2-damaged (1,000 mg/ml) adenovirus was plated on HeLa cells pretreated with 0.1 µg/ml of the same compound.

Discussion

The experiments described here were designed to identify human tumours deficient in the repair of alkylation damage. Of the human primary cell cultures examined, which were derived from normal and tumour tissues, only one ovarian carcinoma was shown to be defective in host-cell reactivation of MNU-damaged DNA of adenovirus 3. Although an insufficient number of tumours was examined, our finding is of interest in that it suggests that repair-deficient human tumours are not rare. Such repair-deficiency occurs not only in ovarian carcinomas, as was demonstrated by DAY and collaborators (3), who examined a large series of established human cell strains, prepared from normal and tumour tissues, and found 23% to be deficient in reactivating alkylation-damaged adenovirus 5. These included glioblastomas, lung, colon and epidermoid carcinomas and melanoma, which are all repair-defective to the action of different alkylating agents. In our study, primary and low-passage tumour cell cultures were used, implying the involvement of mixed popolation of tumour and normal cells.

Since repair deficiency does not occur in any of the normal human cell strains tested to date (3), it is reasonable to conclude that primary cultures, wich contain various proportions of normal cells, will display variations in the degree of host-cell reactivation of damaged viruses. Thus, a primary culture of ovarian carcinoma was less defective in repairing alkylation damage than an established cell strain of glioblastoma (U-105MG). Moreover, a primary culture of astrocytoma showed a diminished capacity to reactivate MNU-damaged adenovirus 3 as compared with KB and melanoma cells (Fig. 1). We cannot state whether this was due to the heterogeneity of the cell population or wether it is an intrinsic property of this tumour. Despite certain drawbacks, therefore we have shown that primary and early-passage cell cultures may be useful in screening repair-defective human tumours. However, many more human tumours should be tested for host-cell reactivation of alkylation-damaged viruses in order to establish the distribution and frequency of tumours defective in the repair of alkylation damage. In addition, it would be of great importance to determine whether or not repair-defective tumours and their cell cultures are more susceptible to the toxic effects of alkylating agents. Since there are indications that this might be so (3, 4), we believe that our experimental model system could be useful for predicting which chemotherapy to use in the treatment of human tumours.

Summary

We examined the host cell reactivation of N-methyl-N-nitrosourea damaged Adenovirus 3 by cell cultures derived from the following human tumour and normal tissues: ovarian, cervical carcinomas, glioblastomas, melanomas, normal ovary, skin. The plaque forming ability of alkylating agent treated virus was determined on each of these cell types in culture. Of the tested cell cultures only one ovarian carcinoma was found to be defective in reactivation of alkylation-damaged DNA of Adenovirus 3. This supports the notion that repair deficient human tumours are not rare and that this experimental system could be useful for chemotherapy predictive testing of human tumours.

References

1. BOCKSTAHLER, L. E. and LYTLE, C. D.: Radiation enhanced reactivation of nuclear replicating mammalian viruses. Photochem. Photobiol. *25* (1977), 477—482
2. BRDAR, B. and BAN, J.: Inhibition of viral RNA synthesis by 1-methyl-1-nitrosourea. Biochim. Biophys. Acta *606* (1980), 285—291
3. DAY III, R. S., ZIOLOWSKI, C. H. J., SCUDIERO, D. A., MEYER, S. A. and MATTERN, M. R.: Human tumour cell strains defective in the repair of alkylation damage, Carcinogenesis *1* (1980), 21—32
4. KORNBLITH, P. L. and SZYPKO, P. E.: Variations in response of human brain tumours to BCNU in vitro. J. Neurosurg. *48* (1978), 580—586
5. LYTLE, C. D., DAY III, R. S., HELLMAN, K. B. and BOCKSTAHLER, L. E.: Infection of UV-irradiated Xeroderma pigmentosum fibroblasts by herpes simplex virus: Study of capacity and Weigle reactivation. Mut. Res. *36* (1976), 257—264
6. NAGY, B., BAN, J. and BRDAR, B.: Fibrinolysis associated with human neoplasia: Production of plasminogen activator by human tumours. Int. J. Cancer *19* (1977), 614—620
7. SARASIN, A. R. and HANAWALT, P. C.: Carcinogens enhance survival of UV-irradiated simian virus 40 in treated monkey kidney cells: Induction of a recovery pathway? Proc. Natl. Acad. Sci. USA *75* (1978), 346—350

[1] Radiochemotherapy Dept., Bellaria Hospital, [2] Neurosurgical Dept., Bellaria Hospital, [3] Immunological Unit, Malpighi Hospital, Bologna, Italy

Effects of Surgical and Radio-Chemotherapeutic Treatment on the Immunological Pattern in Malignant Glioma Patients

L. Cacciari[1], E. Beltrandi[3], M. A. Bucci[3], R. Parente[1], F. Spagnolli[1] and F. Servadei[2]

Summary

Patients with primary encephalic neoplasias have a variety of immunological disorders, and patients who undergo to radio-chemotherapeutic treatment for all kinds of solid tumour show a significant impairment of the immunological response. This report concerns the immunological pattern of a homogeneous group of 45 patients with supratentorial malignant gliomas, who underwent surgery and an established radio-chemotherapeutic protocol, involving bischloroethyl nitrosourea. We determined the subpopulations of B and T lymphocytes and their in vitro reactivity to mitogenic lecithins. Immunological determinations were carried out before surgery, after surgery, and during and after the radio-chemotherapeutic treatment. In comparison with healthy controls, glioma patients were found to have significant impairment of cell-mediated immunological parameters; the impairment was not increased during treatment.

Introduction

Patients with anaplastic glioma (glioblastoma, astrocytoma grades 3/4) have a very short life expectancy (several months), regardless of surgical, radiotherapeutic and/or chemotherapeutic treatment. They appear to have altered immunological parameters: reduction in peripheral blood lymphocytes (15, 26), reduction in rosette-forming T-cells (5) and impaired response to various mitogens (6, 19). Therapeutic irradiation, alone (9, 18, 22) or in combination with chemotherapy (17), appears to depress lymphocyte function in patients with such tumours. The aim of our study was to determine the changes induced by radio-chemotherapy in the immunological pattern of glioma patients.

Material and methods

We examined 45 patients (23 men, 22 women) with a mean age of 52, ranging from 31 to 68 years. Each had a histologically determined supratentorial anaplastic glioma, for which they underwent surgery. 28 patients were also treated by radio-chemotherapy, as follows: eight days after surgery, a "one-week" protocol was instituted in which 100 mg/m^2 bichloroethyl nitrosourea (BCNU) were given on days 1 and 7 and whole-head irradiation through bilateral opposing parts with 3 Gy/day X-rays on days 2—6. This protocol was repeated 3 and 10 weeks later. The treatment was a standard one for glioma patients, slightly modified on the basis of recent reports (7, 11, 27).

For immunological monitoring, peripheral blood samples were taken two weeks after surgery, at the end of the first week of therapy, again at the end of the second week, and, for cases followed up for three months at least, at the end of the third week of radio-chemotherapy. When the samples were taken, the patients were not receiving any drug.

Lymphocytes were separated from freshly heparinized peripheral blood, as described by Boyum (1), and counted. For determination of erythrocyte-antibody-complement rosettes (EAC rosettes), a suspension of sheep red blood cells (SRBC) was incubated with rabbit anti-sheep-red-blood-cell diluted 1:2000. Fresh human complement, diluted 1:20, was added and the suspension incubated. Equal volumes of the prepared sheep cells and isolated lymphocytes were mixed, incubated and centrifuged. The percentage of EAC rosettes was calculated as described by Kaplan and Clark (14), and provides an estimate of the number of B-lymphocytes.

To determine total rosettes, SRBC were treated with the sulfhydryl reagent 2-aminoethylisothiouronium bromide. The percentage of lymphocytes binding more than two SRBC was determined as above, and reflects, to some extent, the total number of T-lymphocytes.

The blastogenic responses of lymphocytes to various mitogens (phytohaemagglutinin-P; concanavalin A and pokeweed mitogen (PHA, ConA, PWM)) were evaluated by incorporation of ^{3}H-thymidine in vitro.

Results and discussion

Our patients had fewer lymphocytes than a group of healthy, age-matched controls; however, the difference was not statistically significant, and there is not any significant further modification of the total number of lymphocytes after radio-chemotherapy. The percentages of EAC rosette-forming cells (the so-called 'B-pool') (Fig. 1) were also within the normal range of values, both preoperatively and after radio-chemotherapy (10,16). However, both the number of total rosette-forming cells (the so-called 'T-pool') (Fig. 2) and in-vitro responses to different mitogens (Fig. 3—5) were altered before treatment to a statistically significant degree. The impairment of lymphocyte response

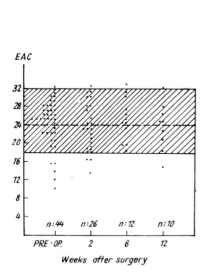

Fig. 1

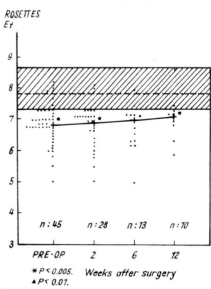

Fig. 2

Fig. 1. Levels of erythrocyte-antibody-complement (EAC) rosettes before (PRE-OP) and 2, 6 and 12 weeks after surgery in lymphocytes from patients with malignant glioma.

Fig. 2. Levels of total rosette-forming cells (E_t) before (PRE-OP) and 2, 6 and 12 weeks after surgery in lymphocytes from patients with malignant glioma.

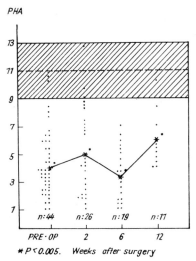

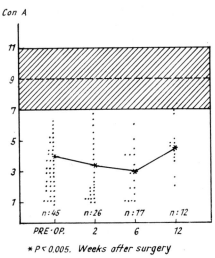

Fig. 3

Fig. 4

Fig.3. Blastogenic response to phytohaemagglutinin (PHA) of lymphocytes from patients with malignant glioma, before (PRE-OP) and 2, 6 and 12 weeks after surgery.

Fig. 4. Blastogenic response to concanavalin A (Con A) of lymphocytes from patients with malignant glioma, before (PRE-OP) and 2, 6 and 12 weeks after surgery.

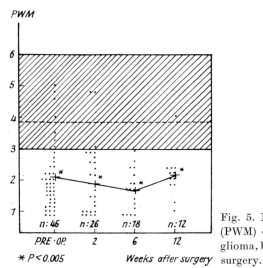

Fig. 5. Blastogenic response to pokeweed mitogen (PWM) of lymphocytes from patients with malignant glioma, before (PRE-OP) and 2, 6 and 12 weeks after surgery.

in glioma patients has been correlated with the presence of serum blocking factors (4, 17). Such factors decrease one week after surgery (3), resulting in improved lymphocyte reactivity and cell-mediated immunity after the resection of a tumour mass (29). In our patients, who also underwent radio-chemotherapy, the lymphocyte responses did not show such improvement; indeed, the mean values 2, 6 and 12 weeks after surgery do not differ from those at the end of the treatment period. There is general agreement that lymphocyte function is depressed by radio- and chemotherapy. However, although radiotherapy of solid tumours affects the ability of lymphocytes

420

to replicate (a 45% decrease in the response to PHA (2) and a 48—64% depression in transformation tests (21)), even when irradiation does not cover the mediastinal (thymic) area (9, 18, 22, 24, 25, 28), this effect does not appear to be as pronounced in patients treated only to the head (23). Chemotherapy depresses the lymphocyte response to mitogens (in vitro, a 71% decrease when compared with pretreatment cultures (13)) by affecting the T-pool of cells, whereas the B-pool remains almost unchanged (8); however, with chemotherapy widely fractionated into two or more periods, the immunological functions remain at levels that are close to normal (12).

We conclude that patients with malignant intracranial tumours have an altered immune status, which does not appear to be affected by combined irradiation and BCNU therapy. It is possible that the resection of the tumoral mass, which is known to improve immunological parameters, may counteract the depression, however slightly, induced by the combined treatment.

References

1. BOYUM, A.: Separation of leucocytes from blood and marrow. Scand. J. Clin. Lab. Invest. 21 (1968), 1—109

2. BRAEMAN, J.: Lymphocytes response after radiotherapy. Lancet II (1973), 683—688

3. BROOKS, W. H., NETZKY, M. G., NORMANSELL, D. E. and HOROWITZ, D. A.: Depressed cell-mediated immunity in patients with intracranial tumours. J. Exp. Med. 136 (1972), 1631—1647

4. BROOKS, W. H., CALDWELL, H. D. and MORTARA, R. H.: Immune response in patients with gliomas. Surg. Neurol. 2 (1974), 419—423

5. BROOKS, W. H., ROSZMAN, T. L. and ROGERS, A. S.: Impairment of rosette-forming T lymphocytes in patients with intracranial tumours. Cancer 37 (1976), 1869—1873

6. BROOKS. W. H., LATTA, R. B., MAHALEY, M. S., ROSZMAN, T. L., DUDKA, L. and SKAGGS, C.: Immunobiology of primary intracranial tumours. Part 5: Correlation of a lymphocyte index and clinical status. J. Neurosurg. 54 (1981), 331—337

7. CACCIARI, L., LOSTIA, G., PIAZZI, M. and TESTONI, M.: Terapia radiante ed antiblastica delle neoplasie cerebrali primitive. Osped. della Vita 3 (1979), 27—47

8. CAMPBEL, A. C., HERSEY, P., HARDING, B., HOLLINGSWORTH, P. M., SKINNER, J. and McLEN-NAN, I. C. M.: Effects of anticancer agents on immunological status. Br. J. Cancer. 28, Suppl. 1 (1973), 254—261

9. CHEE, C. A., ILBERY, P. L. T. and RICHINSON, A. B.: Depression of lymphocyte replication ability in radiotherapy patients. Br. J. Radiol. 47 (1974), 37—43

10. GEROSA, M., AMADORI, G., SEMENZATO, C., RAUMER, R., CISOTTO, P., PEZZUTO, A., GASPA-ROTTO, G. and CARTIERI, A.: Immunobiology of pediatric intracranial tumours. Acta Neurochir. 50 (1979), 49—54

11. GUTIN, P. and WILSON, C. B.: Modern concept in brain tumours therapy. Summary of symposium. Surg. Neurol. 8 (1977), 392, 396

12. HASKELL, C. M.: Immunologic aspects of cancer chemotherapy. Ann. Rev. Pharmacol. Toxicol. 17 (1977), 179—195

13. HERSH, E. M. and OPPENHEIM, J. J.: Inhibition of in vitro lymphocyte transformation during chemotherapy in man. Cancer Res. 27 (1967), 98—105

14. KAPLAN, M. E. and CLARK, C.: An improved rosetting assay for detection of human T-lymphocytes. J. Immunol. Meth. 5 (1974), 131—135

15. MAHALEY, M. S., BROOKS, W. H., ROSZMAN, T. L., DANEL, D. B., DUDKA, L. and RICHARDSON, S.: Immunobiology of primary intracranial tumours. Part I: Studies of the cellular and humoral general immunocompetence of brain tumours patients. J. Neurosurg. 46 (1977), 467—476

16. MAHALEY, M. S., STEINBOK, P., ARONIN, P., DUDKA, L. and ZINN, D.: Immunobiology of primary intracranial tumours. Part IV: Levamisole as an immune stimulant in patients and in the ASV glioma model. J. Neurosurg. *54* (1980), 220—227

17. MARKOE, A. H.: The effects of combined radiation therapy and chemotherapy on immune responses. Prog. Exp. Tumour Res. *25* (1980), 219—228

18. RABEN, M., WALACH, N., GALILI, U. and SLESINGER, M.: The effect of radiation therapy on lymphocyte subpopulation in cancer patients. Cancer *37* (1976), 1417—1421

19. ROSZMAN, T. L. and BROOKS, W. H.: Immunobiology of primary intracranial tumours. Part III: demonstration of a qualitative lymphocyte abnormality in patients with brain tumours. Clin. Exp. Immunol. *39* (1980), 395—402

20. RUSSEL, D. S. and RUBINSTEIN, L. J. (1977): Pathology of the Nervous System, London, Edward Arnold, p. 448

21. SLATER, J. M., NGO, E. and LAN, B. H. S. (1976): Effect of therapeutic irradiation on the immune response. Am. J. Roentgenol. *126* (1976), 313—320

22. STEWART, C. C. and PEREZ, C. A.: Effect of irradiation on immune responses. Radiology *118* (1976), 201—210

23. STJERNSWARD, J., JONTAL, M. and VANKY, F.: Lymphopenia and change in distribution of human B and T lymphocytes in peripheral blood induced by irradiation for mammary carcinoma. Lancet *II* (1972), 1352—1356

24. STRATTON, J. A., BYFIELD, P. E., BYFIELD, J. E. and SMALL, R. C.: Comparison of the acute effects of radiation therapy including or excluding the thymus on the lymphocyte subpopulation of cancer patients. J. Clin. Invest. *56* (1975), 88—97

25. TARPLEY, J. L., POTVIN, C and CHERETIEN, P. B.: Prolonged depression of cellular immunity in cured laryngopharyngeal cancer patients treated with radiation therapy. Cancer *35* (1975) 638—644

26. THOMAS, D. G. T., LANNINGAN, C. B. and BEHAN, P. O.: Impaired cell-mediated immunity in human brain tumours. Lancet *II* (1975), 1389—1390

27. WALKER, M. et al. (cooperative study): Evaluation of BCNU and/or radiotherapy in the treatment of anaplastic gliomas. J. Neurosurg. *49* (1978), 334—343

28. WAZA, W. M., PHILLIPS, T. L., WAZA, D. W., ANNAN, A. J. and SMITH, V.: Immunodepression following radiation therapy for carcinoma of the nasopharynx. Am. J. Roentgenol. *123* (1975) 482—485

29. ZHIALY, M. M., BRITTON, S., BROSMAN, S. and FAHEY, L. I.: Critical evaluation of lymphocyte function in urological-cancer patients. Cancer Res. *36* (1976), 132—137

Department Hematology and Oncology, Free University Berlin, Klinikum Charlottenburg, Berlin (West)

Control of Megacaryocyte Differentiation in Healthy and Leukemic Patients

B. M. Bombik, S. Serke and H. Gerhartz

Introduction

Among the differentiating cell systems of the bone marrow the megacaryopoiesis is least understood. While erythropoietic and granulocytic cell systems in tissue culture are well established, and even long term cultures are described by Dexter et al (1), megacaryocyte cultures in vitro were difficult to obtain. However, it would be desirable to understand better megacaryocyte formation and the factors and co-factors involved, since numerous hematological disorders including the leukemias are accompanied by thrombocytopenia.

In this report we compare in vitro results of megacaryocyte colony formation during different stages of leukemic patients with a control group of normal and healthy donors.

Materials and methods

The plasma clot technique described by Mac Leod et al (2) with the modifications given by Vain-chenker et al (3) was used. The final 1.0 ml Petri dish volume contained: 0.2 ml AB-serum, 0.1 ml bovine serum albumin, fraction V, 0.1 ml 1-asparagine, 0.3 ml α-medium, 0.1 ml bovine plasma, 0.1 ml cells ($= 5 \times 10^6$) and 0.1 ml erythropoietin ($= 6$ units/assay).

Human bone marrow was obtained by aspiration into a heparinized syringe from either healthy donors lacking any hematological disorder and then leukemic patients. The cells were diluted twice with α-medium, and were layered over ficoll-metrizoate (lymphoprep. 1.077 g/ml), and centrifuged 40 minutes at 400 g.

Thereafter, the buffy coat was washed three times in α-medium. After a trypan blue exclusion test, the cells from this mononuclear cell layer were incubated at a concentration of 6×10^6 cells at 37. 5°C in a 5% CO_2-atmosphere for 14 days.

The cell cultures were stained with dimethoxybenzidine and hematoxylin (Harris-Lillie). Cells with a polylobulated nucleus, perinuclear eosinophilia and over 30 μ in diameter were considered to be megacaryocytes. There was a clear morphological difference to macrophages.

Erythropoietin used in the culture system was a step III preparation from phenylhydrazine treated sheep (Connaught Lab., Canada).

Results

Under the conditions described, we obtained approximately 15 to 35 megacaryocytic colonies with an average number of 20 colonies from healthy donors (Fig. 3/I), the large spread presumably due to considerable variations of stem cells contained in the

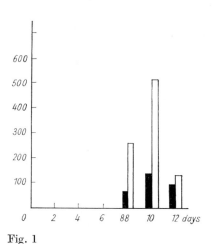

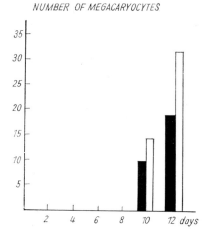

Fig. 1

Fig. 2

Fig. 1. Number of erythroid bursts with erythropoietin added at 0—24—48 hours, and epo added at 0—24—48—72—96 hours.

Fig. 2. Number of megacaryocytes, epo at 0—24—48 hours added to the test system epo added at 0—24—48—72—96 hours after initial incubation.

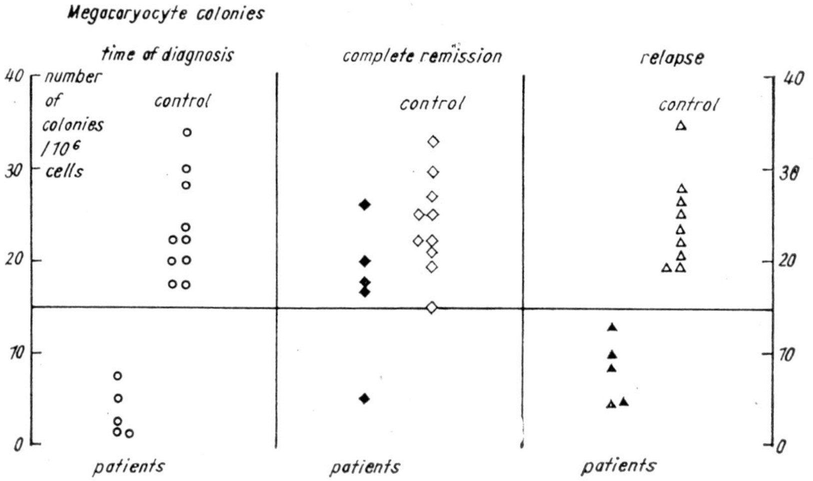

Megacaryocyte colonies

Fig. 3. Megacaryocyte colony formation under various conditions.

mononuclear cell layer, and also depending upon experimental conditions. Figure 1 demonstrates the number of erythroid bursts with erythropoietin (epo) added at different times.

Figure 2 however, shows the formation of megacaryocytes as a function of epo added to the tissue culture system at subsequent hours over a prolonged period of time. In all the following experiments we used the epo addition within a 24 hours intervall as Figure 2 demonstrates.

Compared to healthy donors, on the other hand, the bone marrow from five patients with acute leukemias (ALL and ANLL) showed little megacaryocytic colony formation.

After reaching clinically a complete remission, the ability of forming megacaryocyte colonies is with all but one exception restored, as Figure 3/II demonstrates. We routinely checked the bone marrow every 6 to 8 weeks for its ability to form megacaryocyte colonies.

Gradually the number of megacaryocyte colonies declined, while the hematological parameters, e. g. hemoglobin content, the number of leucocytes and platelets were still normal, and also the cell morphology including cytochemistry did not show any signs of a relapse.

Eventually, the megacaryocyte formation ceased. At that time the relapse was also hematologically full established (Fig. 3/III).

Discussion

Thrombocytopenia is a frequent symptom of a variety of systemic and hematological disorders, including the leukemias. Its pathophysiology is not well understood. Infiltration of the bone marrow by tumour cells may account as well as biochemically active molecules, e. g. membrane bound proteolytic enzymes, and a defective stem cell differentiation.

Our in vitro system yields some valuable information with respect to megacaryopoiesis. At the time of diagnosis there is little megacaryocyte colony formation in vitro, hence the argument of tumour cell infiltration and thus reducing formation of megacaryocytes does not hold. We consider the possibility that the presence of certain molecules inhibits the megacaryocyte formation, and possible malfunction of stem cell differentiation. Experiments are under way to investigate further this question.

With regard to the clinical situation, however, we are able to follow closely the course of the disease. While at the time of clinical remission the megacaryocyte formation returns to normal, a considerable time before hematological parameters turn away, the in vitro megacaryocyte formation declines, thus hinting the imminent relapse of the disease. Therefore, this test is not only of prognostic value, but might bear also therapeutic consequences, e. g. when to start a new round of induction therapy and also questions the value of maintenance therapy.

References

1. DEXTER, T. M. and TESTA, N. G. (1976) in: Methods in Cell Biology, Vol. XIV, P. 387, eds. Prescott, D. M., London, New York, Academic Press
2. MAC LEOD, D. L., et al.: Blood *44* (1974), 517
3. VAINCHENKER, W. et al.: Blood Cells, Vol. 5, No. 1 (1979), 25

[1] Department of Haematology and Oncology, Klinikum Charlottenburg, Free University, Berlin, and

[2] Institute of Pharmacy, Free University, Berlin (West)

Cytotoxic T Lymphocytes: Various Effects on Human Myeloma Cells

G. Hagner[1], B. M. Bombik[1], W.-D. Voigt[2] and H. Gerhartz[1]

It is generally accepted that neoplastic transformation may induce modifications of the plasma membrane. These include altered expression of normal cell surface antigens or the expression of novel antigens. From studies in animal tumours there is increasing evidence that these novel ("tumour-associated") antigens may be associated with gene products of the major histocompatibility complex (MHC) (1, 2) and thus be recognized by cytotoxic T cells (CTL) (3). In man, numerous attempts have been made to generate in vitro CTL which should be capable of lysing autologous transformed cells. In acute leukaemias, e. g., coculture experiments between remission lymphocytes and autologous or allogeneic blast cells did not prove to be successful. Despite stimulation in mixed lymphocyte-tumour cultures (4), cytotoxic responses against the autologous leukaemia cells were absent in most cases (5, 6). One new and promising approach to this problem came from Bach et al (7). They postulated that allogeneic sensitization of lymphocytes to a pool of irradiated normal cells from 20 unrelated donors might produce CTL which destroy autologous virus transformed or neoplastic cells. This was concluded from observations in man, where pool-sensitized cells lysed virtually any cell carrying foreign histocompatibility antigens (8) and from the well established fact that many experimental tumours express antigens cross-reacting with normal allogeneic histocompatibility antigens (9, 10, 11). The cited authors demonstrated the efficacy of this concept in several Epstein-Barr virus transformed lymphoblastoid cell lines (12) and in 2 cases of hairy cell leukemia (13). In a previous study, we had observed specific antileukaemic cytotoxicity of various degrees in 2 patients with acute promyelocytic leukaemia mediated by the autologous pool-primed lymphocytes (G. Hagner and B. M. Bombik, in preparation). It was obviously correlated to the state of the disease, as leukaemic relapses occurred a short period after disappearance of cytotoxicity.

It was the aim of this study, to evaluate the effect of pool-primed cells on the malignant plasma cells in patients with multiple myeloma of light-chain types IgG_{Kappa} (IgG_K) and IgG_{Lambda} (IgG_L). CTL were also induced by "specifically" sensitizing the patients' peripheral lymphocytes to the autologous or to several allogeneic myeloma cells in various combinations. The cytotoxicity was tested in a standard ^{51}Cr release assay. As targets we used the tumour cells and, as a control, the peripheral lymphocytes of these patients. In parallel experiments, we pretreated the stimulating cells or the target cells for a short time with neuraminidase and determined its influence on the degree of cytotoxicity.

Our results strongly suggest that there exist antigenic differences between a patient's lymphocytes and his myeloma plasma cells. In addition, there is evidence that on IgG_K and IgG_L myeloma cells distinct tumour-associated antigens are expressed.

426

Materials and methods

We obtained bone marrow samples from the iliac crests of 9 unrelated patients with multiple myeloma either at the time of diagnosis or at least 4 weeks after completion of a course of chemotherapy. By means of immunoelectrophoresis we diagnosed IgG_K myeloma in 5 patients and IgG_L myeloma in 4 patients. There were no significant differences between the two groups with respect to age or haematological parameters. Most of the patients had advanced disease and all had extensive marrow infiltration of more than 40% plasma cells. The bone marrow was separated by density gradient centrifugation (14). The resulting cell suspensions consisted of more than 80% myeloma cells. These cells were cryopreserved and stored in liquid nitrogen. Mixed cultures were set up in 10 ml volumes of supplemented medium between the patients' ficoll-hypaque separated lymphocytes and equal numbers (6×10^6) of stimulating cells. The latter included lymphocytes from the myeloma patients, myeloma plasma cells or pooled normal lymphocytes. The stimulating cells had been thawed and ^{60}Co irradiated (25 Gy) immediately prior to use. Lymphocytes pooled from 20 unrelated donors were obtained from Biotest Diagnostics. We used an identically composed supplemented medium (RPMI 1640/20 mM Hepes (Seromed), 25% inactivated human serum (Serva), 100 U/ml penicillin , 100 µg/ml streptomycin, 4 mM L-glutamine) for mixed cultures, the ^{51}Cr release assay and all washing procedures. In some experiments were pretreated the stimulating cells and/or the target cells with VC-Neuraminidase (Behring-Werke). This was done by incubation 10^7 cells with 40 U of the enzyme for 1 hr at 37 °C. Subsequently they were washed three times. The mixed cell cultures were incubated at 37 °C for 7 days in a humidified 5% CO_2 atmosphere and fed on day 2, 4 and 6. The primed cells were recovered and then dispensed in various dilutions into the wells of microtitration plates (Linbro). Cryopreserved cells which served as targets were thawed 24 hours before testing and cultured in supplemented medium. 5×10^6 to 1×10^7 cells were labeled with 200 to 400 µCi ^{51}Cr (Na_2 $^{51}CrO_4$; Amersham) for one hr at 37 °C in a total volume of 1 ml. After three washings and appropriate dilution, the labeled target cells were added to the effector cells, resulting in ratios of effector (E) to target cells (T) varying from 1:1 to 20:1. After short centrifugation (100 g; 4 min) the microtrays were incubated for 6 hours at 37 °C. The supernatants were harvested by means of a disposable collection system (Titertek Skatron). The degree of cytolysis was expressed as % specific ^{51}Cr release (% SR), according to the formula:

$$\% \text{ SR} = \frac{\text{experimental release} - \text{spontaneous release}}{\text{maximum release} - \text{spontaneous release}}.$$

Following this procedure the maximal ^{51}Cr release from 1×10^4 cells ranged between 800 and 3,800 cpm and the spontaneous release never exceeded 25%.

Results

Sensitization of the patients' lymphocytes to the *autologous* myeloma cells elicited only low levels of cytotoxicity against the autologous tumour cells. The mean value of specific ^{51}Cr release, calculated from 6 different patients was $6.5 \pm 7.1\%$ (E:T = 10:1), and the maximum values did not exceed 12%. IgG_K and IgG_L cells did not significantly differ with respect to their stimulating capacity. Both mediated only irrelevant cross-killing of allogeneic myeloma cells.

When we cultured the patients' lymphocytes together with *allogeneic* myeloma cells of type IgG_K, they exhibited in no case cytotoxicity against the stimulating cells and they did not kill the autologous myeloma cells, neither of type IgG_K nor of type IgG_L. Lysis of third-party myeloma cells could not be demonstrated. Neuraminidase pretreatment of the stimulating IgG_K cells slightly enhanced the killing potential of the responding cells. Similar levels of cytotoxicity were observed after priming with

427

allogeneic lymphocytes from the IgG$_K$ myeloma patients. In contrast, sensitization to allogeneic myeloma cells of type IgG$_L$ was more effective. It gave, in most cases, rise to CTL capable of destroying tumour cells of the same origin as the stimulating cells. In addition, these primed cells were highly cytotoxic for the autologous myeloma cells both of type IgG$_L$ and IgG$_K$, and they extensively killed third-party myeloma cells of the two light-chain types. In two patients we tested this unique property of IgG$_L$ myeloma cells to induce cross-reacting cytotoxic responses on several occasions before or during chemotherapy. The results were well reproducible and chemotherapy did not significantly affect the cytolytic activity of the effector cells. Thus, it is excluded that the immunological status of the responder plays a major role in this phenomenon. MLC and CML tests between the patiens' lymphocytes were used as controls. They were positive in all combinations, without striking differences. Thus, we ruled out the possibility of shared histocompatibility antigens between certain patients.

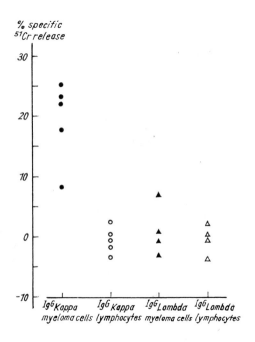

Fig. 1 presents data from our pool-sensitization experiments. Pool-sensitized cells specifically lysed the autologous tumour cells in 4 of 5 patients with IgG$_K$ myeloma. The specific ^{51}Cr release ranged between 17.7 ± 1.5% and 25.4 ± 3.2%. These data are based on E:T ratios of 10:1 There was no concomitant killing of the autologous lymphocytes. In IgG$_L$ myeloma, cytotoxicity against the autologous tumour cells could not be detected in 3 of 4 cases, and was low (6.3 ± 1.2%) in one case. The killing rate of IgG$_L$ myeloma cells increased, when they were pretreated with neuraminidase, but never reached the levels observed in IgG$_K$ cells. The patients' pool-sensitized cells destroyed, as expected, allogeneic myeloma plasma cells, but, in general, the degree of cytolysis was not high (8.9 ± 5.3%). Here again, killing of IgG$_K$ myeloma cells was more pronounced than that of IgG$_L$ cells. Responder lymphocytes from IgG$_K$ and IgG$_L$ myeloma patients gave comparable results. As a rule, the allogeneic

428

Table 1.

Generation of cytotoxic T lymphocytes in patients with IgG$_{Kappa}$ and IgG$_{Lambda}$ myeloma

Mixed cultures Cytotoxicity/^{51}Cr labelled target cells

	K$_O$	K$_N$	(K)	K$_{All/O}$	K$_{All/N}$	(K)$_{All}$	L$_{All/O}$	L$_{All/N}$	(L)$_{All}$
(K) — pool	++	++(+)	—	+	+(+)	++(+)	(+)	+	++(+)
(K) — K$_{All/O}$	—	—	—	—	—	—	—	—	—
(K) — K$_{All/N}$	(+)	(+)	—	(+)	ND	ND	—	—	—
(K) — (K)$_{All}$	(+)	(+)	—	(+)	+	+++	ND	ND	ND
(K) — L$_{All/O}$	++	++(+)	—	+(+)	++	—	++	++(+)	(+)
(K) — (L)$_{All}$	—	ND	—	—	ND	ND	ND	ND	+++

	L$_O$	L$_N$	(L)	L$_{All/O}$	L$_{All/N}$	(L)$_{All}$	K$_{All/O}$	K$_{All/N}$	(K)$_{All}$
(L) — pool	—	(+)	—	(+)	+	++(+)	+	+(+)	++(+)
(L) — L$_{All/O}$	+(+)	++	—	+(+)	++	ND	+(+)	+(+)	—
(L) — (L)$_{All}$	—	—	—	ND	ND	+++	ND	ND	ND
(L) — K$_{All/O}$	—	—	—	—	—	—	—	—	(+)
(L) — (K)$_{All}$	—	—	—	ND	ND	ND	(+)	+	+++

(L), (K), L$_O$, K$_O$, L$_N$, K$_N$ = autologous lymphocytes (L), (K); untreated myeloma cells L$_O$, K$_O$, and neuraminidase treated myeloma cells L$_N$, K$_N$ in patients with IgG$_{Lambda}$ (L) or IgG$_{Kappa}$ (K) myeloma. (L)$_{All}$, (K)$_{All}$, L$_{All/O}$, K$_{All/O}$, L$_{All/N}$, K$_{All/N}$ = allogeneic lymphocytes and myeloma cells of IgG$_L$ or IgG$_K$ myeloma patients.
— to +++ = mean values (%) of specific ^{51}Cr release at E:T ratios of 10:1, based on at least 3 experiments, where — = 0 to 5 ,(+) = 5 to 10, + = 10 to 15, +(+) = 15 to 20, ++ = 20 to 25, ++(+) = 25 to 30, +++ = more than 30

myeloma cells were less susceptible to lysis than the corresponding lymphocytes. These differences were diminished, particularly in IgG$_K$, after treatment of the myeloma cells with neuraminidase. Table 1 gives a general view of our data.

Discussion

Our study has shown that cytotoxic responses against human myeloma cells can be produced in various ways. These responses are mediated by cells, since lytic activity was not found in supernatants of mixed cultures. Pool-sensitized cells as well as lymphocytes sensitized to allogeneic myeloma cells may become cytotoxic for autologous and allogeneic myeloma plasma cells. In contrast to others (14), we did not find significant amounts of cytotoxicity after stimulation with autologous myeloma cells, but this may be due to different testing systems. The cytolysis appears to be confined to T cells. It was completely abolished, when the effector cell population was depleted of SRBC rosette forming cells (data not shown). There is evidence that MHC antigen linked structures are involved in the mechanism of lysis, since neuraminidase, which is known to react with MHC antigens, enhanced the degree of lysis in many combinations.

Our data suggest that there exist antigenic differences between IgG$_K$ and IgG$_L$ cells with respect to their capacity of inducing CTL, when used as allogeneic stimulators in

MLC, and with respect to recognition and lysis by CTL, when used as targets in CML. IgG_L cells can induce allogeneic stimulation to lysis of both IgG_L and IgG_K cells. IgG_K cells are not effective as stimulators. This finding may be explained by an additional stimulating antigen expressed on IgG_L, but not on IgG_K cells, and by common cross-reacting target structures on IgG_K and IgG_L cells. An alternative explanation is the activation of T helper cells by allogeneic IgG_L cells, and of T suppressor cells by IgG_K cells. However, different immunoresponsiveness of the patients cannot be totally excluded. On the other hand, IgG_K cells are preferentially destroyed by autologous pool-sensitized lymphocytes. This suggests that IgG_K cells express antigenic determinants, which are not shared by the corresponding patients' lymphocytes, but cross-react with normal alloantigens present in the stimulating pool. These antigens may be absent or repressed on IgG_L cells. This observation is in accord with findings in murine myeloma tumours (15) and favours the hypothesis that some human myeloma antigens may be presented as inappropriately expressed normal alloantigens.

References

1. BOURGUIGNON, L. Y. W., HYMAN, R., TROWBRIDGE, I. and SINGER, S. J.: Proc. Natl. Acad. Sci. USA 75 (1978), 2406—2410
2. CALLAHAN, G. N., ALLISON, J. P., PELLEGRINO, M. A. and REISFELD, R. A.: J. Immunol. 122 (1979), 70—74
3. ZINKERNAGEL, R. M. and DOHERTY, P. C.: Adv. Immunolog. 27 (1979), 51—177
4. LEVENTHAL, B. G., HALTERMAN, R. H., ROSENBERG, E. B. and HEBERMAN, R. B.: Cancer Res. 32 (1972), 1820—1825
5. SONDEL, P. M., O'BRIEN, C., PORTER, L., SCHLOSSMAN, S. F. and CHESS, L.: J. Immunol. 117 (1976), 2197—2203
6. LEE, S. K. and OLIVER, R. T. D.: J. Exp. Med. 147 (1978), 912—922
7. BACH, M. L., BACH, F. H. and ZARLING, J. M.: Lancet I. (1978), 20—22
8. MARTINIS, J. and BACH, F. H.: Transplantation 25 (1978), 39—41
9. INVERNIZZI, G. and PARMIANI, G.: Nature 254 (1975), 713—714
10. WRATHMELL, A. B., GAUCI, C. L. and ALEXANDER, P.: Br. J. Cancer 33 (1976), 187—194
11. GARRIDO, F., SCHIRRMACHER, V. and FESTENSTEIN, H.: J. Immunogenet. 4 (1977), 15—27
12. ZARLING, J. M. and BACH, F. H.: J. Exp. Med. 147 (1978), 1334—1340
13. ZARLING, J. M., ROBINS, H. I., RAICH, P. C., BACH, F. H. and BACH, M. L.: Nature 274 (1978), 269—271
14. PAGLIERONI, T. and MACKENZIE, M. R.: Blood 54 (1979), 226—237
15. RUSSELL, J. H., GINNS, L. C., TERRES, G. and EISEN, H. N.: J. Immunol. 122 (1979), 912—919

Istituto di Farmacologia dell 'Università di Bologna, Italy

Analysis of AHH Inducibility Ratios and Distribution in Human Lymphocytes by TLC-Radioisotopic Assay

G. Cantelli Forti, G. Aicardi, N. M. Trieff, E. Speroni, T. Rossi and G. L. Biagi

Aryl hydrocarbon hydroxylase (AHH) is an inducible enzymatic complex of microsomal cytochrome P-448-dependent mixed function oxygenases (1), which metabolizes polycyclic aromatic hydrocarbons (PAHs), drugs, steroids, etc. (2). It is present in various mammalian tissues and organs (3) and in white blood cells (4—7), which are of particular interest for human investigation. This enzymatic complex converts PAHs into various more polar metabolites, some of which have carcinogenic activity (8).

The health-related significance of the AHH assay is that PAHs such as benzo(a)pyrene (BP) are ubiquitous in nature, and are present, for example, in tobacco smoke, in various foods, such as smoked and charcoal-broiled meats and fish from polluted waters, and particularly in urban air due to pollution from petrochemical factories and other combustion sources (9).

All PAHs undergo biotransformation by AHH into hydroxylated metabolites, including phenols, dihydrodiols, epoxides, hydroxymethyl derivatives and various quinones. Of the metabolites of BP, diols and diolepoxides are thought to bind readily to DNA and are considered to be the most carcinogenic of the metabolites (8).

Nevertheless, the relationship between AHH activity, or inducibility, in human lymphocytes and environmental cancer is not well established. A number of reports have documented the possible role of the AHH complex in provoking chemical carcinogenesis in man (5, 10—12); and various authors have indicated that AHH activity and the BP present in smoke are principal risk factors in the development of lung cancer, particularly bronchogenic carcinoma (10, 13—14).

Using a thin-layer chromatographic(TLC)-radioisotopic assay, which is capable of detecting and measuring several BP-metabolic fractions, we have examined the distribution of the AHH inducibility ratios in the lymphocytes of a normal population of 131 subjects, randomly selected, both smokers and non-smokers, males and females, and with positive and negative family histories of cancer. In particular, we examined the relationship between inducibility ratio (I/C), and three independent variables: sex (SX), smoking (SM) and familial cancer history (FCH). In addition, the various TLC regions were tested for mutagenicity, using the microbial test system of Ames et al (15).

Material and methods

Human lymphocytes obtained from normal volunteers were separated (16) and cultured by means of a sterile technique according to Gurtoo et al (17). Half of the cultures from each donor were induced by addition of 5 µl of a 5 mM acetone solution of 3-methylcholanthrene (3-MC); the remaining cultures were kept as control and received 5 µl solvent. The purification and preparation of the BP and ³H-BP mixture added as substrate to each lymphocyte culture have already been reported (18).

The enzymatic assay in an aqueous buffer was performed as described in the literature (17, 19), and the reaction was stopped with 4 ml acetone:hexane (1:3). However, instead of using fluorimetric determination, a TLC separation was carried out: The hexane phase was evaporated and the residue taken up in 100 µl pure benzene, and the mobile phase was spotted on silica-gel G precoated plates (Merck). After development, the TLC plate was inspected under ultra-violet light and the silica-gel G layer divided into five areas, including those of the BP substrate and of its metabolites.

The areas were scraped off by the Stripmix technique (20) and counted for the tritiated compounds or used for the Ames test. For the latter test, the areas were extracted with 10 ml pure benzene. After vortexing, the samples were filtered and the benzene removed under a gentle stream of nitrogen. The residue was dissolved in 400 µl dimethylsulfoxide (DMSO) and sterilized through a Millipore FH membrane filter; and 100 µl of this solution were used for the Ames test (15). In the assay, 200 units of β-glucuronidase and 10 units of sulfatase were added to the top agar of each dish. All operations were carried out under yellow light.

Results

Table 1 shows the frequency of occurrence of four metabolic fractions in the 131 individuals studies. The nature of the metabolites in these four TLC fractions has not been characterized; however, a comparison between our R_f values and those of SIMS (21) and BAIRD (22) provides some idea of their probable identity.

Table 1.

R_f values and frequencies of occurrence of the principal fractions of benzo(a)pyrene (BP) separated by thin-layer chromatography from 262 human uninduced and 3-methylcholanthrene-induced lymphocyte samples and detected under ultra-violet light (253.7 nm)

Fraction		Frequency (%)	R_f value	± SE	Confidence limits (P < 0.05)	Presumed metabolites (21, 22)
B	B_a	100	0.905	0.022	0.900 0.910	Benzo(a)pyrene
	B_b	58	0.832	0.002	0.828 0.837	Unidentified
M_1	M_{1a}	92	0.728	0.004	0.720 0.736	Unidentified (quinone ?)
	M_{1b}	58	0.673	0.002	0.668 0.678	Unidentified (quinone ?)
M_2	M_{2a}	45	0.532	0.009	0.528 0.536	6-OH-benzo(a)pyrene
	M_{2b}	82	0.370	0.003	0.365 0.367	Phenol: 5-OH-benzo(a)-pyrene (?)
H		52	0.248	0.002	0.245 0.252	3-OH-benzo(a)pyrene
F		100	0.073	0.00001	0.073 0.073	7,8-dihydro-7,8-dihydroxy-benzo(a)pyrene (?) and other dihydrodiols
BP standard		—	0.911	0.006	0.898 0.923	
3-OH-BP standard		—	0.246	0.002	0.242 0.251	

Table 2 gives a detailed characterization of the inducibility ratios of the study group of 131 individuals. Most were in the 40—50 year age bracket; 88% were men, 61% were smokers and 24% had a family history of cancer.

A multiple regression analysis was carried out. (The numerical codes for positive and negative smoking history, sex, positive and negative FCH are reported in footnotes a—c of Table 3.) The only significant equations, with their correlation coefficients (r), variance (r^2) and F values from multiple regression analysis, are given in Table 3. Thus, the I/C in the M_1-TLC fraction correlated significantly ($p = 0.05$) with FCH.

Table 2.
Mean inducibility ratios of the entire study population and of subsets

Groups	No.	Mean inducilibity ratios (1/C) $\times$ 100 $\pm$ SE by thin-layer chromatography metabolic fraction			
		M_1	M_2	H	F
Entire population	131	173.95 $\pm$ 12.07	122.45 $\pm$ 5.08	124.30 $\pm$ 3.09	115.67 $\pm$ 2.086
Males	115	178.65 $\pm$ 13.52	123.51 $\pm$ 5.73	121.49 $\pm$ 2.81	116.51 $\pm$ 2.30
Females	16	144.40 $\pm$ 20.48	116.52 $\pm$ 6.04	143.82 $\pm$ 14.24	110.46 $\pm$ 4.08
Smokers	80	168.88 $\pm$ 13.86	127.58 $\pm$ 7.95	129.30 $\pm$ 4.73	117.49 $\pm$ 2.78
Non-smokers	51	182.09 $\pm$ 22.24	114.40 $\pm$ 3.70	116.44 $\pm$ 2.50	112.82 $\pm$ 3.11
Negative FCH[a]	99	189.08 $\pm$ 15.58	125.10 $\pm$ 6.00	125.70 $\pm$ 3.92	113.32 $\pm$ 2.69
Positive FCH	32	124.98 $\pm$ 7.61	114.26 $\pm$ 9.39	119.96 $\pm$ 3.60	117.97 $\pm$ 3.00
Male smokers	70	174.04 $\pm$ 15.34	127.72 $\pm$ 9.01	124.90 $\pm$ 4.22	118.46 $\pm$ 3.04
Male non-smokers	45	185.83 $\pm$ 25.17	116.96 $\pm$ 4.21	116.2 $\pm$ 2.80	113.47 $\pm$ 3.48
Female smokers	10	138.90 $\pm$ 33.03	125.64 $\pm$ 8.35	159.16 $\pm$ 21.60	110.98 $\pm$ 6.57
Female non-smokers	6	154.10 $\pm$ 7.33	101.30 $\pm$ 2.91	118.25 $\pm$ 3.64	164.6 $\pm$ 1.88
Pos. FCH, smokers	20	121.93 $\pm$ 11.42	121.31 $\pm$ 14.58	120.44 $\pm$ 5.43	119.54 $\pm$ 4.62
Pos. FCH, non-smokers	12	130.07 $\pm$ 7.49	102.50 $\pm$ 5.54	119.15 $\pm$ 3.49	115.35 $\pm$ 2.31
Neg. FCH, smokers	60	183.05 $\pm$ 17.95	129.67 $\pm$ 9.47	132.26 $\pm$ 6.01	114.16 $\pm$ 3.60
Neg. FCH, non-smokers	39	198.10 $\pm$ 28.59	118.05 $\pm$ 4.39	115.61 $\pm$ 3.10	112.04 $\pm$ 4.01
Male smokers, pos. FCH	16	132.90 $\pm$ 12.16	123.75 $\pm$ 18.29	117.67 $\pm$ 6.59	117.69 $\pm$ 5.03
Male smokers, neg. FCH	54	188.27 $\pm$ 19.07	129.08 $\pm$ 10.44	127.04 $\pm$ 5.10	118.69 $\pm$ 3.66
Male non-smokers, pos. FCH	9	116.60 $\pm$ 3.49	100.73 $\pm$ 7.40	116.73 $\pm$ 4.40	115.87 $\pm$ 3.11
Male non-smokers, neg. FCH	36	203.13 $\pm$ 30.86	120.00 $\pm$ 4.62	116.07 $\pm$ 3.35	120.00 $\pm$ 4.62

[a] FCH, familial cancer history

The I/C in the H-TLC fraction correlated significantly with SM ($p = 0.05$), SX ($p = 0.05$) and with SM + SX ($p = 0.05$). The F test showed that equation (4), in which SM and SX are independent variables, is a significant improvement over equation (3), in which SX is the only independent variable in terms of explaining a higher fraction of the variance (r^2) of I/C.

With regard to equation (1), relating the I/C in fraction M_1 to FCH, the negative slope indicates that subjects with a positive FCH have a lower inducibility ratio than do those with a negative FCH with respect to the M_1 fraction.

Table 3.
Significant multiparameter regression equations of inducibility ratio (I/C) for various thin-layer chromatography fractions *versus* smoking history (SM)[a], sex (SX)[b] and familial cancer history (FCH)[c]

Fraction	Regression equation	Eq. No.	n	r	F
M_1	I/C = −6.684 FCH + 268.539	(1)	131	0.195	5.116*
H	I/C = −1.286 SM + 142.169	(2)	131	0.179	4.228*
	I/C = 2.295 SX + 96.249	(3)	131	0.214	6.156*
	I/C = −1.270 SM + 2.274 SX + 114.142	(4)	131	0.276	4.284*[d]
	I/C = −1.328 SM + 2.514 SX − 0.884 FCH + 124.384	(5)	131	0.295	1.449[e]

[a] Smoker = 10, non-smoker = 20
[b] Male = 11, female = 21
[c] Positive FCH = 22, negative FCH = 12
[d] $F_{2,127}$ obtained by comparison with equation (3). The F test showed that equation (4) is a significant improvement over equation (3) in terms of increasing r.
[e] $F_{3,127}$ obtained by comparison with equation (4). The F test showed that equation (5) is not a significant improvement over equation (4) in terms of increasing r.
* Significant at p = 0.05

Table 4.
Mutagenic activities of benzo(a)pyrene thin-layer chromatographic fractions as determined in the AMES test

Fraction	Salmonella typhimurium TA 100		Salmonella typhimurium TA 98	
	his* revertants	Revertants spontaneous	his* revertants	Revertants spontaneous
B	268	1.7	62	1.4
M_1	241	1.5	115	2.6
M_2	567	3.5	282	6.4
H	1202	7.4	621	14.1
F	1568	9.7	674	15.3
his spontaneous revertants	162	—	44	—

Equation (2), relating I/C to SM in the H fraction, also has a negative slope, indicating that SM decreases when I/C increases: Thus, a smoker should have a higher inducibility ratio in the H fraction than a non-smoker, which is indeed the case. Equation (3), relating I/C to SX in the H fraction, suggests that, as the number of females increases, the I/C for the H fraction also increases. Equation (4) predicts that with decreasing SM and increasing number of females there will be an increase in the inducibility ratio in the H-TLC fraction. Hence, it is predicted that the subset with the highest I/C in the H-TLC fraction is smoking women. When I/C was regressed against

434

SM, SX and FCH, there was no increase in the significance of the regression (equation 5).

In order to determine the mutagenicity of the metabolites, TLC fractions of pooled, induced and uninduced lymphocyte cultures incubated with BP were tested by means of the Ames test. The results obtained with *Salmonella typhimurium* strains TA98 and TA100 are reported in Table 4. Fractions F, H and M_2, with relative ratios of 15.3, 14.1 and 6.4 in TA98 strain and 9.7, 7.9 and 3.5 in TA100 strain, were the most mutagenic.

Discussion and conclusions

Under our experimental conditions, we can conclude that in terms of potential risk of individuals exposed to BP and other PAHs, the correlation between inducibility ratio (I/C) and the variables SX and SM in the H-TLC fraction is more highly significant than that between I/C and FCH in the M_1 fraction. The F fraction, to which particular attention must be given, showed no significiant increase in I/C ratio but was the most mutagenic in the AMES test. Various workers have observed that one step in the transformation of PAH precarcinogens to ultimate carcinogens involves the oxidation of a dihydrodiol intermediate to a dihydrodiol epoxide (23). Hence, the presence of closely related compounds or derivatives, such as epoxides, in the F- or H-TLC fraction, may account for the mutagenicity and/or carcinogenicity of BP.

There have been reports that AHH inducibility is subject to seasonal variation (24) and that there is a slight increase in women who use oral contraceptives (25). The present study is in line with a limited number of investigations relating cigarette smoking and sex to AHH inducibility.

The higher AHH inducibility in the H-TLC fraction of smokers is compatible with the findings of JETT et al (26) that cigarette smokers have a higher level of metabolism of BP than do non-smokers. In our study, the rather small (n = 16) population of women showed a higher AHH inducibility in the H-TLC fraction than men, primarily in the smoking population. Multiparameter regression analysis showed a significant correlation (p = 0.05) between inducibility ratio in the H fraction and SX and SM (Table 3). While the sample is small, female smokers (n = 10) appeared to be at greatest risk, in that they had a higher AHH inducibility than male smokers. This is of special concern in view of the fact that women are showing a rapid increase in the rate of lung cancer (27).

It is particularly interesting that the correlation between inducibility ratio and SX and SM is seen in the H-TLC fraction, since substantial bacterial mutagenicity can be demonstrated in that fraction.

Acknowledgement

We are grateful to AVIS, Blood Donors of Bologna, for their kind co-operation; to the Fulbright Commission for Educational and Cultural Exchange between Italy and the United States; and to the CNR — Italian National Commitee for Research — for their generous support (of N. M. TRIEFF).

References

1. GORTOO, H. L., PARKER, N., PAIGEN, B., HAVENS, M. B., MINOWADA, J. and FREEDMAN, H. J.: Induction, inhibition and some enzymological properties of aryl hydrocarbon hydroxylase in fresh mitogen-activated human lymphocytes. Cancer Res. *39* (1979), 4620

2. CONNEY, A. H.: Pharmacological implications of microsomal enzyme induction. Pharmacol. Rev. *19* (1967), 317

3. NEBERT, D. W. and GELBOIN, H. V.: The in vivo and in vitro induction of aryl hydrocarbon hydroxylase in mammalian cells of different species, tissues, strains, and development and hormonal states. Arch. Biochem. Biophys. *134* (1969), 76

4. BUSBEE, D. L., SHAW, C. R. and CANTRELL, E. T.: AHH induction in human leukocytes. Science *178* (1972), 315

5. KELLERMANN, G., LUYTEN-KELLERMANN, M. and SHAW, C. R.: Genetic variation of AHH in human lymphocytes. Am. J. Human Genet. *25* (1973), 327

6. CANTRELL, E., ABREU, M. and BUSBEE, D. L.: A simple assay of aryl hydrocarbon hydroxylase in cultured human lymphocytes. Biochem. Biophys. Res. Commun. *70* (1976), 474

7 BAST, Jr., R. C., OKUDA, T., PLOTKIN, E., TARONE, R., RAPP, H. J. and GELBOIN, H. V.: Development of an assay for aryl hydrocarbon (benzo(a)pyrene) hydroxylase in human peripheral blood monocytes. Cancer Res. *36* (1976), 1967

8. YANG, S. K., ROLLER, P. P. and GELBOIN, H. V. (1978): Benzo(a)pyrene metabolism: mechanism in the formation of epoxides, phenols, dihydrodiols, and the 7,8-diol-9,10-epoxides. In: JONES, P. W. & FEUDENTHAL, R. I., eds., Carcinogenesis, Vol. 3, Polynuclear aromatic hydrocarbons, New York, Raven Press, p. 285

9. ANDELMAN, J. B. and SUESS, N. J.: Polynuclear aromatic hydrocarbons in the water environment. Bull. WHO *43* (1970), 479

10. KELLERMANN, G., SHAW, C. R. and LUYTEN-KELLERMANN, M.: Aryl hydrocarbon hydroxylase inducibility and bronchogenic carcinoma. New Engl. J. Med. *289* (1973), 934

11. BRANDENBURG, J. H. and KELLERMANN, G.: Aryl hydrocarbon hydroxylase inducibility in laryngeal carcinoma. Arch. Otolaryngol. *104* (1978), 151

12. FRAUMENI, J. F., Jr.: Respiratory carcinogenesis: an epidemiological appraisal. J. Natl. Cancer Inst. *55* (1975), 1039

13. TOMIGANS, R., POTT, F. and DEHNEN, W.: Polycyclic aromatic hydrocarbons in human bronchial carcinoma. Cancer Lett. *1* (1976), 189

14. WARD, E., PAIGEN, B., STEENLAND, K., VINCENT, R., MINOWADA, J., GURTOO, H. L., SARTORI, P. and HAVENS, M. B.: Aryl hydrocarbon hydroxylase in persons with lung or laryngeal cancer. Int. J. Cancer *22* (1978), 348

15. AMES, B. N., DURSTON, W. E., YAMASAKI, E. and LEE, F. D.: Carcinogens are mutagens: a simple test system combining liver homogenates for activation and bacteria for detection. Proc. Natl. Acad. Sci. USA *70* (1973), 2281

16. GOLDROSEN, M. H., GANNON, P. J., LUTZ, M. and HOLYOKE, E. D.: Isolation of human peripheral blood lymphocytes: modification of a double discontinuous density gradient of ficoll hypaque. J. Immunol. Meth. *14* (1977), 15

17. GURTOO, H. L., BEJBA, J. and MINOWADA, J. (1975): Properties, inducibility and an improved method on analysis of aryl hydrocarbon hydroxylase in cultured human lymphocytes. Cancer Res. *35* (1975), 1235

18. TRIEFF, N. M., CANTELLI FORTI, G., SMART, V. B., KEMPEN, R. R. and KILIAN, D. J.: Appraisal of fluorimetric assay of aryl hydrocarbon hydroxylase in cultured human lymphocytes. Br. J. Cancer *38* (1978), 335

19. FREEDMAN, H. J., PARKER, N. B., MARINELLI, A. J., GURTOO, H. L. and MINOWADA, J.: Induction, inhibition and biological properties of aryl-hydrocarbon hydroxylase in a stable human B-lymphocyte cell line, RPMI-1788. Cancer Res. *39* (1979), 4612

20. CANTELLI FORTI, G., TRIEFF, N. M., RAMANUJAM, V. M. S. and KILIAN, D. J.: Spray technique for applying Stripmix (cellulose acetate) to TLC plates for tritiated organic compounds. Anal. Biochem. *80* (1977), 319

21. SIMS, P.: The metabolism of benzo(a)pyrene by rat liver homogenates. Biochem. Pharmacol. *16* (1967), 613

22. BAIRD, W. M., DIAMOND, L., BORUN, T. W. and SHULMAN, S.: Analysis of metabolism of carcinogenic polycyclic hydrocarbons by position-sensing proportional counting of thin-layer chromatograms. Anal. Biochem. *99* (1979), 165

436

23. BERGER, G. D., SMITH, I. A., SEYBOLD, P. G. and SERVE, M. P.: Correlation of an electronic reactivity index with carcinogenicity in polycyclic aromatic hydrocarbons. Tetrahedron Lett. *3* (1978), 231

24. RICHTER, A., KADAR, D., LISZKA-HAGMAJER, E. and KALOW, V.: Seasonal variation of aryl hydrocarbon hydroxylase inducibility in human lymphocytes in culture. Res. Commun. Chem. Pathol. Pharm. *19* (1978), 453

25. NASH, D. R. and STEINGRUBE, V. N.: Induction of arylhydrocarbon hydroxylase by lymphocytes from women taking oral contraceptives. Contraception *20* (1970), 297

26. JETT, J. R., STOBO, J. D. and MOSES, H. L.: Aryl hydrocarbon hydroxylase activity in subpopulations of peripheral blood mononuclear cells. Cancer Res. *38* (1978), 1979

27. ACS: Cancer statistics. Cancer J. Clin. *30* (1980), 23

Institute of Toxicology and Chemotherapy
German Cancer Research Center, Heidelberg, FRG

Antitumour Actitivy of New Nitrosoureas on Yoshida Sarcoma Ascites Cells In Vivo

M. Habs, H. Habs, G. Eisenbrand and D. Schmähl

Introduction

The chemotherapeutic response of tumours to a large number of nitrosoureas has been investigated in different experimental models. BCNU (1,3-bis(2-chloroethyl)-1-nitrosourea), CCNU (1-(2-chloroethyl)-3-cyclohexyl-1-nitrosourea), and MeCCNU (1-(2-chloroethyl)-3-(4-methylcyclohexyl)-1-nitrosourea) are established drugs in clinical use. MeCCNU is considered the nitrosourea of first choice for gastrointestinal tumours. The first part of this report is concerned with the effect of newly synthesized nitrosoureas compared with these established drugs on Yoshida sarcoma ascites cells implanted into the wall of the descending colon of rats. The model used seems to be suited to identify nitrosoureas which are capable to reach the rat colon in a therapeutically sufficient amount. It is used for prescreening, and only active compounds will then be tested in more sophisticated and probably more reliable animal tumour models, such as, for instance, autochthonous colon cancers. The second part of our presentation describes the effect of pretreatment with disulfiram on the acute toxicity and antitumour activity of 1-(2-hydroxyethyl)-3-(2-chloroethyl)-3-nitrosourea (HECNU).

Colon tumour studies

Animals and tumour induction

A total of 1023 male Sprague-Dawley rats were used in a series of eight experiments. Yoshida sarcoma in ascites form was maintained in the same strain of rat by serial i. p. injection of 0.5 ml ascites fluid. 3×10^6 cells were injected into the colon wall as previously described. In these earlier studies cell numbers of $\geq 1.5 \times 10^6$ were shown to result in 100% tumour takes. The chemotherapeutic treatment was carried out on the 8th day after implantation of the tumour cells.

Chemicals

BCNU and MeCCNU were supplied by the Drug Development Branch, Division of Cancer Treatment, National Cancer Institute, Bethesda, MD, U.S.A. Cyclophosphamide was obtained from Asta-Werke, Bielefeld, (F.R.G.) The other nitrosoureas were synthesized according to published methods. Cremophor EL as obtained from Badische Anilin- and Soda-Farbik, AG Ludwigshafen (F.R.G.). Water-insoluble compounds were dissolved in Cremophor EL/ethanol/physiologic saline (20:20:60 vol. %). Water-soluble substances were dissolved in physiologic saline.

Table 1 lists the structures, chemical names, and abbreviations of all compounds tested. Table 2 gives the experimental design of the eight individual experiments.

All test compounds were administered i. p. The nitrosoureas were applied at approximately equitoxic doses corresponding to about 80% of the acute LD_{50} values observed in healthy rats of the same strain over a 28-day observation period.

Investigation of therapeutic activity

Each experiment involved an untreated control group and a varying number of treated groups. Individual survival times were counted asd ays after tumour inoculation. At the time of death a record of whether an animal was tumour-free or not was made. All animals alive on day 120 after tumour inoculation were killed. Animals that according to macroscopic examination had no tumour at the end of the experiment were regarded as cured. Since in a number of control rats, too, no tumours were seen after

Table 1.
Compounds tested

Structure[a]	Chemical name	Abbreviation used
	Cyclophosphamide = 2-bis-(β-chloroethyl)-amino-oxo-2-oxa-2-λ^5-phospha-3-aza-cyclohexane	CP
Cl—CH$_2$—CH$_2$—CNU	1.3-bis-(2-chloroethyl)-1-nitrosourea	BCNU
CH$_3$—◯—CNU	1-(2-chloroethyl)-3-(4-methyl-cyclohexyl)-1-nitrosourea	MeCCNU
	2-[3-(2-chloroethyl)-3-nitroso-ureido]-D-glucopyranose	Chlorozotocin
OH—CH$_2$—CH$_2$—CNU	1-(2-hydroxyethyl)-3-(2-chloroethyl)-3-nitrosourea	Hydroxyethyl-CNU
CH$_3$—SO$_2$—O—CH$_2$—CH$_2$—CNU	2-[3-(2-chloroethyl)-3-nitroso-ureido]-ethylmethanesulfonate	Hydroxyethyl-CNU-MS
H$_2$N—C(=O)—CH$_2$—CNU	1-(2-chloroethyl)-1-nitroso-3-(methylenecarboxamido)-urea	Acetamido-CNU
◯(N)—CH$_2$—CNU·HCl	[1-(2-chloroethyl)-1-nitroso-3-(methylene-3-pyridilium)-ureido]-chloride	Picolyl-3-CNU · HCl
CNU—CH(COOH)—CH$_3$	1-(2-chloroethyl)-1-nitroso-3-(1-carboxyethyl)-urea	α-alanine-CNU
CNU—N◯O	1-(2-chloroethyl)-1-nitroso-3-(4-morpholino)-urea	Morpholino-CNU

Structure	Name	Abbreviation
CNU—N (2,6-dimethylmorpholino, CH₃, O, CH₃)	4-[1-(2-chloroethyl)-1-nitroso]-3-[4-(2,6-dimethylmorpholino)]-urea	Dimethylmorpholino-CNU
CNU—N (piperidino)	1-(2-chloroethyl)-1-nitroso-3-(1-piperidino)-urea	Piperidino-CNU
CNU—(CH₂)₂—CNU	1,1'-ethylene-bis-3-(2-chloroethyl)-3-nitrosourea	BCNU-ethane
CNU—(CH₂)₄—CNU	1,1'-tetramethylene-bis-3-(2-chloroethyl)-3-nitrosourea	BCNU-butane
CNU— (methylenedioxybenzyl, O—CH₂, O)	1-(2-chloroethyl)-1-nitroso-3-(3,4-methylenedioxybenzyl)-urea	Methylenedioxybenzyl-CNU
CNU—CH₂— (pyridyl, N)	1-(2-chloroethyl)-1-nitroso-3-(methylene-3-pyridyl)-urea	Picolyl-3-CNU

[a] $CNU = NHCON(NO)CH_2CH_2Cl$

120 days, the differences in cures between controls and treated animals rather than absolute numbers are reported. Differences in survival were evaluated statistically by individual comparisons between treated rats and controls using a non-parametric log-rank test. Numerical evaluation was performed using a computerized system. The results of the present chemotherapy experiments are summarized in Table 3.

Discussion

The tumour model used has been discussed previously (HABS, 1981).

Established clinical N-nitrosoureas

The experiments in which BCNU, MeCCNU, and chlorozotocin were administered at a high single dose confirmed that tumour-bearing animals are less resistant to the toxicity of nitrosoureas than healthy animals. Of the three clinically used nitrosoureas, the best results were obtained with chlorozotocin, its most effective dose being 17 mg per kg.

Newly developed N-nitrosoureas

Of the water-soluble test compounds, hydroxyethyl-CNU, picolyl-3-CNU · HCl, morpholino-CNU, dimethylmorpholino-CNU, and piperidino-CNU proved to be active. The present investigation confirmed the assumption that the cytostatic activity of nitrosoureas is not merely a function of water-solubility because the water-soluble compounds acetamido-CNU and α-alanine-CNU were practically ineffective. Among

440

Table 2.
Experimental design

No. of experiment	Substance tested	Dose (mg/kg)	Number of animals	Solvent Surfactant	Physiol. saline
1	Untreated control	—	28	—	
	CP	70	30		+
	BCNU	25	30	+	
	MeCCNU	45	29	+	
	BCNU-ethane	45	29	+	
	BCNU-butane	35	28	+	
	Hydroxyethyl-CNU	25	33		+
	Hydroxyethyl-CNU-MS	22	27		+
2	Untreated control	—	27	—	
	CP	70	30		+
	Acetamido-CNU	14	30		+
	Methylenedioxybenzyl-CNU	35	30	+	
	Picolyl-3-CNU	25	30	+	
	Picolyl-3-CNU · HCl	25	30		+
3	Untreated control	—	28	—	
	CP	70	30		+
	α-alanine-CNU	40	30		+
	Morpholino-CNU	28	30		+
	Piperidino-CNU	15	30		+
	Chlorozotocin	20	30		+
4	Untreated control	—	19	—	
	Hydroxyethyl-CNU	12	20		+
	Hydroxyethyl-CNU	17	20		+
	Hydroxyethyl-CNU	22	20		+
5	Untreated control	—	30	—	
	Dimethylmorpholino-CNU	45	30		+
	Hydroxyethyl-CNU	3 × 7	20		+
	Hydroxyethyl-CNU	21	20		+
6	Untreated control	—	18	—	
	Chlorozotocin	3 × 7	20		+
	Chlorozotocin	12	20		+
	Chlorozotocin	17	20		+
	Chlorozotocin	21	20		+
7	Untreated control	—	19	—	
	α-alanine-CNU	3 × 11	19		+
	α-alanine-CNU	33	20		+
8	Untreated control	—	15	—	
	CP	70	15		+
	Methylenedioxybenzyl-CNU	35	15	+	
	Picolyl-3-CNU · HCl	25	14		+
	Morpholino-CNU	28	15		+
	Piperidino-CNU	15	15		+

Table 3.
Results of chemotherapeutic treatment wih the test compounds

Substance	Dose (mg/kg)	M days	% M	p	tf_{120} No. (%)	D_{120} %	tf_{1-120} No. (%)	D_{1-120} %	Initial number of animals
Expt. 1:									
Untreated control	—	46	100		7 (25)	—	7 (25)	—	28
CP	70	> 120	> 260	+	15 (50)	25	21 (63)	38	30
BCNU	25	74	160		13 (43)	18	14 (47)	22	30
MeCCNU	45	60	130		10 (33)	8	15 (52)	27	29
BCNU-ethane	45	39	84		8 (28)	3	12 (41)	16	29
BCNU-butane	35	> 120	> 260		13 (46)	21	14 (50)	25	28
Hydroxyethyl-CNU	25	23	50		6 (18)	−7	16 (48)	23	33
Hydroxyethyl-CNU-MS	22	40	87		8 (30)	5	12 (44)	19	27
Expt. 2:									
Untreated control	—	22	100		6 (22)	—	6 (22)	—	27
CP	70	> 120	> 545	+	17 (57)	35	24 (80)	58	30
Methylenedioxy-benzyl-CNU	35	80	366	+	14 (47)	25	15 (50)	28	30
Picolyl-3-CNU	25	28	130		6 (20)	−2	7 (23)	1	30
× HCl	25	27	125		11 (37)	15	12 (40)	18	30
Acetamido-CNU	14	23	107		4 (13)	−9	6 (20)	−2	30
Expt. 3:									
Untreated control	—	17.5	100		8 (29)	—	8 (29)	—	28
CP	70	> 120	> 686	+	20 (67)	38	23 (77)	48	30
α-Alanine-CNU	40	17.5	100		8 (27)	−2	16 (53)	24	30
Morpholino-CNU	28	> 120	> 686	+	19 (63)	34	21 (70)	41	30
Piperidino-CNU	15	> 120	> 686	+	15 (50)	21	15 (50)	21	30
Chlorooztocin	20	35	200		9 (30)	1	18 (60)	31	30
Expt. 4:									
Untreated control	—	14	100		3 (15)	—	3 (15)	—	19
Hydroxyethyl-CNU	12	27	193		7 (35)	20	7 (35)	20	20
Hydroxyethyl-CNU	17	92	657	+	9 (45)	30	9 (45)	30	20
Hydroxyethyl-CNU	22	20	143		4 (20)	5	11 (55)	40	20
Expt. 5:									
Untreated control	—	19	100		6 (20)	—	6 (20)	—	30
Dimethylmor-pholino-CNU	45	71	374	+	12 (40)	20	14 (47)	27	30
Hydroxyethyl-CNU	3 × 7	35	187		5 (25)	5	8 (40)	20	20
Hydroxyethyl-CNU	21	58	308		6 (30)	10	7 (35)	15	20
Expt. 6:									
Untreated control	—	16	100		3 (16)	—	3 (16)	—	18
Chlorozotocin	3 × 7	22	140		6 (30)	14	7 (35)	19	20
Chlorozotocin	12	22	140		4 (20)	4	5 (25)	9	20
Chlorozotocin	17	60	379	+	8 (40)	24	10 (50)	34	20
Chlorotozocin	21	27	171		4 (20)	4	5 (25)	9	20

Fortsetzung Tabelle 3.

		M	$\%M$	p	tf_{120}	D_{120}	tf_{1-120}	D_{1-120}	
Expt. 7:									
Untreated control	—	14	100		1 (5)	—	1 (5)	—	19
α-Alanine-CNU	3 × 11	31	221		1 (5)	0	3 (16)	11	19
α-Alanine-CNU	33	17	125		1 (5)	0	5 (25)	20	20
Expt. 8:									
Untreated control	—	10	100		0	—	0	—	15
CP	70	40	400	+	1 (7)	7	1 (7)	7	15
Methylenedioxy-benzyl-CNU	35	17	170	+	0	0	0	0	15
Picolyl-3-CNU · HCl	25	15	150		0	0	0	0	14
Morpholino-CNU	28	18	180	+	0	0	0	0	15
Piperidino-CNU	15	16	160	+	1 (7)	7	2 (13)	13	15

M = Median survival time
$\%M$ = Median life expectancy of treated animals vs. controls $M_{treat.}/M_{untreat.} \times 100$
p = Probability of error $< 5\%$ (log-rank test comparison of survival time)
  + indicates that the survival time of treated animals is different from the controls
tf_{120} = Animals surviving day 120 without tumour
D_{120} = Difference (%) between tf_{120} of treated and untreated animals
tf_{1-120} = Animals dying without tumour over the whole experimental time, i.e., tf_{120} + animals dying of toxicity
D_{1-120} = Difference (%) between tf_{1-120} of treated and untreated animals

the water-soluble compounds tested, methylenedioxybenzyl-CNU and BCNU-butane proved to be most active. BCNU-ethane and picolyl-3-CNU exerted only marginal activity at the administered doses.

In the present tumour model hydroxyethyl-CNU, chlorozotocin, morpholino-CNU, piperidino-CNU, dimethylmorpholino-CNU, methylenedioxybenzyl-CNU, and BCNU-butane reached the distal colon at chemotherapeutically effective concentrations. Their administration induced a remarkable increase in the proportion of tumour-free animals alive at the end of the observation period (120 days) and a significant increase in survival time except for BCNU-butane.

The volume-doubling time of tumours was estimated to be approximately 19 h during the log-phase of tumour growth in the present tumour model. It is thus not likely that a tumour would be found in animals that had been relapse-free for more than 100 days if they were observed for a longer period (Habs, 1981).

Some of the compounds tested in the present tumour model have also been tested in other models with regard to their anticancer activity. Remarkable differences in the ranking of the chemotherapeutic activity of these compounds were seen among these models. However, the predictive value of such test models for clinical application schemes is still limited.

Compounds which proved to be inactive in the colon tumour model are either not capable of reaching the distal colon at effective concentrations or do not act cytostatically on Yoshida ascites cells.

Combination therapy study

In animal experiments, pretreatment with disulfiram (DSF) has been shown to decrease the acute and chronic toxicity of various N-nitroso compounds (Wattenberg,

1978; SCHMÄHL et al, 1971). Based on this previous information it was decided to investigate the effects of DSF on the acute toxicity of HECNU and further to determine whether such possibly enhanced detoxification interferes with the cytostatic chemotherapeutic action of this compound.

Toxicity experiment

Lethal toxic effects were recorded over a 28-day observation period. The fatal response to several geometrically spaced (expanding factor 1.15) individual doses of HECNU injected i. p. was compared to the effect of identical doses applied 2 h after treatment with DSF. DSF was administered by gavage at a dose of 1,000 mg/kg to 2-week-old male rats that had not received any food overnight. Each dose was represented by a treatment group of 8 rats. Deaths were recorded every 2 h during day-time. For animals dying at night the approximate time of death was estimated at necropsy.

Chemotherapy experiment

Cells (1×10^7) were implanted i. p. at a volume of 1.0 ml/animal. Treatment was carried out in the same way as in the toxicity experiment except that HECNU was injected i. v. Three days after transplantation the rats were treated with geometrically spaced doses (expanding factor 1.2) of HECNU ranging from 15 to 61.8 mg/kg. Half of the animals were pretreated with orally administered DSF at a dose of 1,000 mg/kg 2 h prior to HECNU treatment.

Results

Treatment with DSF (1,000 mg/kg p. o.) 2 h prior to i. p. injection of HECNU reduced the acute toxicity of HECNU by 50% in male Sprague-Dawley rats. The LD_{50} was raised from 36 to 54 mg/kg. The DSF pretreatment also resulted in improved clinical appearance and weight gain. After i. p. transplantation of 1×10^7 Yoshida sarcoma ascites cells, untreated rats had a median survival time of 8 days. The maximum survival time was increased to about 14 days in rats treated with HECNU alone. Pretreatment with DSF resulted in identical or slightly higher life expectancy and thus in a reduction of the toxic side effects of HECNU without reducing its anti-tumour potency (HABS and HABS, 1981).

References

1. HABS, M. (1981): Methoden, Ergebnisse und Probleme der experimentellen Chemotherapie. In: Maligne Tumouren — Entstehung, Wachstum, Chemotherapie, SCHMÄHL, D. (ed.) pp. 455 to 498, Editio Cantor, Aulendorf
2. HABS, H. and HABS, M.: Effect of the pretreatment with disulfiram on the toxicity and anti-tumour activity of 1-(2-hydroxyethyl)-3-(2-chloroethyl)-3-nitrosourea in Sprague-Dawley rats. Cancer Letters 13 (1981), 63—69
3. SCHMÄHL, D., KRÜGER, F. W., IVANKOVIC, S. und PREISSLER, P.: Verminderung der Toxizität von Dimethylnitrosamin bei Ratten und Mäusen nach Behandlung mit Disulfiram. Arznei.-Forsch. 21 (1971), 1560—1566
4. WATTENBERG, L. W. (1978): Inhibitors of chemical carcinogenesis. In: Advances in cancer research, Vol. 26, KLEIN, G., WEINHOUSE, S. (eds.), pp. 197—226, Academic Press, New York

Gustav-Embden-Center of Biological Chemistry, J.-W.-Goethe-University Frankfurt/Main, FRG

The Mode of Action of Cyclophosphamide[1]

H. J. Hohorst. L. Bielicki and G. Voelcker

Alkylating agents which exert their cytotoxic reaction by a uniform attack on all nucleophilic centers available to them in a cell would appear to be a most unsuitable object for the study of the problem of cancerotoxic selectivity of cytostatic agents. Not only this simple theoretical consideration would lead to that conclusion: both the long history of research on the mechanism of action of alkylating cytostatics as well as the numerous and more or less fruitless efforts to develop alkylating cytostatics with higher cancerotoxic selectivity by reducing their alkylating activity (e. g., by drug latency) point in that way. In fact, a proportional relation appears to exist between alkylating activity and cytotoxic action, as postulated in 1953 by Ross (1) and as demonstrated in our own studies on the cytotoxic specificity of N-mustards (2, 3). At least one class of latent alkylating cytostatics, namely cyclophosphamide and its oxazaphosphorinane analogues, however, show a high degree of selectivity in vivo, as represented by a high therapeutic index (4), despite the fact this cytotoxic reaction is also the result of alkylations.

The apparent deviation of cyclophosphamide from the proportionality rule described above, together with the felicitous finding that cyclophosphamide is a very stable compound and is metabolized relative slowly by well identified single steps, represented a challenge to our group to study its cancerotoxic selectivity.

The metabolism of cyclophosphamide (Fig. 1) can be divided into three major steps: activation, deactivation (detoxication) and toxication. Activation is catalysed by mixed-function hydroxylases in the liver, which yield 4-hydroxycyclophosphamide (4-OH-CP) as a primary activated metabolite. Because of the hemiaminal group at carbon 4 of the oxazaphosphorinane ring, 4-OH-CP is a very reactive but not yet alkylating molecule (2). It shows about the same high cancerotoxic selectivity as cyclophosphamide when given in vivo; but, in contrast to the latter, it also has a high cytotoxic activity and specificity against tumour cells in vitro (2, 3).

4-OH-CP is in equilibrium with its ring opened tautomer, aldophosphamide, and can be deactivated enzymatically by an NAD-dependent aldehyde hydrogenase in the liver to yield 4-ketocyclophosphamide and carboxyphosphamide, the two urinary detoxicated excretion products (5). It can be also deactivated non-enzymatically by reaction with thiol-compounds, including protein thiols, to yield relatively stable 4-(SR)-sulfidocyclophosphamides (2, 6, 7). In the third step, toxication, the alkylating moiety, phosphoric-acid-diamide mustard (PAM), is released from 4-OH-CP by spontaneous β-elimination of acrolein (8). This toxication is the rate-limiting step for

[1] This study was carried out with the support of the Deutsche Forschungsgemeinschaft Bonn—Bad Godesberg

445

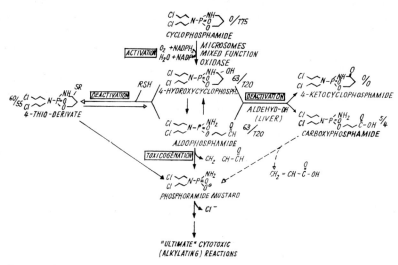

Fig. 1. Metabolic activation, deactivation and toxication of cyclophosphamide. The figures represent cytotoxic specificity: cancerotoxic selectivity ratio.

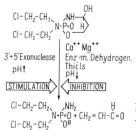

Fig. 2. Factors which modulate the spontaneous toxication of activated cyclophosphamide.

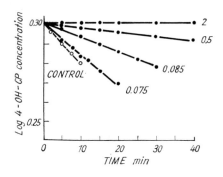

Fig. 3. Effect of Ca++ ions (mM concentrations as indicated) on the toxication of 4-hydroxycyclophosphamide (4-OH-CP) (2 mM). The concentration of 4-OH-CP in phosphate-buffered saline, pH 7 at 37 °C, was measured by the nitrobiphenyl assay.

the whole metabolic sequence and can be controlled by a number of modulators, as shown in Figure 2.

Generally speaking, any reaction on the hemiaminal (aldehydogenic) group at carbon 4 of the oxazaphosphorinane ring can modulate the toxication of activated cyclophosphamide, including increase or decrease of pH, complexing with earth-alkali ions (Fig. 3), and enzymatic dehydrogenation or non-enzymatic reaction with thiols. When, for example, a protein-thiol-like bovine serum albumin is reacted with 4-OH-CP (Fig. 4), the rate of toxication is reduced by factor of six compared with the toxication rate of 4-OH-CP in the absence of thiols (7).

446

In comparison with its toxication, the conversion of 4-OH-CP by thiols to 4-(S-protein)-sulfidocyclophosphamide [4-(SR)-sulfido-CP] is very fast; and the sulfido derivative is even more stable in vivo, where an excess of protein and non-protein thiols is present in the cells. Thus, 4-OH-CP cannot be toxicated to the ultimate alkylating moiety, PAM. In other words, all or most of the activated cyclophosphamide that permeates into cells from the blood is trapped as deactivated 4-(SR)-sulfido-CP. Only that small portion of the unaltered 4-OH-CP that is excreted in the urine after cyclophosphamide treatment (9) can be toxicated, and is the cause of the urotoxicity seen with this treatment (10).

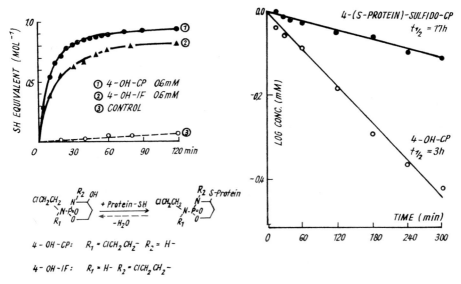

Fig. 4. Decrease in titratable SH groups after addition of 4-hydroxycyclophosphamide (4-OH-CP) to bovine serum albumin (BSA) (0.6 mM BSA at pH 7, 37 °C), and rate of toxication of 4-OH-CP and 4-(S-protein)-sulfidocyclophosphamide. Toxication was determined by measuring the decrease in alkylating capacity of 1 mM solutions of the compounds in phosphate-buffered saline, pH 7, at 37 °C.

Up to this point, the metabolism of cyclophosphamide involves no reaction that could lead to cancerotoxic selectivity. The question therefore arises of how the 4-(SR)-sulfido-CP trapped in the cellular compartment can be reactivated and/or toxicated. A simple reversal of the thiol reaction by hydrolysis of 4-(SR)-sulfido-CP, to yield 4-OH-CP again would appear to be very unlikely; and we therefore sought another mechanism for toxication. During pharmacokinetic studies with 4-OH-CP, we observed an unexpectedly high decomposition of activated cyclophosphamide in rat serum (Fig. 5). The effect was found to be associated with serum protein and to be heat-sensitive; it was observed not only with 4-OH-CP but also with 4-(SR)-sulfido-CP, and in the latter case, free, titratable sulfhydryl groups (Fig. 6) of the protein component, acrolein and alkylating material were released.

In studies of the nature of the proposed enzyme, we found that phosphodiesterases from various sources could toxicate both activated cyclophosphamide and 4-(SR)-sulfido-CP (Table 1). Only those phosphodiesterases (exonucleases) which hydrolyse the phosphodiester-bond in the 3'5' direction were found to split the posphodiester bond of the activated oxazaphosphorinane ring. 3',5'-Cyclo-AMP-phosphodiesterase

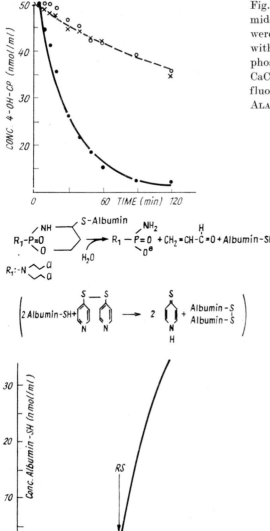

Fig. 5. Toxication of 4-hydroxycyclophospha-
mide (4-OH-CP) by rat serum. 50 µM 4-OH-CP
were incubated with 1 mg/ml rat serum (o) or
with 0.14 mg/ml phosphodiesterase (×) in 0.07M
phosphate-buffered saline containing 50 µM
CaCl$_2$, pH 7, at 37°C. 4-OH-CP was determined
fluorometrically, according to the method of
ALARCON and MEIENHOFER (15).

Fig. 6. Toxication of 4-(S-protein)-sulfidocyclophosphamide by rat serum. 4-(S-protein)-sulfi-
docyclophosphamide was preparaed from bovine serum albumin and 4-hydroxycyclophosphamide
according to the method of COELCKER et al (16) and 1.4 mg/ml were incubated in phosphate
buffer, pH 7 at 37 °C with 0.2 mg/ml 4,4'-dithiopyridine. Free SH groups were determined pho-
tometrically at 324 nm according to the method of GRASETTI and MURRAY (17) before and after
adding 50 µl rat serum.

belongs to this group of enzymes, which confirms the finding of TISDALE (11) that
4-OH-CP interacts with 3',5'-Cyclo-AMP-binding proteins. Moreover, SCHMALL (12)
in our laboratory, observed that a simultaneous inhibition of 3',5'-cAMP-phospho-
diesterase with an increase of 3',5'-cAMP-levels in L1210 cells of mice was the earliest
event after injection of cyclophosphamide. Generally, however, the toxication of 4-
OH-CP or 4-(SR)-sulfido-CP by 3',5'-exonucleases seems to be rather low. Much

448

higher activities were found with 3′,5′-exonucleases linked to DNA polymerases, as shown in Table 2 for the DNA polymerase I from *Escherichia coli*. As an example of an eucaryotic enzyme, we isolated a purified DNA polymerase δ (13) from erythroid hyperplastic rabbit bone marrow: this enzyme has similar characteristics with respect to DNA polymerase and 3′,5′-exonuclease activity as the *E. coli* enzyme; it also actively splits the phosphodiester bond of activated cyclophosphamide. Although many details remain to be clarified, including the possible action on the DNA polymerase of PAM released by the exonuclease part of the enzyme, we assume that these types of enzyme are the missing link in the thiol-hypothesis, explaining the cancerotoxic selectivity of cyclophosphamide.

Table 1.
Toxication of 4-hydroxycyclophosphamide by various phosphodiesterases[a]

Enzyme	Specific activity nmol/min:mg protein
Phosphodiesterase I from snake venom (EC 3.1.4.1.) Exonuclease 3′—5′	4.2
Phosphodiesterase II from calf spleen (EC 3.1.16.1) 5′—3′ Exonuclease	0.0
Exonuclease III from *E. coli* (EC 3.1.4) specific for double-stranded DNA	0.0
Nuclease P_1 from *Penicillium citrinum* (EC 3.1.4 —) 3′—5′ Exonuclease; DNA and RNA	2.3
DNAse I from bovine pancreas (EC 3.1.21.1) Endonuclease	0.0
3′,5′-Cyclic AMP phosphodiesterase from bovine heart (EC 3.1.4.17)	0.7
Ribonuclease I from bovine pancreas	0.0
Rat serum	5.2

[a] Toxication of 4-hydroxycyclophosphamide (1 mg/ml) by the enzymes (0.5 mg/ml) was measured in 0.07 M phosphate-buffer, pH 6, 37 °C, by high-performance liquid chromatography of acrolein released.

Future studies should be directed to investigating whether there is a correlation between the activity of 3′,5′-exonuclease/DNA polymerase measured in normal and neoplastic cells and the sensitivity of those cells to the cytotoxic effects of cyclophosphamide or 4-OH-CP. Because of considerable technical difficulties, we have not yet been able to demonstrate this for a broader spectrum of cells and tissues. However, some observations indicate that such a correlation exists, as, for example, the highly toxicogenetic action of human lymphocytes on 4-OH-CP (Table 3). CHEN et al (14) were able to demonstrate that lymphogenic cells from several mouse myelomas that are very sensitive to CP show a high activity of DNA polymerase-linked 3′,5′-exonuclease.

As a working hypothesis of the mode of action of cyclophosphamide and an explanation for its selective cytotoxicity, the following sequence of reactions may be envisaged:

(1) Cyclophosphamide is activated by mixed-function hydroxylases in the liver to yield 4-OH-CP, a non-alkylating activated metabolite, which spontaneously releases phosphordiamide mustard as the ultimate alkylating agent.

Table 2.
Toxication of 4-hydroxycyclophosphamide by DNA polymerase-associated 3′,5′-exonuclease[a]

Enzyme	Specific activity nmol/min/mg protein
DNA polymerase I 3′,5′-exonuclease EC 2.7.7.7 from E. coli	31.3
DNA polymerase δ 3′,5′-exonuclease from rabbit bone marrow	97.0
Phosphodiesterase I 3′,5′-exonuclease EC 3.1.4.1 from snake venom	4.2

[a] Toxication was determined as described in the footnote to Table 1.
  DNA polymerase δ was prepared and purified according to the method of BYRNES et al (13).

Table 3.
Toxiciation of 4-hydroxycyclophospha-
mide by human lymphocytes[a]

Lymphocytes charge	Activity nmol acrolein min/mg protein
I	22.0
II	67.0
III	50.0
IV	34.0
V	28.0
Human plasma	0.56

[a] Human blood lymphocytes obtained by phlebotomy from normal subjects were prepared and purified by the one-step sodium metrizoate/ficoll centrifugal procedure.

(2) The release of the alkylating moiety from activated cyclophosphamide can be controlled by various cellular constituents.

(3) Protein thiols deactivate 4-OH-CP and bind it to stable 4-(SR) sulfido-CP within the cell.

(4) 3′,5′-Exonucleases, which are intimately linked to DNA polymerases, can split the phosphodiester bond of 4-(SR)-sulfido-CP to yield the ultimate alkylating, cytotoxic agent.

References

1. Ross, W. C. J.: The chemistry of cytotoxic alkylating agents. Advances in Cancer Res. *1* (1953), 397
2. HOHORST, H. J., DRAGER, U., PETER, G. and VOELCKER, G.: The problem of oncostatic specificity of cyclophosphamide (NSC-26271): studies on reactions that control the alkylating and cytotoxic activity. Cancer Treat. Rep. *60* (1976), 309

3. Brock, N. and Hohorst, H. J.: The problem of specificity and selectivitiy of alkylating cyto-statics: studies on N-2-chloroethylamido-oxazaphosphorines. Z. Krebsforsch. *88* (1977), 185

4. Arnold, H., Bourseaux, F. and Brock, N.: Neuartige Krebschemotherapeutika aus der Gruppe der zyklischen N-Lost-Phosphamidester. Naturwissenschaften *45* (1958), 64

5. Backe, J. E., Feil, V. J. and Zaylskie, R. G.: Characterization of the major sheep urinary metabolites of cyclophosphamide, a defleecing chemical. J. Agric. Food Chem. *19* (1971), 788

6. Draeger, U., Peter, G. and Hohorst, H. J.: Deactivation of cyclophosphamide (NSC 26271) metabolites by sulfhydryl compounds. Cancer Treat. Rep. *60* (1976), 355

7. Voelcker, G., Wagner, T. and Hohorst, H. J.: Identification and pharmacokinetics of cyclophosphamide (NSC 26271) metabolites in vivo. Cancer Treat. Rep. *60* (1976), 415

8. Connors, T. A., Cox, P. J., Farmer, P. B.‘ Foster, A. B. and Jarman, M.: Some studies of the active intermediates formed in the microsomal metabolism of cyclophosphamide and iphosphamide. Biochem. Pharmacol. *23* (1974), 115

9. Wagner, T., Heydrich, D., Voelcker, G. and Hohorst, H. J.: Comparative study on human pharmacokinetics of activated ifosfamide and cyclophosphamide by a modified fluorometric test. J. Cancer Res. Clin. Oncol. *96* (1980), 79

10. Brock, N., Stekar, J., Pohl, J., Niemeyer, U. and Scheffler, G.: Acrolein the causative factor of urotoxic side-effects of cyclophosphamide, ifosfamide, trofosfamide and sufosfamide. Arzneim. Forsch., *29* (1979), 659

11. Tisdale, M. J.: Interaction of cyclophosphamide and its metabolites with adenosine 3′,5′-monophosphate binding proteins. Biochem. Pharmacol. *26* (1977), 1469

12. Schmall, M. (1978): Inaugural-Dissertation beim Fachbereich Biochemie und Pharmazie der J.-W.-Goethe-Universität Frankfurt am Main

13. Byrnes, J. J., Downey, K. M., Black, V. U. and So, A. G.: A new mammalian DNA poly-merase with 3′ to 5′ exonuclease activity: DNA polymerase δ. Biochemistry *15* (1976), 2817

14. Chen, Y.-C., Bohn, E. W., Planck, S. R. and Wilson, S. H.: Mouse DNA polymerase; subunit structure and identification of a species with associated exonuclease. J. Biol. Chem. *254* (1979), 11678

15. Alarcon, P. H. and Meienhofer, J.: Formation of the cytotoxic aldehyde acrolein during in vitro degradation of cyclophosphamide. Nature New Biol. *233* (1971), 250—252

16. Grasetti, D. R. and Murray, jr. I. F.: Determination of sulfhydryl groups with 2,2′- and 4,4′-dithiodipyridine. Arch. Bilchem. Biophys. *119* (1967), 41—49

Names and Addresses of Authors

Dr G. Atassi
Laboratory for Experimental
    Chemotherapy and Screening
Institut Jules Bordet
1, rue Héger-Bordet
1000 Brussels
Belgium

Dr C. Auclair
Laboratoire de Biochimie
    Enzymologique
Unité INSERM 140
Institut Gustave Roussy
Rue Camille Desmoulins
94800 Villejuif
France

Dr J. Ban
Laboratory for Experimental
    Cancerology
Central Institute for Tumours and
    Allied Diseases
Ilica 197
41000 Zagreb
Yugoslavia

Dr F. Boccardo
Istituto Scientifico per lo
    studio e la cura dei Tumori
v. le Benedetto XV, 10
16132 Genova
Italy

Professor W. A. Boggust
Department of Experimental Medicine
Cancer Research Unit
University of Dublin
Trinity College
St. Luke's Hospital
Rathgar
Dublin 6
Ireland

Dr B. M. Bombik
Klinikum Charlottenburg
Free University of Berlin
Department of Hematology and
    Oncology
Spandauer Damm 130
1000 Berlin 19
Federal Republic of Germany

Professor P. K. Bondy
Associate Chief of Staff for Research
    and Development
Veterans Administration
Medical Center
West Spring Street
West Haven, CT 06516
USA

Dr B. Brdar
Central Institute for Tumours and
    Allied Diseases
Ilica 197
41000 Zagreb
Yugoslavia

Dr L. Cacciari
Divisione di Radiochemioterapia
Ospedale Bellaria
Via Altura 3
Bologna
Italy

Dr A. H. Calvert
Department of Biochemical Pharmacology
Institute of Cancer Research
Block E
Clifton Avenue
Belmont
Sutton, Surrey SM2 5PX
United Kingdom

452

Dr G. Cantelli FORTI
Istituto di Farmacologia
  dell'Universita di Bologna
Via Zamboni 33
40126 Bologna
Italy

Dr M. J. CLEARE
Johnson Matthey Research Centre
Blount's Court
Sonning Common
Reading RG4 9NH
United Kingdom

Dr E. CSÁNYI
Institute for Drug Research
P.O. Box 82
1325 Budapest
Hungary

Dr D. A. L. DAVIES
Department of Surgery
University of Cambridge Clinical
  School
Addenbrooke's Hospital
Hills Road
Cambridge CB2 200
United Kingdom

Dr L. DE RIDDER
Department of Radiotherapy
  and Nuclear Medicine
University Hospital
De Pintelaan 185
B-9000 Ghent
Belgium

Dr B. F. DEYS
Laboratoire d'Histologie-
  Embryologie-Cytogénétique
Université de Nice
Faculté de Médecine
Chemin de Valombrose
06100 Nice
France

Dr K. ELGJO
Institute of Pathology
University of Oslo
Rikshospitalet
Oslo 1
Norway

Dr I. FRESHNEY
Department of Oncology
University of Glasgow
1 Horselethill Road
Glasgow G12 9LY, Scotland
United Kingdom

Dr T. GIRALDI
Istituto di Farmacologia
Universita degli Studi di Trieste
Via Valerio 32
34100 Trieste
Italy

Professor H. GRUNICKE
Institut für Medizinische Chemie
  und Biochemie der Universität
  Innsbruck
Fritz-Pregl-Strasse 3
6020 Innsbruck
Austria

Dr M. HABS
Institute of Toxicology and
  Chemotherapy
German Cancer Research Center
Im Neuenheimer Feld 280
6900 Heidelberg 1
Federal Republic of Germany

Dr G. HAGNER
Department of Hematology and Oncology
Klinikum Charlottenburg
Free University of Berlin
Spandauer Damm 130
1000 Berlin 19
Federal Republic of Germany

Dr E. HEISE
Central Institute for Cancer Research
Lindenberger Weg 80
1115 Berlin-Buch
German Democratic Republic

Dr P. HILGARD
Bristol-Myers International
  Corporation
Clinical Research, Europe
185 Chaussée de la Hulpe
1170 Brussels
Belgium

Dr H. J. Hohorst
Center for Biological Chemistry
Theodor-Stern-kai 7
6000 Frankfurt-am-Main 70
Federal Republic of Germany

Mrs A. L. Jackman
Department of Biochemical Pharmacology
Institute of Cancer Research
Block E
Clifton Avenue
Belmont
Sutton, Surrey SM2 5PX
United Kingdom

Professor K. Kolarić
Head, Department of Chemotherapy
Central Institute for Tumours and
    Allied Diseases
Ilica 197
41000 Zagreb
Yugoslavia

Dr W. Krafft
Department of Gynaecology and
    Obstetrics
Erfurt Medical Academy
Gorkistraße 6
5020 Erfurt
German Democratic Republic

Dr K. Krolick
Department of Microbiology
University of Texas
Southwestern Medical School
Dallas, TX 75235
USA

Dr J. Krušić
Central Institute for Tumours and
    Allied Diseases
Ilica 197
41000 Zagreb
Yugoslavia

Professor K. E. Kuettner
Chairman, Department of Biochemistry
Rush-Presbyterian-St Luke's
    Medical Center
1753 West Congress Parkway
Chicago, IL 60612
USA

Professor K. Lapis
1. Institute of Pathology and
    Experimental Cancer Research
Semmelweis Medical University
Ulloi út 26
1085 Budapest VIII
Hungary

Dr L. Lenaz
Bristol-Myers Company
International Division
345 Park Avenue
New York, N.Y. 10154
USA

Professor C. Maltoni
Director
Istituto di Oncologia "Felice Addarii"
Viale Ercolani 4/2
40138 Bologna
Italy

Dr M. M. K. Mareel
Laboratory of Experimental Cancerology
Department of Radiotherapy and
    Nuclear Medicine
University Hospital
De Pintelaan 135
9000 Ghent
Belgium

Dr M. Micksche
Institut für Krebsforschung
    der Universität Wien
Borschkegasse 8a
1090 Wien
Austria

Dr G. L. Neil
Research Manager
Experimental Biology Research
The Upjohn Company
Kalamazoo, MI 49001
USA

Dr E. S. Newlands
Department of Medical Oncology
Charing Cross Hospital
Fulham Palace Road
London W6 8RF
United Kingdom

Dr M. Nuti
Department of Health and Human Services
Public Health Service
National Cancer Institute
National Institutes of Health
Bldg. 37, Rm. 1A07
Bethesda, MD 20205
USA

Dr I. Padovan
Head, Department of Head and Neck Surgery
Dr M. Stojanovic University Hospital
Vinogradska 29
02-034 Warsaw
Poland

Dr Z. Paszko
Institute of Oncology
15 Wawelska
02-034 Warsaw
Poland

Dr S. Perez-Cuadrado
Chief of Department of Immunopathology
Istituto Nacional de Oncologia
Ciudad Universitaria
Madrid 3
Spain

Professor A. Piffanelli
Istituto di Oncologia "Felice Addarii"
Viale Ercolani 4/2
40138 Bologna
Italy

Professor A. Pihl
Norsk Hydro's Institute for Cancer
    Research
Radiumhospitalet
Montebello
Oslo 3
Norway

Dr C. J. Rutty
Department of Biochemistry and
    Pharmacology
Institute of Cancer Research
Royal Cancer Hospital
Block E
Clifton Avenue
Belmont
Sutton, Surrey SM2 5PX
United Kingdom

Dr G. Sava
Istituto di Farmacologie e
    Chimica Farmaceutica
Universita di Trieste
34100 Trieste
Italy

Dr H. G. Schleich
Institute of Cell and Tumour Biology
German Cancer Research Center
Im Neuenheimer Feld 280
6900 Heidelberg 1
Federal Republic of Germany

Dr K. Sikora
Ludwig Institute for Cancer Research
Medical Research Council Centre
Hills Road
Cambridge CB2 2QH
United Kingdom

Dr. G. Stathopoulos
Hippokration Hospital
Athens
Greece

Professor S. Stirpe
Institute of General Pathology
University of Bologna
Via S. Giacomo 14
40126 Bologna
Italy

Professor J. Sugár
Director
Research Institute of Oncopathology
Ráth György u. 7
1122 Budapest
Hungary

Dr I. Számel
National Institute of Oncology
Ráth. Gy. u. 7–9
1525 Budapest Pf. 21
Hungary

Dr K. Takeda
Experimental Therapeutics
Roswell Park Memorial Institute
Department of Health
State of New York
666 Elm Street
Buffalo, N.Y. 14263
USA

Professor St. Tanneberger
Director, Robert Rössle Institute
Central Institute for Cancer Research
Lindenberger Weg 80
1115 Berlin-Buch
German Democratic Republic

Professor S. D. Vesselinovitch
Department of Radiology
University of Chicago
950 East 59th Street
Chicago, IL 60637
USA

Dr O. Wildermuth
31265 Lilac Road
Valley Center, CA 92082
USA

Dr F. Workman
MRC Clinical Oncology and
    Radiotherapeutics Unit
The Medical School
Hills Road
Cambridge CB2 2QH
United Kingdom

Professor H. Wrba
Institut für Krebsforschung
    der Universität Wien
Borschkegasse 8a
1090 Wien
Austria

Dr L. R. Zacharski
Chairman, Cooperative Studies
Dartmouth Medical School
Veterans Administration
White River, UT 05001
USA

Index

Abrin 134, 136, 138, 139
Accelerated emergence of lesions 283
A-chain 147
Achievement of screening 359
Acquired resistance 342
Action of transglutaminase 261
Additive effect 131
Adenovirus 414, 415
Adhesion 37
Adhesiveness 35
ADJ/PC 6 tumour 215, 217, 409
Administration of cis-DDP 288
Adoptive transfer 150
Adriamycin 292, 294, 296
Advantages of N-methylolmelamine
    (CB 10-375) over PMM 187
Age of patients 106
Agglutinin 134
AHH (aryl hydrocarbon hydroxylase)
    assay 431
AHH (aryl hydrocarbon hydroxylase)
    inducibility 431, 433
Alkylating agents 120, 122, 189
Alternatives to Hexamethylmelamine (HMM)
    180
Amine oxidase 74, 77, 81
Analogies 341
Analysis of cytostatic effects 349
Analysis of cytotoxic effects 349
Androgen receptor (AR) 104
Animal models 379
Animal tumours for selecting and evaluating
    active drugs 382
Antagonists to the biosynthesis of polyamines
    264
Anthracycline 231
Antibacterial activity 301
Antiblastic dugs 339, 376, 392
Antibodies 127, 136
Antibody A-chain immunotoxin 149
Antibody-drug synergy (ADS) 132

Anti-cancer drugs 159
Anticoagulant 38
— agents 63
— treatment 63
Antifolate-CB 3717 361
Anti-invasion factor (AIF) 15, 19
Anti-immunoglobulin antibodies 147
Anti-invasiveness of microtubule inhibitors
    47, 49
Anti-invasive properties 23
Antileukemic action 309
Antimetabolites 189
Antimetastatic agents 58
— effect 71, 251
— potential 24
Antimicrobial activity 300
— assay 303, 305
Antineoplastic drugs 58
Antiplatelet agents 63
Antiproliferative activity 19
Anti-tumour activity 126, 233, 250, 438
Antitumourigenic activity 287, 289
Antithrombotic agents 63
— therapy 65
Antiviral activity of pyrmidinones 247, 248
Appraisal of screening methods 359
Arabinofuranosylcytosine (Ara C) 277, 279
Artifical metastases 59
Aryl hydrocarbon hydroxylase (AHH) 431
Astrocytoma 355,
— cells 414
Autologous lymphocytes 428
Autologous tumour cells 428
Azimexon 175
BALB/c mice 129, 150, 217
Barriers 15
Basement membrane 19, 35, 38
Basophilic foci 282
B-cell tumour, BCL_1 147, 148
BCNU (1.3-bis-(2-chloroethyl)-1-nitrosourea)
    439, 440, 441, 442

BDF$_1$ mice 218
Biochemical properties of abrin and ricin 134
Biochemical techniques 321
Biological parameters in drug sensitivity 342
Biological response modifiers 237
Biological significance 393
Blastogenic response to concanavalin A (Con A) of lymphocytes 420
Blastogenic response to phytohaemagglutinin (PHA) of lymphocytes 420
Blastogenic response to pokeweed mitogen (PWM) of lymphocytes 420
Bleomycin 354
Blood-brain barrier 287
Blood platelets 36
B16 melanoma 26, 250, 251
Bone marrow 427
Bone marrow transplantation 151
Bradytrophic tissues 20
Brain tumour 42, 376, 377, 378, 385
Breast cancer 87, 99, 104, 106, 108, 318, 319

Calf uterus cytosol 93, 97
Cancer cell surface 111
Cancerostatic lectins 134
Cancerostatic properties of abrin and ricin 136
Cancerotoxic selectivity 446
Carcinogenesis 285
Carcinogenic effects 201
Carcinogenic index 298
Carcinogenicity 292, 391
Carcinoma of uterine cervix 253
Cartilage 15
CBDCA (cyclobutane dicarboxylate derivative) 220
C57Bl/6 mice 130
CB 3717 (N-4(N-((2-amino-4-hydroxy-6-quina-zolinyl)methyl)prop-2-ynylamino)-benzoyl)-L-glutamic acid) 361, 404, 405, 406, 408, 409
Cell cycle 70, 83
— communication 113, 115, 117
— culture technique 317, 320
— infiltration 369
— kinetics 84, 347
— kinetic parameters 332
— locomotion 35
— motility 35
— multiplication 123
— proliferation 349
— surface 119
— surface properties 134
—surface receptors 70, 116
Cervical carcinoma cells 414

Cessation of tumour growth 138
Chalone 83
Chalone-like properties 80
Characteristic of patients 195
Characteristics maintenance 329
Chemical reactivity 161
Chemosensitivity 349
Chemosensitization 170
Chemotherapeutic agents 142
— — experiments 334
— sensitivity 214
— treatment 442
— validity 335
Chemotherapy/immunotherapy 33
Chlorambucil 121, 129, 131
Chlorozotocin (2-(3-(2-chloroethyl)-3-nitroso-ureido)-D-glucopyranose) 439, 440, 441, 442
Chondrocytes 18, 20
Chromosome number 347
Chronic toxicity 391
Circulating cancer cells 35
Cis- and trans-isomers activity 216
Cis-dichlorodiammine platinum (cis-DDP) 214, 287
Clinical activity of selected drugs 360
Clinical evaluation 379
— implications of polyamines 263
— relevance and value 53, 316, 366
— schedules (VP 16-213) 210, 211
— studies 364
— trials of human interferon 241, 242
Cloning ability 321
— efficiency 349
Clonogenic assay 333, 352, 353, 356
Clonogenicity 357
Clonogenic tumour cells 310
CMF administration (BONADONNA et al. 1976) 204
CMF treatment (HABS et al. 1981) 204
CNU-derivatives (N-nitroso-(2-chloroethyl)-urea) 205, 207
Coagulation hypothesis 63
Collagenase inhibitory activity 18
Colony formation 189, 423, 424
Colorectal tumour 328, 332, 334, 335, 369, 370, 372, 438
Combination 190, 191, 192, 291
Combination therapy 26, 138, 443
Comparative pharmacology of HMM and PMM 186
Complement 129
Complete remission 424
Concanavalin A 134
Concentration-dependent effects 280

Confrontation 47
Conjugates 145, 152
Connective tissue barriers 19
Contraindication for Vitamin A 272
Control of megacaryocyte differentiation 423
Control of tumour growth 275
Contact inhibition 35, 116
Conventional organ culture assay 323
Correlation 374
Correlation coefficient 353
Cycloheximide 120
Cyclophosphamide 130, 202, 204, 310, 445, 450
Cytochrome P448-dependent function 431
Cytolysis degree 427
Cytoplasmic immunoglobulin 276
Cytoplasmic microtubule complex 50
Cytoreductive therapy 153
Cytosine arabinoside 131
Cytostatic drugs 201
Cytostatic sensitivity 366
Cytotoxic agents 59
Cytotoxic and antitumoural activities of ellipticine 160
Cytotoxicity 166
Cytotoxic specifity 446

Degradation of polyamines 75, 76, 77
Deoxyuridine 406
Desacetyl vinblastine amide sulphate 23
Detachment of cells 35
Development of new drugs 157
Develepment of Nitroimidazoles 166
Diethylnitrosamine (DEN) 282, 284
Differentiation-inducing agents 280
Diffusion 113
Dimethyl sulfoxide 277
Dihydrofolate reductase (DHFR) 404, 407
Disappearance of tumour 138
Dissemination 34
Disturbance of the microtubule complex 49, 53
Disulfiram (DSF) 443
DM-COOK(p-(3,3-dimethyl-1-triazeno)benzoic acid potassium salt) 56, 58, 309, 310, 311
DNA synthesis of breast cancer 322
Dose-dependent effect 26, 393
Dose-response curves 343, 344, 361
Doubling time of endothelial cells 19
Drug-antibody complex 128
Drug-induced effects 201, 275, 280
Drug metabolism 362
— selection 361
— selection parameters 380
— sensitivity 342
— sensitivity assay 350

— resistance 345
DTIC (dimethyltriazene) 139, 309, 310, 311

Effectiveness of endocrine therapy 109
Effect of abrin and ricin 138
Effect of alkylating agents 120, 122
Effect of antiblastic drugs 376
Effects of gonadectomy 282
Effects of retinoids 274
Effector cells 427
Ehrlich ascites tumour cells 120, 122
Elektroreduction potential 300, 302
Ellipticine derivatives 159, 160, 162
EL4 lymphoma 130
Endocrine therapy 104, 108
Endothelial cell growth inhibitor 20
Endothelial cell surface 37
Enzymes 15, 38
Epidermal growth inhibitor 83
ER (estradiol receptor) status 88, 90, 91
Erythrocyte-antibody-complement (EAC) rosettes 419
Erythrocyte rosettes 276
Erythropoietin 275, 424
Estradiol receptor (ER) 87, 89, 91, 96
Estradiol receptor assay (ER) 93, 99
Estrogen receptor (ER) 101, 104, 106
Evaluation of active drugs in animals 379
Evaluation of correlation rate 366
Evaluation of keratinization 274
Evaluation of new agents 363
Experimental evaluation of antiblastic drugs 391
Experimental model 40
Experimental systems for testing drugs 381
Experimental tumours 380
Extracerebral tumour lesions 290
Extravasation 37

Familial cancer history 434
Feeder layer 352, 353
Fibrinolytic agents 38
Fibroadenomas 383
Fibromas 383
Fibrosarcoma 137
5-Fluorouracil 80, 137, 204, 335, 352, 355
Forestomach epithelial tumours 384
Forestomach squamous carcinoma 388
Free interval 90

Gap junctions 115
Generation of reactive molecular species 159
Genotypic variations 70
Glioma 496/5352

Glucocorticosteroid receptor (GR) 104
Glucose-6-phosphatase 283
Glycolipids 134
Glycoprotein 15, 116, 134
Gonadectomy 282
G_1 phase 19, 83
G_2 phase 83
Granulocytes 275
Growth delay 335
— inhibition 138
— rate of xenografts 333
— regulation 274

H(a)ematopoietic cell differentiation 275
Head tumour 194, 256
HeLa cell cultures 78, 80
Hepatoma cells 189, 344
Hepatocarcinogenic dose 282
Hepatocellular carcinoma 282, 284
Hexamethylmelamine (HMM) 182, 185
High risk breast cancer 318, 319
Histocompatibility antigens 426
Histopathology 222, 369
Host-cell reactivation 416
Hosts for human tumour xenografts 327
Homing effect 127
Homogeneity 320
Hormone-chemotherapy 319
Hormone receptor assays 104
Hormone receptors 85
— therapy 102
Human malignant melanoma 139
Hybrid cells 346
Hypotension 211
Hypothesis 18, 38, 63
Hypoxic drug contact 167
Hypoxic radiosensitization 166

ICRF-159 74
Identification card
— brain tumours 385
— forestomach epithelial tumours 384
— liver angiosarcomas 384
— mammary tumours 382
— nephroblastoma 385
Ig-producing cells 374
Imexon 174
Immune competence 393
— modulation 249
— modulator 393
— rejection 127
— response 127, 145, 374
Immune-suppressed animals 327
Immunoblasts 395

Immunoglobulin-producing cells 369
Immunological pattern 418
Immunomodulating agents 173
Immunoperoxidase technique 66, 69, 369, 370
Immunopharmakology 177
Immunotherapy 33
Immunotoxin 153
Induction during embryogenesis 113
Individualized surgical adjuvant chemotherapy 318
Inhibition of DNA synthesis 232, 279
— of growth 50, 153
— of invasion 48
— of protein synthesis 135, 143, 149
— of RNA synthesis 232
— of ruffling activity 52
— of thymidylate synthetase 408
Inhibitor of transaldolase activity 192
Inhibitory effect 23, 25
Initiation of carcinogenesis 285
Interaction 36
Inter-assay difference 395
Intercellular junctions 113, 115
Interferon 239, 252, 256
Interferon induction 241, 246, 247
Instability 320
Invasion 15, 23, 33, 40, 47
Invasion and tumour vascularization 34
Invasiveness in vitro 43
In-vitro assay of invasion 47
In-vitro cytotoxicity 182
In-vitro-in-vivo correlation 361
In-vitro model 42, 47
In-vitro response 361
In-vitro techniques 315
In-vitro testing 366
In-vivo tests 327
Italian Quality Control Programme (1980) 94, 96

KB cells 414, 415

Laboratory assessment of therapeutic activity 313, 379
Latency period of xenografts 333
Leucemic patients 423
Leucocytes 253, 393
Lewis lung carcinoma 25, 35, 198
Life-time experiments 202
Limitation of screens 359
Limits of clinical chemotherapy evaluation 380
Lipid-protein membrane 113
Lipophilicity 169
Liver angiosarcomas 339, 340, 384, 389

Liver lesions 284
Liver metastasis 389
Localization of metastases 39
Local regulators 20
Locomotion 20, 113
Long-term bioassays 292, 376
Long-term tissue cultures 316
Loss of directional migration 52
L1210 tumour cells 218, 223, 361, 362, 405, 406, 407, 408
Lung cancer 273
Lycurim (LY) 189
Lymphatic system 35
Lymphocyte response 394, 450
Lymphocytes 114, 419, 431
Lymphokines 275
Lytic effects 35

Macromolecular complexes 15
Macrophages 275, 277
Macrophage-depleted cell suspension 74
Macrophage-like cells 279
Madison 109 lung carcinoma 29
Mammary tumours 382
— adenocarcinoma 386, 387
— carcinoma 66, 383
— fibroadenoma 386
— fibroma 386
— fibrosarcoma 387
Malignant glioma 418, 419
Malignant plasma cells 426
Marcellomycin 231, 233
Marker expression 276
Marker for therapeutic success 401
Matrix-degrading enzymes 15, 20
MeCCNU (1-(2-chloroethyl)-3-(4-methylcyclo-hexyl)-1-nitrosourea) 356, 439, 440, 441, 442
Mechanism of action 15, 138, 232, 240, 309
Mechanism of cross-link formation 262
Medison 109 lung carcinoma 29
Medulloblastoma 377, 378, 390
Medulloepithelioma 377
Megacaryocytes 423, 424
Melanoma cells 414
Melphalan (phenylalanine mustard) 130
Membrane fluidity 119, 122
Membrane immunoglobulin 276
Membrane viscosity 124
Meningioma cells 414
Menopausal status 88
Metastases 23, 33, 40, 55, 71
Metastasis formation 59
— localization 39
— models 198

Metastatic brain tumours 287, 289
— cascade 40
— lymph nodes 90
Metabolic activation 446
— deactivation 446
— toxication 446, 447, 448, 449, 450
Methotrexate 204, 405, 407, 409
3-Methylcholanthrene-induced lymphocytes 432
Micropinocytosis 115
Microtitration assay 350, 351, 357
Microtubule assembly — disassembly 49
Microtubule inhibitors 47, 48
Migration 37
Mithramycin 353
Mitostatic drugs 55
ML-1 cells (human myeloblastic leukemia) 275, 276, 277, 278, 279
MNU (N-methyl-N-nitrosourea) 414
Models for long-term bioassays 339, 376
Mode of action of cyclophosphamide 445
Molar conductance 219
Monoclonal antibodies 66, 70, 127
Movement 115
Multiparameter regression equations 434
Mutagenic activity 300, 301, 303, 305, 434
Myeloma cells 426, 427, 428, 429
Myelosuppression (reversible) 211

Na$^+$/K$^+$-ATPase 119, 121, 124
Natural inhibitors 15
Natural resistance 15, 342
N-demethylation of pentamethylmelamine (PMM) 185
Neck tumour 194, 256
Neovascularization 19
Nephroblastoma 385, 390
Neuronal cells 376
Neurocseretion 114
Neurotoxicity 168, 196
Nitrogen mustard (HN$_2$) 121, 123
5-Nitroimidazole derivatives 300, 302
Nitroimidazoles (METRO; MISO) 166
Nitrothiazole derivatives 303
N-Nitrosoureas 438
N-Nitrosoureido derivative (GYKI-13324) 198
Nodal involvement 89
Non-specific toxicity 153
Novikoff-hepatoma cells 233
NPT 15392 175
Nude mice 138, 327

Oestradiol see Estradiol
Oestrogen see Estrogen

OK-432 176
Orchidectomy 283, 285
Organ culture 47, 317, 320
Ornithine decarboxylase 259, 265
Ovarian carcinoma 366, 401, 402, 403, 415
Ovariectomy 283, 285
Oxydative activation 161

Pattern of reactivity 69
Pentamethylmelamine (PMM) 182, 185, 362
Phagocytic activity 279
Pharmacological properties of abrin and ricin 135
Pharmacokinetics 185, 186, 263
Phase I studies and trials 183, 184, 220, 221, 223, 235, 362
Phase II 194, 287
Phenotypic variations 70
Philadelphia chromosome 276
Phosphamide mustard 121
Physical conditions of in-vitro systems 321
Phytoagglutinin 134
Plant lectin 147
Plaque-forming ability 414, 415
Plasma-cell cytoplasmic immunoglobulins 369, 370, 372
Plasma membrane 126
Plasma thymidine levels 363
Plasmin 17
Plasmocytoma 215, 217, 409
Plating efficiency 343
Platinum complexes 221
P388 Leuk(a)emia 30, 310, 345
Poliovirus 415
Polyadenylic: polyuridylic acids (poly A:U) 176
Polyamine levels 264
Polyamine oxydation 71
Polyamines 258
Polymorphonuclear leucocytes 37
Pre-activation 321
Preclinical studies 220
Prediction conclusions 316
Prediction of drug sensitivity 315, 316, 319
Preoperative Chemotherapy 59
Prerequisites of human-equivalent animal models 381, 382
Pretreatment 443
Prevention of dissemination 311
Primary invasion 15, 34
Progesterone receptor (PR) 102
Progesterone receptor assay 99
Progestin receptor (PR) 104, 107
Prognostic value 70, 374

Proliferation 20
Proliferation rate 78, 79, 265
Prolongation of the life-span 309
Promotion of carcinogenesis 285
Prooxidant compounds 159
Prophylactic treatment 26
Proteinases 15
Proteoglycan 15, 18
Protection tests 129
Protein synthesis 350
Proteolytic enzymes in chemotherapy 226
Proteolytic enzymes in metastases 226
Proteolytic enzymes in oncology 225
Proteolytic enzymes in radiation therapy 227
Pseudopodial extensions 117
Pulmonary metastasis 298, 340, 341, 387, 389, 390
Putrescine 71, 72, 81, 259
Putrescine oxydation product 74
Pyrazofurin (PF) 189
Pyrimidinones 245, 246

Quinazoline antifolate 404

Radio-chemotherapeutic treatment 418
Radioimmunoassay 69
Radiosensitization and cytotoxicity 166
Reactivation of adenovirus 3 by tumour cell cultures 413, 415
Receptor level 105, 109
Recognition 113, 117
Recommendations 208
Regeneration of putrescine 259
Regulation of cellular processes 113
Regulatory action 117
Relapse 424
Remissions 287
Repair deficiency 416
Requirements for in-vitro assays 321
Resistance 15, 342
Resistocell 393
Responder lymphocytes 428
Response of colorectal tumour 335
Response rate 287
— of proliferating cells 344
— of resting cells 344
— to cis-platinum 290
— to phytohaemagglutinin (PHA) and re-sistocell (RSTL) in vitro 395, 396, 397, 398
Retinoids 269
Rhabdomyosarcoma 296, 298
Ribonuclease activity 401, 402, 403
Ribosome-inactivating proteins 142
Ricin 134, 136, 138

Ricin A-chain 147
Risk-benefit analysis 201
Risk-benefit assessment of cancer chemotherapy 380
Rodent tumours 359
Rosette-forming cells 419
Routes of dissemination 39
Ruffling membrane 52

Sarcomas 294
Saturation density 356
Schedule of treatment 25
Screening methods 359
Secondary invasion 34
Selective activity 166
— antimetastatic agent 59
— inhibition of invasion 38
— targeting 147
Sensitivity to Vitamin A 271
Sensitized cells 426, 428
Serum ribonuclease 401, 402, 403
Sex hormonal environment 282
Short-term tissue incubation 316, 320
Signals 113, 116
Simultaneous occurrence of steroid receptors 108
Skin cells 414
Skin tumours 256
Slice organ culture assay 322, 323
Smokers 433, 434
Smoking history 434
Spermidine 71, 73, 81, 259
Spermine 71, 73, 81, 259
Specialized membrane structure 116
Splenectomy 154
Spontaneous metastases 59
Sprague-Dawley rats 203, 204, 292, 294, 339, 340, 376, 377, 378, 382, 384, 386, 388, 390
"Stem cell" assay 349
Steroid hormone receptors 105
Steroid receptor assay 99
Steroids 356
Stimuli during embryogenesis 115
Strand breaks in DNA 210
Structure activity 215, 218, 223
Surface receptor 278
Surgical treatment 418
Survival 136, 190, 319, 362, 372, 374, 415
Survival time 72, 90, 129, 131, 136, 273, 310, 405
Surviving fraction 343, 352, 354, 356, 405, 409
Survivors 136, 405
Synaptic junctions 115

Synergistic effects 127, 131, 139
Synergistic interaction 189

Take rate of xenografts 327, 328
Target cells 114, 427
Target for alkylating agents 119
Targets for therapy 24, 33, 35, 111
Target of antimetastatic treatment 59
TdR incorporation 405, 408
Teratogenic effect of Vitamin A 272
Therapeutic activity 379, 391, 439
Therapeutic effects of interferon 254
Therapeutic response assessment 333
Thin-layer chromatography (TLC) fractions 431, 432, 433, 434
Thioproline   (4-thiazolidine-carboxylic acid) 194
Thrombosis 37
Thrombocytes 135
Thrombus formation 63
Thymidylate synthetase 407
Thymidylate synthetase inhibitor 404
TLC -radioisotopic assay 431
TLX/5 lymphoma 183, 361, 362, 409
T-lymphocytes 424, 429
Total lymphoid irradiation 153
Toxicity of Vitamin A 271
Toxic selectivity 164
Toxicological parameters 234
Trasylol 17
Treatment of lung cancer 273
Treatment of malignancy 151
Trenimon 120
Tubulin 50
Tumour blood vessels 35
— cell arrest 37
— — emboli 37
— — heterogeneity 39
— — surface 37
— drug-host interaction 324
— drug response in vitro 323
— growth 71
— products in xenografts 331
— prophylaxis 274
— staining intensity 67
— stem cell assay 360
— specific antiserum 130
— volume doubling time 334, 335
— volume measurements 333
— weights 72

UdR incorporation 405
Urea levels (platinum complexes) 221

Value for prediction of therapy effectiveness 104
Vinca alkaloids 24
Vincristine (VCR) 140, 343, 345, 355
Vincristine distribution 345
Vincristine-resistent P388 cells 346
Vincristine-sensitive P388 cells 346
Vincristine uptake 345, 346
Vindesine (VDS) 23
Vinyl chloride 339, 376
Vitamin A 269
Vitamin A derivatives 270

Vitamin A precursors 270
VP 16-213 210, 211

Walker 256 tumour 36
Warfarin 64
Wistar rats 206

Xenografts 327
Xenografts' use 362

Yoshida sarcoma ascites cells 438

Appendix

Antineoplastic agents and drugs

Abrin 134, 136, 138

Adriamycin 292, 294, 296

Alkylating agents 120, 122, 189

Anthracycline 231

Antiblastic drugs 339, 376, 392

Antimetabolites 189

Antimetastatic agents 58

Anthithrombotic agents 63

Arabinofuranosylcytosine (Ara C) 277, 279

Azimexon 175

BCNU (1.3-bis-(2-chloroethyl)-1-nitrosourea) 439, 440, 441, 442

Bleomycin 354

CBDCA (cyclobutanedicarboxylate derivative) 220

CB 10-375 (N-methylolmelamine) 187

CB 37 17 (N-4(N-((2-amino-4-hydroxy-6-quinazolinyl)methyl)prop-2-ynylamino)-benzoyl)-L-glutamic acid) 361, 404, 405, 406, 408, 409

Chemotherapeutic agents 142

Chlorambucil 121, 129, 131

Chlorozotocin (2-(3-(2-chloroethyl)-3-nitroso-ureido)-D-glucopyranose) 439, 440, 441, 442

Cis-dichlorodiammine platinum (cis-DDP) 214, 287

CNU derivatives (N-nitroso-(2-chloroethyl)-urea) 205, 207

Cycloheximide 120

Cyclophosphamide 130, 202, 204, 310, 445, 450

Cytosine arabinoside see Arabinofuranosylcyto-sine

Cytostatic drugs 201

Cytotoxic agents 59

Desacetyl vinblastine amide sulphate 23

Diethylnitrosamine (DEN) 282, 284

DTIC (dimethyltriazene) 139, 309, 310, 311

Ellipticine derivatives 159, 160, 162

5-Fluorouracil 80, 137, 204, 335, 352, 355

Hexamethylmelamine (HMM) 182, 185

HN_2 (nitrogen mustard) 121, 123

ICRF-159 74

Imexon 174

Lycurim (LY) 189

MeCCNU (1-(2-chloroethyl)-3-(4-methylcyclo-hexyl)-1-nitrosourea) 356, 439, 440, 441, 442

Melphalan (phenylalanine mustard) 130

Methotrexate 204, 405, 407, 409

Mithramycin 353

MNU (N-methyl-N-nitrosourea) 414

Nitroimidazole derivatives 166, 300, 302

Nitrothiazole derivatives 303

N-Nitrosoureas 438

N-Nitrosoureido derivative (GYKI-13324) 198

OK-432 176

Pentamethylmelamine (PMM) 182, 185, 362

Phosphamide mustard 121

Poly A:U (polyadenylic:polyuridylic acids) 176

Pyrazofurin 189

Pyrimidinones 245, 246

Quinazoline antifolate 404

Ricin 134, 136, 138

Thioproline (4-thiazolidine-carboxylic acid) 194

Trasylol 17

Trenimon 120

Vinca alkaloids 24

Vincristine (VCR) 140, 343, 345, 355

Vindesine (VDS) 23

VP 16-213 210, 211

Enzymes 15, 17, 20, 38

Amine oxidase 74, 77, 81

Aryl hydrocarbon hydroxylase (AHH) 431

Dihydrofolate reductase (DHFR) 404, 407

Glucose-6-phosphatase 283

Immunoperoxidase 66, 69, 369, 370

Thymidylate synthetase 407, 408
Transaldolase 192
Ornithine decarboxylase 259, 265
Proteinases 15
Ribonuclease 401, 402, 403

Experimental models
ADJ/PC6 tumour 216, 217, 409
Animal models 379
Astrocytoma 355, 414
BALB/c mice 129, 150, 217
B-cell tumour (BCL$_1$) 147, 148
BDF$_1$ mice 218
B16 melanoma 26, 250, 251
Brain tumours 42, 376, 377, 378, 385
C57 Bl/6 mice 130
Ehrlich ascites tumour cells 120, 122
EL4 Lymphoma 130
HeLa cell cultures 78, 80

Hepatoma cells 189, 344
KB cells 414, 415
Lewis lung carcinoma 25, 35, 198
L1210 cells 218, 223, 361, 362, 405, 406, 407, 408
Melanoma cells 414
Meningioma cells 414
Madison 109 lung carcinoma 29
ML-1 cells (human myeloblastic leukemia) 275, 276, 277, 278, 279
Novikoff-hepatoma cells 233
Nude mice 138, 327
P 388 leukemia 30, 310, 345
Sprague-Dawley rats 203, 204, 292, 294, 339, 340, 376, 377, 378, 382, 384, 386, 388, 390
TLX/5 lymphoma 183, 361, 362, 409
Walker 256 tumour 36
Wistar rats 206
Yoshida sarcoma ascites cells 438